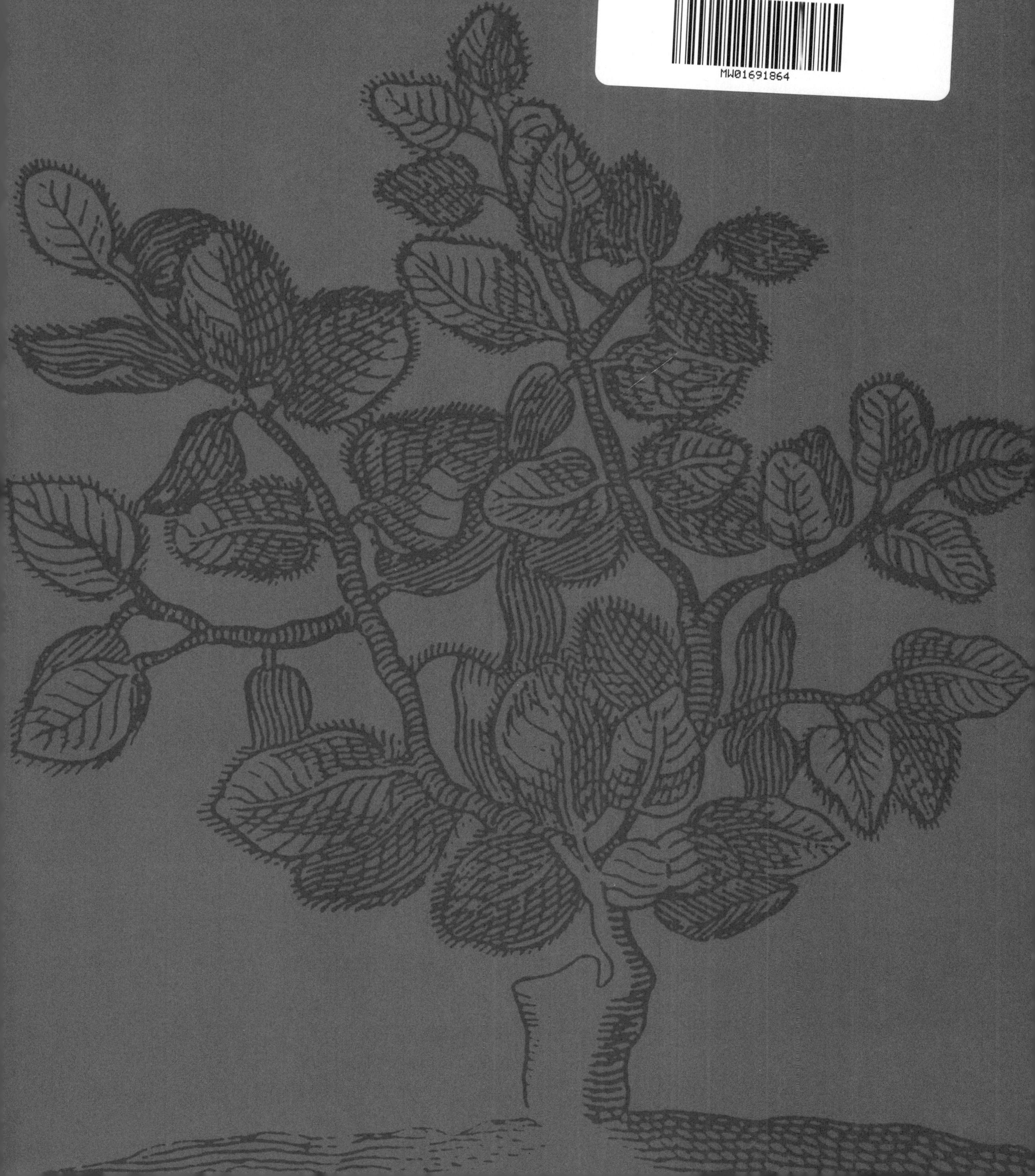

MEDICINE
A HISTORY OF HEALING

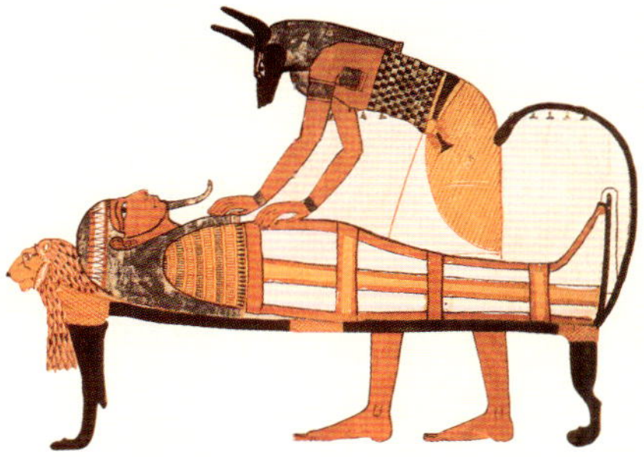

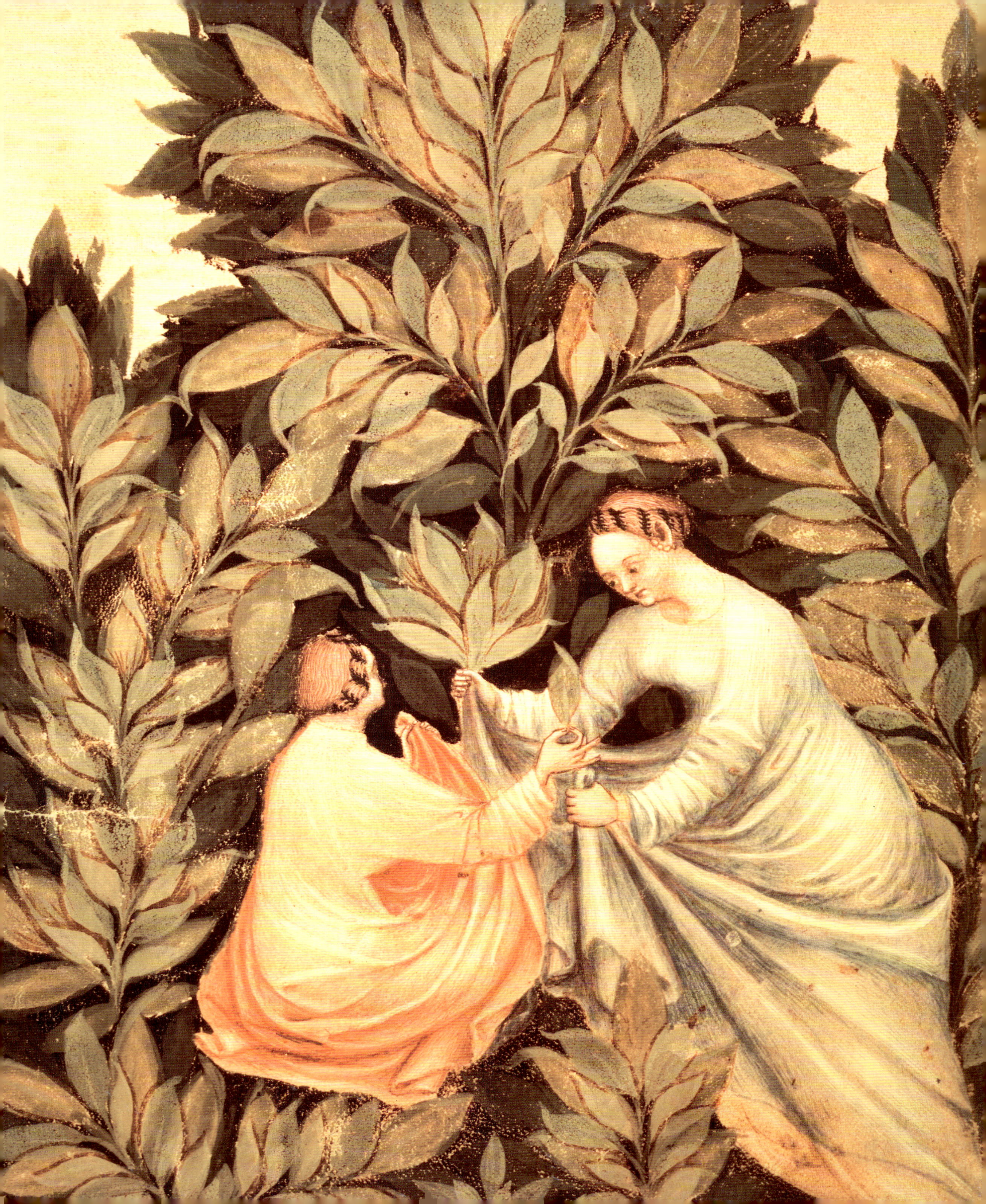

MEDICINE
A HISTORY OF HEALING
ANCIENT TRADITIONS TO MODERN PRACTICES

consultant editor

ROY PORTER

BARNES & NOBLE
BOOKS
NEW YORK

This edition published by BARNES & NOBLE, INC.,
by arrangement with THE IVY PRESS LIMITED

1997 BARNES & NOBLE BOOKS

M 10 9 8 7 6 5 4 3 2 1

ISBN 0-7607-0619-0

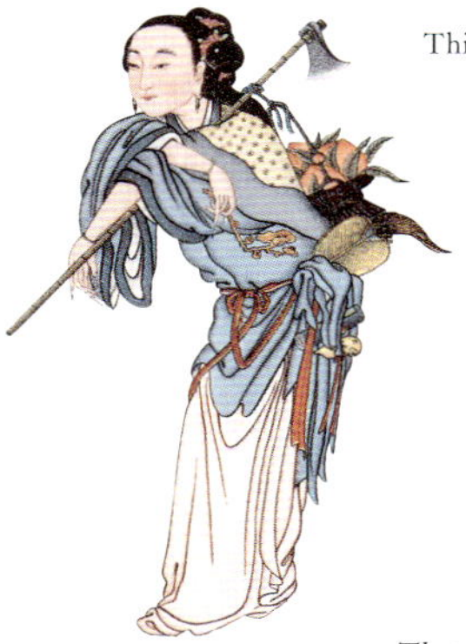

This book was conceived, designed and produced by
THE IVY PRESS LIMITED

Art director: **Peter Bridgewater**
Designer: **Jane Lanaway**
Page layout: **Chris Lanaway**
Commissioning Editor: **Philip de Ste Croix**
Managing Editor: **Anne Townley**
Picture research: **Vanessa Fletcher**
Illustrations: **Lorraine Harrison**

Printed and bound in China

The publishers wish to thank the following for the use of pictures

Archiv für Kunst und Geschichte, London: 12TL, 31TL, 47B, 58, 113T, 125B (Eric Lessing/Österreiche National Bibilothek), 135B – portrait of the German surgeon Theodor Billroth by Adelbert Seligmann – (Eric Lessing, Belvedere Gallery, Vienna) 144T, 146TL, 162B (Eric Lessing/Musée d'Orsay), 172, 196TL, 200 (Wyeth Laboratories), 219T (Bayer AG). **The Bridgeman Art Library:** 12TR (British Museum), 13 (Noortman London), 15, 28 (Cheltenham Art Gallery), 30 (Musée des Beaux Arts, Marseilles), 38 (Bonhams), 42TL (Museum of History of Science), 48M (Coram Foundation), 64R (Assistance Publique, Paris), 68T, 69 (Bibliothèque Nationale, Paris), 71 (Eton College), 75, 78T (Bibliothèque Nationale, Paris), 78B (Vatican Museums and Galleries), 92-3, 95 (Musée des Beaux Arts, Besançon), 100-1 (National Museum of India), 119 (Bibliothèque Nationale, Paris), 122 (Vatican Museums and Galleries), 123 (Bibliothèque Nationale, Paris), 124 (Santa Maria, Barcelona), 127T (Palazzo Pitti), 139T (Royal College of Surgeons), 145 (Musée St Omer), 153 (Bibliothèque Nationale, Paris), 156 (Museo La Desano, Venice), 158 (Prado), 169 (Colnaght & Co), 192 (University of Bologna), 197 (Christies), 198T (Harriet Winter Antiques). **The Bridgeman Art Library/Lauros-Giraudon:** 17. **The Chiropractor Association:** 189T. **Corbis:** 54R, 57, 182R, 188, 206T (UPI). **Mary Evans Picture Library:** 56T, 64, 113B, 162, 168M. **E. T. Archive:** 13TL, 16M, 24T, 24B, 27T, 29, 44T, 47L, 54T, 57B, 68B, 72B, 73, 79, 82T, 82B, 87T, 89, 94TR, 102, 129T, 131B, 140T (the Endell Street Military Hospital by Francis Dodd), 142, 160T, 163, 164-5, 166, 185, 198B, 211B. **Mark Garanger:** 48R. **The Homeopathy Society:** 116. **The Hutchison Library:** 12BR (Sarah Errington), 117B (Felix Greene), 205T (Felix Greene), 212 (N. Durrel-McKenna), 218-19 (N. Durrell-Mckenna). **Hulton Getty:** 165T and M, 190. **The Image Bank:** 44B (Larry Gatz), 61 (Bill Varie), 66T (Larry Gatz), 134 (Jay Freis), 141 (Andre Gallant), 206B (G & M David de Lossy), 209BR. **Images Colour Library:** 103B, 201T, 207T. **The National Library of Wales:** 25B and R. **The Royal College of Surgeons:** 136, 139T. **The Royal Society of Medicine:** 132T and M. **The Science Photo Library:** 42B, 49B, 53B (Hank Morgan), 65 (Will and Deni McIntyre), 92BL (Mark de Fraeye), 104TR (Mark de Fraeye), 106 (Françoise Sauze), 142B (Ron Sutherland), 143 (John Greim), 144 (Scott Camazine) 167T (Damien Lovegrove), 201B (Matt Meadows, Peter Arnold Inc.), 202T (Richard Lowenberg), 202M (Henny Allis), 203T (Henny Allis), 204TL (Tim Maylon & Paul Biddle), 204B (David Campione), 209BL, 214B (Damien Lovegrove), 217TL (Simon Fraser). **The Science Photo Library/Jean Loup Charmet:** 14B, 21M, 41, 53T, 98R, 114T, 114B, 125, 155M, 187. **St Christopher's Hospice:** 195. **Tony Stone Associates:** 189B. **The Wellcome Centre Medical Photographic Library:** 18MR, 20T, 21T, 26B, 31BR, 32M, 33L, 33R, 35TR, 36, 37T, 37MT, 37B, 39, 40T, 43, 50T, 51T, 51B, 59B, 60L, 72T, 74T, 91B, 93T, 94M, 97B, 98T, 100L, 110T, 111TL, 111R, 112, 115T, 118T, 129L, 130T, 131M, 135L, 135T, 136R, 144TL, 149, 150, 152TR, 157T, 159, 160B, 171B, 177B, 179T, 180B, 182L, 184, 192B. **Zefa Picture Library:** 45, 59T (Wartenberg), 66B, 93B (Holdsworth), 97T, 107M, 117TR, 167M, 170L, 181, 196B, 202B, 203B, 207B (Boutin), 208BR, 209T, 214-15 (Stockmarket), 215, 217B (H. Sochurer), 217TR, 219B. The map on pages 86–7 is adapted, by permission of Oxford University Press, from an original published in *The Spice Trade of the Roman Empire* by J. Innes Miller (OUP, 1969).

The publishers wish to thank the authors and the
University of Kansas Medical Centre for supplying material for use in this book.

Frontispiece: Two women picking sage, 15th century manuscript
(Bridgeman Art Library/Bibliothèque Nationale, Paris)

*Every effort has been made to trace all copyright holders and obtain permissions.
The editor and publishers sincerely apologise for any inadvertent errors or omissions
and will be happy to correct them in any future editions.*

CONTRIBUTORS

ROY PORTER (CONSULTANT)
Roy Porter is Professor in the Social History of Medicine at The Wellcome Institute for the History of Medicine, London, and has taught previously at the University of Cambridge and at UCLA in the United States. Among his many influential books are *Mind Forg'd Manacles: Madness in England from the Restoration to the Regency; A Social History of Madness; Health for Sale: Quackery in England, 1660–1850; Doctor of Society: Thomas Beddoes and the Sick Trade in Late Enlightenment England; London: a Social History;* and (co-authored with Dorothy Porter) *In Sickness and in Health: the British Experience, 1650-1850* and *Patient's Progress.*

ROBERTA BIVINS – Roberta Bivins is a Research Fellow at The Wellcome Institute for the History of Medicine in London. She graduated from Columbia University with a degree in the history and language of science, and gained a Ph.D from Massachusetts Institute of Technology with a thesis concerned with acupuncture and the cross-cultural transmission of medical knowledge.

JOHN CULE – John Cule has practised clinical medicine both as a family general practitioner and as a hospital psychiatrist. He is currently joint editor of *Vesalius,* the journal of the International Society for the History of Medicine. He has been President of the International Society for the History of Medicine (1992–1996), President of the British Society for the History of Medicine (1985–1987), and President of the History of Medicine Society of Wales (1978–1980). He was made an Emeritus Member of the American Osler Society in 1990. In 1996 he was elected an Honorary Fellow of the Royal Society of Medicine. He is the author and editor of many books and papers on the history of medicine.

JOHN CRELLIN – John K Crellin holds British qualifications in both medicine and pharmacy. He also holds a Ph.D in the history and philosophy of science. For many years he has been especially interested in self-care with a particular interest in the place of complementary medicine. His present position is John Clinch Professor of the History of Medicine, Memorial University of Newfoundland, Canada.

ANN DALLY – Ann Dally has been a Research Fellow at The Wellcome Institute for the History of Medicine in London since 1990. She qualified as a doctor in 1953, and worked first as a general practitioner and medical journalist, then specialized in psychiatry. Her most recent published works are *Women Under the Knife (1991)* and *Fantasy Surgery (1996).*

HAROLD ELLIS – Since 1993 Professor Harold Ellis has been Clinical Anatomist at the United Medical & Dental School (Guy's Campus) of Guy's and St Thomas's Hospitals in London. He was made Emeritus Professor of Surgery at the University of London in 1989. He has published numerous books, papers, and chapters in textbooks on sugery. His most recent published book is *Operations That Made History.*

PAUL LERNER – Paul Lerner is currently a Post-doctoral Research Fellow at The Wellcome Institute for the History of Medicine in London. His previously published works include *'Hysterical Men': War, Memory and German Mental Medicine, 1914–1926* and *Traumatic Pasts: History, Psychiatry and Trauma in the Modern Age, 1870–1930* (co-edited with Mark S Micale, *1997*). He is currently working on a book dealing with psychiatry in German daily life in the twentieth century.

MIKE SAKS – Professor Mike Saks is Head of the School of Health and Community Studies at De Montfort University, Leicester in England. His recently published books are *Alternative Medicine in Britain (1992), Professions and the Public Interest: Medical Power, Altruism and Alternative Medicine (1995)* and *Health Professions and the State in Europe* (with T Johnson and G Larkin, *1995*).

PHILIP WILSON – Philip K Wilson is an assistant professor of the history of science at Truman State University in Kirksville, Missouri, USA. He recently edited a five-volume series entitled *Childbirth: Changing Ideas and Practices in Britain and America 1600 to the Present (1996).* He is currently working on a book tentatively titled *A Profession of Craftsmen: Daniel Turner, Surgery and Surgery Reform in Augustan London.*

ACKNOWLEDGEMENTS – *Philip Wilson, the author of Chaper Seven Healers in History, would like to acknowledge with thanks the help of the following people: Lisa Fagnani, Gretchen Krueger, Kelly McConnell, Patrick Reed, Chris Wolf, Brian Yochim, and Sarah Zapf for exemplary research assistance; The Rev. Orel Newbrey for information regarding spiritual healing; Tim Barcus for photographic needs; and Susan B. Case, Rare Books Librarian, Clendening History of Medicine Library, University of Kansas Medical Center for unflagging assistance with primary sources.*

CONTENTS

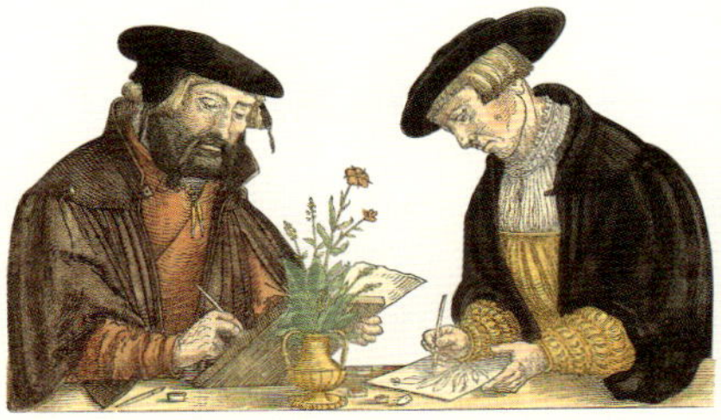

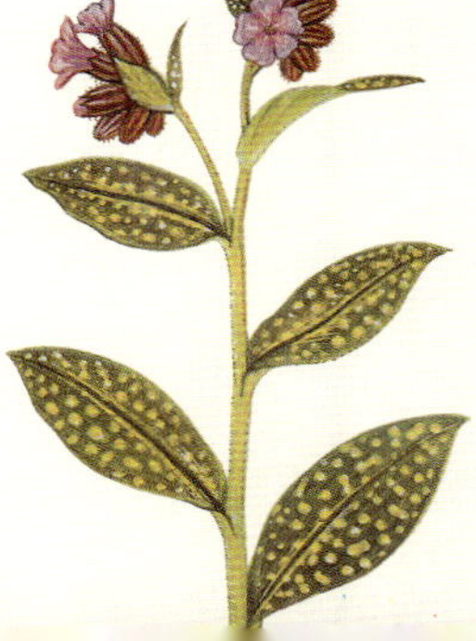

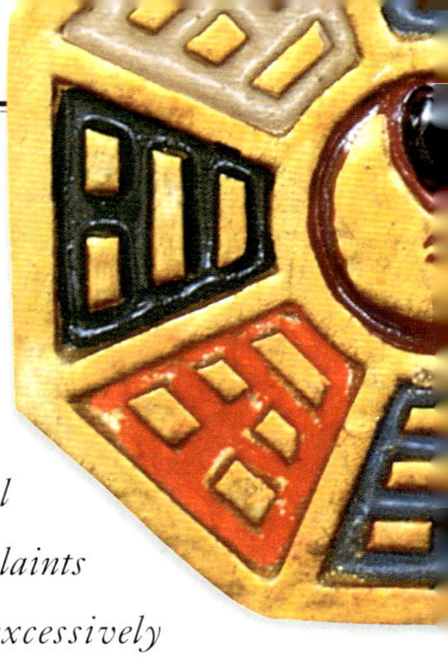

FOREWORD

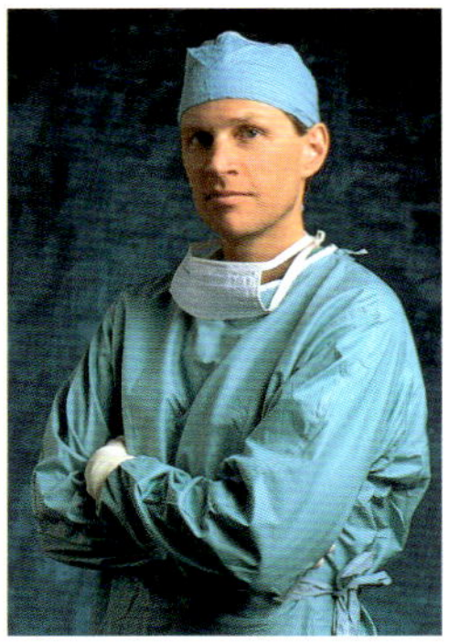

ABOVE Western medicine faces a dilemma – despite its successes, the public often views it with suspicion.

We live in strange times. Medicine, at first glance, is moving from triumph to triumph. It is little more than half a century since antibiotics were introduced, only 30 years since the first heart transplant. The first test-tube baby was born just 20 years ago, now there have been thousands; something approaching half a million coronary-bypass operations and a slightly lower number of operations to dilate the coronary arteries (angioplasties) are performed each year in the United States alone, giving sufferers from heart conditions and survivors from heart attacks the enviable prospect of a longer lease on life.

Everywhere more and more money is being spent on health – something like 14 per cent of the Gross National Product in the USA *and not very much less in other major industrial states – and life expectations are rising. Medical science and clinical practice are achieving ever more breakthroughs; surgeons are doing the impossible, and the consequences seem to be showing in the growing number of survivors – people hale and hearty well into their eighties and even nineties.*

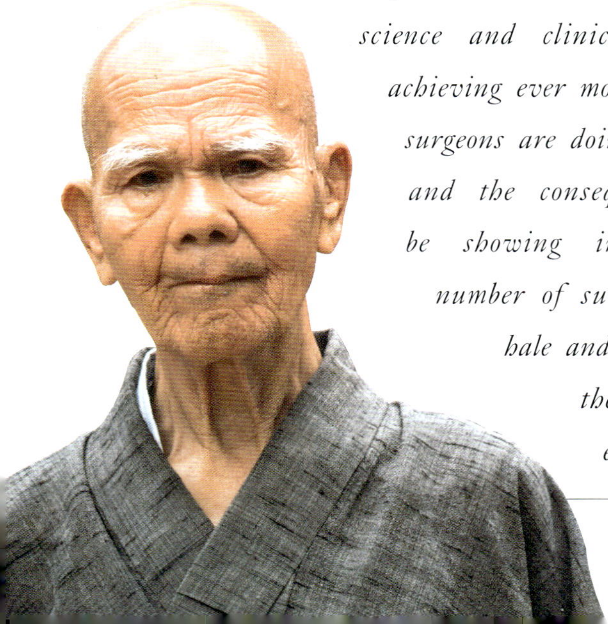

BELOW Medicine has extended human lifespan significantly; is this a triumph or a cause for concern?

Yet these are, paradoxically, also times of growing and vocal dissatisfaction with medicine. The complaints are familiar. It has become excessively technological, impersonal, alien and forbidding. Machines, regulations, bureaucracy, a proliferation of tests, unintelligible jargon, and ethico-legal paraphernalia are rapidly replacing the old friendly family doctor; the one who actually came out on calls when you were sick, and listened to you rather than hastening to fix an appointment to see a specialist in three weeks' time.

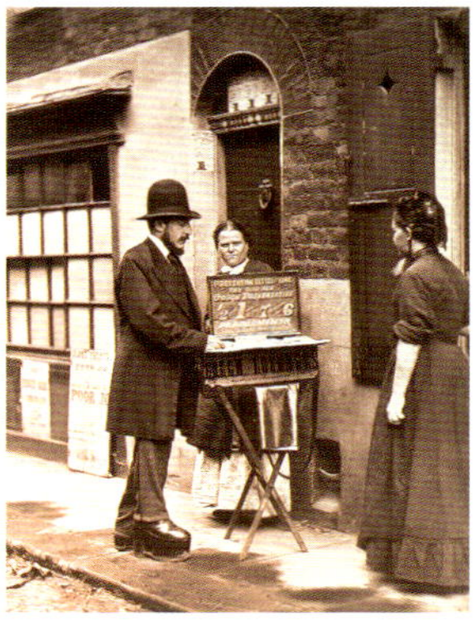

ABOVE Health for sale. Not all physicians are philanthropists; the history of medicine must recognize its commercial aspect.

Somehow the more medicine achieves, the less it satisfies. And this seems to show in the figures. By any objective standard, people in the West are now healthier than ever they have been. Yet they also report more incidence of sickness than ever, and visit the doctors nearly half again as often as they did 50 years ago. We live in times preoccupied by the fear of disease, be it AIDS *or some other new 'hot virus'. Worse still, we live in fear of medicine, or at least bio-scientific research. The prediction that a human clone is genetically possible within a few years has been greeted not with delight, but with shock and horror.*

If medicine is at a crossroads, and perhaps has lost its way, the relevance of this book is underlined. This is a work that directly and implicitly addresses the current dilemmas of medicine through examining the historical movements that have led up to the present. Written by experts in various fields of medical history – half of them experienced and eminent doctors in their own right – its chapters focus on

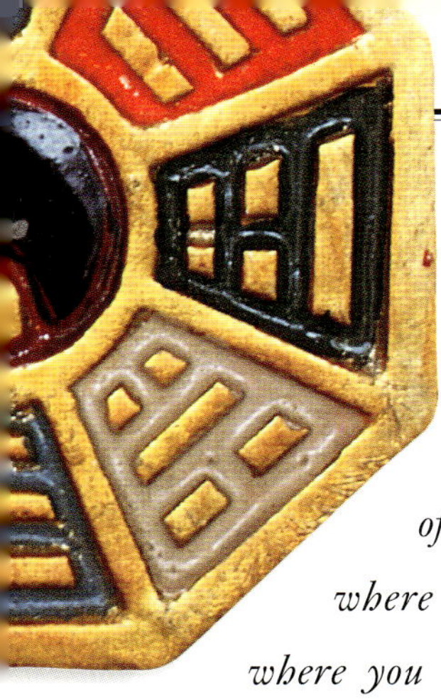

particular departments of medicine, for example surgery and psychiatry, and explore progress and its predicaments, developments and difficulties. It has often been said that it is impossible to know where you should be going unless you know where you have just come from, and in what field could that be truer than medicine? With the mentally ill, for instance, should we be pursuing 'community care'? Or should we be going back to the old standby of institutionalizing them in an 'asylum'? How could we possibly tell unless we have some historical grasp of what both community care and the asylum were like in the past? History can here illuminate the present and point to the future.

This book is far from being just another history of medicine, from the ancient Greeks to the present. For one thing, it is genuinely international and cross-cultural in its scope. It devotes considerable space to the kinds of medicine anthropologists usually study, and also to the great non-Western healing traditions – the Islamic, the Chinese, the Indian. Only the blindest and most bigoted high-tech doctor would now claim that all these traditions have nothing to teach Western physicians and Western patients. Ordinary people have been finding out for themselves, flocking in increasing numbers to practitioners of acupuncture, shiatsu and Zen alongside more Western alternative therapies like aromatherapy, Alexander technique, homeopathy, iridology and herbalism. And, perhaps a bit belatedly, Western physicians have been catching up. Apparently 40 per cent of family doctors in the UK now refer some of their patients to complementary therapists, and many themselves now practise acupuncture. No single tradition, this book shows, has a monopoly upon effective medicine.

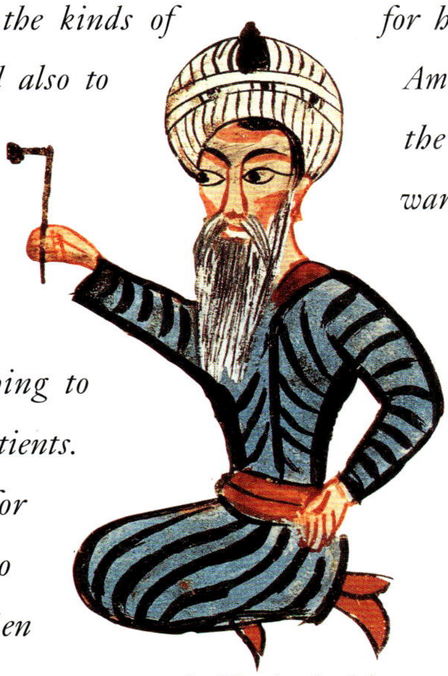

ABOVE An Islamic physician – medicine encompasses a wealth of non-Western healing traditions.

Moreover, this book is not narrowly about medicine but (as the title suggests) is about healing; it is not simply about the progress of science but about healing as an art. Medicine may be largely a body of knowledge, but healing is a personal skill. What makes a good healer? Is it a gift? Is it a matter of personality? Is it something that can be taught and learned? And what is happening to the art of healing in our own time? Is it really true that as medicine progresses, healing declines? Or should we simply be looking for healing talents and traditions in different places? Among the psychotherapists, among nursing staff, in the hospices (one of the most genuinely heart-warming developments of the last 30 years).

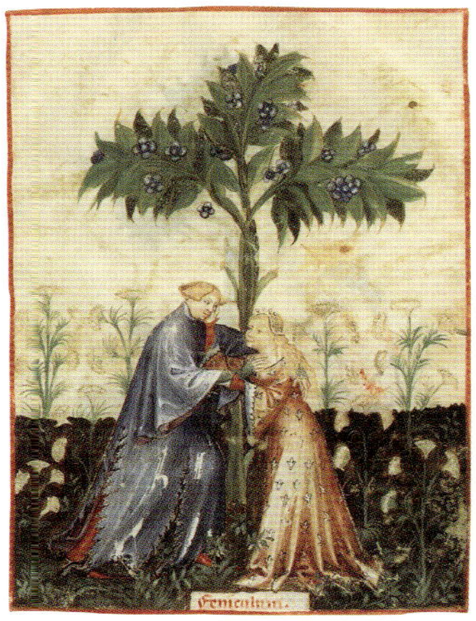

ABOVE Herbalism has a history that is as long as the practice of medicine itself. Herbs were used in ancient Egypt and China.

These are the issues addressed in this book. It offers a wealth of intriguing, often shocking, and sometimes amusing information, skilfully interpreted. It also offers much food for thought, or rather for medicine to chew over. Will we be able to develop a medicine that is sufferer-friendly, a medicine appropriate to our needs, a medicine we can afford? The historical insights offered by this book can help make our judgments better informed.

ROY PORTER *London, 1997*

	10,000–2000 BC	2000–500 BC	500–300 BC	300–100 BC	100 BC–AD 100	AD 100–300	AD 300–500	AD 500–700
WORLD MEDICINE	Written evidence of Egyptian medicine in ancient texts	Laws of Hammurabi in Babylon *(1948–1905)* Ayurvedic medicine founded in India *Ebers Papyrus* in Egypt *(c.550)* Traditional Chinese medicine established Homer describes medicine as 'the noble art' in the *Iliad*	Doctrine of humours propounded by Empedocles in Greece *(500–430)* Medical school founded in Cyrene *(429)* Hippocratic school of medicine flourishing in Greece	School of Alexandria marks development of medical education *(c.310–250)* Arrival of Greek physicians in Rome *Huangdi Neijing* written in China *(c.200)* *Yoga Sutra* of Patanjali written in India	*Nanjing* written in China during 1st or 2nd centuries Celsus writes *De medicina (c. AD 25)*	*Mei Ching* composed by Wang Shu-ho *(280)* Plague in Rome kills 5,000	Evidence of medicine practised in Mayan culture of Mesoamerica Oribasius compiles works of Galen as *Synopsis* Earliest surviving texts of *Caraka Samhita* and *Susruta Samhita (end 5th century)*	Greek medicine spreads into Arab world through the work of Arab translators of medical texts
HEALERS	Yellow Emperor, legendary founder of Chinese medicine *(2698–2598)* Imhotep in Egypt *(c.2980)*	Caraka alive in India during first millennium BC Siddhartha Gautama, the Buddha *(c.563–c.483)*	Hippocrates of Kos *(460–377)* Empedocles *(c.490–c.430)* Bian Que *(407–310)*	Zhang Zhongjing *(fl. 200)*	Asclepiades of Bithynia *(fl. 1st century)* Aulus Cornelius Celsus *(fl. 25)* Dioscorides *(c.40–c.90)*	Hua Tuo *(?190–265)* Galen of Pergamum *(?131-201)* Ge-Hong *(284–364)*	Oribasius of Byzantium *(?325–?403)*	Paul of Aegina *(625–690)*
SCIENCE								
HERBALISM	Herbal medicines used in Mesopotamia In China legendary emperor Shen Nong *(3494)* discovers herbal medicine Evidence of Egyptian medicinal use of herbs	*Ebers Papyrus (c.1550)* lists use of medicinal herbs in Egypt	Books in the *Hippocratic Corpus* list hundreds of medicinal herbs	Medicines and herbs traded between East and West via spice routes	*De compositione medicamentorum* lists opium as medical drug Dioscorides writes *De materia medica (c.50)*	*Shen Nong Bencao Jing* appears in China		*Codex vindobonensis*, early herbal *(512)*
SURGERY	Evidence of needles and trephination in Stone Age Mummification practised in Egypt	Laws of Hammurabi describe early surgery in Mesopotamia Earliest surviving surgical text – *Edwin Smith Papyrus* from Egypt *(c.1600)*	Surgery practised in India, as described in *Susruta Samhita* *Hippocratic Corpus* give details of surgery in Greece		Celsus describes surgery in Rome	Galen becomes surgeon to gladiators *(158)* Hua Tuo pictured operating on arm of Chinese general		Paul of Aegina describes current surgical practices
PSYCHIATRY								
WORLD HISTORY	First farmers settle land *(c.9000)* First cities in Mesopotamia *(3500)* Egyptian civilization established *(c.3000)* Indian civilization established *(c.2500)*	Civilization in China *(1600)* Rome founded in 753 BC	Peloponnesian War *(431–404)* Alexander the Great invades Asia *(334)*	Rome at war with Hannibal and Carthage Hannibal defeated at Zama *(202)* Romans destroy Carthage *(146)*	Julius Caesar assassinated *(44)* Romans invade Britain *(43)* Christianity established	Jewish rebellion against Rome *(132)* Three Kingdoms period in China *(220–280)*	Rise of Mayan civilization in Middle America *(c.300)* Goths sack Rome *(410)* Anglo-Saxons conquer Britain *(450)*	Byzantine conquest of Italy *(535)* and North Africa *(534)* Death of Mohammed *(632)* – start of Arab expansion

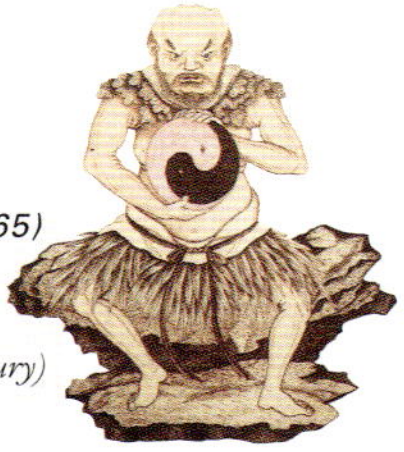
HUA TUO *(?190-265)*

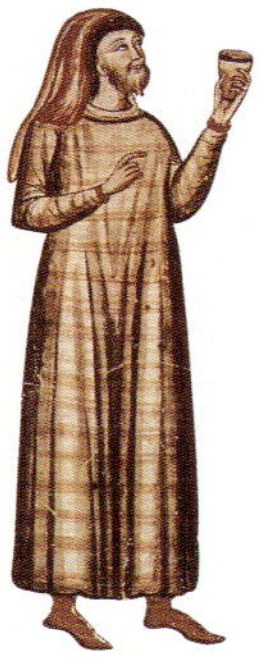
HIPPOCRATES OF KOS *(460–377)*

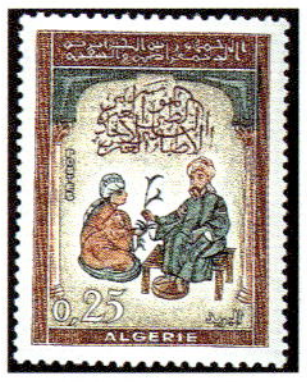

DIOSCORIDES *(c.40–c.90)*

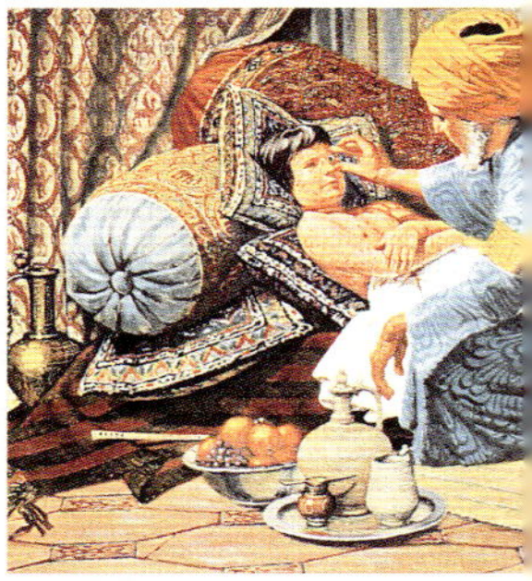
RHAZES *(c.864-925)*

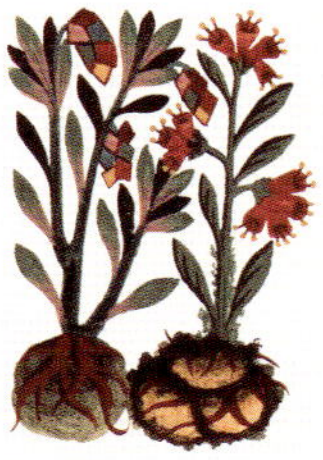
HEALING HERBS

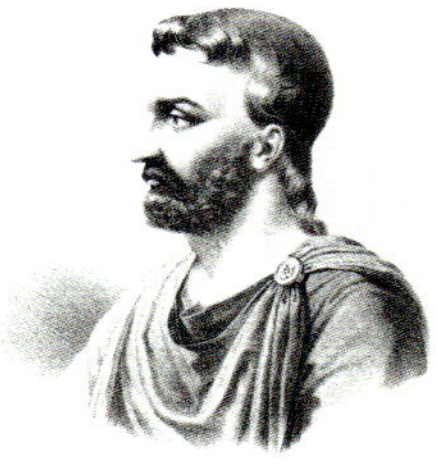
CELSUS *(fl. 25)*

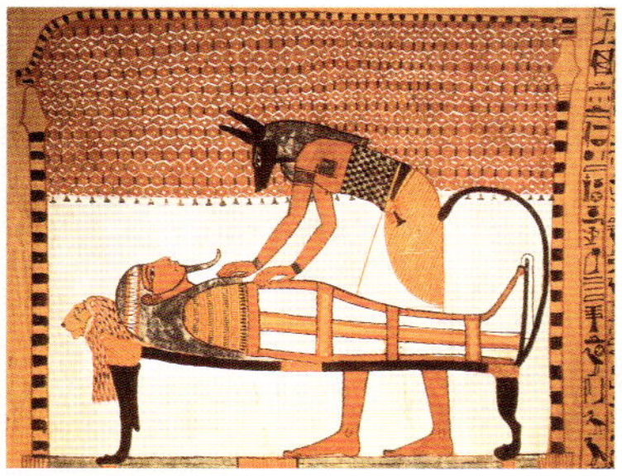
MUMMIFICATION IN EGYPT

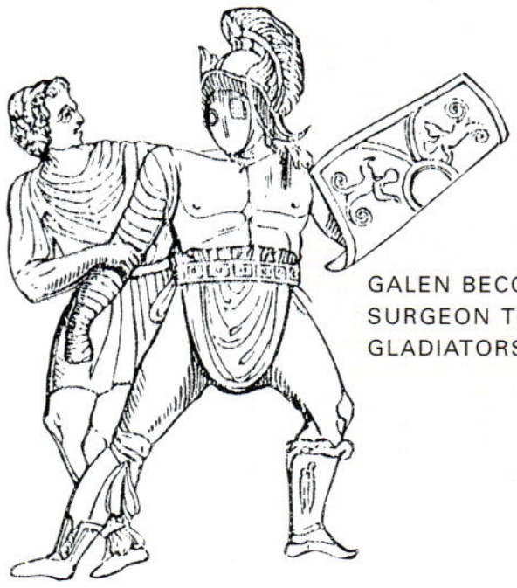
GALEN BECOMES SURGEON TO THE GLADIATORS *(158)*

LIFE OF CHRIST

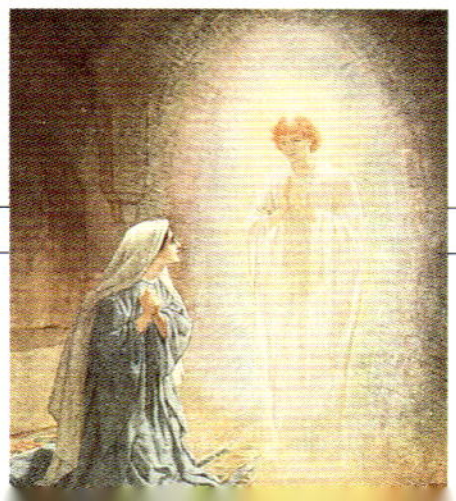

AD 700–900	AD 900–1100	AD 1100–1300	AD 1300–1500	AD 1500–1600	AD 1600–1700	AD 1700–1750	AD 1750–1800
	Dao Yin exercises integrated into the Chinese medical canon Medical school at Salerno in Italy thriving *(1050)* Many Arabic translations of Greek texts are now translated into Latin	Medical school at Montpellier in France founded University of Padua founded *(1222)* Medicine introduced at University of Bologna *(late 13th century)*	Great Plague ravages Europe *(1346–47)* Syphilis epidemic in Europe *(1496–1500)*	Influenza pandemic in Europe *(1510)* Paracelsus questions the traditional authority of Galen and Avicenna and burns their books *(1527)* Establishment of anatomy theatres *(1550)*	William Harvey discovers of the circulation of the blood in 1616 Athanasius Kircher suggests micro-organisms as cause of infectious disease Thomas Sydenham working on classifying disease entities *(1670s)*	Herman Boerhaave establishes teaching of clinical method at Leiden Development of hospitals in Europe First university department of obstetrics *(1726)* in Edinburgh	Benjamin Franklin and Thomas Bond found first hospital in USA *(1752)* Giovanni Morgagni publishes *De sedibus et causis morborum... (1761)* Edward Jenner vaccinates patient against smallpox *(1796)*
Rhazes *(c.864–925)*	Haly Abbas *(d. 994)* Avicenna *(980–1037)* Albucasis *(936–c.1013)* Trotula *(fl. 11th century)* Hildegard of Bingen *(1098–1179)*	Averroës *(1126–1198)* Moses Maimonides *(c.1135–1204)* Arnold of Villanova *(1235–1311)*	Guy de Chauliac *(c.1300–1368)* Thomas Linacre *(1460–1524)* Girolamo Fracastoro *(c.1478–1553)* Paracelsus *(1493–1541)*	Li Shi-zhen *(1517–1593)* Andreas Vesalius *(1514–1564)* Ambroise Paré *(1510–1590)* William Harvey *(1578–1657)*	René Descartes *(1596–1650)* Thomas Sydenham *(1624–1689)* Marcello Malpighi *(1628–1694)* Herman Boerhaave *(1668–1738)* Giovanni Battista Morgagni *(1682–1771)*	Franz Anton Mesmer *(1734–1815)* John Hunter *(1728–1793)* Edward Jenner *(1749–1823)* Benjamin Rush *(1745–1813)* Philippe Pinel *(1745–1826)*	Samuel Hahnemann *(1755–1826)* Franz Joseph Gall *(1758–1828)* Samuel Thomson *(1769–1843)* Philippe Bozzini *(1773–1809)* Dominique-Jean Larrey *(1766–1842)*
				Andreas Vesalius publishes *De humani corporis fabrica (1543)* Girolamo Fracastoro publishes work on contagious illnesses *(1546)*	Sanctorius invents clinical thermometer *(1609)* William Harvey publishes *De motu cordis (1628)* Robert Hooke's *Micrographia* published *(1665)*	Post-mortem examinations advance understanding of disease	Antoine Lavoisier isolates and defines oxygen *(1775)* Linnaeus introduces his classification of diseases *(1763)*
Arab contributions to herbal medicine passed to the West through translated texts *(9th–12th centuries)*	Norman invaders introduce spicers into Britain	Medicines dispensed by monks from plants grown in monastery herb gardens Pharmacy develops as a specialist practice in the West	First apothecary shop in London *(1345)*	Otto Brunfels' *Herbarium vivae eicones (1530)* Leonhard Fuchs' *De historia stirpium (1542)* Li Shi-zhen's *Great Herbal* compiled in China *(1552–78)* John Gerard's *Herball (1597)*	Medicinal plants imported into Europe from the New World Nicholas Culpeper's *Herbal (1652)* Quinine from Peru used to treat malaria in Europe	Medicine chests stocked with herbs and drugs sold for use in the home in Europe	Anton Störck demonstrates use of poisonous plants as remedies *(1760s)* William Withering publishes account of his use of digitalis to cure dropsy *(1776)*
	One volume of Albucasis' collection of works devoted to surgery	*Surgery* by Roger of Palermo published *(c.1170)* Influential schools of anatomy at Salerno and Montpellier	Guido de Vigevano's *Anatomia (1345)* *Chirurgia magna* by Guy de Chauliac *(1363)*	Vesalius corrects anatomical mistakes of Galen Ambroise Paré eschews use of boiling oil to cauterize wounds *(1537)* Barber-Surgeons Company founded in England *(1540)*			John Hunter lectures on theory and practice of surgery *(1771)* Dominique-Jean Larrey introduces *ambulances volantes (1793)*
			Insane asylums established at Seville *(1409)* and Padua *(1410)*	St Mary of Bethlehem hospital (Bedlam) founded in London *(1547)*			William Battie publishes *Treatise on Madness (1757)* Philippe Pinel liberalizes treatment of the insane in Paris *(1790s)*
Muslim invasion of Spain *(711)* Collapse of first Mayan civilization *(850)*	Vikings settle in Greenland *(985)* and reach America *(1000)* Norman conquest of Britain *(1066)* Gunpowder invented in China *(1044)*	Crusades *(1095–1291)* Inca dynasty founded in Peru *(1200)* Marco Polo arrives in China *(1275)* Mongols sack Baghdad *(1258)*	Ming dynasty founded in China *(1368)* Johann Gutenberg uses type to print books *(1440–1455)* Turks capture Constantinople *(1453)* Columbus discovers New World *(1492)*	Reformation in Northern Europe *(1517–1521)* Mughal dynasty founded in India *(1526)* Spanish overthrow Aztec empire *(1521)* Francis Drake circumnavigates world *(1577–1580)*	First English settlement in America *(1607)* End of Ming dynasty in China *(1644)* Pennsylvania founded *(1681)*	War of the Spanish Succession *(1710–1713)* Ephraim Chambers publishes influential *Cyclopaedia (1728)* Industrial Revolution begins *(c.1750)*	James Watt invents steam engine *(1765)* James Cook lands in Australia *(1770)* American Declaration of Independence *(1776)* French Revolution *(1789–1799)*

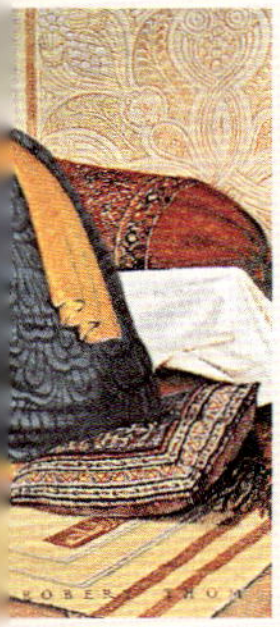

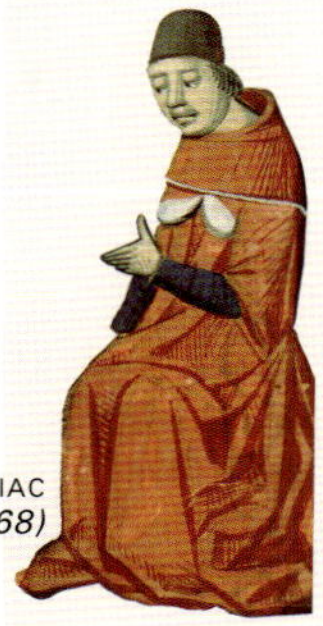

GUY DE CHAULIAC *(c.1300-1368)*

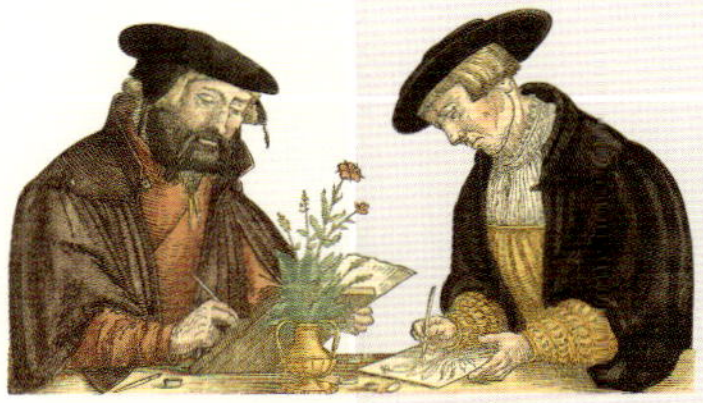

LEONHARD FUCHS (LEFT)

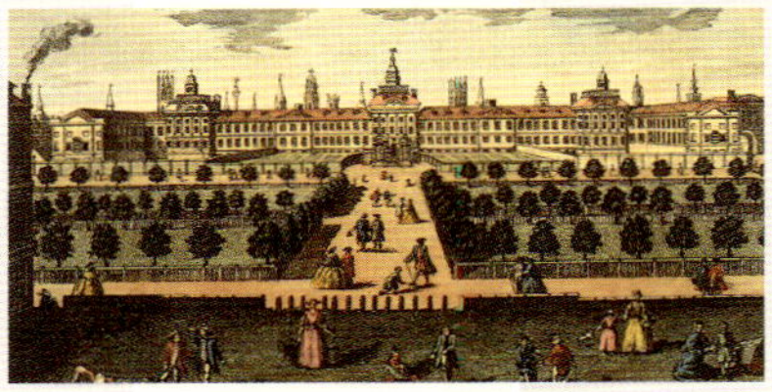

ST MARY OF BETHLEHEM HOSPITAL

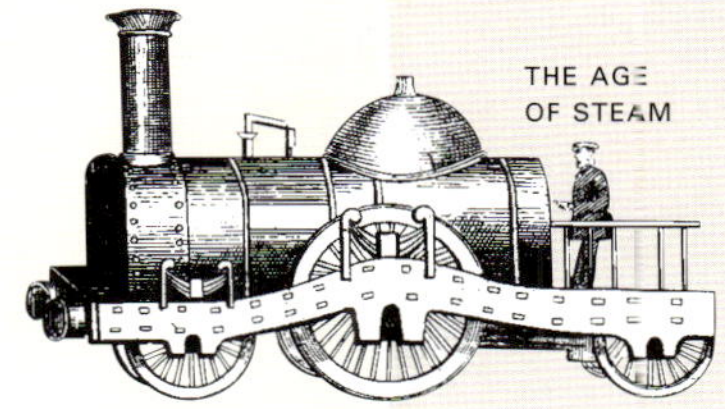

THE AGE OF STEAM

	AD 1800–1815	AD 1815–1830	AD 1830–1850	AD 1850–1860	AD 1860–1870	AD 1870–1880	AD 1880–1890	AD 1890–1900
WORLD MEDICINE	Rise of specialist hospitals *(through 19th century)*	First publication of *Lancet* medical journal in England	Introduction of anaesthesia *(1840s)* American Medical Association founded *(1847)* Ignaz Semmelweiss establishes principles of asepsis *(1849)*		International Red Cross founded *(1864)* Louis Pasteur shows that germs cause decay *(1861)*	Rise of specialism in Western medical practice Thermometers used in clinical diagnosis	Robert Koch announces discovery of tubercle bacillus *(1882)*	Ronald Ross discovers parasite responsible for malaria *(1897)* Aspirin introduced on the market by Farbenfabriken Bayer *(1899)*
HEALERS	Edwin Chadwick *(1800–1890)*	Ignaz Semmelweiss *(1818–1865)* Louis Pasteur *(1822–1895)* Jean-Martin Charcot *(1825–1893)* Florence Nightingale *(1820–1910)* Joseph Lister *(1827–1912)*	Robert Koch *(1843–1910)* William Osler *(1849–1919)* Daniel D. Palmer *(1845–1913)* Wilhelm Roentgen *(1845–1923)*	Paul Ehrlich *(1854–1915)* Sigmund Freud *(1856–1939)*	Sir Frederick Gowland Hopkins *(1861–1947)* Marie Curie *(1867–1934)* Harvey Cushing *(1869–1939)*	Carl Jung *(1875–1961)*	Harold Gillies *(1882–1960)* Margaret Sanger *(1883–1966)* Alexander Fleming *(1881–1955)* Elizabeth Kenny *(1886–1952)* Marie Stopes *(1880–1958)*	Frederick Banting *(1891–1941)* Gerhard Domagk *(1895–1964)* Charles Best *(1899–1978)* Howard Florey *(1898–1968)*
SCIENCE	MFX Bichat publishes *General Anatomy...* *(1801)*	RTH Laënnec invents stethoscope *(1816)*		Hermann Helmholtz invents ophthalmoscope *(1851)* Rudolf Virchow publishes *Die Cellularpathologie* *(1858)*	Carl Wunderlich publishes *On the Temperature in Disease* *(1868)* Science of bacteriology develops	First cystoscope developed *(1877)*		Wilhelm Roentgen announces discovery of X-rays *(1895)* Viruses discovered *(1890s)*
HERBALISM		Alkaloids begin to be isolated from plants *(1817)* *In vacuo* evaporation used in preparation of plants by John Barry *(1819)* Thomsonian medicine established in USA *(1820s)*		Albert Niemann isolates cocaine from the leaves of a Peruvian shrub *(1860)*				
SURGERY	Ephraim McDowell performs first elective abdominal operation *(1809)*		Anaesthesia (ether) first used by Crawford Long during surgery *(1842)* Inhalation method of anaesthesia established *(1846–7)*	Nikolai Pirigov publishes *Klinische Chirugie* *(1854)*	Joseph Lister conducts first operation with antiseptic *(1865)*		First successful gastrectomy by Theodor Billroth *(1881)*	
PSYCHIATRY	Benjamin Rush writes first American textbook on psychiatry *(1810)*		First school for mentally retarded founded in Massachusetts *(1847)*		Association of German alienists founded *(1864)*	Jean-Martin Charcot working with hysterics at Salpêtrière *(1870s)*	Hypnosis used to treat mental illness *(1880s)*	Sigmund Freud formulates theory of hysterical neurosis *(1895)*
WORLD HISTORY	Louisiana Purchase *(1803)* Napoleon defeated at Waterloo *(1815)*	First passenger-carrying steam railway *(1825)* Louis Daguerre invents photography *(1829)*	Slavery abolished in the British Empire *(1830)* First Opium War between England and China *(1840–1842)*	Crimean War *(1853–1856)* Charles Darwin publishes *The Origin of Species* *(1859)*	American Civil War *(1861–1865)*	Alexander Graham Bell invents telephone *(1876)* Thomas Edison invents electric light bulb *(1879)*	First motor cars invented	Boer War *(1899–1902)*

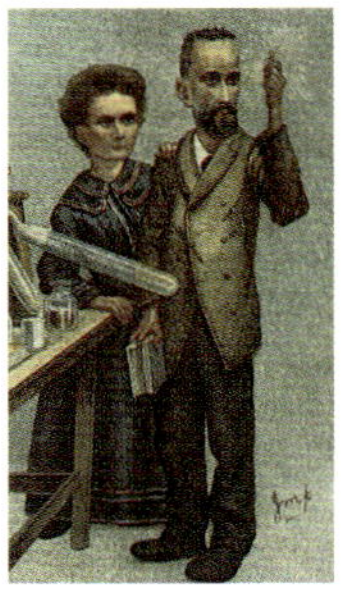
MARIE CURIE
(1867–1934)

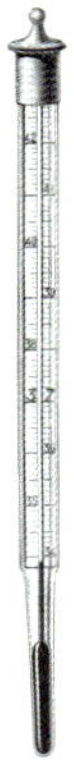

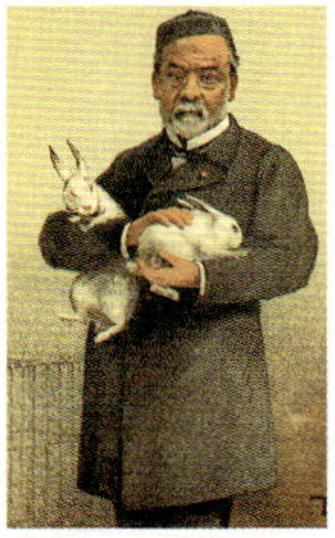
LOUIS PASTEUR
(1822–1895)

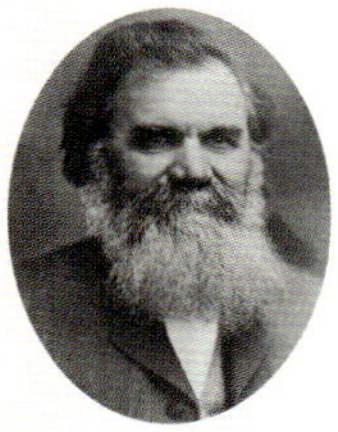
DANIEL D PALMER
(1845–1913)

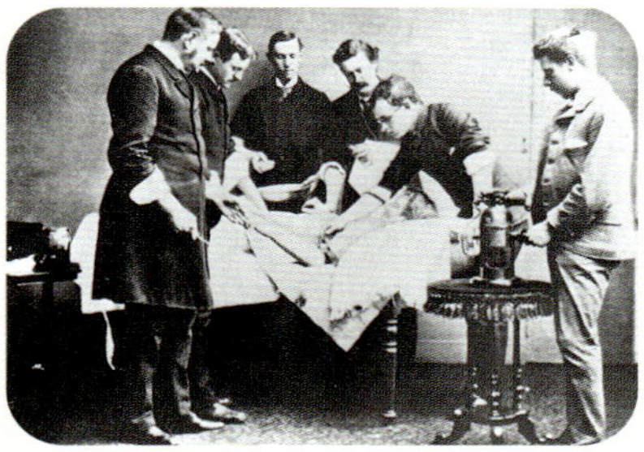
USE OF ANTISEPTIC IN 1860s

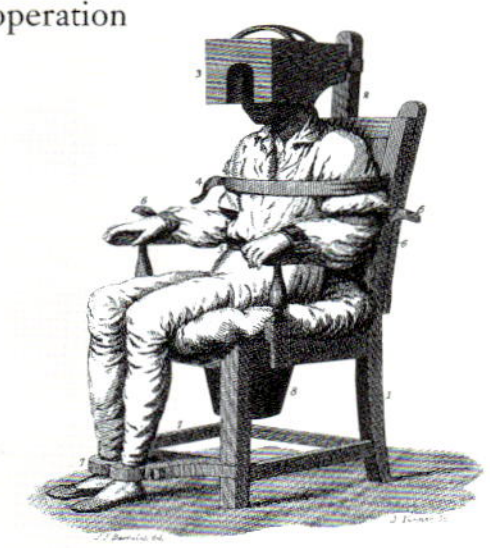
RUSH'S RESTRAINT CHAIR

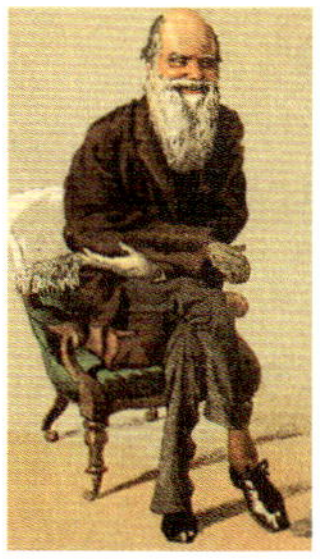
CHARLES DARWIN

HYPNOSIS
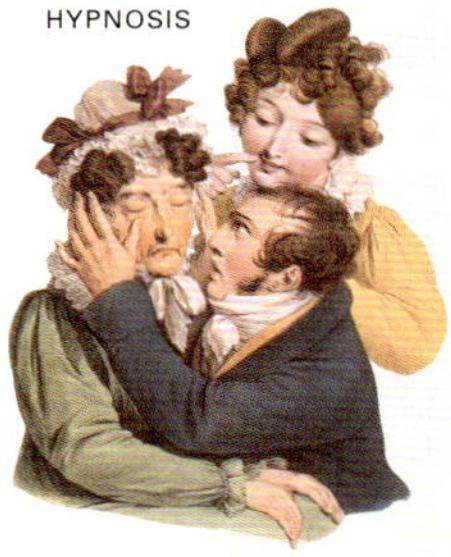

EDISON INVENTS LIGHT BULB
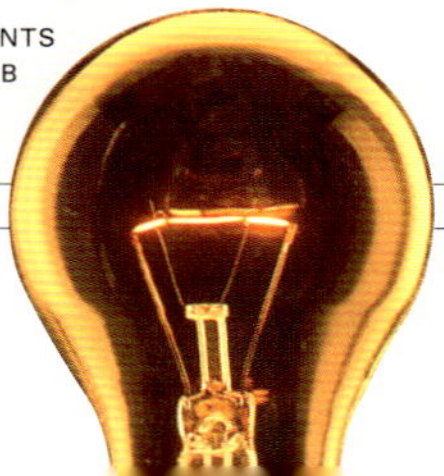

AD 1900–1910	AD 1910–1920	AD 1920–1930	AD 1930–1945	AD 1945–1960	AD 1960–1970	AD 1970–1980	AD 1980–PRESENT DAY
Discovery of main blood groups makes blood transfusions possible *(1901)* Barbiturates introduced *(1903)* Marie Stopes opens first birth-control clinic in England *(early 1900s)*	Paul Ehrlich discovers first 'magic bullet' drug – salvarsan – to treat syphilis *(1910)* Influenza pandemic kills 15 million *(1918–1919)*	Leon Calmette inoculates children against TB with BCG. *(1924)*	Anti-malarial drug, atebrin, discovered *(1932)* Sulphonamide drugs discovered *(1935)* Selman Waksman discovers anti-tuberculosis drug, streptomycin *(1943)* Antibiotics used to treat bacterial infections	Structure of DNA elucidated by Wilkins, Crick and Watson *(1953)* Polio vaccine discovered by Jonas Salk *(1955)* DDT widely used to control mosquitos transmitting malaria	Measles vaccine introduced *(1963)* Hospice movement for care of terminally ill introduced by Dame Cicely Saunders *(1967)*	First test-tube baby born *(1978)*	First clinical description of AIDS *(1981)*
Ernst Chain *(1906–1979)* Gregory Pincus *(1903–1967)*	Jonas Salk *(1914–1995)* Peter Medawar *(1915–1987)* Maurice Wilkins *(1916–)* Francis Crick *(1916–)*	Christiaan Barnard *(1922–)* James Watson *(1928–)*					
Marie Curie publishes *Researches on Radioactive Substances* *(1903)* ECG tests introduced by Wilem Einthoven	Vitamin B isolated *(1917)*	Frederick Banting and Charles Best discover insulin *(1921)* Alexander Fleming discovers pencillin *(1929)*	First kidney dialysis machine invented by Willem Kolff *(1938)* Howard Florey and Ernst Chain establish clinical use of pencillin *(1941)*	Contraceptive pill developed by Gregory Pincus *(1951)* First clinically useful ultrasound images *(1950s)*		CAT scanners developed *(1970s)*	Magnetic resonance imaging (MRI) developed *(1980s)*
	Chemical industry develops – pharmaceutical industry produces drugs that supplant herbs in general market		Edward Bach develops Bach flower remedies *(1930s)*			*Barefoot Doctor's Manual*, a Chinese herbal, published in the West Herbal 'renaissance' develops in the West, embracing diverse systems and practices of healing from around the world	
	Harold Gillies organizes unit for facial plastic surgery during World War I American College of Surgeons founded *(1913)*		First leucotomy performed by Egas Moniz *(1935)* Penicillin used to treat wound infection *(1940s)*	Heart/lung pump first used in open-heart surgery *(1953)* First resection of aortic aneurysm *(1951)* First kidney graft *(1954)*	First heart transplant by Christiaan Barnard *(1967)*		Keyhole surgery developed *(1986)*
Emil Kraepelin publishes *Lectures in Clinical Psychiatry* *(1901)*	Eugen Bleuler proposes the term 'schizophrenia' *(1911)* to replace dementia praecox		ECT used to treat depression Frontal leucotomy introduced for treatment of psychiatric disease *(1935)*	Psychotropic drugs used to treat schizophrenia and depression *(1950s)*			The antidepressant drug Prozac is licensed by the US Food and Drug Administration *(1987)*
First powered flight by Wright brothers *(1903)*	World War I *(1914–1918)* Albert Einstein publishes *General Theory of Relativity* *(1916)*	Soviet Union established *(1922)*	Adolf Hitler comes to power in Germany *(1933)* World War II *(1939–1945)* US explodes first atomic bomb *(1945)*	Soviet Union launches Sputnik I, first satellite *(1957)*	Cultural Revolution in China *(1966–1976)* Cuban Missile Crisis *(1962)* First man on the Moon *(1969)*	Oil crisis following Yom Kippur War *(1973)*	IBM Personal Computer (PC) introduced *(1981)* Collapse of Soviet Union *(1991)* Internet revolutionizes personal access to information

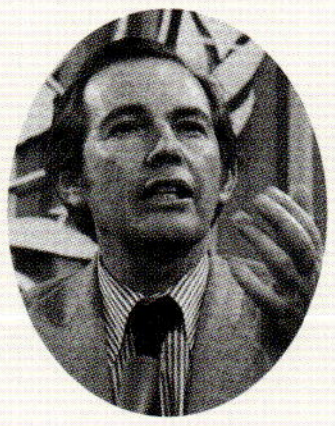
CHRISTIAAN BARNARD *(1922-)*

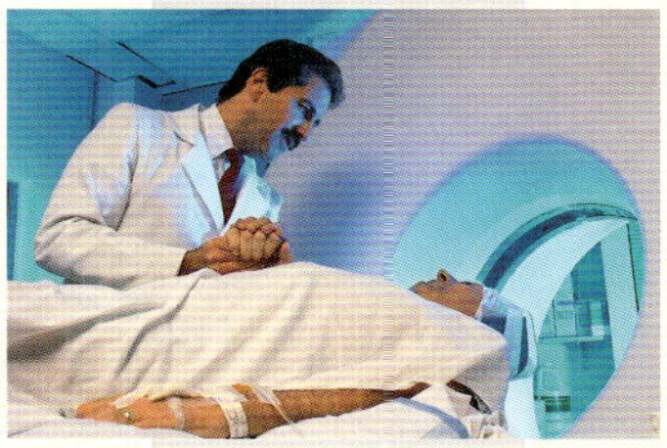
CAT SCANNER

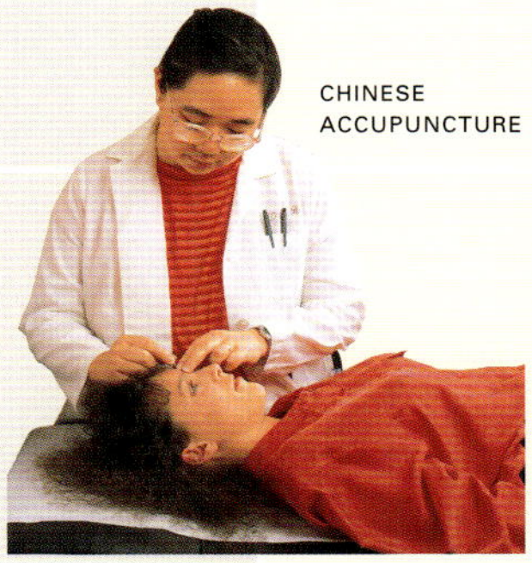
CHINESE ACCUPUNCTURE

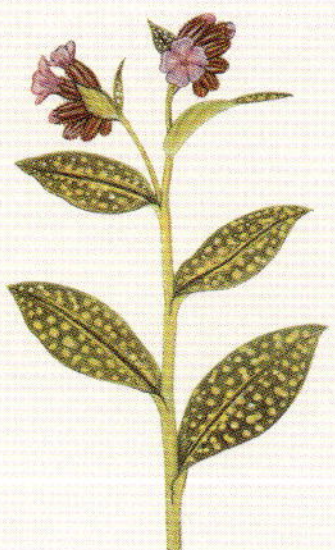
FLOWER REMEDIES

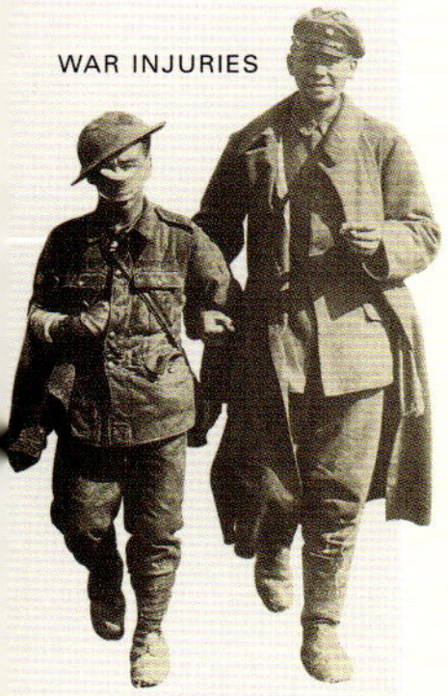
WAR INJURIES

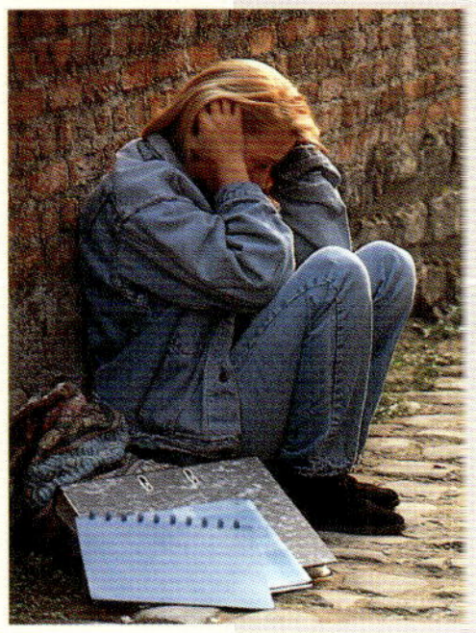
DEPRESSION

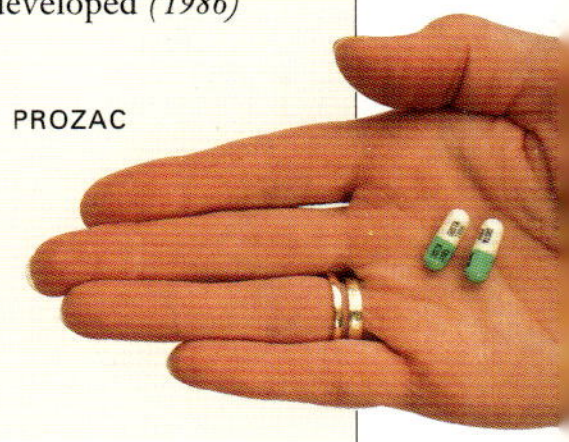
PROZAC

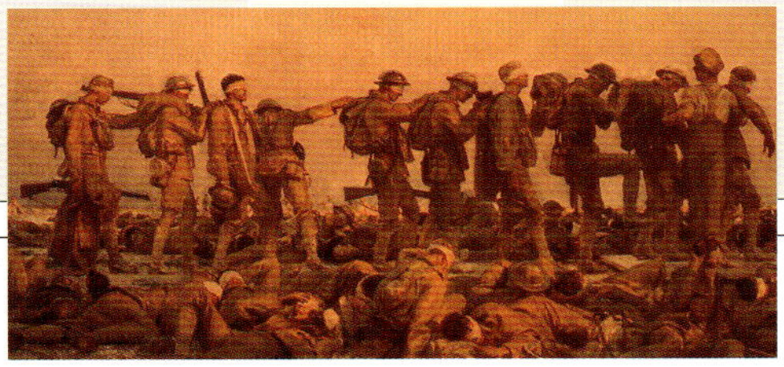
WORLD WAR I

CHAPTER ONE

THE HISTORY OF MEDICINE

FROM ITS ANCIENT ORIGINS TO THE MODERN WORLD

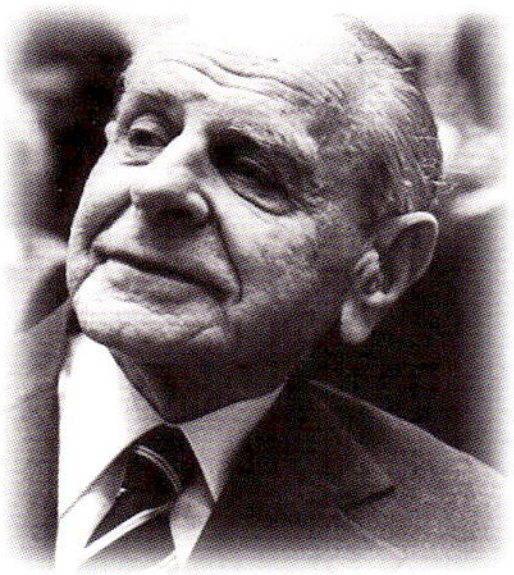

ABOVE Karl Popper, the distinguished twentieth-century philosopher of science.

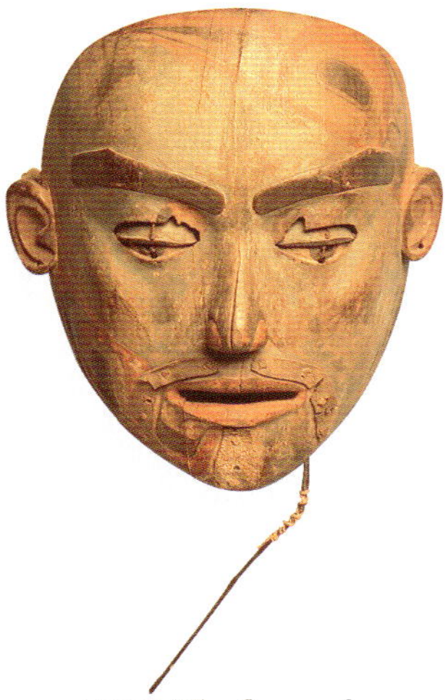

ABOVE The figure of the shaman occupies a significant place in the history of primitive medicine. This mask is from the Haida culture of north-west America.

MEDICINE AND SURGERY *today cover a multitude of special disciplines. To follow the world history of each requires the tracing of many separate routes through time. Different cultures, from their very beginnings, have established their own special ways in the care of the sick. Scientific and alternative medicine have followed different paths at different speeds. Rational treatment ultimately depends upon properly understanding the true nature of disease. The philosopher Karl Popper, who has clarified much scientific thought, said that the advance of knowledge consists, mainly, in the modification of earlier knowledge. And so it is in the art of healing.*

It is as well, at the beginning, to enquire where does modern medical knowledge start? Has the science of modern medicine and surgery anything to do with the primitive beliefs of our early forefathers? Do you believe that a totemic object associated with witchcraft, such as an African nail effigy resembling a human pincushion, has anything to do with the history of medicine? Do aromatherapy and cardiac surgery have a common ancestor?

What purpose did the nail effigy serve? It suggests the European magical practice of sticking pins into a wax doll to cause harm to an enemy. This can have little to do with the real cause and effect of injury and disease. Rationally, we argue that sticking nails into a manikin does not cause injury; and neither would pulling them out cure it. But such an explanation could well fit the ideas and firmly held beliefs of its users. There could, therefore, be accepted reason for the practice. But it has no scientific future. It is an attempt to provide harm by association, known as sympathetic magic. There are other traces of it to be found in Europe in the Middle Ages, when surgeons sought to cure wounds – with no success – by treating only the weapons that caused them, using an ointment known as a weapon salve.

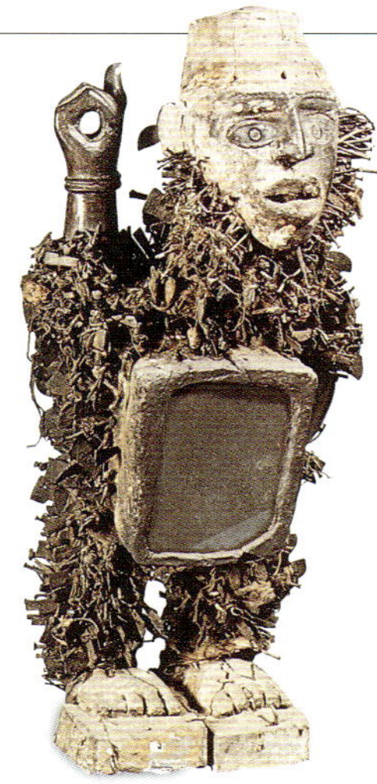

ABOVE A dramatic nail effigy like this, which comes from Africa, suggests a belief in sympathetic magic. Ill health is ascribed to the influence of external powers.

RIGHT A Dinka witchdoctor from Sudan – a modern exponent of an ancient art.

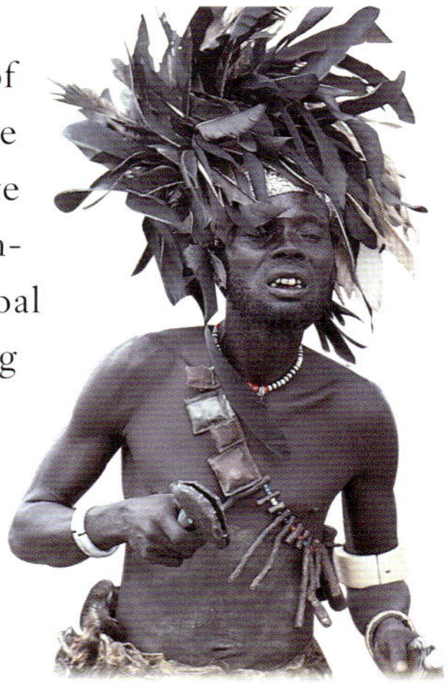

Using the same line of argument, neither can we believe that the elaborate rituals associated with divining bones, hallowed by tribal tradition, before throwing them and interpreting the pattern of their fall, are the origin of clinical diagnosis. Have they a place in medical history?

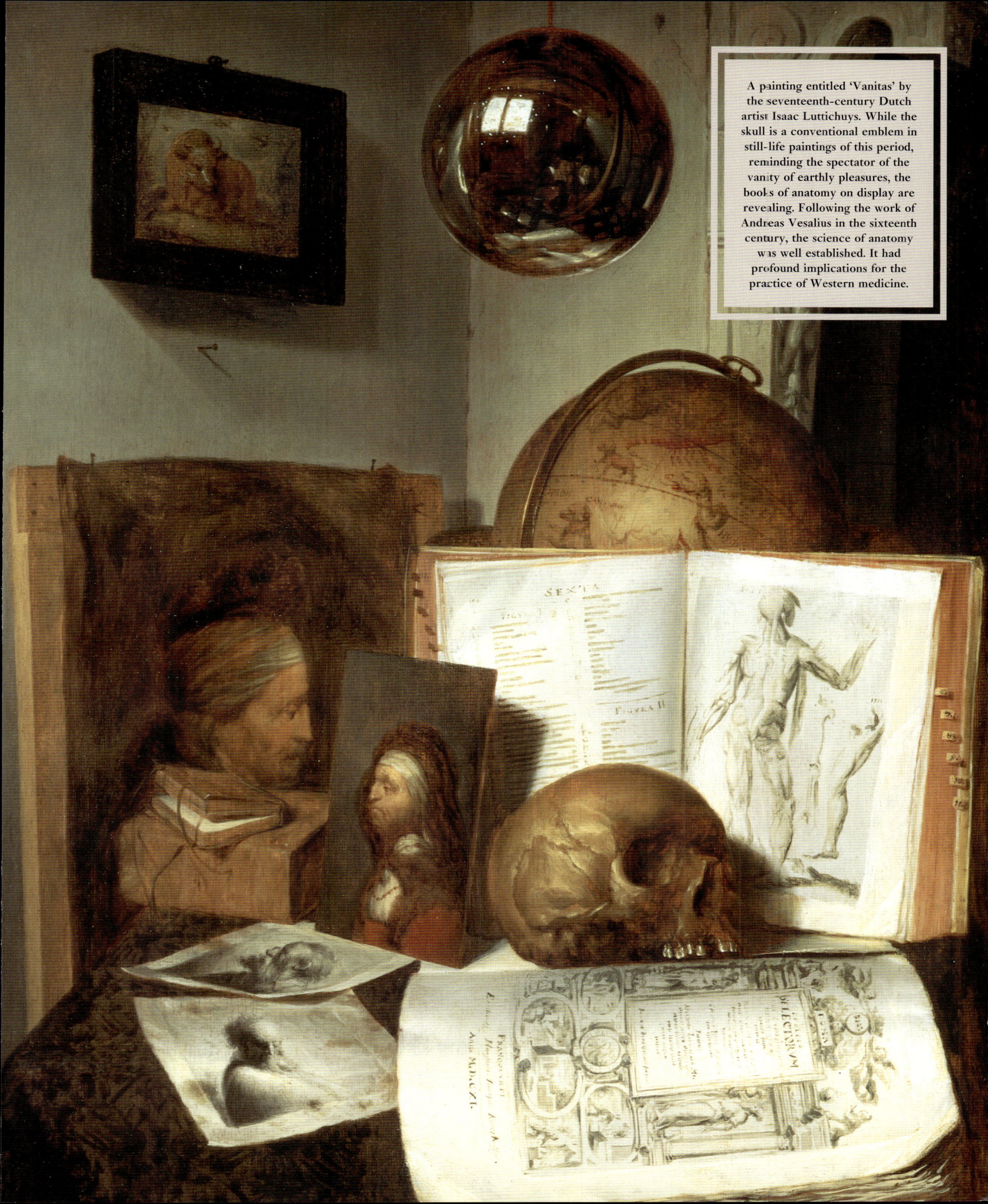

A painting entitled 'Vanitas' by the seventeenth-century Dutch artist Isaac Luttichuys. While the skull is a conventional emblem in still-life paintings of this period, reminding the spectator of the vanity of earthly pleasures, the books of anatomy on display are revealing. Following the work of Andreas Vesalius in the sixteenth century, the science of anatomy was well established. It had profound implications for the practice of Western medicine.

THE MEDICINE MAN'S DIAGNOSIS

In the terms of primitive society, the medicine man, who manipulated this type of model of sickness and health, was a carefully selected practitioner. Carefully selected for his ability to explain disease, as well as other natural phenomena, in terms well understood by the patient, even though they have no scientific basis as we in the West would understand it today. He did more than treat illness. He also needed to explain misfortune in terms understood by his patients and to treat its consequences. Ill luck was an accepted part of his practice, but it was ill luck that was thought to have an attributable cause.

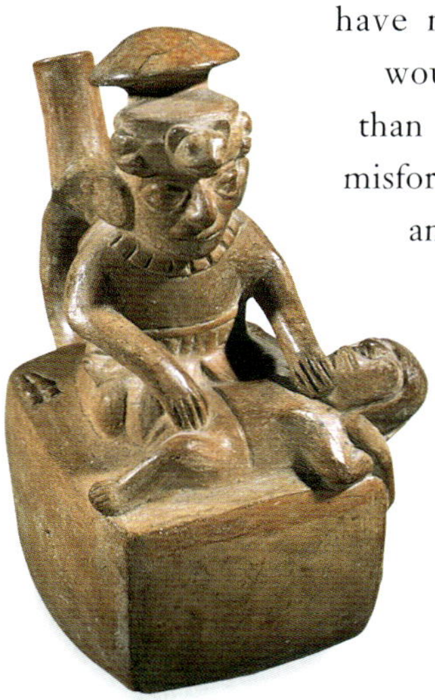

ABOVE This pottery jar from the Mochica culture of northern Peru *(c.200 BC to AD 600)* shows a doctor or shaman figure examining a woman patient.

The medicine man used the current tribal interpretations of natural happenings to arrive at a diagnosis. They provided an explanation of the cause of illness or misfortune. The advice often included prophylaxis, i.e., how to prevent a recurrence. The displeasure of the spirits, the ghosts of the dead, or the gods of nature were accepted as sound reasons for punishment of human beings, and such manifestations of displeasure required expert handling. Punishment for the offence could take the form of an attack of illness. We would probably dismiss such explanations of an event as superstitious; they are untestable in scientific terms. Yet they were acceptable to the tribal code of beliefs. They were sometimes complex. The medicine man was the final arbiter.

There have been many different types of therapists who performed a similar role in different countries around the globe. Many still existed in the nineteenth century and some may be found even in the twentieth century. The Native American medicine man is perhaps the best known. But other examples include the Siberian shaman, the African witch doctor, the English leech, even the Welsh *dyn hysbus* (or magician) and the ubiquitous seer. Different countries have also developed their own simple folk remedies by dint of trial and experience.

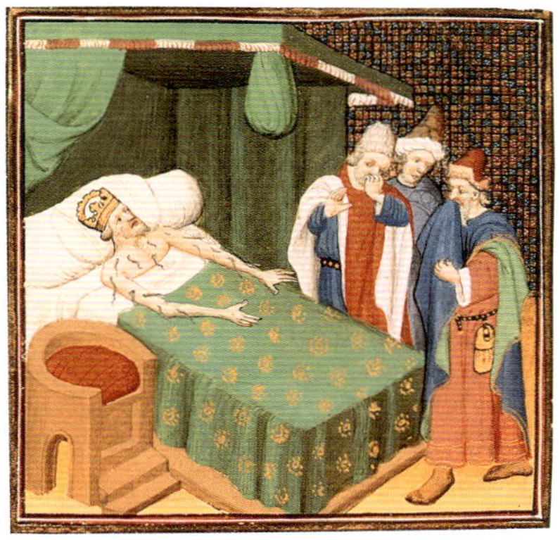

ABOVE Blood-letting was thought to draw off corrupt matter from the body. This illustration shows leeches applied to the Roman emperor Galerius by his physicians.

In a way, the role of the medicine man resembled that of the lawyer more than the doctor. He was trained to acknowledge tribal precedents and thus, to be a successful practitioner, he had clearly to understand his peoples' customs. He was not an innovator. His methods were not open to question. Because he looked only *outside* the human body for the cause and cure of disease, his role differed from that of the modern family doctor.

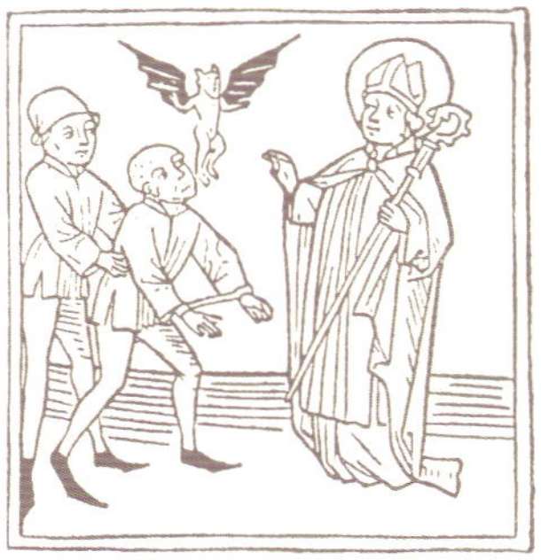

ABOVE In the past, treament of the mentally ill often involved the casting out of demons, which the Christian church termed exorcism.

Ideas of demons and possession of the body and mind by evil spirits have been a common and enduring feature in human civilization. As late as the seventeenth century, the practice of orthodox European doctors was not so advanced that possession by demons could be regarded as superstitious folly. Indeed the ritual of exorcism was encouraged by the Catholic Church.

EARLY IDEAS OF MEDICAL TREATMENT

As a general principle, therapy seems appropriate if the patient accepts an explanation of its purpose and rationale. When illness was believed to result from the displeasure or anger of the spirits, or because of the trangression of their laws, then appeasement or propitiation of the spirits was called for. This is rational behaviour if one accepts a belief in spirits, and if everyone further accepts that the remedies will work.

This acceptance of the prevailing belief in the efficacy of tried-and-tested methods accounts for the power of empirical remedies, more commonly known as 'tried remedies'. It is a class of medical treatment on which orthodox and unorthodox practioners have relied for centuries, and many still do.

To understand the history of medicine it is important to understand the meaning of the frequently used term *empiricism.* This is succinctly defined by *The Oxford English Dictionary* as 'The theory which regards experience as the only source of knowledge.' It formed the accepted practice of the Graeco-Roman School of empiricists who stated that 'illness was cured by medicine, not by argument'. The term empiricism has since been used pejoratively as describing the 'ignorant practice of a quack doctor'. However, this latter observation perpetuates an injustice to the origins of the term. The difficulty is in knowing when and how a remedy may be both 'tried' and effective. Prejudice naturally affects such judgements.

Many folk remedies have maintained their reputation for effectiveness, to be handed on from generation to generation, on the word of the village elders. Often, the detail changes. Reliance on the old-fashioned home doctor's 'cold cures' of goose grease rubbed on the chest with an old sock, or the magical removal of warts brought about by burying bacon at the crossroads, have in recent times been replaced by belief in proprietary remedies. Advertisements extolling the remedial powers of pills and potions, showing countless satisfied users, have long been a common feature of newspapers and magazines. Advertisements on our television screens are in a way modern substitutes both for them and the older rural quack doctor.

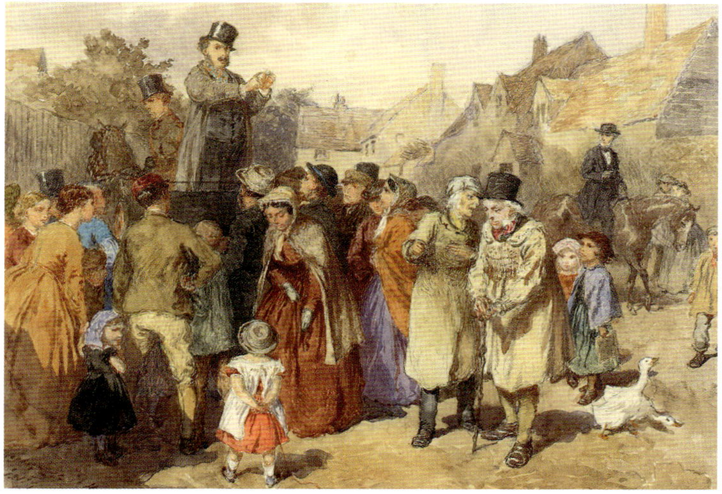

ABOVE The quack doctor – here painted by Charles Green *(1840–1898)* – trades on popular belief in the efficacy of what he is selling. Traditionally people like to place their trust in the empirically tried remedy.

Faith in the efficacy of a treatment plays a large part in feeling better. Confidence in a remedy is reinforced by word-of-mouth repetition, when everyone tells everyone else in everyday conversation that they simply know it works. In the past, compliance in accepting nasty medicine and undergoing heroic surgery was generally ensured when patients were warned of the dire consequences to their health that might follow if they refused. The acceptance of the presently prevailing beliefs are comfortably reassuring to the sick.

In the light of these observations, it is easier for us to understand how, in order to make a diagnosis, the early medicine man quite reasonably looked around and about, in accordance with his precepts, for signs of the spirits' or the gods' displeasure and advised on how best the wrath could be propitiated.

ANGLO-SAXON SUPERSTITION

The Anglo-Saxon of the tenth century, in seeking the cause of disease, would sometimes conduct a search for elf shot, which was imagined to be a shower of arrows with which elves were believed to produce attacks of sudden illness in humans. Elves were well known as mischievous bringers of ill luck. No offence was necessary to invite a shower of elf shot. Naturally, it was not easy to demonstrate actual signs of its use by producing evidence of the missiles themselves, though in more recent times Neolithic arrowheads have been regarded as elf-arrows or elf-bolts by people living in localities where they are found. Belief in elves was widespread in northern Europe at this time.

People have a basic need to explain personal misfortune, whether it comes in the form of an accident or illness. Why did it happen to me? And they need confidence in accepting explanations as to how to avoid or overcome it. Popular 'folk' explanations are not always supported by sound science. This is understandable, for there has been a continuity in our behaviour and our beliefs since the very earliest times that owes more to our inherited emotions than to what we, as men and women, have learned from philosophers. We might concur with the archaeologist, Grahame Clarke, who is of the opinion that 'To the peoples of the world generally... I venture to think that Palaeolithic Man has more meaning than the Greeks.'

This primitive but confident attitude to disease and its treatment fulfilled a fundamental human need. It may even explain the expressed preference of many people in the late twentieth century for 'alternative' rather than scientific medicine. It is paradoxical that a decline in patient confidence in doctors in recent years has accompanied remarkable improvements in many therapies and in rates of curing previously fatal diseases. Primitive medicine, therefore, has a justifiable place in a general history of our attitudes to medicine, treatment and disease.

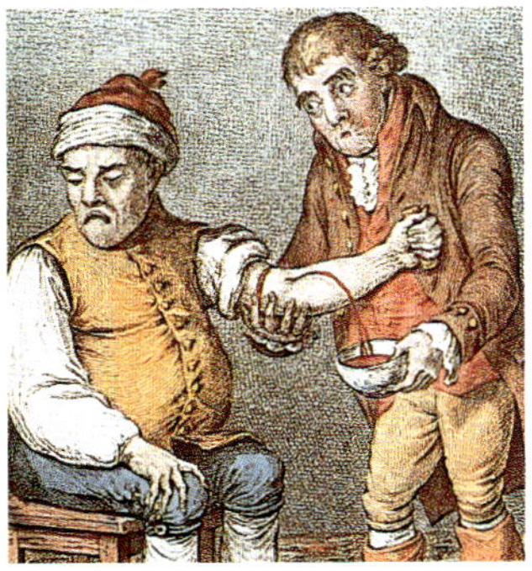

ABOVE **Blood-letting – a therapy whereby a vein is opened to drain off a quantity of blood – has a long medical history.**

From the earliest civilizations essentially until the eighteenth century, we shall see that medical practice remained basically simple; confidently, but mistakenly, adding enemas, purges and bleedings on a material plane, while continuing to accept the possibility of miraculous healing on a spiritual one.

PRIMITIVE SURGERY

There has been a tendency for historians to regard the surgeon as the poor relative of the physician, not necessarily in the financial sense, but certainly in the intellectual. This slur may have arisen because his work was frequently regarded as requiring more manual than mental skill. There is little concrete evidence of the results of surgery in prehistoric times. The soft tissues on which it was used have perished. But there are skeletal survivals from the past which indicate that surgery did take place, and parallel procedures observed in contemporary primitive cultures indicate its possible nature.

The surgeon's most valuable and readily available instrument is his own hand. In the course of time its simple use in the manipulation of fractures and dislocations was extended by the addition of a knife, which facilitated amputations or the removal of arrow heads in wounds. Knives were frequently made from sharpened shells and stones. Wounds needed protection and the likely dressings were mosses and leaves. Needles made of bone, with an eye for thread, have been found in Palaeolithic deposits. So the apparatus for suturing (or stitching up wounds) was available, although we can never be sure when it was first used to close wounds and arrest haemorrhage. An ingenious method of suture has been observed in modern primitive tribal cultures whereby the edges of the wound are drawn closely together and ants or termites are then applied to the wound, so that their powerful jaws secure the flesh. Once attached, the body of the termite is then severed, allowing only the jaws to remain firmly in place to hold the wound shut. Perhaps Palaeolithic man used a similar technique?

The practice of circumcision is another age-old form of simple surgery which does have an hygienic basis. An even older and more dramatic surgical operation, for which there is prehistoric fossil evidence, is revealed by our earliest ancestors' skill in trephining the skull to remove a round piece of bone from it. It is possible to do this with flint instruments, either by gradually scratching through the skin and bones of the skull, getting gradually deeper and deeper; or by drilling a series of small holes in a circle in the skull and then cutting the small bridges between to remove a disc of bone.

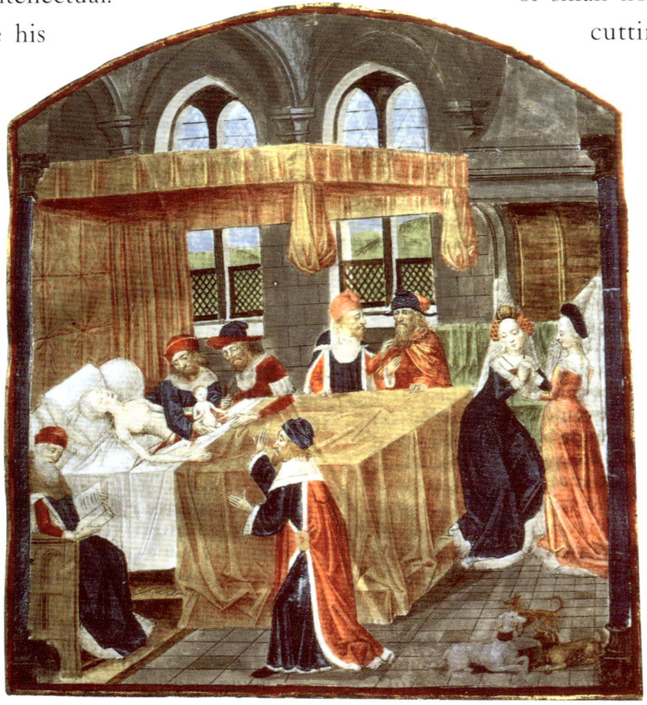

ABOVE **A fifteenth-century French illustration of birth by Caesarean section. Until the nineteenth century, the likelihood of the mother surviving such an operation was remote.**

The real purpose of this seemingly dangerous and terrifying experience is unknown. There have been many proffered explanations. The most commonly accepted suggestion is that it was done so that the piece of bone removed from the skull might be used as a talisman or amulet. The number of trephined skulls that have been found demonstrate the frequency with which it was performed. The fact that the edges of the bony hole in some examples show callous formation indicates the survival of the patient or victim. The occurrence of skulls with multiple holes shows that some probably survived to undergo futher trephination. Others have suggested that the practice was therapeutic, either to remove a depressed fracture, to try to cure mental illness, or more theoretically to relieve headache!

The history of Caesarean section for surgical delivery of the unborn child is also of great antiquity, with accounts of its even being performed by the mother herself. It got its name from the Roman *Lex Caesarea* which stipulated that a foetus had to be removed from a dead pregnant woman and buried separately.

EARLY HISTORICAL EVIDENCE OF MEDICINE AND SURGERY

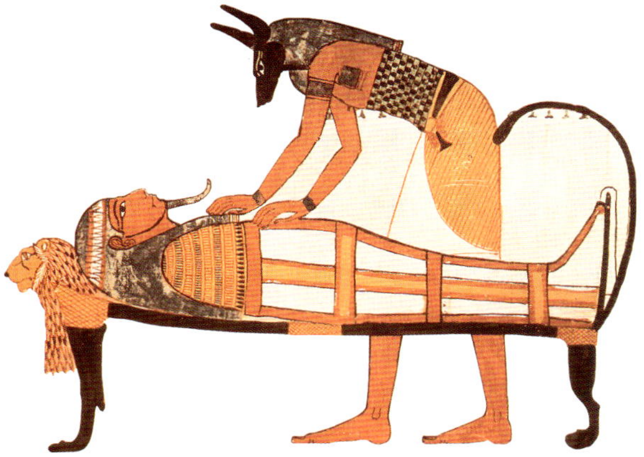

ABOVE A wall painting from the tomb of Sennedjem (XIXth Dynasty, *c.1320–1200 BC)* showing the god Anubis embalming the body of a pharaoh. Although the supernatural played a large part in Ancient Egyptian medicine, there is also evidence of an organized medical profession.

EGYPT

The name most frequently recalled in accounts of Ancient Egyptian medicine is that of Imhotep, the grand vizier (or high government official) of King Zoser, who reigned about 2980 BC. A man of many parts (he was the reputed architect of the large pyramid of Sakkara), Imhotep was greatly revered as a physician and was later deified as the god of medicine. Temple sleep, known as incubation, in which the god appeared to the patient in a dream and indicated the appropriate treatment, became one of the rites of his worship. Similar rites developed in the later Greek worship of the god Aesculapius.

The Ancient Egyptian texts that have survived, dating from about 2000 to 1200 BC, refer to even earlier periods. One of the most important is the Edwin Smith Papyrus of about 1600 BC. The name is that of its discoverer, an American Egyptologist, who discovered it at Luxor in AD 1862.

MEDICINE IN BABYLON AND ASSYRIA

There is more evidence of early medicine found in the cuneiform writing preserved on baked clay tablets from ancient Babylon and Assyria. These early civilizations developed in Mesopotamia (in what is now known as Iraq) from around 3500 BC onwards. The most well known account is found in the Laws of Hammurabi *(1948–1905 BC)*, Hammurabi being a ruler of Babylon. They were written on a pillar or slab, known as a stele, eight feet (2.4m) long. Among a variety of laws dealing with social conditions and economic regulations are some detailing the responsibilities of the physician. These showed that the profession was highly regulated and contained clauses that inflicted severe punishment on the unsuccessful surgeon, including the loss of his hand as a penalty for surgical incompetence.

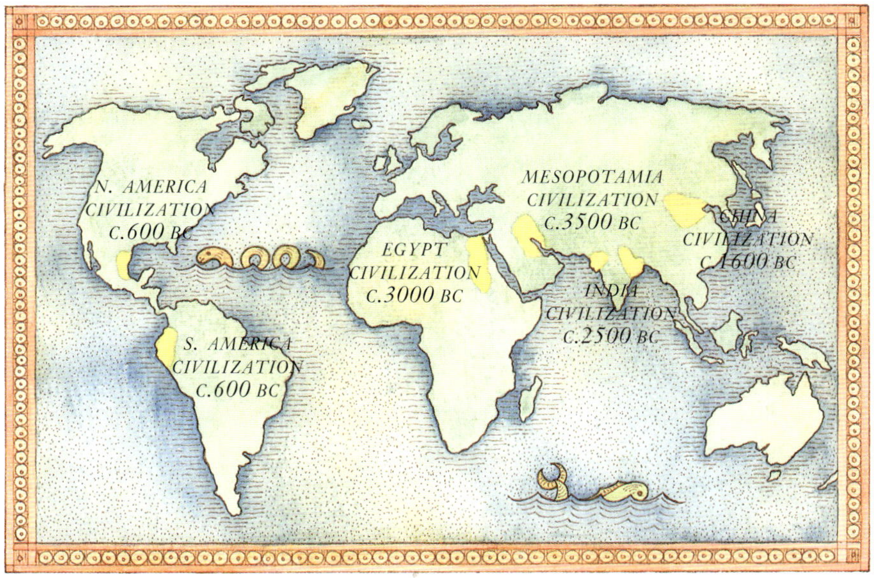

BELOW This map shows the first civilizations for which written evidence of medical practices exists. Our understanding of medicine in prehistoric times remains largely guesswork.

The Ebers Papyrus, dating from the sixteenth century BC, contains even older prescriptions for the treatment of various diseases. It was discovered in a tomb near Luxor. The papyri show that both medicine and surgery were extensively practised, with evidence of specialization in certain disciplines. Many prescriptions are listed; these are made up from hundreds of different substances including minerals, plants, and animal byproducts. The treatments for bone fractures are given in detail. An interesting addendum appears in some documents to the effect that the practitioner divides his advice on treatment into three parts: an ailment or injury that he will treat, one that he will contend with and one that he will not treat.

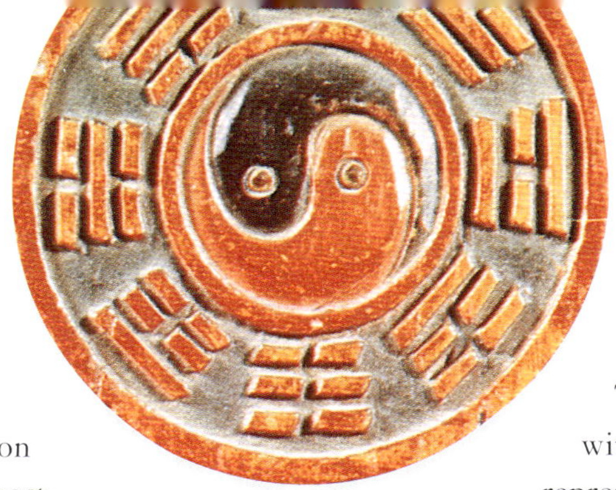

ABOVE The Chinese symbols of the opposed but complementary principcles of *Yin* and *Yang* are surrounded by trigrams that represent natural phenomena.

INDIA

Early Hindu medicine belongs to the Brahman period *(800 BC–AD 1000)* and the famous medical textbook *Su´sruta Samhitā* contains a materia medica of some 760 medicinal plants. There is a large section on surgery, describing 101 instruments, 'the most important of which is the hand'. The use of the cautery, of leeches, excision, aspiration, and suturing are described. The instructions are detailed and cover operations for anal fistula, tonsillectomy, lithotomy and Caesarian section. The operation for rhinoplasty (plastic surgery on the nose) was devised presumably to restore the noses of adulterers, who had lost them as punishment.

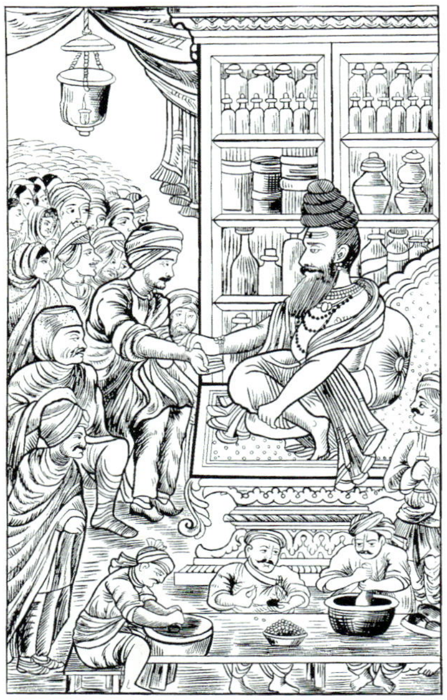

ABOVE An undated drawing of Su´sruta, one of the founders of Indian medicine. Although hard to date precisely, the classic text entitled *Su´sruta Samhitā* or *Su´sruta's Compendium* is thought to have been composed in Benares in around the second century AD.

There are two great names in the early period. Caraka lived during the millennium before Christ and Su´sruta in the millennium after. Their dating has not been precisely determined. Su´sruta was predominantly a surgeon and his book gives instructions for anatomical dissection and its use in improving surgical technique.

The earlier Caraka described himself as an interpreter of Atreya , the 'father of Indian medicine', who was, according to tradition, the son of Atri, an earthly manifestation of the important Hindu god Brahma. The *Caraka Samhitā* is predominantly a medical treatise and is regarded as a classic text of Hindu medicine.

A third name of note from ancient Indian medicine is that of Vagbhata, whose chief work was the *Astranga Sangraha,* which encompasses medicine, surgery and midwifery. There is also uncertainty about his date, which has been placed variously between the second century BC and the seventh century AD.

CHINA

Chinese medicine developed on lines not dissimilar to those of the early Greeks, which will be discussed shortly. The tradition is much older, however, with the classic text-book, *Huangdi Neijing,* representing the medical teaching of China in the time of the legendary founder of Chinese medicine, the Yellow Emperor, Huangdi *(2698–2598 BC).* This has been interpretively translated as *The Yellow Emperor's Inner Canon,* probably composed in this form around 200 BC. Ancient Chinese theories continued to be refined and developed over many centuries; some of them bear many remarkable resemblances to those of the Greeks, later declaimed by the physician Galen.

They considered life and death and the meaning of 'life-force'. The Chinese postulated that all states of being, characteristics and physical phenomena could be categorized as either *Yang,* which was formless and existed conceptually in an association with light, heaven, heat and masculinity, or *Yin,* which corresponded to darkness, earth, cold and femininity. Diagnosis of illness would involve identifying excesses of yin and yang in the patient, and systems of healing aimed to rebalance his or her inner yinyang energy. It is a complex concept and not easily reduced to a simple explanation. The reader should turn to Chapter Four for a more detailed treatment of the subject.

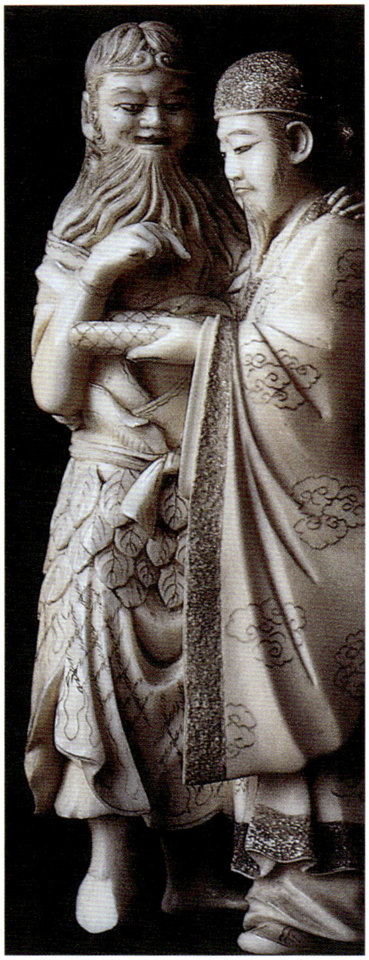

ABOVE An ivory figure depicting the legendary founders of Chinese medicine, Huangdi, the Yellow Emperor, and Shen Nong. The *Huangdi Neijing* is one of the seminal texts in the history of traditional Chinese medicine.

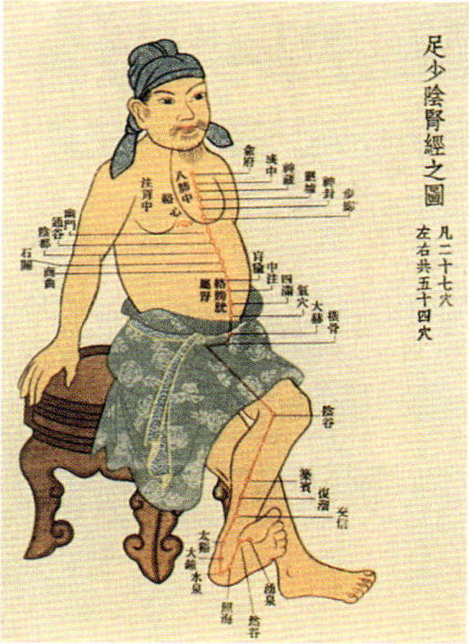

ABOVE An illustration dating from the Ming Dynasty *(1368–1644)* showing acupuncture points located on one of the meridians along which qi is thought to flow.

Chinese acupuncture is undoubtedly and deservedly amongst the oldest effective therapies, and its success is related to the extraordinary ability of the ancient Chinese to keep detailed records. Acupuncture is a system of treatment with needles. It is based on the notion that the vital life-force, or *qi,* flows through a system of channels, or meridians, through the body. Blockages or disturbances in the flow of qi may produce symptoms of illness in the body; the acupuncturist aims to stimulate the flow of qi by inserting needles in specific acupoints on the appropriate meridian to correct imbalances noticed during diagnosis. It is often the case that these acupoints are physically at some distance from the part of the body in which the symptoms are manifested.

In the *Neijing,* 295 acupoints are identified. For the benefit of the twentieth century practitioner, efforts were later made to reduce these to a more manageable, but necessarily less precise, number of between twenty and fifty! The textbooks that explained and illustrated the locations of the various meridians and their acupoints were known as acutracts.

Today the efficacy of acupuncture seems increasingly to have a scientific explanation. Patients may also gain confidence from the fact that orthodox acupuncture requires a long, expensive and traditional apprenticeship. Many years of study are required for the pupil to learn the acupoints and relate them to all the indications of illness detailed in the traditional and classical method.

The Chinese also have long experience of medicinal herbs. Books such as the *Shen Nong Bencaojing (Classic of Roots and Herbs of Shen Nong)* appeared as early as the third century AD. Shen Nong was venerated as the Father of Chinese Medicine, and this was the first extant book on materia medica; it contains some 365 herbs and drugs. The herbal tradition reached its peak some thousand years later. Li Shi-zhen compiled his *Great Herbal* of 52 volumes between 1552 and 1578 AD. Interestingly, the modern drug ephedrine had its origin in *ma huang,* a Chinese herb of great antiquity. The complexities of Chinese herbal medicine are difficult to summarize briefly. The reader is again directed to Chapter Four, where they are explained in more detail.

THE AMERICAS

Our knowledge of medical practices in the ancient civilizations of Southern America relates mainly to the Mayas in the fourth century AD and the later cultures of the Aztecs and Incas, which flourished until the sixteenth century. Medicine in its early days had primarily a religious and magical flavour, but was to develop much further than that of Native American cultures to the north. By the time of the Spanish Conquest, Francisco Hernandez *(1517–1587)* was able to record some 3,000 Aztec herbs used in medicine. Many of these compilations are to be found in the sixteenth-century *Codex barberini* held in the Vatican Library. It has been suggested that the surgical skills of the Aztecs may have benefited from the anatomical knowledge gained in their macabre pursuits of human sacrifice.

The ancient Peruvians also possessed an extensive materia medica from which we have inherited quinine, cocaine and curare, among many other medicines. As with the ancient Egyptians, mummification of the dead was practised.

GREEK MEDICINE

The beginnings of true medical science in the West were laid when the reliance on superstition that underpinned tribal medicine was replaced by civilized and rational curiosity about the cause of illness. The great pursuit of metaphysics, or of thinking about the essence of things and principles of being, ushered in a variety of medical theories and with them a demand for a choice of doctor. This had not been possible in earlier societies where 'a second opinion' was not possible.

The growth of civilized thought allowed for argument on medical cause and cure. This stimulated a fair degree of contention, which, paradoxically, often has the effect of reducing popular confidence in the practitioner.

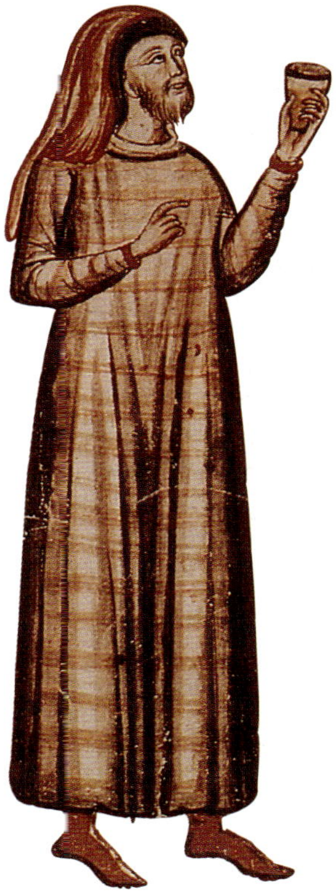

ABOVE A medieval representation of Hippocrates of Kos. He based his medical practice on careful bedside observation, and recognized the importance of keeping records of case histories. He also established a set of ethical standards for the medical profession which inspired the Hippocratic oath.

As western civilization developed, so new ideas arose among the Greek doctors. Hippocrates of Kos flourished between 460 and 377 BC. He is rightly regarded as the 'father of Western medicine', acknowledged for his interest in the whole patient. He developed and taught his concept of *physis,* meaning that one must consider the human being as an organic unity, which must be observed and treated as a whole, and which could be influenced by the environment.

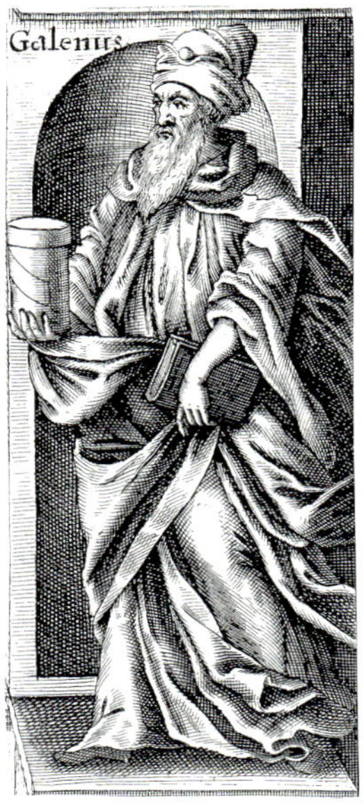

ABOVE The humoral theory propounded by Hippocates was taken up and elaborated at a later date by the famous physician Galen. He stressed the importance of critical days in the course of acute diseases.

THE FOUR HUMOURS

An important Greek idea concerning the cause of disease had developed out of the humoral theory of Empedocles, the Sicilian philosopher *(c.500–430 BC).* It was developed by Hippocrates, and consolidated by Galen, as will be mentioned later. It eventually was absorbed into medieval medicine, and its influence even extended into the nineteenth century. This was the doctrine of the four humours. In the first place Empedocles argued that everything was made from four elements: earth, air, fire and water, with their associated qualities of dryness, coldness, warmth and wetness. From these elements and qualities derived the idea of the four humours (or fluids) of black bile, yellow bile, blood and phlegm, with their associated melancholic, choleric, sanguine and phlegmatic temperaments. It was believed that the balance of these humours in the body determined physical states of health.

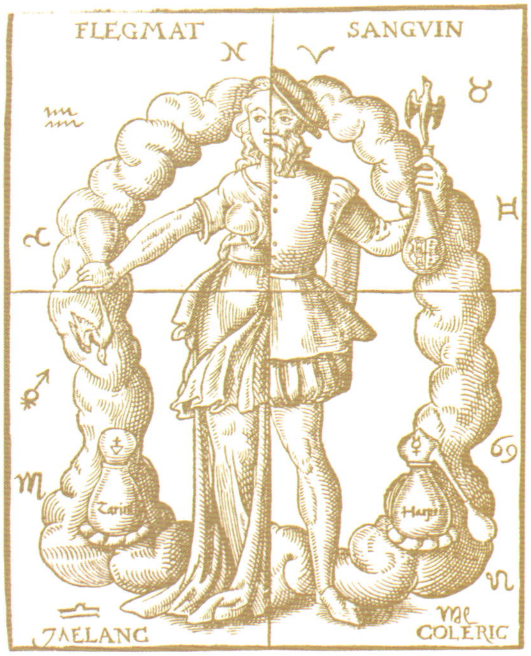

ABOVE A sixteenth-century engraving that relates the four humours to astrological signs of the Zodiac.

Perfect health was enjoyed when there was a perfect balance of the humours, known as a *crasis* or *eucrasia.* An imbalance of one or more humours resulted in *dyscrasia.* There was a natural physical tendency toward recovery and self-healing via a process known as *pepsis* or coction.

The Hippocratic School extolled the idea of *vis medicatrix naturae,* i.e., the power of nature to cure itself, and thus the belief that there was a natural tendency for things to get better on their own. This tendency could be aided by providing a beneficial environment for the patient and by improving physical function with a regimen of suitable diet and exercise. In extreme cases further aids to recovery could be sought, and stubbornly offending humours removed with the help of blood-letting and purgatives, and with the application of sudorifics to induce sweating, and diuretics to increase urination.

CLINICAL PROGNOSIS CAME BEFORE CLINICAL DIAGNOSIS

Hippocrates of Kos had taught ancient Greek doctors to recognize which changes in the physical appearance of the patient were of serious consequence and which were not. These skills constitute the art of prognosis, rather than fulfilling the more exact requirements of diagnosis. Prognosis foretells the outcome or future course of a disease, and is learned by observation and experience. Diagnosis, on the other hand, is the art of determining the nature of the disease.

The description of the face in serious illness, often portending death, is still known as the Hippocratic facies, and is indicative of his powers of direct physical observation. In his own words, the worst countenance to be seen in acute disease showed 'a sharp nose, hollow eyes, collapsed temples; the ears cold, contracted and their lobes turned out; the skin about the forehead being rough, distended and parched; the colour of the whole face being green, black, livid or lead-coloured.'

Empedocles also taught that respiration took place through the pores of the skin as well as through the lungs, so that if you thought a condition was caused by closed pores, you sought a remedy to open them. And if you thought it due to open pores, you sought to close them.

The thinking man – and just thinking is what metaphysics really signifies – was evidently now concentrating on the patient's body. The causes and effects of disease were being sought in the body itself, rather than in magic or external powers. Nevertheless, it was also appreciated by masters such as Hippocrates that external factors in the environment played a part. This change of emphasis brought the first glimpses of a realization of the fundamental concepts of the nature of disease. Arguably, by the time of Galen in Rome in the second century AD, the historical foundations of both alternative and scientific medicine in the West had been laid. Another enduring influence of the teachings of Hippocrates can be identified in the way the ethical relationship of doctor to patient has been immortalized in the Hippocratic Oath; a simple statement of the ethical code governing medical professional relationships with the patient. Contrary to popular belief, however, it is not universally part of the ritual of medical graduation today.

THE INFLUENCE OF GREEK MEDICAL IDEAS

Remarkably little is known of the life of Celsus (lived around *AD 25*), a Roman who lived about the same time as Christ, and who wrote an important medical treatise in Latin called *De medicina (On medicine)*, using the valuable earlier Greek works as his sources. These included the extant Hippocratic *corpus,* a collection of medical books containing the teaching of all the Hippocratic School of thought, and probably the lost works of Asclepiades, Heracleides, and Erasistratus as well as a surgeon known as Meges of Sidon. The *prooemium* (or preface) to the treatise has been described by W.G. Spencer, who provided the Engish translation for the Loeb Classical Library, 'as a most fair and judicious summary of the history of [Greek] medicine.' One of the things for which Celsus is best remembered in medical practice is that he left us the four signs of inflammation by which this condition is still confidently recognized today: *dolor, rubor, calor et tumor,* or pain, redness, heat and swelling.

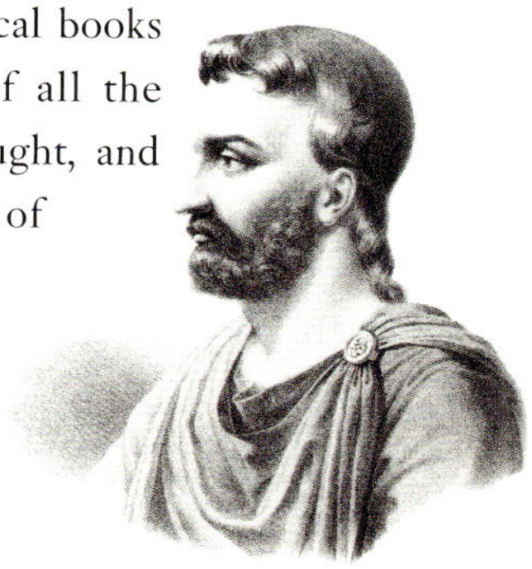

RIGHT Celsus was a Roman writer who lived during the first part of the first century AD. His influential work *De medicina* was essentially a compilation in Latin of earlier sources, particularly those of the Hippocratic school. It includes detailed descriptions of surgical practice, including the use of the ligature and an operation for cataracts.

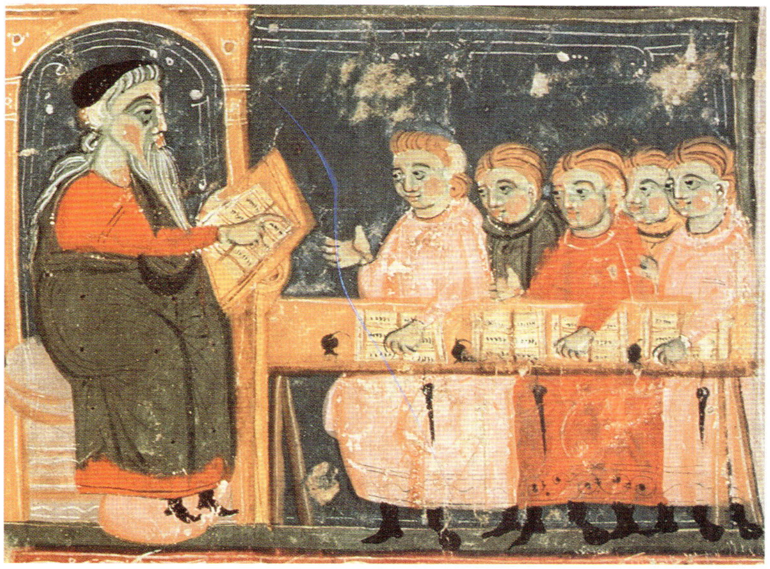

BELOW The teachings of Hippocrates exerted their influence across centuries of Western medical history. This medieval manuscript illumination shows a teacher instructing his pupils in the Hippocratic aphorisms.

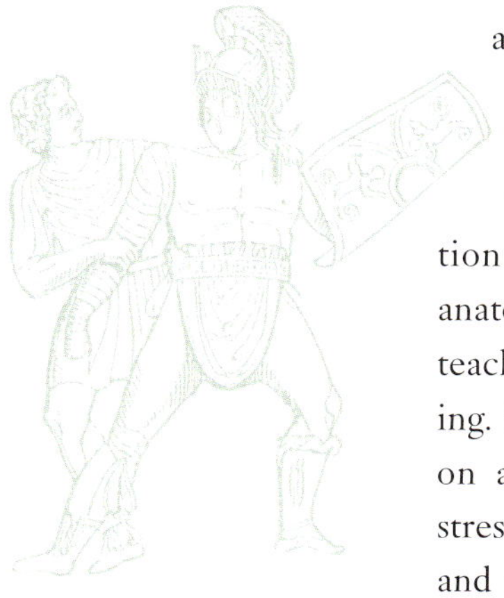

ABOVE A great figure in medical history, Galen began work as a doctor to gladiators in Pergamum.

The name in Greek medicine that influenced and bestrode European practice for centuries was that of Galen *(AD ?131–201).* He was born at Pergamum in Asia Minor in about the year 131 AD. His first medical appointment was as surgeon to the gladiators there. He later went to Rome where he took no pains to conceal his contempt for his fellow practitioners. He nevertheless built a great reputation for himself and wrote extensively on anatomy, physiology and practical medicine. His teaching dominated the revival of medical thinking. He himself claimed to have written 125 books on a variety of subjects. His medical writings stressed the humoral theory, which he elaborated, and the Hippocratic doctrine of critical days. In acute diseases, it was taught that the rebalance of the humours tended to take place on particular days by a process known as *crisis.*

This process is particularly evident in the resolution of lobar pneumonia and was regularly seen and taught. It even persisted into the twentieth century, before the discovery of antibiotics provided an effective treatment for the condition. Clinical recovery of an acutely fevered patient with distressed breathing, and who might be comforted only with expert nursing, could be dramatically sudden. Galen viewed it as likely to occur on uneven days in the course of the illness, usually the fifth or seventh. The concept was still important centuries later, when the great Canadian physician Sir William Osler *(1849–1920)* regarded the crisis as very variable, rarely likely to happen before the third or after the twelfth day.

Oribasius *(?325–?403)* was the physician to the Emperor Julian in the 4th century AD and also one of the last great compilers of classical Greek texts. Oribasius made the works of Galen available for the medical practitioners of the Byzantine Empire in his extensive compilation known as his *Synopsis.*

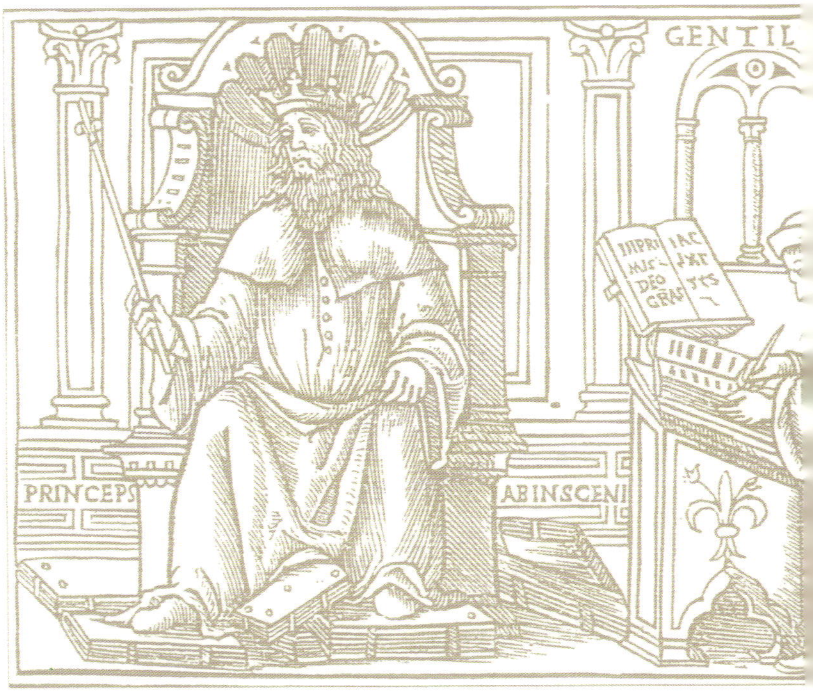

ROMAN MEDICINE

The Romans were great soldiers, and one of the natural consequences of battle was an increased demand for practical doctors. War, as is its wont, advanced the care of the wounded, and encouraged the provision of hospitals and medical officers in the field. The need for practical health care, however, is not necessarily conducive to the wider speculations that generate scientific advance. The historian Pliny's *Natural History* is contemptuous of the superstitious nature of Roman medical practice. For instance, Cato the Censor *(234–149 BC)* wrote *De agri cultura*, an agricultural book on the medical care of cattle and slaves, with special attention being devoted to the former. His principal remedy was cabbage, both raw and cooked, to be taken internally and applied to wounds and sores. If the slave was not cured by means of the cabbage panacea, Cato advised, amazingly, that 'he be got rid of'. The arrival of Greek physicians in Rome in about the third century BC certainly improved the outlook for the human patients, at least!

The fact that the Roman army itself had a competent medical service is supported by the evidence of the hospitals built throughout the Roman Empire, particularly to care for the needs of soldiers in the field. Scribonius Largus *(fl. AD 47)*, author of *De compositione medicamentorum*, a work on medicaments, was the medical officer who accompanied Emperor Claudius to Britain in AD 43. It is thought he may have been a Greek. He has left us one of the earliest statements of the Hippocratic Oath. His list of drugs indicates the use of opium.

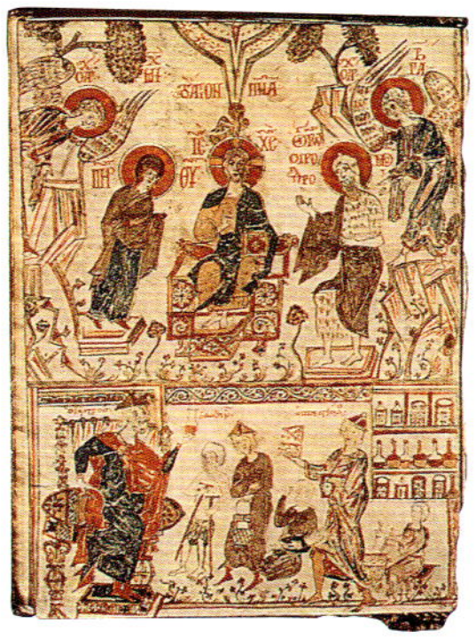

ABOVE After the fall of the Roman Empire, Islamic culture kept the flame of learning alive. This is the Byzantine doctor Myrepsos.

THE ARAB INFLUENCE

The prophet Mohammed *(AD 571–632)* effected a world change; it was brought about by the establishment of the religion of Islam. Within a century of his death Arab powers had conquered half the known world. The Arabic language of the Koran became as important to this empire as Greek and Latin were to the West.

The heretical sect of Nestorian Christians had already fled from their medical school at Edessa in the Byzantine Empire at the end of the fifth century. Their far-flung missionary activity had stimulated in them an interest in the medical scholarship of India and China. To this tradition they were able to add their own Greek medical learning. They established a famous and important school of learning at Gondisapor in Persia.

The Arabs captured Gondisapor in AD 636. Far from suppressing the inhabitants, they encouraged the growth of its university. The Nestorian Christians and the Jews and Arabs continued to translate influential Greek medical works into Syriac, with the benefit of their acquired Indian, Chinese and Persian medical knowledge. Greek medicine thus spread through Syria into Persia and so to the rest of the Arab world.

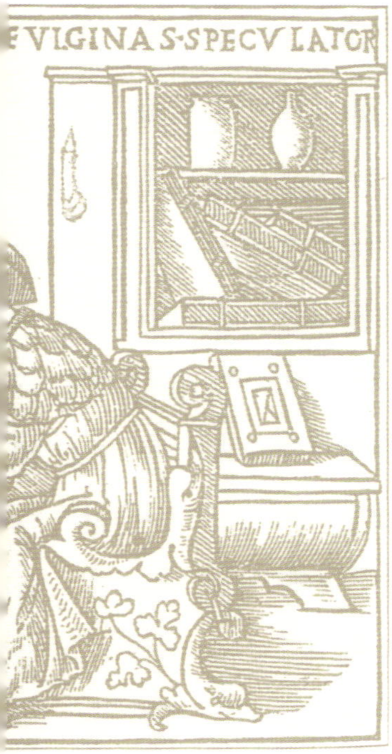

ABOVE Avicenna's *Canon of Medicine* was a highly influential text in the medieval curriculum.

Arab medicine, so-called because of the language in which it was written down, greatly influenced the medical thinking of the West from the twelfth to the fifteenth centuries. The great names of this movement included Rhazes *(c. AD 864–925)*, Haly Abbas *(d. AD 994)* and Avicenna (ibn Sina) *(AD 980–1037)*. The largest of Rhazes' works, *al-Hawi,* known in Latin as *Liber continens* or a compendium, is said to show him as a follower of Hippocrates in theory and Galen in practice. The Arabs played an important part in teaching the art of prescribing. The ninth book of *al-Hawi* deals with pharmacology and therapeutics. Avicenna, known by his contemporaries as 'the prince of physicians', is captured for us in his dispensary in the splendid illuminated copy of his *Canon of Medicine* in the University of Bologna Library in Italy. The fifth book of Avicenna's influential *Canon* is devoted to materia medica.

Spain at this time formed part of the Umayad Emirate in the Moorish or Saracen Empire. Cordoba became the capital city of the Western Caliphate in the tenth century. Albucasis *(936–c.1013)*, the great surgeon of Islam, was born near Cordoba in 936 and Averroës *(1126–1198)* in Cordoba in 1126. These two, and Averroës' pupil Maimonides *(1135–1204)*, wrote extensively on medicine and surgery using many Greek sources. The physician Avenzoar, born in Seville in 1091, also had great influence on European thought.

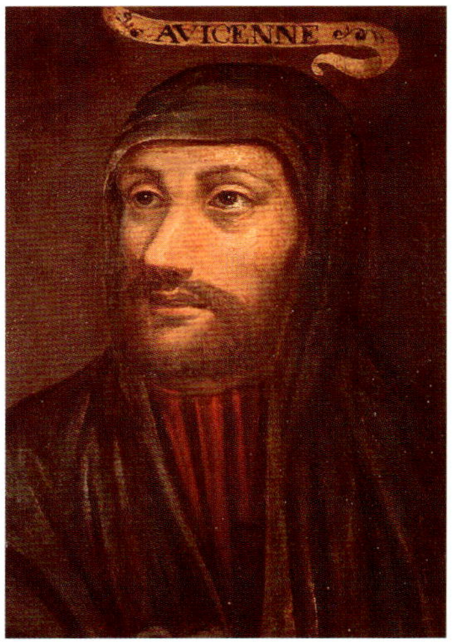

RIGHT The map shows the extent of Islamic influence at the start of the eleventh century.

LEFT The great eleventh-century Persian philosopher and physician Avicenna (ibn Sina). His *Canon of Medicine* was first translated into Latin in the twelfth century.

LEPROSY

The Hebrew Bible is a great source for early medical history, but the story of one disease associated with both the Old and New Testaments has resulted in much confusion and distress to its victims. The Hebrew name *tsara'ath*, a Biblical term which does not refer at all to the modern disease known as leprosy or Hansen's disease, by a complicated process was mistakenly translated as leprosy. How this happened makes an intriguing study of historical detection and translation. It links us with the history of medicine from Biblical times to the present.

The confusion came about through mistakes made by the Jewish and Arabic translators of the Bible from Greek sources, who occasionally became muddled. As a result, the condition of spiritual uncleanness of *tsara'ath,* which was a matter for investigation and treatment by the priests, became associated through translators' errors with the mutilating deformities of leprosy. Scholars have recognized and corrected this erroneous interpretation and as a result the modern hospital for lepers in Jersualem, once known as the Hospital for the *Tsara'Atish,* has recently had its name changed to the Hospital for Hansen's Disease. Leprosy today has become eponymously known as Hansen's disease, named after the Norwegian Armauer Hansen *(1841–1912)*, the discoverer of the bacillus *Mycobacterium Leprae* that causes it.

Leper houses, full of real lepers, abounded in the Middle Ages, and the classical leonine face of lepromatous leprosy is there to be seen in countless medieval representations.

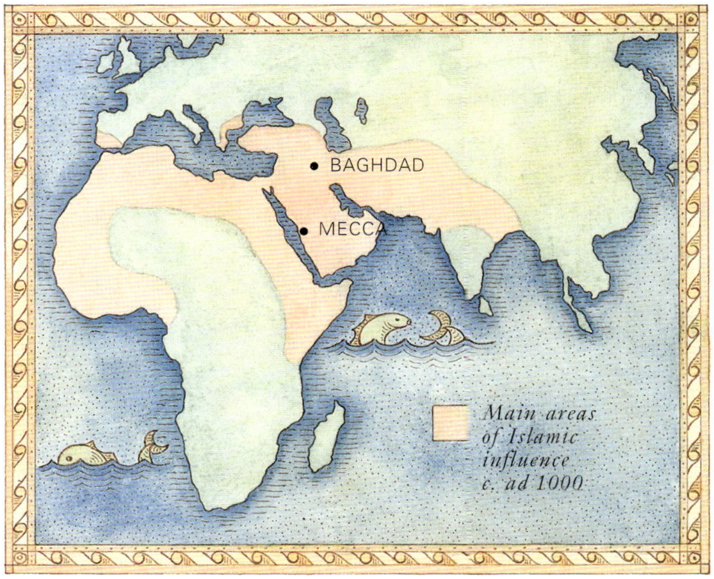

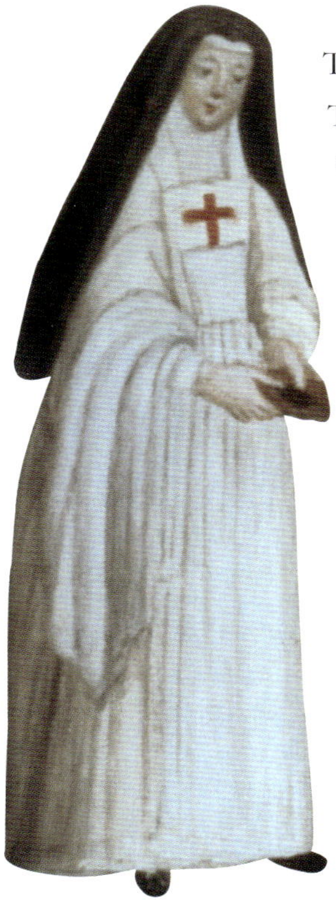

ABOVE The practical care of the sick in Europe in the Middle Ages was often undertaken by members of the Church. It expressed the Christian virtue of *caritas* in a demonstrable form.

THE CHRISTIAN CHURCH

There existed meanwhile another religious force with a powerful influence on Western medical development. In the Byzantine Empire, the early Church itself was not without blame in suppressing the freedom of thought that had been the glory of classical Greece, in order to preach its own dogma. The Church wisely absorbed many pagan gods and rituals into its own liturgy. Old pagan festivals had been part of the common life of the new Christians for generations past. They were enjoyable and could be adapted for use in the new ceremonies.

It is now disputed whether the Church's ingenuity had much effect in discouraging medical science by substituting 'theological pathology' and 'theological therapy' for the magical medical rituals of its pagan predecessors. Bones of saints and holy water became accepted remedies that recalled the magical role of the African figurine described at the beginning of this chapter. Did the supernatural explanation of illness, with the Church's authority, stifle the opportunity for the advance of the secular medical ideas taught by Hippocrates? Centuries earlier he had clearly indicated how important it was to seek natural, rather than supernatural, causes for illness. His essay on epilepsy decried any description of it as 'the sacred disease'. We may legitimately ask how far the ideas implicit in exorcism and the casting out of devils are removed from the African witch doctor's ideas of aetiology?

At a time when theology was regarded as the 'queen of the sciences', the Church ruled men's and women's lives in a way that is inconceivable in modern society. The historian Charles Homer Haskins, writing of the rise of the universities, states that 'Paris was pre-eminent in the Middle Ages as a school of theology... the supreme subject of medieval study'.

At this time Paris was an important university and its example, and the importance it attached to theology, was to become a model for other teaching establishments.

The Church's adaptations of practices dating from the pre-Christian era for its own rites were not exclusively taken from those of pagan origin. An accommodation had eventually to be reached as well with the lessons that had been learned from progressive Greek ideas as expounded in the influential writings of the classical philosophers. Greek thinking, revealed in the philosophy of Plato and his pupil Aristotle, could not be permanently ignored. It therefore became integrated by the Fathers of the Church into its religious philosophy.

Fortunately, Aristotle had trained as a physician and this was reflected in his analytical method and respect for fact as a basis for doctrine. In this way, he influenced Galen, whose works in turn influenced the schools of medieval medicine. However, the reverence for the authority of Galen paradoxically came to enforce an enduring rigidity in medical thinking that was to persist for centuries to come.

Overall, the Church was a source of great support in the practical care of the sick, the poor and the needy. It extolled the virtue of *caritas,* love for one's neighbour, and sympathetic, practical charity in a sense that has no translation into a single English word.

The monastery and its infirmary set the example in this respect,

BELOW A fresco *(1443)* by Domenico di Bartolo from the Santa Maria della Scala Hospital, Siena, showing a monk treating a sick man. Monastic infirmaries were effectively the hospitals of the Middle Ages.

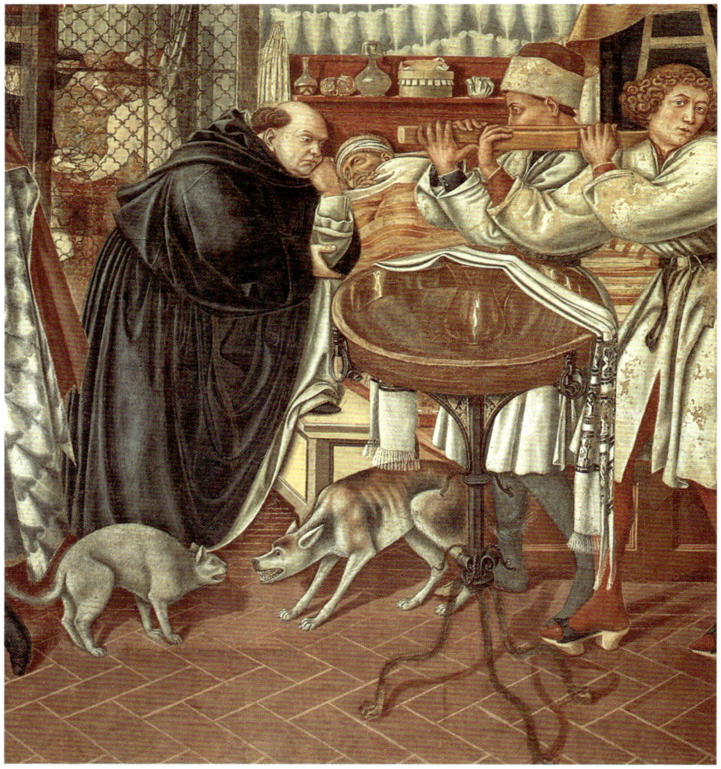

helping the sick and poor. The denial of charity, of *caritas,* was regarded as the unforgivable sin. Its practice was the dominant virtue. Even today, it is a concept of great relevance to the successful practice of medicine.

However, things do not always work out according to prevailing ideas of morality. Practice does not always follow precept. Medieval medicine contained a mixture of pagan superstition and Christian prejudice, but beneath the surface it is just possible to see portents of the beginnings of medical science. Abstract philosophy was still the mainstay of medicine, rather than direct observation of nature and the search for accurate description of illness and experiment in treatment. The empirical testing of hypotheses, which is the basis both of science and of modern medicine, was still to come.

ASTROLOGY AND SURGERY

Astrological ideas were also an important factor in European medical thought. Astrology itself was of much older provenance even than the ideas of the Greeks. The Babylonians had plotted the courses of planets during the reign of Nebuchadnezzar, between 664 and 562 BC. Claims have been made for the discovery of astrological symbols of even greater antiquity in the Sumerian kingdom during the third millennium BC. And the practice of astrology would survive both the upheavals in thought brought about by the Renaissance and even the twentieth-century scientific revolution.

In the Middle Ages, astrological medicine played a large part in diagnosis and treatment, despite astrology's uncomfortable association with magic – and magic was proscribed by the Church. It relied on the proposition that the *macrocosm* of the planets in the Universe governed the *microcosm* of the internal parts of man. This idea had an inherent popularity. In the prevailing climate of opinion, it was a theory that could be generally accepted as rational. Astrologers produced tables and drew figures to illustrate its application, and to enable it to be taught as a method of medical practice.

Another mainstay of medieval therapy was blood-letting. Surgeons and barber-surgeons were skilled at it. An illustration in the Mostyn manuscript shows the sites and indications for bleeding, including the well-known joke (even then) indicating the armpit with the comment 'If you bleed here the patient will die from laughing'. The medical historian Vivian Nutton has commented that venesection (blood-letting) and astrology had both been controversial issues since 'Galen had rejected astrological medicine as mumbo-jumbo'. How it survived this criticism and the Church's antagonism to become a cornerstone of medieval medicine is unclear. And it continues to defy all reason by making rich all sorts of forecasters and fortune-tellers of health and wealth even today.

Such doctrines flourished in the fifteenth century, despite the Church's religious doubts about their proper place in the scheme of things. At this time illness was still thought to result from an improper balance of the humours. Excess of one or lack of another required the appropriate rebalancing with a dose of a suitable medicine, chosen to correct the deficiency. This practice required a knowledge of the humoral nature both of the illness and of the remedy. Galen's theories were to remain as the basis of diagnosis and treatment for many centuries to come.

ASTROLOGICAL MEDICINE IN WALES

Such was the popularity of astrology, the word reached as far as Wales. Welsh copyists made texts, that would have been read by others than those primarily engaged in medical practice. Medicine was not the prerogative of an elite. The illustrations shown here are taken from the beautiful fifteenth-century Welsh language Mostyn Manuscript 88 (*AD 1488–1489*) and seem intended for a general readership.

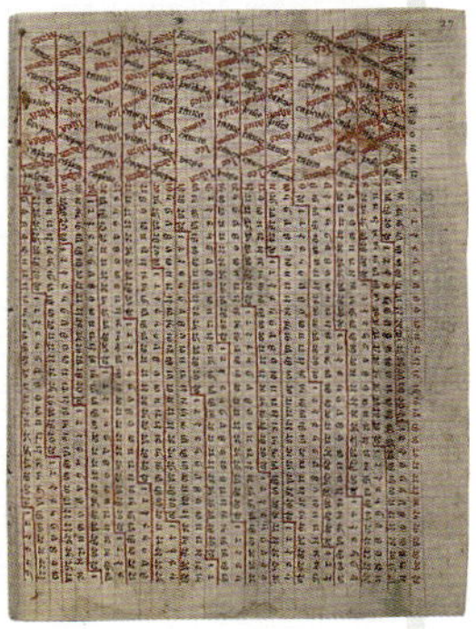

The interpretation of the Zodiac man for use in particular cases of diagnosis was aided by a circular ready-reckoner, which 'computerized' the calculations.

The Mostyn manuscripts include instruction in other ancient principles, besides those associated with astrology. They reveal what was accepted contemporary practice, giving for example a treatise on urine with a coloured guide to urine gazing.

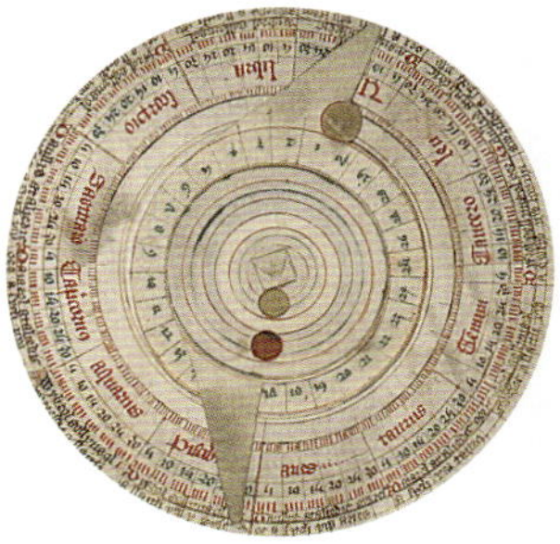

ABOVE AND LEFT Two illustrations from the Welsh Mostyn Manuscript showing (left) a rotating calculator and (above) tables used in astrological medicine, which recognized a link between zodiacal signs and specific parts of the human body.

MEDICINE IN THE MIDDLE AGES

The Middle Ages was essentially a world of competing schools of medical thought extolling simple symptomatic 'cures'. Modern diagnoses depend upon the later concept of the specificity of disease, the recognition of individual illnesses. In the Middle Ages, signs and symptoms had not been grouped into entities. Signs of illness are what the doctor finds on physical examination – Hippocrates used them in his art of prognosis. Symptoms are what the patient complains of; e.g., pain and depression, or coughs and sneezing. They cannot always be seen or felt by the medical examiner, but they are of great importance to the sufferer. There is an adage taught to medical students: 'Listen to the patient. He is telling you what is the matter.' The patient describes the symptoms and only he or she knows them, so the doctor must take heed.

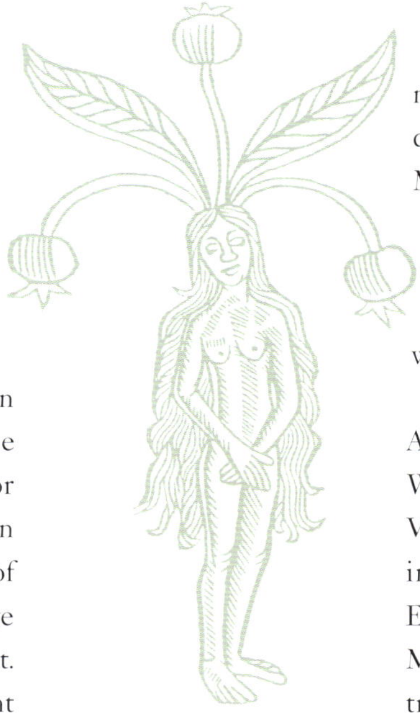

ABOVE Said to resemble the human form, the root of the mandrake plant was credited with remarkable powers in times past. The Book of Genesis tells how Leah procured them to make herself fertile so as to bear a son to Jacob.

HERBAL REMEDIES

Medieval physicians had more limited knowledge of medical processes than we have today. Of necessity, they treated the presenting signs of the malady, those obvious manifestations such as lumps or sores, without any appreciation of the fact that they formed part of a collection of signs and symptoms that together constituted a particular single illness. As therapists, they were beholden to relieve the symptoms of which the patient complained. The patients really knew best whether or not they were relieved. There always is, rightly and naturally, an insistent popular demand for practical therapy, because treatment is of greater import to the patient than diagnosis. The patient can actually experience it and can complain if it does not work. The cough can be cured or the lump removed. And the sooner, the better.

The Greeks, as we have seen, had recommended following rules regarding exercise and diet, and these continued to be valued in the Middle Ages. In the matter of drugs, the common substance most capable of exploitation, of easy description, collection and application was the herb, later known as the Galenical simple. This was the medicine of the Middle Ages.

One of the very earliest herbals, that of Juliana Anicia, daughter of the Roman Emperor of the West, is the *Codex vindobonensis (AD 512)*, now in Vienna. This contains the naturalistic plant drawings of Crateus, physician to Mithridates VI Eupator *(c.115–63 BC)*, a king of Pontus in Asia Minor, which are combined with the sixth-century translation of the *De materia medica* of the first-century AD Greek surgeon Dioscorides, which is regarded as the first Western herbal.

The illustrations are accompanied by instructions. One illustration shows the shrub *Vitex agnus-castus*, popularly known as the Chaste tree. This may have been used for the treatment of mental illness, as it was said to help the 'lethargicull and phreneticull', for depression and hypomania.

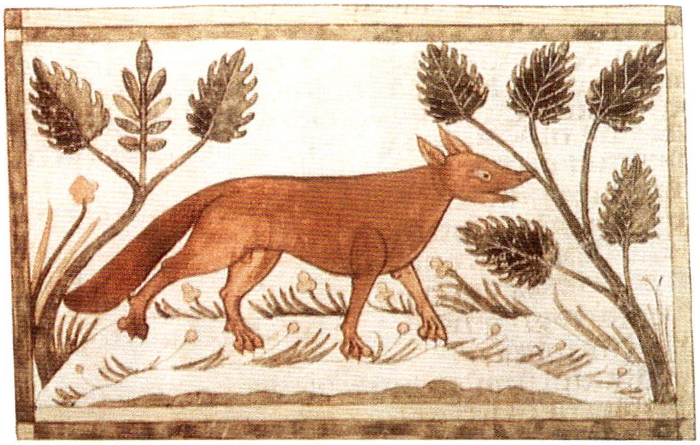

ABOVE Animal as well as plant remedies were used in the Middle Ages. This illustration from *Medicina de quadrupedibus* by Sextus Placitus relates to products obtained from foxes.

In the Middle Ages, the materia medica was to be found in the herbal manuscript. Good ones were not easy to get. They were rare and very expensive. The classical ones were therefore copied for ease of reference. These became the new 'tried remedies', backed by the authority of their age and tradition. Anglo-Saxon and later examples contained animal as well as plant remedies. As an example of the persistence of their influence, the use of fox fat as an ointment is still mentioned by Theophilus Redwood in his authoritative publication *Gray's Supplement to the Pharmacopoeia* of 1847.

The Anglo-Saxons have often been denigrated as 'pirates' and are not renowned for their scholarship and learning. They had inherited a rather confused therapy of ill-digested classical ideas, which, as we have seen, were corrupted in their passage from hand-to-hand since their origin in classical times. The Norman conquerors of Britain sought to educate the Anglo-Saxons, as well as suppressing them. The Normans were particularly strong in Church matters; with the establishment of their monasteries came the beginnings of academic medicine.

The basis of prescribing, as mentioned earlier, was the herb, the Galenical 'simple'; i.e., any herb which was additionally thought to have medicinal value. How was the monk in the 'farmery', as the infirmary was often known, to distinguish the healing herb from the poisonous one, if there was not a spicer readily to hand to give his opinion? How was he to learn the important differences between herbs when there was a shortage of skilled herbalists and herbals to consult? The remedy was to copy and circulate the old drawings. And they were increasingly copied by people who did not know what the original plant looked like.

The Anglo-Norman herbal vividly illustrates one of the pitfalls that stands in the way of the popularizer. The results could be beautiful, but they were often singularly useless as a reliable guide to medicinal plants. The 'Romanesque' or Norman diagrammatic style was magnificent pictorially, although examples have been described as reaching 'the lowest form of illustrational degradation', depending on whether you were seeking art or plant identification. Furthermore, the classical allegories woven into the written descriptions were of little practical help in recognizing the plant. In one example, a drawing of a mythical centaur dominates what should have been a representation of a plant, the centaury. A good drawing is better than a description. Corrupt versions are bizarre and of no practical value.

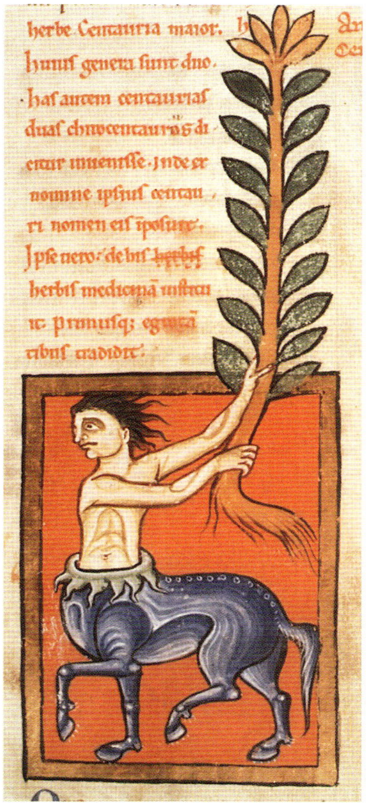

ABOVE This illustration of a centaur in a medieval herbal purports to represent the plant centaury. Such inaccuracies were common.

ARTISTIC LICENCE

Other herbals drawn by ignorant copyists sometimes showed the plant upside down, the roots where stems should have been, and vice-versa. The fact that many of the plants and animals were of foreign origin further added to the difficulties. It was of little use recommending cures derived from lions or tigers, if lions and tigers were not readily available. One example of the comic results of untutored attempts to draw unknown creatures may be seen in some of the pharmaceutical jars and tiles purporting to portray the rhinoceros of the Worshipful Society of Apothecaries of London. The result often resembled an armadillo!

The spicers in England were later to develop, via their association with the London guild known as the Grocers Company, into apothecaries, who practised medicine. The apothecaries on the continent of Europe, by contrast, never changed from the trade of their chemist and druggist forebears. The Moorish figure represented by the sign of the 'Yawner' that frequently is found on Dutch pharmacies is a graphic reminder of the influence of the Moors and the spice trade.

SPICES AND HERBS IN NORMAN TIMES

The Normans brought their spicers to England to preserve their meats. Every winter, in anticipation of the expected shortage of animal fodder, it became necessary to kill off the cattle that would otherwise starve to death. Only the breeding stock, which had to be maintained through the dark months, were kept alive in order to ensure continuity of the supply of meat on the hoof in the springtime. There was, therefore, at the beginning of each winter, a surfeit of meat for a short period. Attempts had to be made to preserve it, if it were to last long enough to be brought to the table and remain edible. As the preserving methods of the time were of dubious quality, the meat could only be enjoyed with the liberal use of spices to enhance, or more probably just disguise, the 'gamey' viands offered at the table. These spicers became the herbal experts.

PARACELSUS AND CHEMICAL REMEDIES

One of the most famous questioners of medical authority was Paracelsus *(1493–1541)*, whose full name was Philippus Aureolus Theophrastus Bombastus von Hohenheim. To this impressive list he chose to add Paracelsus, by which title he is usually known. It is not certain whether he intended by this to proclaim his equality with the first century AD Roman Celsus, or more generally with the great *(para celsus)*, or merely to follow custom and latinize his surname Hohenheim.

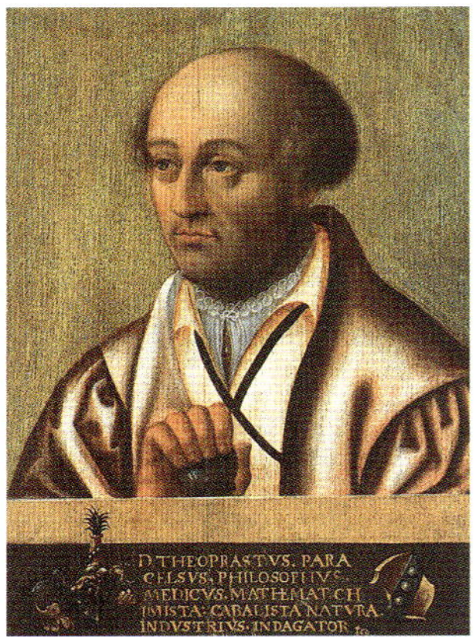

ABOVE Paracelsus, one of the iconoclasts of medical history. Not content with refuting the authority of Galen and Avicenna, he publicly burned their books.

He was born in Switzerland in the year that Columbus returned from his first voyage to the Americas. As a boy of ten years, he had moved with his father to Villach in Carinthia. His father, who also had a medical background, taught in the mining school there, where the young Paracelsus was introduced to the values of chemistry.

Paracelsus was an enigmatic character, flamboyant, quarrelsome and reforming. His somewhat eccentric behaviour prevented his settling down in any one place and gave his life a vagabond flavour. These unfortunate traits did not help his avowed mission to reform medical practice.

In a printed pamphlet outlining his 'programme', which he published in 1527 at Basle, Switzerland, where he stayed no longer than ten months, he promised to free the decayed art of medicine from its worst errors. This sort of language did not endear him to his colleagues in the town, who had invited him to become its municipal physician, which office gave him the right to lecture at the university. He railed against acceptance of the doctrine of the humours and added that if he wanted to prove anything, he would not do so merely by quoting the authorities, 'but by experiment and reasoning thereon'.

His later work was based on his four pillars of the healing art: philosophy in a knowledge of nature, astronomy rather than astrology, chemistry and virtue. In defining virtue he extolled love as the true ground of medicine. He is credited with enlisting the help of chemicals in therapeutics and vigorously opposing polypharmacy, or the prescription of multiple ingredients in a single medicine.

SURGERY IN THE FOURTEENTH TO THE SIXTEENTH CENTURIES

In the fourteenth century, the Plantagenet kings of England had found it convenient to encourage the formation of guilds. These were groups or fraternities of the king's subjects following similar livelihoods and they laid down rules which governed apprenticeships in their trade. The Company of Barbers also practised minor surgery, such as blood-letting and tooth extraction. There was also a Guild of Surgeons, who regarded themselves as of higher status. In 1540, the companies of surgeons and barbers combined as the Barber-Surgeons Company and they existed as such for over 200 years until 1745.

Historian Vivian Nutton has summarized the essential trilogy of classical medicine as dietetics, drugs and surgery. This triad is not exclusively confined to classical times. It is the triad of treatment on which medieval as well as modern therapy is built. The development of surgery requires less metaphysics than the other two. For wounds and lumps, the knife and the suture were the ready answer. War has often been the catalyst in the development of surgery. And even in times of peace, there was never a dearth of violence.

BELOW 'The Barber Surgeon' by Isaac Koedijck. Surgeons tended to be looked down upon by physicians at this period.

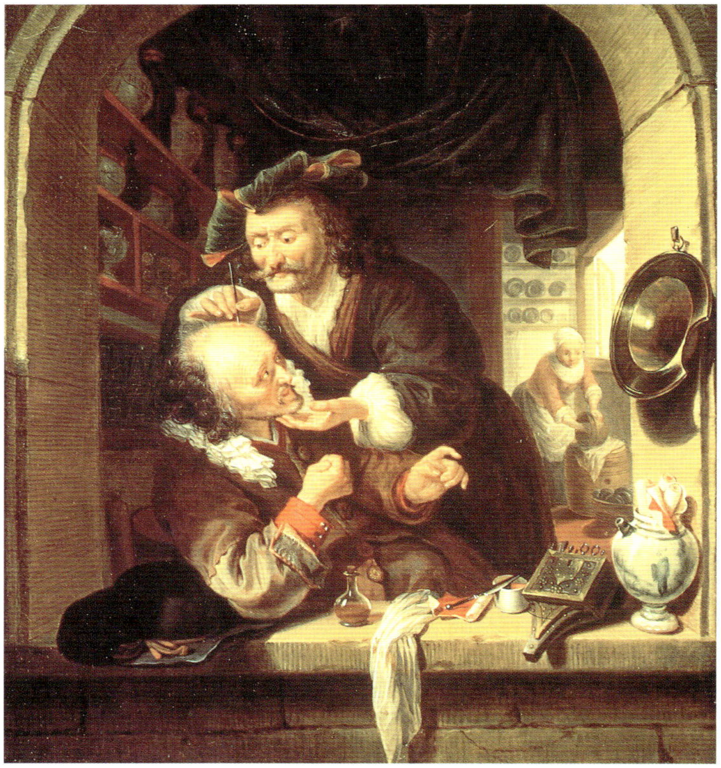

AMBROISE PARÉ

Giovanni da Vigo *(1460–1525)*, surgeon to Pope Giulio II, still recommended the use of boiling elder oil for cauterization of wounds 'poisoned with gunpowder'. Fortunately for the wounded French soldiers on their way to attack Turin in the war between Francis of France and the Holy Roman Emperor Charles V, the medical supplies of elder oil were low. All that was available when the elder oil ran out was a salve of egg yolk, rose water and turpentine.

A French surgeon called Ambroise Paré *(1510–1590)* was extremely anxious that he had been unable to carry out the recommended treatment and feared the worst. To his surprise he found that those who had been given the boiling oil treatment were in a sorry state compared with the rest. While the latter had passed a restful night and their wounds looked well, the wretched men who had suffered the agonies of orthodoxy were sleepless, in pain, and feverish with badly inflamed wounds. Paré determined never to expose them to such suffering again.

Paré was not a university man. His training was as an apprentice to a barber-surgeon in Paris. This may actually have been to his advantage, because in Paris the barber-surgeons performed many major operations and developed special skills, making them superior in surgical practice to those trained at either the Faculty of Physicians or the Surgeons' College of Saint Côme.

He gained experience as resident surgeon at the the Hôtel Dieu, the only Parisian public hospital. He had the advantage of the availability of the published works of Giovanni da Vigo and also of Guy de Chauliac *(1300–1367)* of Montpellier and Bologna, the leading surgeon of the fourteenth century. Paré attached great importance to a knowledge of anatomy and acknowledges his later debt to Vesalius in the preface to his own *Anatomie Universelle (1541)*. His more famous *Apology and Treatise containing the Voyages made into divers places* was published in English as part of Paré's *Works* in London in 1634.

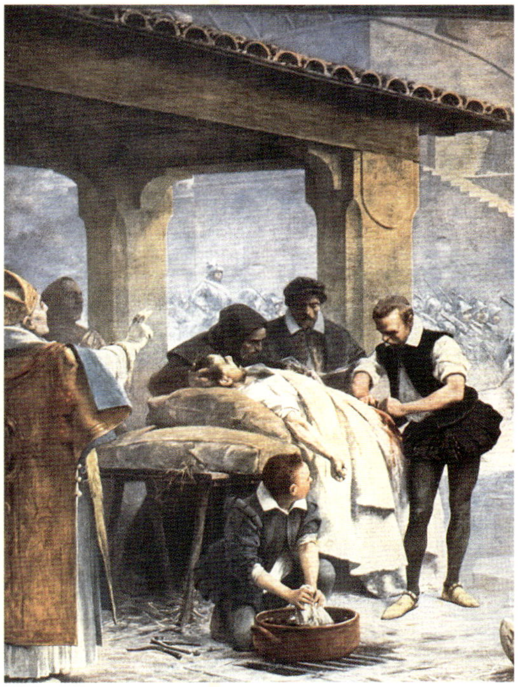

ABOVE A nineteenth - century depiction of the surgeon Ambroise Paré applying a ligature to a wounded soldier at the Siege of Metz.

Guido de Vigevano's *Anatomia* of 1345 demonstrates that clinical methods of examination, such as taking the radial and brachial pulses of the arm, were within the surgeon's province. Surgeons examined the body and palpated the abdomen. Surgeons were aware of the prognostic signs described by the Greeks. They were therefore by no means deserving of their description as merely crude barbaric relatives of the physicians, exploiting the ravages of war and other disasters for the exercise of their craft.

UNIVERSITIES AND THE FLOWERING OF SCIENCE

To trace the influence of the rise of universities on medical teaching, we now need to step back in time again, to eleventh-century Italy. The great individual Arab and Jewish medical translators in North Africa and Spain had been the means of preserving the great medical literature of classical times. In Italy and Sicily, another important communal development was taking place.

In the eleventh century, the first medical school of repute in Europe was founded at Salerno, south of Naples in Italy. This medical university had well established connections with the Islamic world and the East, and in it the medical writings of the ancient Greeks were studied assiduously. Although its foundation was of considerable antiquity, within a few centuries its international influence was to wane in comparison with that of the European universities which succeeded it. Salerno was only ever a school of medicine. Bologna was to become much more.

Our modern schools of medicine have been described as the heirs and successors, not of Athens and Alexandria, but (of the universities and colleges) of Paris and Bologna. The university and its medical school is the lineal descendant of the colleges of medieval Paris and Bologna. The rise of the modern university began in the twelfth century.

An alliance of purpose grew up in the universities of Europe. Increasing scientific conformity in medical teaching eventually enabled its practitioners to establish the beginnings of a recognizable international standard of tuition. Formal licensing and registration of individual medical practitioners came much later. The founding of the universities, which began in the Middle Ages, ensured that the form of medical education essentially changed its style. Earlier teaching had been characterized by individual apprenticeships. Discussions of classical theories and metaphysical arguments on the bodily causes of illness were to be replaced by a more broadly based science, leading to direct observation of the body, which eventually made questioning of accepted medical orthodoxy inevitable, and opened the way for the pursuit of scientific investigation.

Italy was one of the leaders in this movement. The students of Bologna rapidly attracted other students from all over Europe, who formed their own 'universities' there, with the foreign students grouped together as 'nations'.

The University of Padua was founded in 1222 AD as an act of secession from Bologna, following an exodus of its disaffected legal students. Medicine was never the sole reason for the eminence of Padua as an educational institution. It rapidly became a centre of excellence in a wide variety of subjects.

The establishment of universities in Britain came a little later. Oxford, influenced by the foundation of the University of Paris, branched off from its parent stem late in the twelfth century. Cambridge was established a little later. Oxford and Cambridge were formed of corporations of masters or teachers, while Bologna and Padua were essentially student-run establishments. Cambridge received formal recognition as a university by a papal bull of 1318, although by then it had been in existence as a place of learning for at least a century.

The early medical association between the English and Italian medical schools can be traced to the fifteenth century with the arrival in Italy of Thomas Linacre *(?1460–1524)*, who later founded the Royal College of Physicians in England in 1518. He was educated at Oxford, whence he journeyed to Padua, where he proceeded to the degree of doctor of medicine.

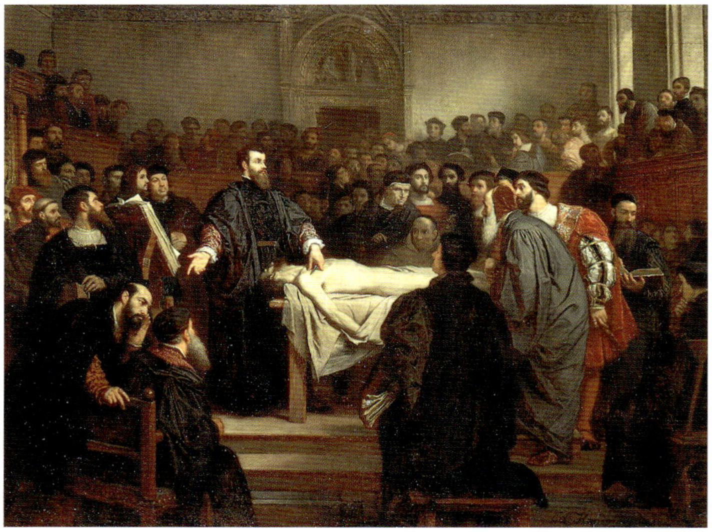

ABOVE A painting by the nineteenth-century French artist Edouard Hamman depicting Andreas Vesalius lecturing at the University of Padua, where he was a professor of surgery and anatomy until 1543.

On his return to Britain in about 1492, by then familiar with the medical activity in the northern Italian universities, he founded lectureships in medicine at both Oxford and Cambridge. In 1540, Henry VIII established the Regius Professorship of Physic at Cambridge. This apparently important step, unfortunately, did not result in the creation of an active medical school there.

Fortunately, it did lead to many of its graduates seeking instruction at Padua in the footsteps of Linacre. A pattern of Italo-Britannic co-operation had been established. In this exchange, John Caius *(1510–1573)* played a large part. He was an outstanding member of the medical school at Cambridge and later became president of the College of Physicians founded by Linacre. In March 1539, he went to Padua to profit from the clinical teaching of Montanus *(1498–1552)*.

John Caius lodged with Andreas Vesalius of Brussels *(1514–1564)*, during which time the latter wrote and illustrated his celebrated books of anatomy, *De humani corporis fabrica*. Vesalius was also revising the Latin translations of certain of Galen's works for the newly planned and elaborate Giunta edition of Galen's *Opera omnia (1541–1542)*. (The Giunta family were important booksellers and publishers.)

Ultimately, a rift developed between Caius and Vesalius, the result of their differing views on the significance of Galen's writings. But in the end, it was Vesalius who was better able to modify his earlier acceptance of Galen's hitherto unchallenged authority, the accepted orthodoxy, when he tested it by comparison with direct observation of nature itself, as seen in the course of human dissection.

Caius believed Galen to be faultless, and thought that any possibility of error must be acknowledged as the result of either miscopying or mistranslation of the original Greek text into Latin. Vesalius was able to refute this assertion, by indicating by practical demonstration anatomical errors in Galen's work which were to be highlighted by publication of the *Fabrica*.

THE RENAISSANCE AND MEDICAL ADVANCE

No other advance in scientific knowledge in the sixteenth century can compare with that signified by the publication of three great works in the 1540s. The first of these was German botanist Leonhard Fuchs' *(1501–1566) De historia stirpium (The history of plants)* in 1542. This work may be considered as marking the foundation of modern botany in terms of the naturalistic drawings of plants it contains. His work emphasized the importance of drawing directly from nature rather than copying from books.

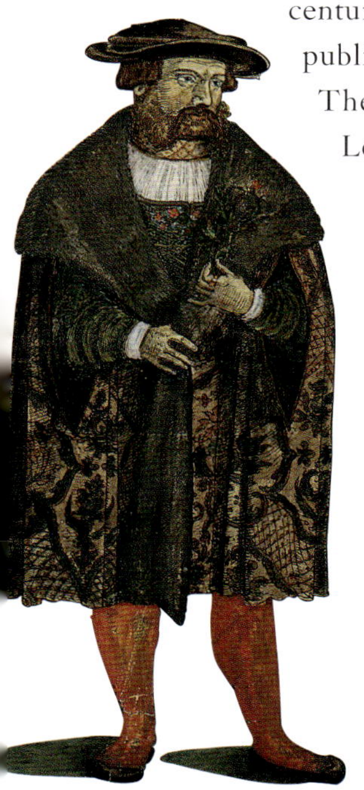

ABOVE Botanist Leonhard Fuchs. His work of 1542, *De historia stirpium*, was significant in that it featured naturalistic drawings of plants and herbs.

In 1543, Andreas Vesalius' *(1514–1564) De humani corporis fabrica (The structure of the human body)*, a highly influential work on human anatomy, was published.

The value of both these works, with their accurate representations of living plants and active human figures, was to free scholars from dependence on written authority and so enable them to work directly from nature.

The third great work, also published in 1543, was Nicolaus Copernicus' *De revolutionibus orbium coelestium (On the revolution of the celestial spheres)*, a work of cosmology that argued that the Sun, rather than the Earth, was at the centre of our planetary system. This was a major blow to the old Aristotelian cosmology that had prevailed through the Middle Ages. Yet despite his destruction of its basis, geocentric astrology continued to flourish, even influencing such great minds as that of William Harvey. Although it was clearly shown that the Earth was not the centre around which the other planets revolved, an idea which formed the very essence of astrological theory, it did not diminish the power of astrologists. This conundrum intrigues the medical historian.

It was the work of Vesalius that transformed the medical importance of Padua, where he was demonstrator of anatomy. The attraction of the university before his time had been primarily that of the law. The Cambridge scholars who had gone there in earlier times did so for its prestige in the arts. It set the scene for the Italian journey of William Harvey, which had a different motive.

By the age of fifteen, William Harvey *(1578–1657)* had already entered the Cambridge College founded by John Caius. He, too, was to experience the sense of the inadequacy of medical education in his English *alma mater.* But Harvey was able to avail himself of the special statutes instituted by Caius, giving permission for Cambridge students to study in either Padua, Verona, Montpellier or Paris. Despite his Galenical bias, Caius understood the need for a wider medical education and made provision for it.

In Harvey's case this was provided by his great teacher, the anatomist Girolamo Fabrizi d'Acquapendente *(1533–1619)*, who had the robust nature of many later professors of that discipline. William Harvey was foremost in scientific trials in establishing the theory of the circulation of the blood by scientific method. Its simplicity in demonstrating the direction of blood flow, which can be seen in the veins of the human forearm and the evidence of the internal arterial and venous systems in animals, gives him a place among the first of medical scientists. Yet he retained astrological ideas long after Copernicus' revelations should have destroyed them. He could not even rid himself of the idea of the value of venesection, hallowed by generations of doctors and surgeons.

William Harvey said, 'For daily experience satisfies us that blood-letting has a most salutary effect in many diseases and is indeed foremost among all general remedies.' It is another example of the power of 'the tried remedy' and the demonstration that even the greatest among us are anxious not to lose the reassurance of convention.

Harvey's demonstration of the circulation had a notable gap. He did not discover how the blood completed its circular journey by

BELOW William Harvey demonstrating his theory of the circulation of the blood to King Charles I. His work *De motu cordis* remains a milestone in science.

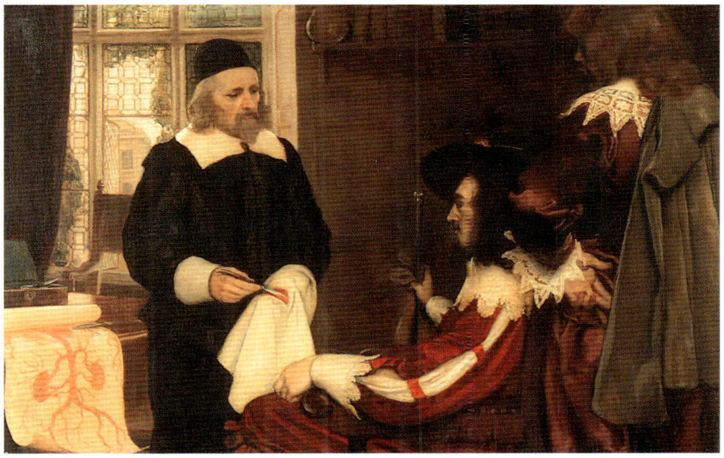

PLAGUES AND PANDEMICS

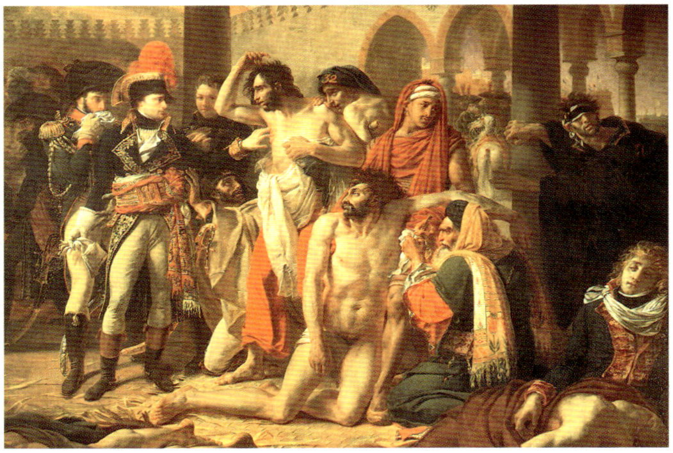

ABOVE Antoine's Gros' painting of Emperor Napoleon courageously visiting plague victims at Jaffa.

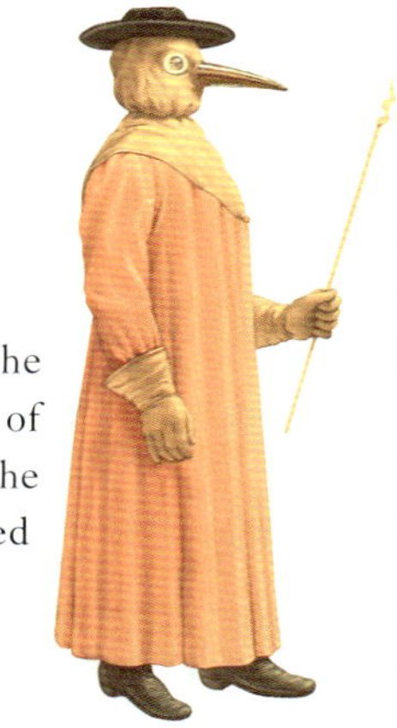

RIGHT Seventeenth-century plague doctors wore this strange costume to ward off infection.

THE PLAGUE

The Great Plagues, the Black Death of the Middle Ages and those bubonic plagues of later years were carried by *Rattus rattus,* the black rat (a somewhat more domesticated species than *Rattus norvegicus,* the sewer rat, and thus more dangerous to human populations), which was the principal intermediate host for the flea *Xenopsylla cheopis.* A bite from this flea was the cause of the transmission of the bacterial infection to humans. It caused the deaths of the millions of plague victims, whose corpses litter the pages of world history.

The plague was feared by governments for the damage it caused to national economics, as well as for its tragic toll of human suffering. Governments went to almost any length to deny its presence. The Emperor Napoleon I moved freely amongst the stricken soldiery at Jaffa to show his belief in its non-infectious nature. He knew its dangers full well, but insisted that the dreaded word plague, or *la peste,* should not be mentioned; and so his physicians had to invent the pseudonym *fièvre à bubons.* Napoleon's courage in such circumstances, and likewise on the battlefield, has been attributed to his conviction that he would die of cancer of the stomach, as did many of his family. Such was his fatalism about this, it was said that he would ask the surgeon Dominique-Jean Larrey to draw the situation of the growth so that he could see it in advance of his demise.

TYPHUS

The other great scourge of armies and civilians was the louse that transmitted the bacteria of typhus. The armies of lice were at least as important as the armies of men in determining the fates of nations. Besides the effects on the actual battle campaigns, for proof of this we have the *cri-de-coeur* of Lenin, when typhus threatened the Russian Revolution, 'If Socialism does not defeat the louse, the louse will defeat Socialism.' When the louse failed, competing politicians tried again.

SYPHILIS

The introduction of syphilis to Europe, which first came to our attention with the work of Fracastorius, has traditionally been associated with the return of the crew of Christopher Columbus to Naples at the end of the fifteenth century. They are blamed for carrying syphilis from the Americas to Europe. This has since been the subject of much controversy. The first illustration of syphilis, drawn by Albrecht Dürer, is given in a pamphlet of 1496 by Theodoricus Ulsenius, city physician of Nuremberg, who attributes its appearance to the malign conjunction of the planets Jupiter and Saturn in 1484.

Since the sixteenth century, the standard treatment had been the dangerous and prolonged dosage of mercury, which led to the oft repeated quip 'a night with Venus leads to a life with Mercury.'

The first great 'breakthrough' in treatment came with the work of Paul Ehrlich *(1854–1915)* in Berlin. He was seeking a method by which he could use arsenic selectively to kill pathogenic trypanosomes (small protozoal organisms) in mice, without damage to the mice. After the six-hundred-and-sixth attempt, he found the answer with salvarsan, an organic compund containing arsenic which he aptly named '606'. The similarity between the trypansome and the treponeme (the spiral bacterium) of syphilis led him to the successful treatment of the latter with the drug.

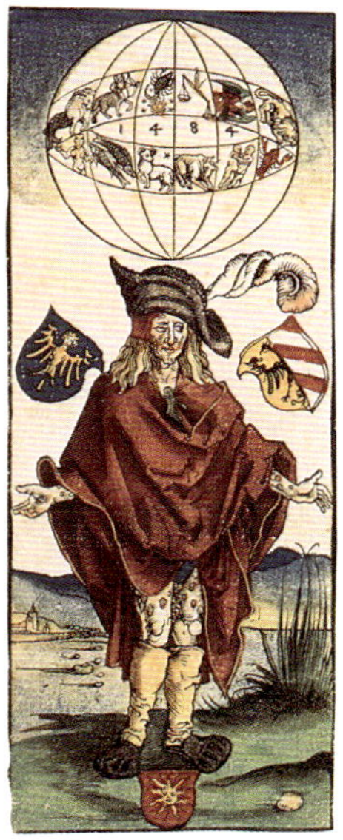

ABOVE Albrecht Dürer's illustration of a syphilitic man covered in chancres. Note the astrological influence suggested by the Zodiac above him.

passing from the arteries to the veins, although he surmised that this must be possible. The revelation was eventually made by the Italian Marcello Malpighi *(1628–1694)* of Bologna and physician to Pope Innocent XII. He used a microscope to demonstrate the structure of the organs and showed the minute capillaries by which the connection was made. His great work was *De pulmonibus (1661),* on the histology of the lungs.

Such basic knowledge of anatomy and physiology greatly improved understanding of how the body worked, yet medical treatment remained woefully defective. It was the pursuit of enquiry, aided by direct observation, into 'natural philosophy', rather than repetitious acceptance of the written *status quo,* that made advance in medical knowledge possible. Medical knowledge, in the twentieth century sense, becomes increasingly recognizable after the Renaissance, as part of the history of science and technology. The greatest influence on medical education in the United States came from the Scottish school at Edinburgh and indirectly from the Dutch school of medicine at Leiden. It was at the latter that the great medical teacher Herman Boerhaave *(1688–1738)* established the teaching of clinical method. The medical department of Harvard University was founded in 1782, two years after the University of Oxford had established its chair of clinical medicine.

MICROSCOPY AND THE GERM THEORY

The terror produced by the great plagues and epidemics of history gave rise to all sorts of speculations concerning their causes and how they spread. It is to Italian physician Girolamo Fracastoro *(c.1478–1553),* whose name was latinized to Hieronymous Fracastorius, that we owe an early formalization of these ideas. He was a graduate of the University of Padua and witnessed a severe plague in his home city of Verona. He is remembered as a poet for his Latin verses on *Syphilis sive morbus Gallicus (Syphilis or the French disease) (1530),* in which he recognized syphilis as a venereal disease. But his greater contribution towards an understanding of the nature of infection is contained in his *De contagione et contagionis morbis et curatione (1546).* This book on 'contagion and contagious illness' was published in Venice and it recognized contagion by contact; contagion by fomites (such as clothing, etc.), and contagion at a distance.

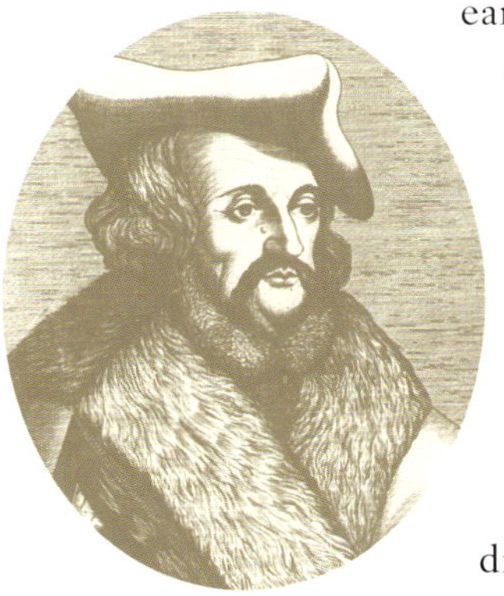

ABOVE Girolamo Fracastoro formulated the doctrine of contagion. His ideas anticipated the discovery of pathogenic organisms.

Contagion at a distance had its origins in the Hippocratic ideas of changes in the air produced by miasms or 'stains' carried on the winds. The miasmatic theory must have influenced Fracastoro's thought. But his work portended the modern recognition of *contagium vivum* or *contagium animatum,* in which minute pathogenic living organisms can be borne on the wind.

The germ theory itself had a long gestation period. It had been invented for centuries before a germ itself was actually seen. Even the Frenchman Pierre Fidele Bretonneau *(1771–1862)* of Tours, who was responsible for the idea of the association of a specific illness with a specific *germe reproducteur,* which he visualized in his mind never actually saw one. Bretonneau's views became more widely known through the work of his pupil the physician Armand Trousseau *(1804–1867).*

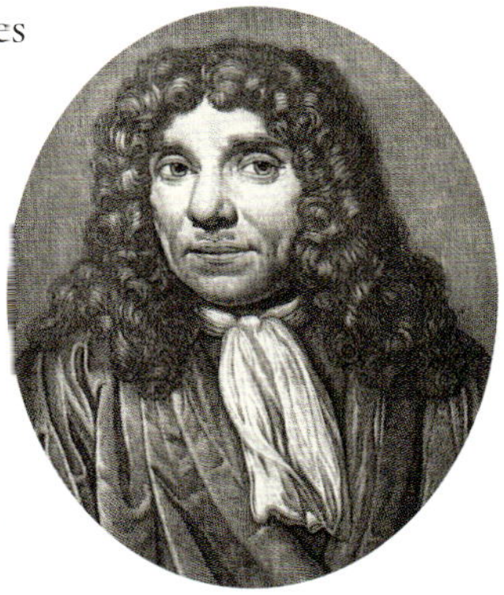

ABOVE Dutchman Antoni van Leeuwenhoek was a pioneer of microscopy. In 1674 he described human red blood cells.

It did not become possible to see germs until the microscope was invented. Robert Hooke *(1635–1703)* included many microsopic drawings in his famous *Micrographia* of 1665, but no illustrations of germs. Improvements in microscopy came with the solar microscope invented by Antoni van Leeuwenhoek *(1632–1712),* which was perfected by J N Lieberkühn in 1739. It was still a crude instrument. The invention of achromatic lenses for the correction of chromatic aberration was made by Chester Moor Hall *(1703–1771),* a barrister of London's Inner Temple, in 1733, and independently by the English optician John Dollond *(1706–1761).*

Leeuwenhoek's microscope and his communciations to the Royal Society in London made the next step in the development of the germ theory possible. Benjamin Marten was inspired to postulate a *New Theory of Consumptions More especially of a Phthisis or Consumption of the Lungs* in 1720. This was essentially an enunciation of the germ theory of disease by 'some certain Species of Animalcula or wonderfully minute living creatures'. He even suggests their specificity and deals in particular with tuberculosis of the lungs. However, his hope that some 'other hand' than his would be able to demonstrate the truth of his theories was not to be realized during his lifetime.

MEDICINE AND SCIENCE

THE SPECIFICITY OF DISEASE

Thomas Sydenham *(1624–1689)*, a practical Englishman who had served as an officer in the Parliamentary Cavalry during the English Civil War, was much concerned with clinical entities – a taxonomy or classification of syndromes, which are collections of signs and symptoms. In the aetiology or causation of epidemic diseases, he suggested there were miasmatic reasons for the preponderance of any particular symptom in any particular season. This observation effectively marked the beginning of clinical science; it gave a glimpse of the effect of the environment on disease.

Scientific medical treatment ultimately depends on improvements in scientific diagnosis – on the discovery of the causation of disease – and this was a long time coming. Hippocrates' contribution to prognosis had resulted from his keen observation of the portent of signs and symptoms. It was not until the seventeenth century that Thomas Sydenham began to group them into disease entities. As he wrote, 'First, it is necessary that all Diseases should be reduced to certain and definite Species, with the same diligence we see it is done by Botanick Writers in their Herbals.' He had quoted the philosopher Francis Bacon on the title page of his book, 'We have not to imagine, or to think out, but to find out what Nature does or produces.'

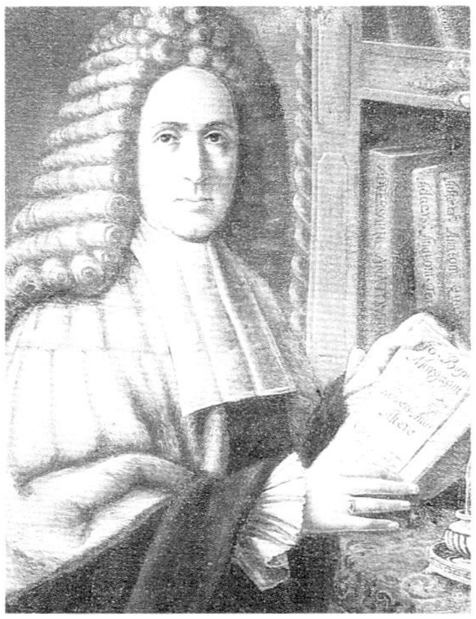

ABOVE Italian pathologist Giovanni Battista Morgagni used his findings from post-mortem examinations to demonstrate a link between a patient's symptoms and the anatomical lesions visible on the body.

The true understanding of the aetiology of disease was yet to come via such men as the Italian Giovanni Battista Morgagni *(1682–1771)*, who provided an anatomic model showing the relationship between disease and the human organs.

Morgagni was another son of Padua. Acknowledging the work already achieved by his forebears, he built on their efforts and related the signs and symptoms of disease in living patients to the results of his examinations of their bodies after death. This was an important systematization and in achieving it he produced the first practical textbook of pathological anatomy, *De sedibus et causis morborum per anatomen indagatis... (The sites and causes of illness as shown by anatomy)*, when he was nearly 80 years of age, in 1761. It was a step that recognized an anatomical model of aetiology (the study of the cause of diseases) in the demonstration of diseased organs post-mortem.

This was the first time that the cause of illness was shown to be localized in the patient's internal anatomical organs, for example in the lungs, the heart and the kidneys. As historian Richard Shryock wrote:

'In pathology [as a whole] the anatomic concept provided the first real model... animalculism [or the belief in minute animal creatures] was another model which could not gain acceptance until after the anatomic approach was gradually adopted... Until anatomy was made the basis of disease identification, the animalcules were viewed as presenting just another competing system in pathology.'

RICHARD SHRYOCK

Later, the Frenchman René-Théophile-Hyacinthe Laënnec *(1781–1826)* demonstrated the ability to link directly the changes occurring in the diseased organs with the clinical signs they produced in the living body by the use of his stethoscope to listen to what was 'going on' inside the chest. Laënnec's auscultation was aided by Auenbrugger's percussion. Leopold Auenbrugger *(1722–1809)* was the son of an inn-keeper and was familiar with the practice of tapping on the side of the barrel to learn how full it was. He taught the use of this technique in percussing the chest wall to demonstrate whether it was resonant, as it is normally, or dull when there is some change in the lungs, such as the presence of fluid in a pleural effusion (the accumulation of fluid in the pleural cavity).

Laënnec and Auenbrugger used simple clinical methods to aid diagnosis that are still used today. Laënnec furthermore linked the physical signs that he found in life with the pathological changes he found after death.

JENNER, PASTEUR AND KOCH

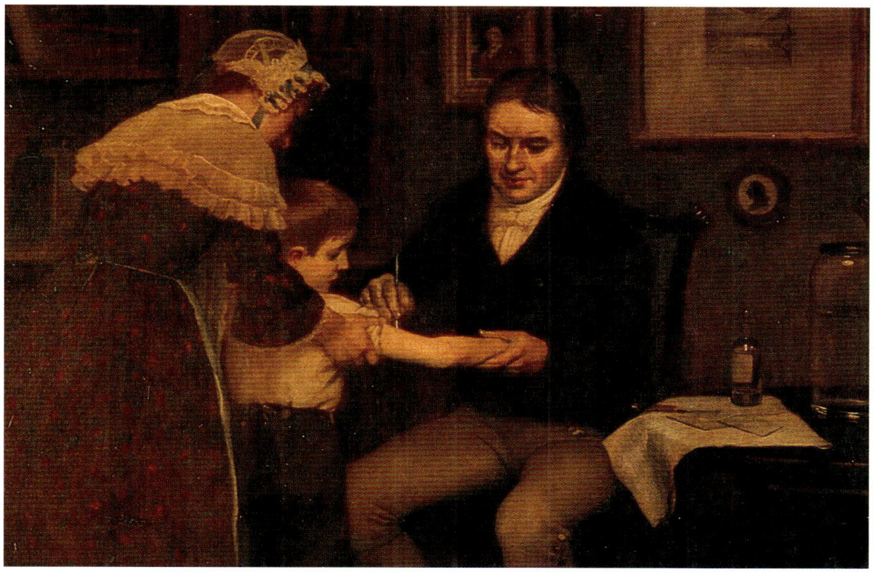

ABOVE 14 May 1796 – Edward Jenner vaccinates James Phipps with fluid taken from a cowpox vesicle on Sarah Nelmes' hand. Six weeks later he inoculated Phipps with smallpox, to which he proved immune.

The Frenchman Louis Pasteur *(1822–1895)* was a chemist and not a physician. As the former, he made contributions to stereochemistry and isomerism, which relates to the atomic structure of chemical molecules in three-dimensional space. His work on fermentation showed the function of small living organisms, the yeasts, in that process. He was also asked to investigate the cause of a disease in silkworms that was devastating the French silk industry, and as a result of his work he recognized the infectious nature of the epidemic and how it might be prevented. He had already worked on anthrax, as well as several other animal infections, before he produced the anti-rabies 'vaccine' – as he called it after Jenner's discovery of the protection against smallpox given by vaccination using cowpox – for which he is best remembered.

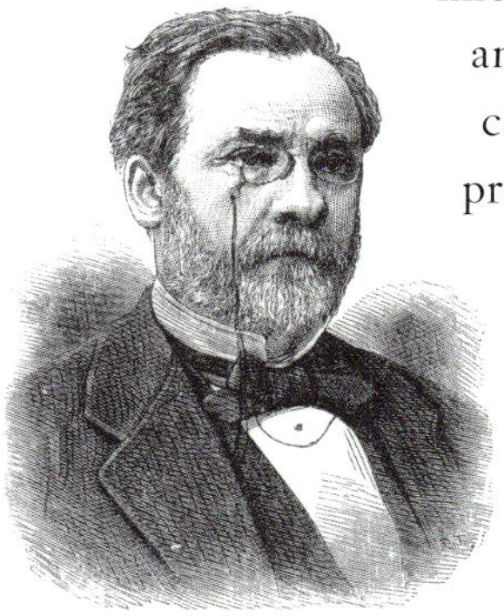

ABOVE Louis Pasteur, the microbiologist and chemist who recognized that micro-organisms were responsible for many infectious diseases.

The English physician Edward Jenner *(1749–1823),* who practised in the town of Berkeley, Gloucestershire, had observed that milkmaids who had caught cowpox from their animals did not develop the major killing and disfiguring disease of smallpox. He put this theory of immunity to the test by artificially infecting patients with material taken directly from the pustules on the sick cow. It was successful – the patients did not develop smallpox – and became known as vaccination (from the Latin for cow, *vacca*).

Throughout the nineteenth century and into the twentieth, the arguments continued as to whether the micro-organisms seen in a sick patient were merely co-incidental with the illness or resulted from the changes brought about by the illness itself. Or, the question was asked, were they the *germes reproducteurs* of Bretonneau? The theory that specific germs could cause specific disease remained a contentious one until the beginning of the twentieth century. The old theories of miasma were modernized by the adoption of new terminology – they were now called 'poisonous effluvia'. Some theorists favoured ideas of contagion, or spread of disease by direct person-to-person contact, that had been suggested many years before. They called themselves contagio-miasmatists.

As late as 1892, Dr Max von Pettenkofer *(1818–1901)* of Bavaria, a distinguished experimental hygienist, still required a 'touch of miasma' in his explanation of the infectivity of cholera. He postulated that an environmental factor in the soil needed to be added to the cholera vibrio, or comma bacillus, which had been isolated as the infective agent of the disease, in order to cause illness.

He was prepared to put his views to the ultimate test and challenged the great proponent of the germ theory, Robert Koch *(1843–1910)*, in a famous letter.

'Herr Doctor Pettenkofer presents his compliments to Herr Doctor Professor Koch and thanks him for the flask containing the so-called cholera vibrios, which he was kind enough to send. Herr Doctor Pettenkofer has now drunk the entire contents and is happy to be able to inform Herr Doctor Professor Koch that he remains in his usual good health.'

MAX VON PETTENKOFER

X+Y=Z

X = *the comma bacillus*

Y = *the soil factor*

Z = *the cholera miasm*

ABOVE Max von Pettenkofer could not accept that cholera had a simple bacterial cause. Instead, he reasoned that there must be some chemical agent in the soil that activated the bacillus.

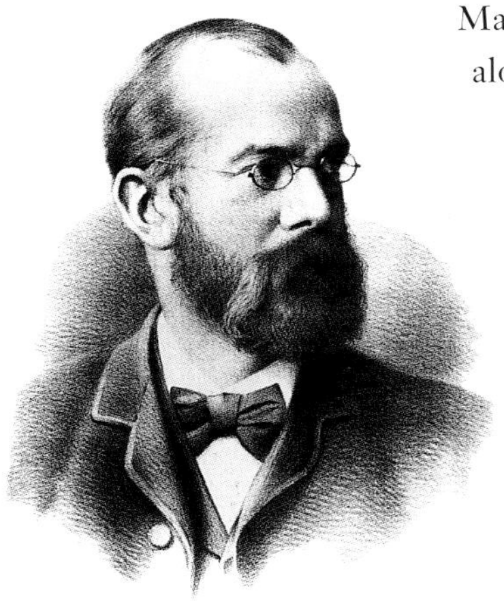

ABOVE The great German bacteriologist Robert Koch who enunciated four criteria – known as Koch's Postulates – necessary to prove that a disease was caused by a particular micro-organism.

Max von Pettenkofer was by no means alone in his spirit of scepticism.

He was already aged 74 when he wrote the letter. He shot himself nine years later.

Robert Koch, the son of a German miner, was 20 years younger than Pasteur. Koch's discoveries of specific bacillary causes for disease, followed by those of his famous pupils, which are now so readily accepted, were by no means generally accepted in the last quarter of the nineteenth century. During this period of scientific discovery, the causative organisms of diseases such as anthrax, cholera, tuberculosis, gonorrhoea, diphtheria, leprosy, typhoid, trypanosomiasis and malaria were revealed by Koch and his followers.

In 1885, Sir John Burdon Sanderson *(1828–1905)* of Oxford had described Koch's work on cholera as 'an unfortunate fiasco'. Sir Charles Sherrington *(1857–1952)* was a young member of a British medical mission which had studied a cholera outbreak in Spain in 1885, and he reported that in his opinion the comma bacillus was not its cause. He thought it was due to a fungus. Indeed, the leader of another British mission to India in 1884 even wrote that he regarded Pettenkofer as 'the greatest living authority on the aetiology of cholera'.

Timothy Richards Lewis *(1841–1886)*, a Welshman, and David Douglas Cunningham *(1843–1914)*, both of great scientific reputation, had spent more than ten years in India studying cholera and had come to the wrong conclusion. They strongly opposed Koch's views. They even committed themselves in their official reports 'that no microbe found in the living blood of any animal was pathogenic.' The resistance to new ideas underlines once more the fact that great scientific discoveries do not necessarily produce great changes in clinical medicine. Empirical beliefs and tried remedies often persist beyond experimental evidence of their frailty.

Koch's paper presented to the Physiological Society of Berlin on 24 March 1882 had summarized his evidence of the infectious nature of tuberculosis. 'All of these facts taken together lead to the conclusion that the bacilli which are present in the tuberculous substances not only accompany the tuberculous process, but are the cause of it. In the bacillus we have, therefore, the actual tubercle virus.'

Koch had isolated the tubercle bacilli from artificially produced lesions in animals, inoculated them into healthy guinea pigs and reproduced tuberculosis just as in the naturally occurring disease. Tuberculosis could henceforth be diagnosed by demonstrating the bacilli in the sputum. It has been said that this paper established clinical bacteriology.

Griffith Evans *(1835–1935)*, a colleague of Lewis and Cunningham, supported Koch's views and summed up the situation succinctly, in his own work on surra, a fatal disease of horses that was creating enormous problems for the British Army in India.

The question suggested by these facts is, whether the presence of the parasite is the cause of the disease, or whether the disease is the cause of the appearance of the parasites. That they are most intimately related to each other, is beyond reasonable dispute. There are some eminent pathologists in India who deny the parasitic origin of specific blood diseases: they say the cause of all such diseases, from smallpox to anthrax fever, is not any organic spore, germ or ova or parasite of any kind, but some purely chemical agent which has never yet been discovered, and that these organisms develop at once in the blood which has been so chemically altered, each chemical virus developing its specific organism, the spores or ova of which are supposed to be in the normal blood ready to develop as soon as chemistry favours them. The organisms themselves, even when developed, are supposed to be harmless…

GRIFFITH EVANS

PUBLIC HEALTH

Concepts of public health had their beginnings early in medical history, as is evidenced by Biblical rules on health and hygiene, and such great architectural works as the building of aqueducts to supply fresh water to Rome, and the removal of waste by means of the great drain, the *cloaca maxima.* In AD 96, Rome was supplied with 250 million imperial gallons (1,136 million litres) of water a day through ten aqueducts, the first of which was designed and built by the Etruscans in 312 BC. These provided 50 gallons (227 litres) each for each member of its population of two million, with plenty of spare for other purposes.

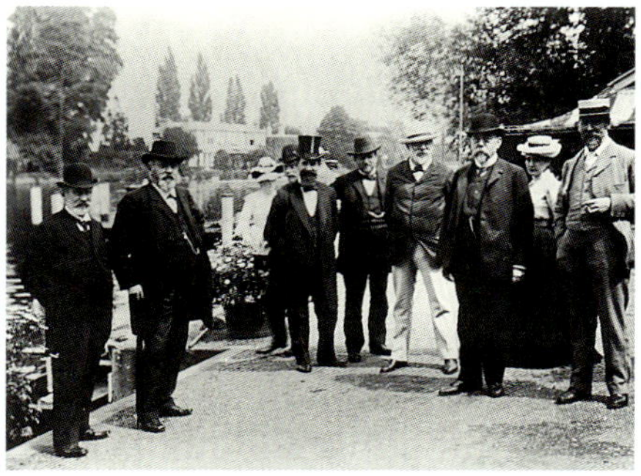

LEFT Members of the International Congress on Tuberculosis in 1901 on a weekend excursion to Maidenhead in England. Paul Ehrlich is on the extreme right and Robert Koch is third from the right.

TREATING TUBERCULOSIS

The Great White Plague of tuberculosis has provided many pages in the history of world medicine. Part of its history has been related under the story of Robert Koch. The traditional treatment since the early nineteenth century had been by rest in suitable climates, particularly on mountains, in spas and in warmer climes. The principle of resting the affected part, in this case the lungs, resulted in the popularity of 'collapse therapy' of the affected lung by injecting air through the chest wall (pneumothorax) or surgically by thoracoplasty (the operation for collapsing a diseased lung). It was not until 1943 in the Department of Microbiology at Rutgers University in New Jersey, USA, that Selman A. Waksman *(1888–1973)* discovered the first effective anti-tuberculous drug, streptomycin. He received the Nobel Prize in Medicine for this work in 1952.

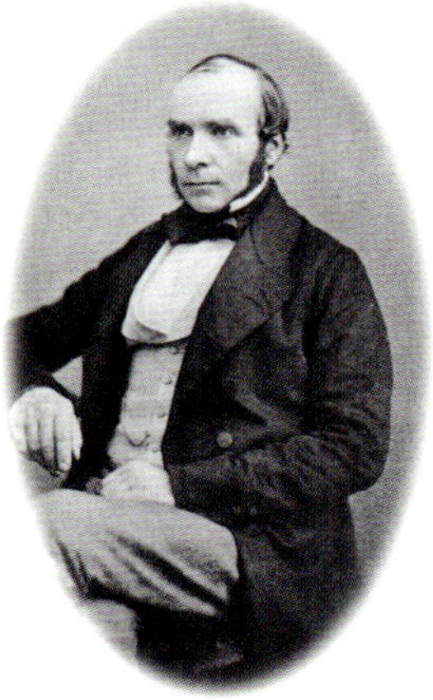

ABOVE John Snow, who was both an eminent hygienist and the anaesthetist who introduced ether to Britain. His removal of the handle from the Broad Street pump controlled the spread of cholera in London in 1854.

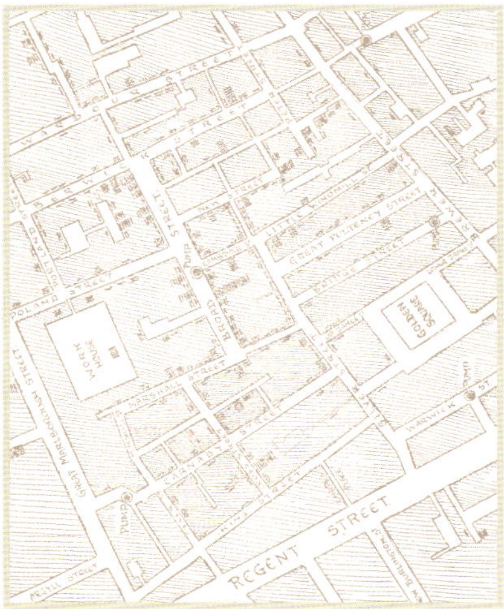

ABOVE John Snow's map of Soho, London, showing the infected water pump in Broad Street that led to the 1854 cholera epidemic. The black lines in the shaded areas represent the number of fatalities in each building.

Principles regarding safe diets and personal hygiene were taught by the great religions. These, reinforced by later miasmatic notions, popularly associated with evil smells, did fortuitously help to prevent the spread of some diseases. Evil smells do indicate poor sanitation and their removal reduces sources of infection.

In England in the nineteenth century, the miasmatic school of thought remained strong. The great civil servant in sanitary engineering Sir Edwin Chadwick *(1800–1890)* and the famous nurse Florence Nightingale *(1820–1910)* clung to the miasmatic theory throughout their long lives; on the whole to the improvement of public health. It became known as the atmospheric or *pythogenic* theory and its supporters concentrated on cleaning up smelly places where people lived or were cared for in hospitals.

Good reasons for associating ill health with contaminated water were already known. John Snow *(1813–1858)* had effectively brought to an end the 1854 cholera epidemic in Soho, London, by demonstrating that only those who drank from the infected Broad Street pump contracted the disease. The source was stopped and the outbreak ended. And there were others, such as William Budd *(1811–1880)* of Bristol, England, who provided further evidence that this was the method by which typhoid and cholera were spread.

A great public health battle ensued in England in the nineteenth century over the cause and cure of epidemics. Edwin Chadwick, the advocate of public health measures who greatly advanced sanitary engineering, maintained to the last his opposition to acceptance of the germ theory.

His formidable opponent, Sir John Simon *(1816–1904)*, the pioneering officer of public health, changed his earlier orthodox medical views on the causation of these diseases as the century moved toward its end. At first, we hear his firmly expessed opinion in 1853 that the typhoid outbreak was due to a 'fog of faecal evaporation' and not to an infected water supply. Within a few years he had changed his mind. By the 1870s he was expressing his unequivocal view that 'the true cause of each metabolic contagion must either be, or must essentially include a specific living organism, able to multiply its kind'. Royston Lambert's biography of Sir John Simon fascinatingly reveals the progress of medical science, shifting from medieval theories of infectivity to modern bacteriology in the span of one man's life.

WOMEN AS PATIENTS AND PRACTITIONERS

There has been much controversy over the place of women in medical history, firstly as patients in a male-dominated profession and then as practitioners in the same environment. Childbirth is basically a normal process and yet in the past it has been responsible for the avoidable deaths of countless women. Why should this have been so? In earlier times the prevalence of mass poverty and inadequate diet resulted in anaemias and vitamin-deficiency diseases such as rickets, causing pelvic deformity. Debilitating illnesses such as tuberculosis caused great physical weakness. Unhygienic living conditions and unhygienic methods of delivery brought about infection.

The Hungarian obstetrician Ignaz Philipp Semmelweis *(1818–1865)* made the perceptive observation that after deliveries by midwives, either at home or in the hospital, the mortality rate of mothers was less than it was when they were attended by medical students. He concluded that two factors were involved. The first was that the midwives paid much greater attention to personal cleanliness. The second was that students made vaginal examinations without washing their hands first, and often came directly to the confinement from the autopsy room.

In 1847, Semmelweis attended the autopsy of a professor who had died from an infection resulting from an injury he had sustained during a post-mortem examination. Semmelweis was impressed by the similarity of the pathological findings with those he had observed in women dead of a puerperal sepsis (infection of the birth canal). He thereupon introduced the regulation in his department that all attendants of the woman in labour must first wash their hands in a solution of calcium chloride. This simple measure reduced, within a year, the frightful mortality previously noted in his department of more than 12 per cent to nil. The principle of asepsis had been established.

Although the name of Semmelweis is rightly ranked among the saviours of women in childbirth, it is sometimes forgotten that an American had written on *The Contagiousness of Puerperal Fever* five years earlier in 1843. This was the great literary figure Oliver Wendell Holmes *(1809–1894)*, who qualified in medicine in 1836. It was he who also first suggested the use of the term *anaesthesia* in a letter to William Morton in 1846.

Unless one recognizes the claim that James Barry *(1797–1865)*, inspector general of the British army medical services in 1858, was female, the first woman to graduate in medicine was an Englishwoman from Bristol. Elizabeth Blackwell *(1821–1910)* succeeded in her ambition at the Geneva

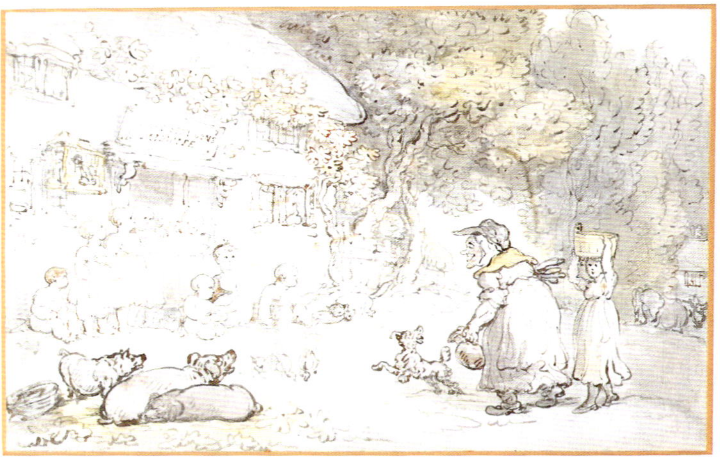

ABOVE A watercolour by the eighteenth-century English caricaturist Thomas Rowlandson entitled 'Mary Spriggens, the Midwife'. For centuries, obstetrics was usually left to women, often with little or no training. Male midwives started to become fashionable in Europe in the eighteenth century.

THE HAZARDS OF CHILDBIRTH

Until the eighteenth century, the practice of obstetrics had been almost exclusively in the hands of female midwives. In the early part of the century, the man-midwife appeared. Little was clearly understood about the mechanics of labour, but obstructed labour was seen to be the cause of frightful, prolonged pain and frequently the death of the mother and child. A surgical remedy was to sacrifice and deliver the baby by perforating the skull and removing the rest piecemeal. This procedure did not always save the mother.

The alternative was to deliver the unborn child with an instrument known as the obstetric forceps. It had been in limited use for over a century and was said to have been invented by Peter Chamberlen *(1560–1631)*, a Huguenot refugee to England. Four generations of Chamberlens had kept its use hidden as a family secret of commercial value. The last of its guardians, Dr Hugh Chamberlen, died in 1728 and left no son and heir to continue the tradition.

The general use of the forceps was initiated by the Scot William Smellie *(1697–1763)*. He used them with moderation and laid down careful rules for their application. His clearer understanding of the mechanism of labour is outlined in his book *Treatise on the theory and practice of Midwifery*, published in 1752. Smellie moved to London, where after a few years he was joined by another Scot, William Hunter *(1718–1783)*, who was also destined to leave his mark as both an obstetrician and anatomist. Men then dominated the midwifery scene until the twentieth century.

Medical School of New York in 1849. She was the first woman in the USA to be acknowledged as a qualified doctor. Her success, despite enormous prejudice from a male-dominated profession, was followed by the foundation of the Philadelphian Women's College of Medicine in 1830. Elizabeth Garrett *(1836–1917)*, who became Mrs Garrett Anderson after her marriage, encountered tremendous opposition before she, too, succeeded in obtaining the diploma of the Worshipful Society of Apothecaries in London in 1865. She was the first woman to qualify in medicine in the UK.

SURGERY IN THE EIGHTEENTH TO TWENTIETH CENTURIES

One of the great figures of eighteenth-century surgery was John Hunter *(1728–1793)*, brother of the obstetrician William. He is regarded as the founder of surgical pathology and assembled the great collection of specimens that were stored in the Royal College of Physicians in London.

It was a period that saw the blossoming of the art of military surgery through the work of medical officers in different and often warring armies. In Britain, George James Guthrie *(1765–1856)* was responsible for the humanizing of the treatment of the wounded; he left important treatises on surgery. He stressed the importance of early amputation of battle wounds, as did his French counterpart Larrey.

Dominique-Jean Larrey *(1766–1842)* was Napoleon's chief military surgeon. His surgical competence was the equivalent of that of Guthrie and he has left great works on military surgery. He advocated the principle of taking the medical officer to the wounded on the battlefield by means of his *ambulances volantes,* the flying ambulances. The third in the great military surgeons of the eighteenth and nineteenth centuries is the Russian Nikolai Ivanovich Pirogov *(1810–1881),* who published his *Klinische Chirurgie* in three parts between 1851 and 1854. He encouraged the female nursing services in the Russian army during the Crimean campaign, while Florence Nightingale was looking after the British troops on the other side. He took early advantage of the introduction of ether as an anaesthetic, and used it extensively during the Crimean War.

The effects of infection and its treatment and prevention were often recognized before its real cause as a consequence of surgery was accepted. In 1867, the British surgeon Joseph Lister *(1827–1912)* was seeking the causes of wound suppuration and gangrene and taught his Glasgow students the dangers of sepsis. In 1867, he published a paper on the antiseptic use of carbolic acid in the treatment of compound fracures; it had eliminated wound sepsis in his wards. The Latvian Ernst von Bergmann *(1836–1907)* also promoted the practice of asepsis in surgery with the use of steam sterilization of instruments.

ANAESTHESIA

The relief of pain has a long history. It can trace its origins to ancient times with the use of anodynes, such as the Greek soporific sponge. In the nineteenth century there was growing familiarity with the effects of opium and of the liberal use and abuse of alcohol. Bitter disputes have arisen over the claims made for the person to be credited with the introduction of the modern inhalational method of anaesthesia. Horace Wells *(1815–1848)*, a dentist from Hartford, Connecticut, had undoubtedly been using nitrous oxide, or 'laughing gas' in his dental practice. His former partner William Thomas Green Morton *(1819–1868)* of Charlton, Massachusetts, who later obtained a medical degree, developed his technique further with the use of ether. His progress was sufficient to permit Dr John Collins Warren *(1778–1856)* of the Massachusetts General Hospital to remove a tumour from the neck of an anaesthetized patient on 16 October 1846. The operation took five minutes. The word of this tremendous boon spread round the world rapidly. The British surgeon Robert Liston *(1794–1847)* amputated a leg under ether in London in December of the same year. On 4 November 1847, the Scottish obstetrician, Sir James Young Simpson *(1811–1870),* who had hitherto been using ether in midwifery practice, changed to chloroform, which had been discovered by the German chemist Baron Justus von Liebig *(1803-1873).*

BELOW The dentist William Morton used ether to anaesthetize his patients. In 1846 he adminstered ether to a man who was then operated on by the surgeon John Collins Warren.

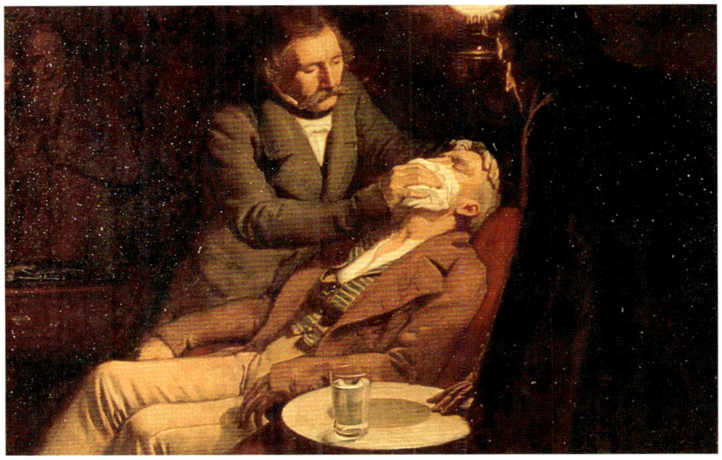

THE RISE OF THE SPECIALIST

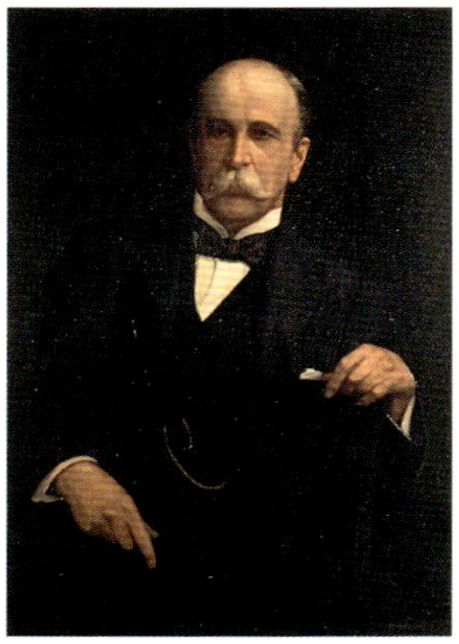

ABOVE Sir William Osler by Roger Eliot Fry. Osler achieved academic distinction on both sides of the Atlantic.

The Canadian William Osler *(1849–1919)* is undoubtedly one of the profession's leading medical heroes. He was an outstanding clinician, who has left the evidence of his skills and understanding in his textbooks on medicine.

In his address to the Paediatric Society in Boston in 1892, William Osler thanked them for choosing 'as your presiding officer one whose work has lain in the wide field of general medicine [which] is an indication that you truly appreciate the relation of the special subject in which you are now interested, and to which this society is devoted'. Until then it had been possible to regard the general physician and surgeon as sufficently experienced to deal with the wide variety of childhood ailments. Osler was saying that at the end of the last century the paediatrician was not recognized as a specialist as such.

He enlarged on this by remarking that in the larger cities the specialist was encroaching on the generalist, 'and this condition, though in many ways to be regretted, is not likely to be changed'. He concluded that 'the rapid increase of knowledge has made concentration of work a necessity; specialism is here and here to stay.'

Although in the nature of things there had always been practitioners with particular skills, the modern concept of the medical specialist did not take root until the middle of the nineteenth century. The emerging new specialist required access to a larger number of patients than did the generalist if he was to achieve financial success within the restrictions imposed by the limited number of patients requiring his special knowledge. And the more specialized the knowledge, the larger the general pool of patients required. The conditions that made such a development possible were established when the improvement in communications meant that a specialist's fame could spread far and wide, and reliable travel facilities enabled patients to reach him. Newspapers and improved road, rail and sea passages provided the necessary conditions.

MENTAL ILLNESS

The history of people afflicted by madness, or possessed by spirits, or accused of witchcraft in which mental illness probably played some part is a long and troubling one. A chapter later in the book is specifically devoted to this subject.

A major description of depression was presented by Robert Burton *(1516–1639)* in his *Anatomy of Melancholy* in 1621. Over a hundred years later, William Battie *(1703–1776)* published his *Treatise on Madness* in 1757, which provided an early textbook on the discipline of psychiatry. The definition of madness caused difficulties.

James Prichard *(1786–1848)* wrote on *Moral Insanity* in 1837 as a 'form of mental derangement consisting in a morbid perversion of the feelings, affections and active powers, without any illusion or erroneous condition impressed upon the understanding'. He added that 'it sometimes co-exists with an apparently unimpaired state of the intellectual faculties'.

In the United States, Benjamin Rush *(1745–1813)* is regarded as the 'father of American psychiatry' and he became director of the first psychiatric department there in the Pennsylvania Hospital. He appropriately contributed the first American textbook on psychiatry, *Medical Inquiries and Observations upon the Diseases of the Mind* in 1810.

The Frenchman Philippe Pinel *(1745–1826)* is credited with the liberalization of the treatment of the insane, transferring them from a prison-like confinement to hospital-type care. In England, Samuel Tuke *(1747–1857)* initiated reform in the management and care of the mentally ill with the example set at his York Retreat, of which he has left an historical account.

The great French neurologist Jean-Martin Charcot *(1825–1893)*, in his demonstrations at the Salpêtrière in Paris, showed the characteristics of patients with hysterical symptoms. His explanations of the behaviour of those under the effects of hypnosis provoked much controversy.

Another neurologist, the Austrian Sigmund Freud *(1856–1939)*, influenced by the growing number of theories relating to psychiatry, developed his new concepts, which resulted in the development of treatment with psychoanalysis.

The history of the treatment of mental illness must also concern itself with the place of institutional care and care in the community, together with the necessity today of balancing the effects of environment on the mental health of the individual and the place of chemical therapy in the treatment of the psychiatric illnesses known as the psychoses, such as schizophrenia and manic-depression.

TECHNOLOGY AND PROGRESS

The advance of technology was further to encourage specialization because of the ability doctors were granted to look below the surface of the skin, inside the body, without the necessity of surgical wounds and their attendant discomforts.

Wilhelm Konrad Röntgen *(1845–1923)* announced his discovery of X-rays in 1895 to a meeting at Würzburg, where he was the chairman of physics. Its use has now advanced from the simple diagnosis of bone fractures and the location of foreign bodies to examination of the internal organs of the body. In 1897, while he was still a student, Walter Cannon *(1871–1945)*, professor of physics at Harvard, used drinkable solution of radio-opaque bismuth as a diagnostic meal to outline the stomach. Röntgen rays, using radio-opaque substances, have since become an essential agent for the examination of the cardiovascular and central nervous systems and the urogenital tract. These techniques have made separate specialties within that of general radiology.

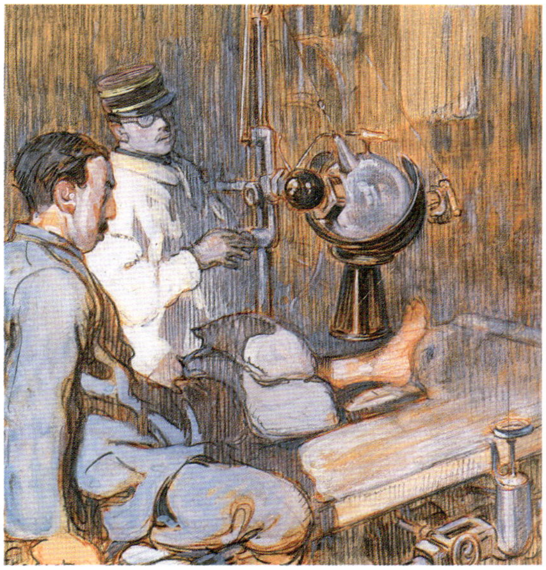

ABOVE X-rays were discovered by Wilhelm Röntgen in 1895. This technology was rapidly put to medical use, as this drawing of a World War I French army radiographer shows.

It was also found that X-rays had a place in the treatment of malignant disease. The Curies, the Pole Marie *(1876–1934)* and her French husband Pierre *(1859–1906)*, discovered the value of radium and its radioactive rays. Marie Curie published her *Researches on Radioactive Substances* in 1903. She herself was to die as a result of her exposure to radiation, as were many other early workers, suffering the dangerous side effects of radium and X-rays.

The problem of trying to see directly inside the body was one that had occupied the minds of doctors throughout the nineteenth century. Bladder stones had been a painful scourge for which patients had been prepared to undergo the frightful operation of lithotomy, in which the bladder was cut open and the stone removed. Diagnosis was confirmed by 'sounding' the bladder with a metal probe. Philipp Bozzini *(1773–1809)* of Frankfurt had first tried to improve on this expedient by looking into the bladder, using reflected light, through an illuminated straight tube in 1805. Not unexpectedly, he met with little success. A J Desormeaux *(d.1894)* of Paris began work in 1805 on producing a sort of pan-endoscope, capable of viewing inside either the trachea, lungs, stomach or bladder. In 1865, he published a work on an improved cystoscope (an instrument for looking inside the bladder). It was not until 1877, when a system of lenses became available, that a Viennese instrument maker, Joseph Leiter, and Max Nitze *(1848–1906)* of Dresden produced the first modern-type cystoscope. Leiter developed the first modern oesophagoscope in 1880.

In the twentieth century and particularly since World War II, surgical technology and medical therapy have advanced so rapidly that it would require as much print as we have already used simply to outline the recent scientific changes. The reader is directed to the next chapter, which examines nineteenth and twentieth century developments in medical science much more fully than is possible here.

The most significant developments include the discovery of antibiotics, which have almost conquered acute infectious diseases, and chemotherapy, which has altered the nature of the attack on malignant disease. Endoscopy has enabled doctors to view most of the body cavities, and new scanning techniques have revealed what X-rays had left unseen. There is now a wholly new promise from the discoveries in cell biology, which were undreamed of by Theodor Schwann *(1810–1882)* when he introduced his 'cell theory' in 1839, and when Rudolf Virchow *(1821–1902)* wrote his work *Cellular Pathlogy* in 1858. The ability to alter the genetic code and so affect inherited diseases has been realized since biologists found in 1953 that nucleic acids, DNA and RNA, were the substance of chromosomes, which determine hereditary factors.

Yet despite these astonishing medical advances, we are left with a paradox. Why is it that despite these vast improvements in therapy, many patients are abandoning orthodox medicine and seeking comfort from the very oldest methods of health care, which are now revived in an assortment of therapies known as 'alternative medicine'? It is a paradox for which the medical historian can offer no simple explanation.

CHAPTER TWO

THE DEVELOPMENT OF WESTERN MEDICAL SCIENCE

THE WEST'S CONTRIBUTION TO HEALING

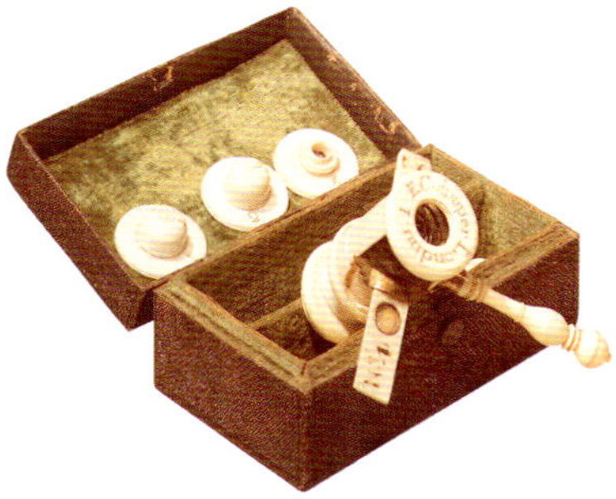

ABOVE The invention of the microscope in the early seventeenth century opened up a new world of study to the medical scientist.

WESTERN MEDICAL SCIENCE *is the medicine that has developed and been practised both generally and officially during the last two hundred years in those industrial nations that are collectively known as 'the West'. Scientific medicine developed against a background of changes in society in the nineteenth century, when new influences in society and religion affected attitudes towards both medicine and the medical profession. These included progressive secularization with the loss of Christian faith, changing beliefs about death, new doubts about the afterlife and greater involvement of doctors, who were increasingly expected to make a diagnosis of the illness based on demonstrable pathology. There was also greater expectation on the part of the patient of treatment or cure of an illness, or at least of alleviation of symptoms and distress.*

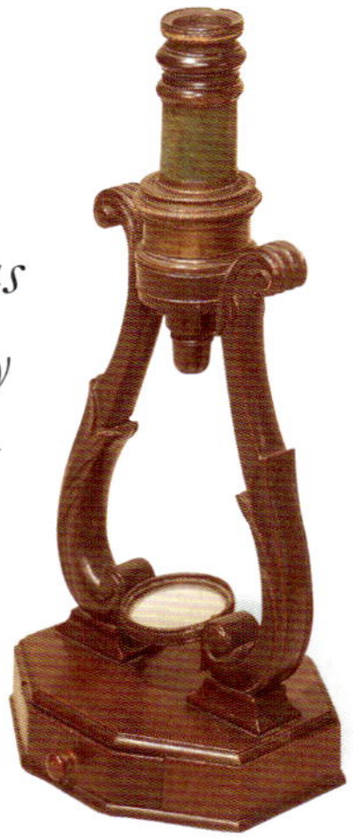

ABOVE A simple monocular microscope dating from the late seventeenth century.

Modern Western medicine, sometimes known as scientific medicine or biomedicine, is based upon whatever its practitioners and patients regard as scientific knowledge, method or practice. The scientific is usually defined as that which is objective, demonstrable, measurable, self-evident and, increasingly, the result of personal observation or high-tech practice. The concept of what is scientific changes over time and varies between individuals and institutions. Scientific medicine values accurate observation and, still more, accurate measurement. It has a single-minded, materialistic approach that, basically, reduces all bodily function and dysfunction to material causes, mechanical mechanisms and structural flaws that can be thought of and studied in isolation from those who suffer from them.

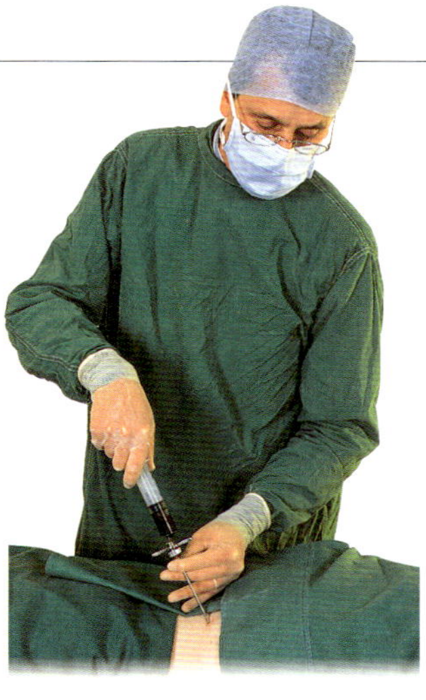

ABOVE Western scientific medicine is often criticized for ignoring the patient in its overriding concentration on the disease.

Medical practitioners have often emphasized (particularly in recent years) that patients are *people* and should be treated as such, but at the same time many modern doctors make it clear that they are more interested in the disease than in the people who have the diseases. Patients complain of feeling valued only as walking stomachs, blood sugars, heart valves or whatever is the seat of their 'disease'. The great physician William Osler *(1849–1919)* was considered to be one of the best scientific doctors. He became Professor of Medicine at Johns Hopkins University, Baltimore and later Professor of Medicine at Oxford. Yet he

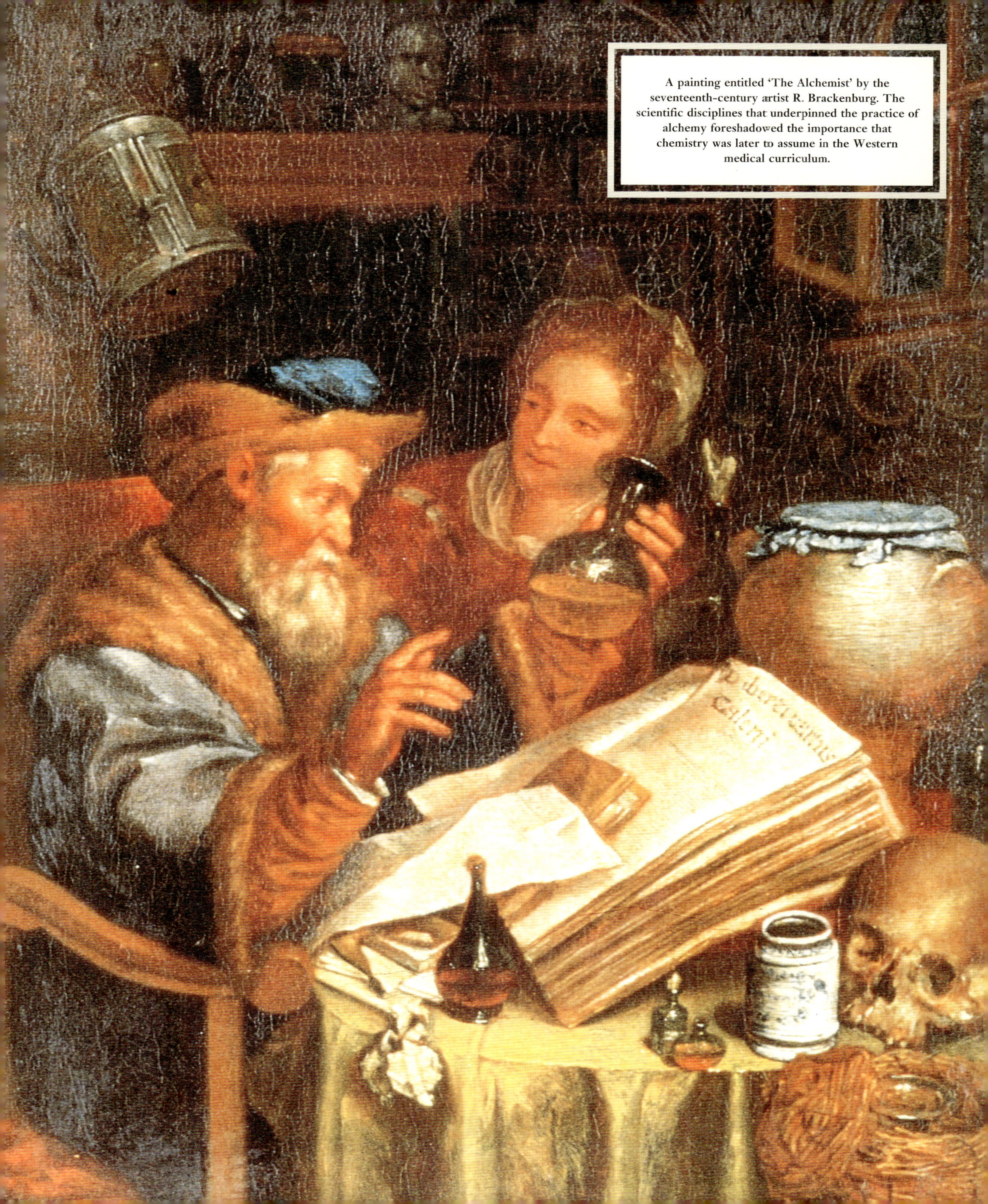

A painting entitled 'The Alchemist' by the seventeenth-century artist R. Brackenburg. The scientific disciplines that underpinned the practice of alchemy foreshadowed the importance that chemistry was later to assume in the Western medical curriculum.

emphasized, 'It is much more important to know what sort of patient has the disease than to know what sort of disease the patient has!' This is not the way most Western medicine is regarded and practised. The emphasis on the 'lesion' (the anatomical abnormality) and the disease has become more conspicuous as investigation and treatment has become more objective and scientific. This depersonalization of the patient is an important reason why so many people are turning to other forms of medicine to seek relief of their symptoms.

This scientific attitude has many advantages and disadvantages. As long as the patient's illness can be successfully accommodated within the boundaries of scientific medicine, it has a good chance of cure or at least alleviation. If it does not, scientific medicine has little to offer and may do harm.

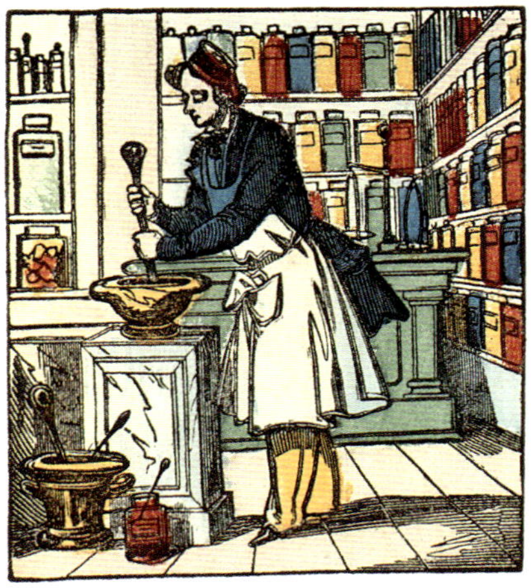

ABOVE **Herbalism is currently enjoying a renaissance in the West as many people are turning to alternative therapies for help.**

Scientific medicine rejects all concepts of 'vitalism', the belief in immaterial spiritual or vital forces to explain natural phenomena. It has no place for 'life forces' or vital principles distinct from physical and chemical processes. In this it differs from other major medical systems, particularly those of the East.

Scientific medicine is a product of the capitalist society it serves. Strongly geared to 'progress', it proclaims and markets spectacular advances in knowledge and practice in specific areas with dramatic 'discoveries' and 'cures'. Sometimes these save people from death or greatly improve the lives of sufferers, but they can also have adverse side-effects that may damage patients.

For instance, the life of anyone who has an abdominal catastrophe, such as acute appendicitis or peritonitis, is more likely to be saved by modern surgery than by any other kind of medicine, and some cases would undoubtedly die without modern surgery. But not every surgical intervention is successful and every operation carries a risk of complications and death.

THE PROS AND CONS OF SURGERY

Responsible surgeons are aware that the history of their subject reveals that many operations, once considered valuable and vital, turned out to be useless or harmful. Another problem relates to the number of operations that are performed on people who are then found not to need them; for instance, those who *might* have acute appendicitis but turn out to have normal appendices. Having undergone an unnecessary operation or having been dismissed as not needing one, patients often find that scientific medicine cannot help them, though they still suffer from the pain.

There are many other examples. Anyone who develops 'heart block' (a failure of the electric circuitry in the heart) is, if untreated, likely to be disabled and in constant danger of sudden death. He or she will gain benefit and probably life from the insertion of a modern cardiac pacemaker, a triumph of medical engineering. But someone whose aberrant heart rhythm reflects anxiety or inner conflict may find no relief from the application of modern science, and may be dismissed with the problem unsolved. What is really troubling them goes undetected, and may manifest itself in other areas of the body.

THE PARADOX OF SCIENTIFIC ADVANCE

Scientific medicine has many means of saving and improving life and these are constantly increasing in number and efficiency. No other system of medicine can perform such feats, but sometimes the treatments are not successful or there are serious obstacles or side-effects. Moreover, those who practise Western medicine find it difficult to accept the fact that, even when the methods they employ are successful in general, they do not always succeed in individual cases.

What are characterized as miracle cures or wonder drugs may save or transform the lives of individuals, but their effect on mortality rates is seldom consistently impressive and there may be long-term side-effects and disadvantages in using them. More lives are saved by improvements in diet, hygiene and living conditions than by one-off miracle drugs.

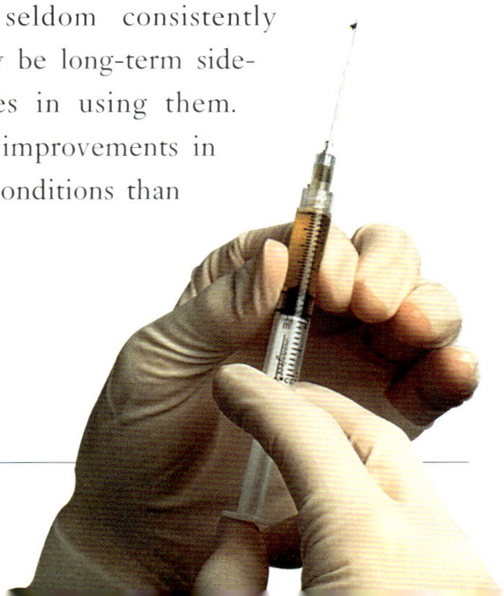

RIGHT **Modern scientific medicine can achieve remarkable results, but there are attendant risks also.**

The advantages and disadvantages of scientific medicine can be clearly seen in the different remedial demands of acute disease and chronic illness. (In medical terms, an *acute* illness is one that begins rapidly, reaches a peak and resolves rapidly. Examples include pneumonia, acute appendicitis and measles and of course medical emergencies such as wounds, fractures, burns and poisoning. A chronic illness comes on slowly, proceeds slowly and resolves slowly, if at all. Examples include osteoarthritis and diabetes (especially diabetes of mature onset). Scientific medicine is, on the whole, more efficient in dealing with acute illness. It is no good telling someone who has had a heart attack or who suffers from an acute abdominal catastrophe that diet, hygiene and living conditions save more lives than scientific medicine.

Many chronic illnesses such as kidney failure, thyroid disorder, pituitary insufficiency, allergy etc., can benefit initially from drugs or surgical intervention, but scientific medicine does not have all the answers. Long-term management of chronic illness needs to address the whole of the patient's life. Nutrition, exercise, family circumstances and financial status are all significant factors and none of these are considered to be in the province of scientific medicine.

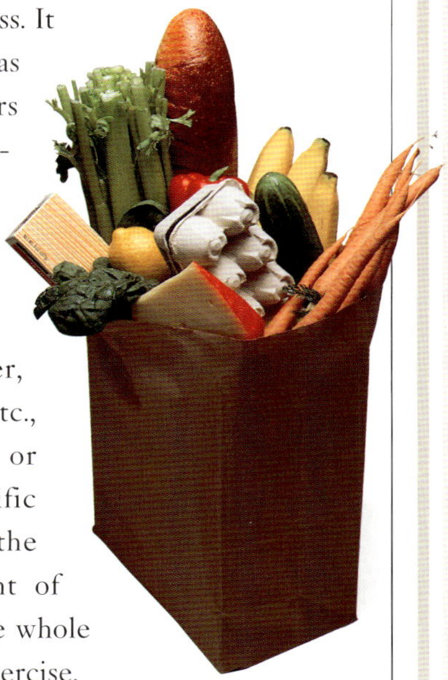

ABOVE 'Prevention is better than cure.' A healthy diet may save as many lives as medical intervention.

THE PROFIT MOTIVE

In capitalist societies medicine is linked with a profit-based pharmaceutical industry. Pharmaceutical companies invest in and develop drugs that are increasingly specific and powerful and save many lives, but they may also extol the benefits of such drugs, often without acknowledging any potentially harmful side-effects. Some doctors go along with this and hand out drugs freely with little indication of potential hazards. Many patients in hospital are there because they have been damaged by 'scientific' treatment. A recent study in a large hospital in the United States found that errors (euphemistically called 'adverse events') occurred in the care of more than 45 per cent of patients. More than one in six of these patients suffered serious consequences, ranging from temporary disability to death.

PREVENTATIVE MEDICINE

An area in which Western medicine has been outstandingly successful is in the prevention of disease, particularly those of an infectious and nutritional nature, and also cancerous and degenerative ones. Sometimes the understanding of the correct treatment is theoretical only, but even when the procedures are not carried out, science has at least shown the way. Outstanding examples of this are vaccines for diseases such as smallpox (now effectively eliminated from the world) poliomyelitis (which could now be eliminated), diphtheria and many others. Other 'triumphs', at least in theory, are the treatments for cholera and tetanus. It is not possible to 'cure' these diseases, but Western medicine has shown how and why they spread and how they could be prevented.

It has also devised ways of keeping sufferers alive until the acute phase of the disease is over. This can be done cheaply in cholera cases through rehydration, and more expensively in tetanus through continuous anaesthesia; similar techniques have recently been devised for meningitis. The discovery of vitamins *(in 1912)* made many deficiency diseases treatable and preventable, often simply and cheaply. These included scurvy, rickets, pellagra, beri-beri, kwashiorkor and many anaemias. Since then an industry in the marketing of vitamins has grown up and many people in the West who have adequate diets are convinced that they require extra vitamins in order to be healthy. The pharmaceutical industry benefits greatly by such beliefs.

Pharmaceutical companies have developed drugs that are capable of effective onslaught on many common and fatal diseases, but regrettably they tend to concentrate on those diseases that are common in rich countries and to ignore those that are common in poor countries where a little 'scientific medicine', applied very cheaply, could save millions of people from lifelong infirmity and death.

Western medicine prides itself on being 'scientific', but is necessarily based on the medical judgment and interventionist skills of the doctor as well as pure 'scientific' evidence. This creates a number of paradoxes. Can personal and clinical 'experience' be 'scientific'? Is the doctor-patient relationship 'scientific' and how does it influence the 'science'? What is the relationship between 'medicine' and 'science' and how has it been influenced by the way in which it developed?

MEDICINE IN THE SIXTEENTH TO NINETEENTH CENTURIES

Western medical science can be conveniently dated from the Scientific Revolution, the transformation of thought *(c.1550–1700)* about nature or the physical world in which the long-standing traditions of the ancient Greeks and Islam were replaced by the findings of modern science. This coincided with the political dominance of Europe in the world and with the advance of capitalism, which was strongly influenced by Protestantism. At first the revolution was most powerfully experienced in mathematics and physical sciences; it emphasized mathematical analysis based on systematic experiments and challenged the idea that man stood at the centre of the universe. At first it retained the idea of a Christian God as Creator and judge; later there was discussion and dispute about this widely-held belief. At least until the mid-nineteenth century the majority of scientists and doctors were believing Christians and they typically used theological arguments alongside their scientific reasoning.

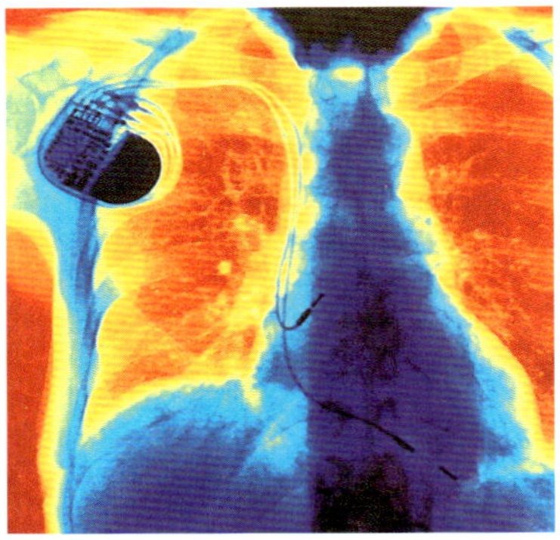

ABOVE Western scientific medicine tends to view the body as a machine. This X-ray of a double chamber heart pacemaker illustrates a mechanical solution to a medical problem.

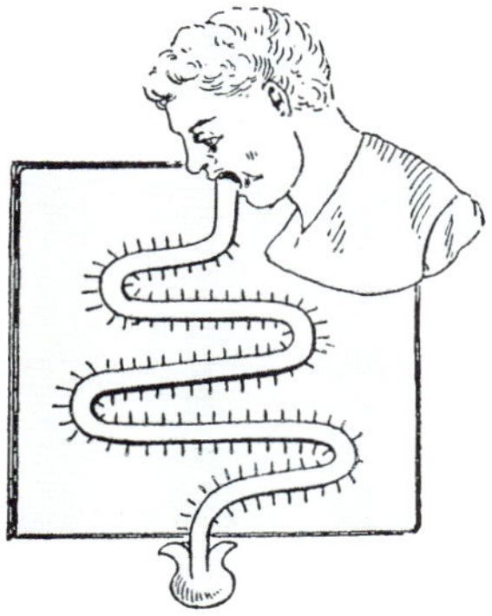

ABOVE Sanctorius *(1561–1636)*, who taught at Padua, was a pioneer of modern physiology. He invented instruments to measure bodily functions, including this early clinical thermometer.

The application of the Scientific Revolution to medicine is usually associated with the British physician William Harvey *(1578–1657)*, who discovered the circulation of the blood, and with the French philosopher René Descartes *(1596–1650)*. Descartes regarded the human body as a machine. Since his time the understanding that there is a division between mind and body – dualism – has been one of the mainstays of Western medicine and to this day is a powerful influence. It is both a strength and a weakness. Unlike most other medical systems, scientific medicine is strongly linked with many inventions, customs and advances that depend on the idea of the body as a machine. Most modern drugs, major surgery, and prostheses (such as artificial limbs and joints, cardiac pacemakers and plastic eye lenses) that have eased and prolonged so many lives have developed as a result of this dualistic hypothesis. It is so strongly embedded in Western culture that its disadvantages tend to be overlooked or ignored. The concept of dualism is also associated with a disregard for symptoms that originate in the mind. Many who believe in it refuse to take psychological factors into account in the diagnosis of illness, and develop an attitude that regards people as merely an aggregation of distinct human parts.

This attitude becomes increasingly pronounced as medicine becomes more divided into specialties and subspecialties. It suits some patients who like to feel that they are in control of their bodies and are content to be relieved of a distressing symptom or to have a painful or damaging part excised or replaced. However, if their disorder is less specific, or is connected with wider aspects of their lives or personalities, the mechanistic approach of Western medicine is rendered unsatisfactory. The tendency of many doctors to concentrate on disease, rather than on the person suffering from that disease, has consequently led many dissatisfied sufferers to seek relief from other complementary therapies, or kinds of medicine.

These new attitudes towards science took several centuries to gain sway over the theory and practice of medicine, which had long been dominated by the doctrine of humours. This held that the Earth is composed of four elements: earth, air, fire, and water, which are reflected in the four major substances of the body: blood, phlegm, yellow bile and black bile. A person's temperament was held to depend on the dominance of one of these humours and illness was due to an imbalance between them. The aim of treatment was to restore the balance.

Doctors who adhered to this doctrine of humours did not have the professional authority enjoyed by later doctors and they were not regarded with the same respect. They were more the patient's equal in knowledge and opinion. Patients had their own theories about how the body worked. Basically there were thought to be two kinds of medical problems: those requiring the immediate evacuation of poisons and those requiring 'tonic' restoration of the body's forces. The patient judged the competence of the doctor and the suitability of the treatment offered. Giving a name to a patient's disorder did not define it in the way it came to do later.

A sick person's condition was thought to follow from a series of errors, many of which were held to be the result of self-neglect. What mattered was not the diagnosis but the symptoms peculiar to the sufferer and the unique disturbance of the humours thought to have produced them. Furthermore, a disease was not regarded as constant; it could turn into another condition. For example, the 'matter' causing pneumonia might shift to produce liver disease, or arthritis could become a disease of the stomach. The physician was expected to maintain the balance of his patron's body, to regulate its fluids, to restore harmony and to keep a balance between the patient's body and the outside world. For this a detailed knowledge of the sufferer's lifestyle was necessary as well as theoretical knowledge of nature's healing powers, of drugs and of physical remedies such as purging and bleeding.

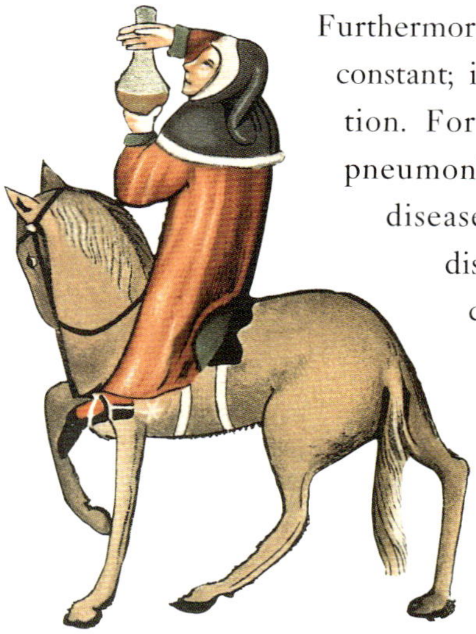

ABOVE Chaucer's Physician practising urine-gazing (uroscopy). Proper chemical analysis of urine did not develop until the eighteenth century.

Taking the history was a lengthy business that was considered essential to the process by which the physician came to know the patient and his or her way of life. Physical examination was much less important than it became later in the history of medical practice. It was conducted mainly visually and was confined to external observation and attention to general appearance, pulse, tongue, and the condition of urine and faeces. There was no such thing as the thorough clinical examination that developed in the nineteenth century, and which was increasingly supported, not to say supplanted, by the laboratory, the X-ray, the CAT scan and other scientific machines and methods.

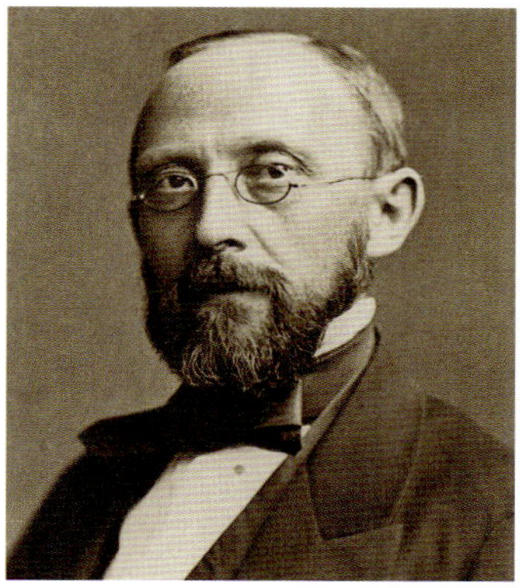

ABOVE The great German pathologist Rudolf Virchow pictured in 1870 when he was in his fiftieth year.

What brought about the change? Medicine reflects its historical and social context and the dominant views and beliefs of the time. The development of Western scientific medicine can be viewed as a result of the Industrial Revolution, an era of change and invention. The change came gradually, prompted by new influences in society and religion. These included the progressive secularization of society, a complicated process. Atheism and agnosticism increased. Some people changed from believing in God to believing in no God. There was increasing comment in the press that was often sceptical or irreligious in nature. Trade and industry developed and increasingly influenced the nature of society. More and more people moved into cities, which grew immensely in size. Life in large cities is naturally quite different from life in the country. Although it also brings its own diseases, and demands different standards of health care, city life makes the development of hospitals possible and can provide the means of studying and understanding disease.

SCIENTIFIC ATTITUDES PREVAIL

The nineteenth century saw the establishment of what we think of as 'scientific' medicine. From about the middle of the century the textbooks and the attitudes they reveal are recognizable as not being very different from modern ones. Before that, medical books were clearly written to address a different mind-set.

Certain doctors began to make systematic attempts to make medicine more comprehensible and more measurable. Examples, among many, include the Frenchman RTH Laënnec *(1781–1826)*, who invented the stethoscope and tried to correlate what he heard in patients' chests with the pathology found at post-mortem. The German Rudolf Virchow *(1821–1902)* worked out a system of medicine based on the cell and insisted that students should always ask, '*Where* is the disease?' His many discoveries and advances included the recognition of leukaemia and descriptions of embolism and thrombosis. Such findings and decriptions were the foundations of modern scientific medicine.

Science and the 'scientific attitude' were developing in parallel with Darwinian ideas about human evolution and such ideas were often seen to conflict with religious teaching. Medicine accordingly became more 'scientific' and sought 'causes' for illness in morbid anatomy and specific diseases, and began to apply statistics to medical situations. Doctors became more involved in illness and death, especially among the middle classes. Death was less associated with sin, divine judgment and hell. People increasingly regarded it as a medical matter, of concern to the doctor, who was increasingly expected to make a diagnosis of the illness based on physical examination, and physical signs, demonstrable pathology, and, preferably, to treat the condition before death occurred. Gradually there was greater expectation of treatment or cure, or at least of alleviation of symptoms and distress, which meant greater participation by the doctor. Doctors' prestige increased along with their social status and the profession recognized the need to be seen as effective.

Traditionally, the medical profession in the West has concentrated on diagnosis and treatment of illness, rather than on the promotion of health and the prevention of disease. In practical terms this was the responsibility of the family doctor, seen as a trusted family friend and helper (to the middle classes). Even though he was not much good at preventing death, he was expected to cope. Knowledge of anatomy and, to a smaller extent, physiology, had increased enormously. Pathology was revealing, and was expected to reveal, why people died, and new laws insisted that the cause of death must be stated. New techniques (such as anaesthesia and radical surgery) brought new dangers – for example, sudden death. Doctors were increasingly expected and obliged to give reasons for what had befallen the patient. For instance, registration of deaths was introduced in England and Wales in 1837.

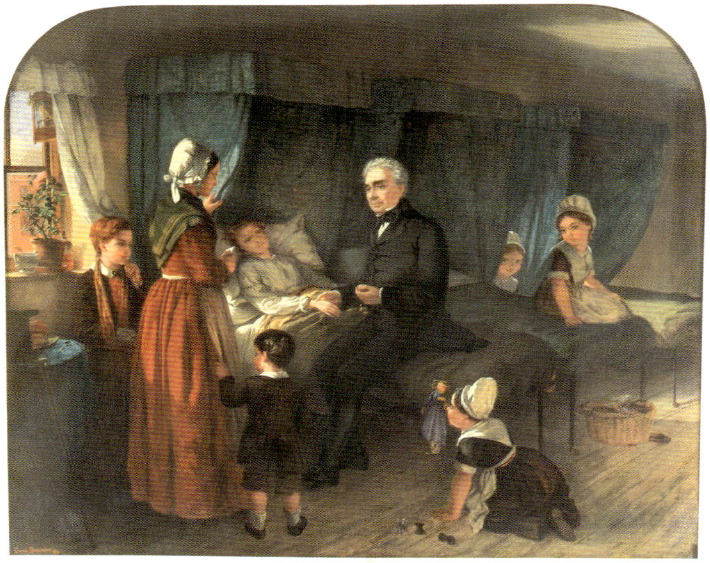

ABOVE 'The Sick Room' painted by Emma Brownlow in 1864. Nineteenth-century doctors favoured well-tried diagnostic techniques like pulse-taking.

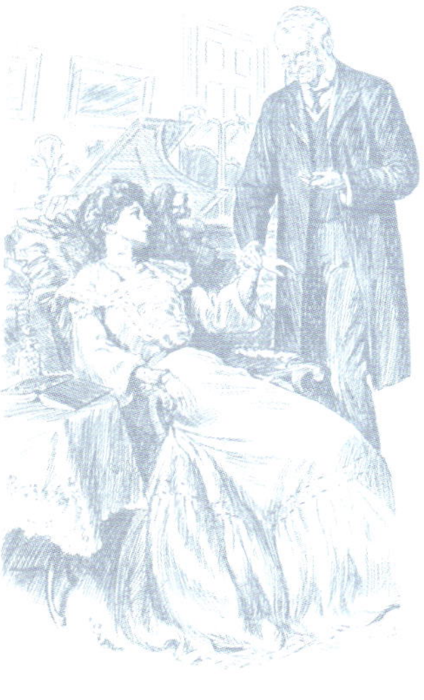

ABOVE The status of the medical profession rose in the nineteenth century. The doctor was part of the established social order.

FOUCAULT'S CLINIC

The French philosopher Michel Foucault *(1929–1984)* thought long and hard about the development of scientific medicine. His book *The Birth of the Clinic. An archaeology of medical perception (1963)* has had considerable influence on medical historians, though many have disagreed with him. He identified what he saw as the mechanisms of power which have developed in Western society since the end of the eighteenth century to explain the development of modern Western medicine. He presented his idea of 'the clinic', by which he meant not only hospitals but also the clinical medicine that developed in them after the late eighteenth century.

Previous medicine had relied largely on the authority of printed books. Part of the process of rejecting the past that was typical of the French Revolution was the rejection of this tradition in favour of direct observation of patients, which Foucault called *le regard,* cleverly translated as 'the gaze'. The gaze is reductionist, analytical and progressively more intense. It develops continuously with new scientific evidence and invention and thereby becomes progressively more penetrating in ever more varied ways. New inventions (such as X-rays, CAT scans, electrocardiographs and methods of genetic analysis) continually reveal new ways of 'seeing', analyzing and judging the human body.

The main features of Foucault's 'clinic' which most influenced the early development of medical science were the establishment of hospitals, clinical examination and the post-mortem examination.

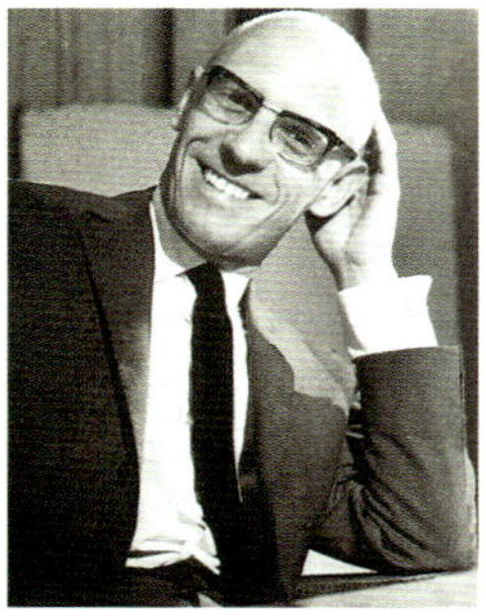

RIGHT French philosopher Michel Foucault, an influential critic of modern scientific medicine.

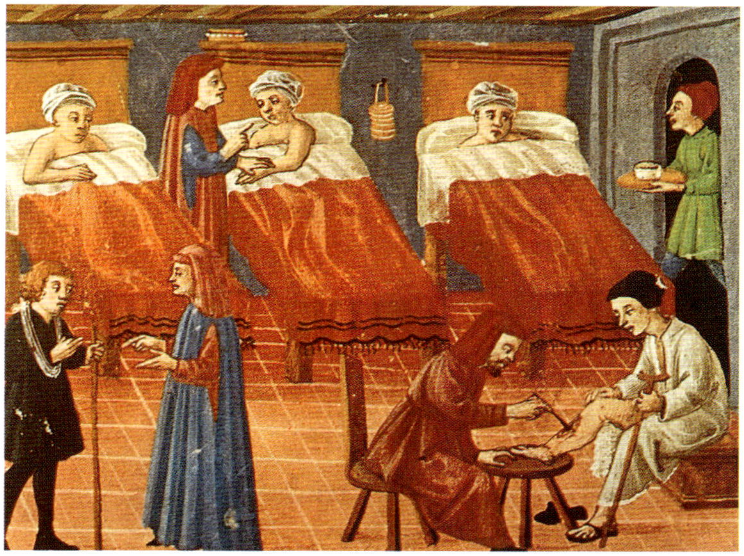

LEFT The medieval hospital was usually a charitable Christian foundation. It provided care and shelter for the sick, but medical treatment was rudimentary.

HOSPITALS

The development of modern hospitals was a fundamental change in caring for the sick that initiated, promoted and supported the development of 'scientific' medicine. The hospital, once a charitable Christian refuge largely for the urban poor, without much medical action or significance, gradually became central to medicine. This hospital movement began in Paris in the eighteenth century. In Britain in the eighteenth century, with the expansion of the middle classes, many general hospitals were established. In the middle of the same century specialist hospitals began to be founded.

The development of modern hospitals was closely bound up with changing ideas of disease. The idea of a hospital that investigated and treated disease rather than simply offering sustenance to the indigent sick developed in Paris after the French Revolution and the political and technological revolution that accompanied it. It acknowledged techniques and concepts unknown in former times. Instead of relying on the authority of books, doctors began to study patients, to analyze differences between them and to delineate separate diseases. Diseases came to be recognized as afflictions that were common to all who suffered from them rather than unique to each individual.

A system developed that was based on observation, physical examination, pathological anatomy, statistics and the concept of the lesion. A lesion is a morbid change (i.e., caused by disease) in the body, which was thought to be the cause of disease and became the object of search in diagnosis. By the middle of the nineteenth century investigations had extended beyond the bedside and living patient, and had moved on to the cadavers in the mortuary and tissue cultures in the laboratory.

When patients died, doctors dissected their bodies for more information and tried to correlate what they found with the symptoms and signs that had been present during life. The delineation of diseases according to lesion rather than as general and humoral phenomena made it possible to locate them in specific places and organs where they could be studied and treated separately.

Hospitals also offered a chance to make statistically viable studies of disease. When many ill people were gathered together, the similarities between certain groups of sufferers became apparent. Doctors began to describe, measure and count these similarities. Their study was based on bedside medicine, which entailed physical examination by hand, eye and ear and, increasingly, with instruments.

In modern times the hospital has gradually changed into a high-tech institution where illness is investigated and treated, accidents and emergencies are dealt with, and invasive (and potentially dangerous) life-saving procedures are carried out under conditions made as safe as possible. It is also the place where doctors, nurses and other professions associated with medicine are trained, where the élite of the medical profession work and where status in the profession is acquired. At the top of the tree in Britain, for example, are the 'teaching hospitals', which are associated with universities and have medical schools attached to them for the training of doctors and other medical staff.

BELOW The role of the hospital changed in the nineteenth and twentieth centuries. Teaching and study became important.

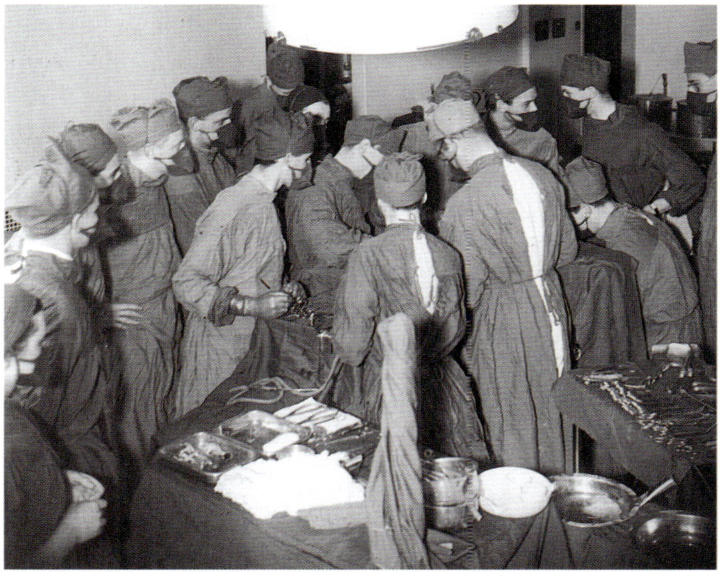

THE RISE OF SPECIALIST HOSPITALS

Hospitals became the institutional basis of professional power, status and prestige. Some doctors who could not gain a foothold in the big hospitals set up their own, often specialist hospitals for eyes, ears, gynaecology and so on. By 1860, London alone had 66 special hospitals. At first these hospitals were criticized and opposed by élite doctors in the big general hospitals, but by the end of the century these doctors were keen to have jobs in them. The status and power of hospitals increased greatly after the introduction of anaesthesia in the late 1840s. It was gradually realized that big surgical operations, like other complicated scientific procedures, were safer when they were carried out in institutions organized for them, and with other skilled people available.

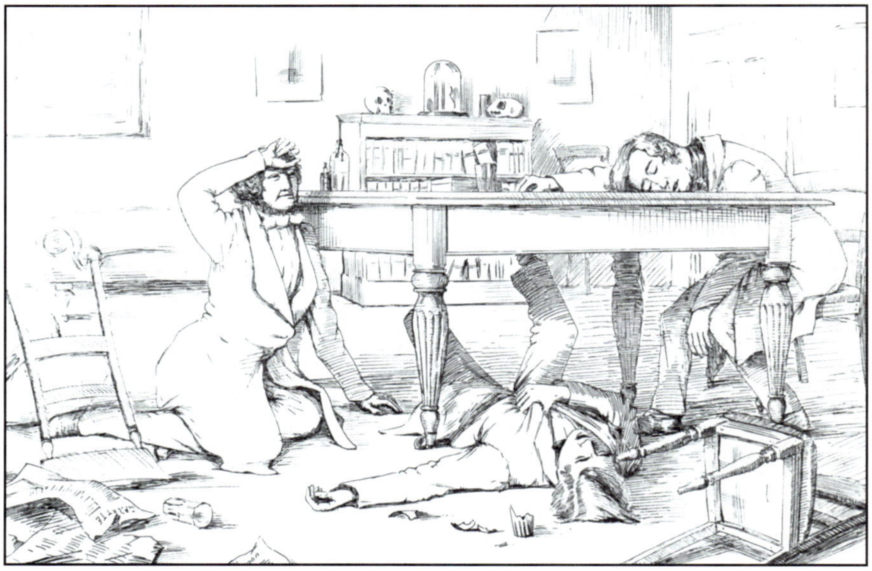

ABOVE In 1847 the obstetrician James Young Simpson and two assistants, James Matthews Duncan and Thomas Keith, experimentally inhaled chloroform to assess its anaesthetic properties. The drawing shows Simpson recovering consciousness.

Medicine practised in an institutional setting has many possibilities not open to those practising in isolation. There are more available patients, who can be grouped and classified. Colleagues with different skills and experience are available for co-operation and discussion.

There were, however, disadvantages, of which the most prominent was infection. Some diseases seemed to arise in the hospitals themselves. These 'hospital diseases' were often fatal and were particularly common in the surgical wards. In the middle of the century they caused enormous anxiety and led to concerted attempts to overcome them. Semmelweis, Pasteur and Lister led the way. Hungarian obstetrician, Ignaz Semmelweiss *(1818–1865)* revealed that puerperal fever, a particularly virulent form of hospital disease, was spread by staff and students who had visited the dissecting rooms before examining their live patients. He did this by close observation in a maternity hospital, comparing wards run by doctors and medical students, who attended post-mortems, with those run by midwives, who did not. Later, Louis Pasteur's work established the existence of germs that caused disease. Joseph Lister *(1827–1912)* introduced antisepsis, which gradually gave way to asepsis (freedom from the presence of micro-organisms), which is still the basis of germ-control in surgery today. Its practice has enabled surgeons to develop and undertake much more complex operations and to perform them much more frequently than hitherto. But infection has remained one of the great dangers of surgery, and sometimes even the most advanced medical units have to be closed because of an outbreak.

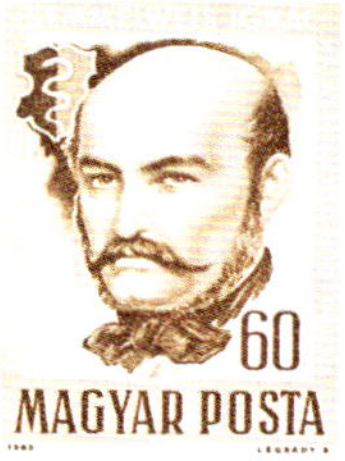

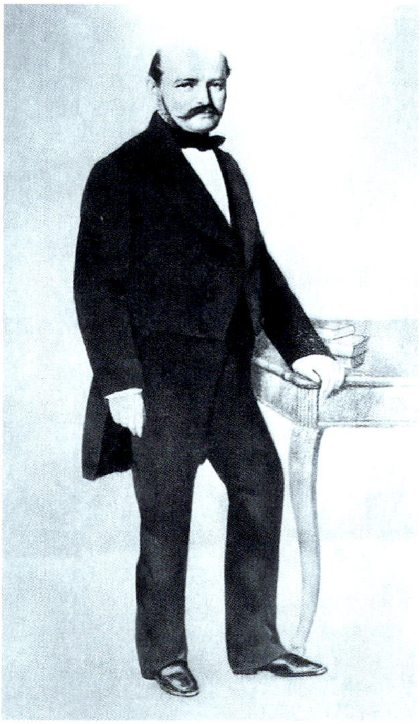

LEFT AND ABOVE Ignaz Semmelweiss' insistence on rigorous standards of hygiene on his hospital wards reduced the mortality rate among his patients dramatically. His views were unacceptable to many of his colleagues and he was forced to leave Vienna. Sustained criticism led to his mental breakdown.

The growth of the hospital movement influenced the fundamental content of medical knowledge. Now interest shifted from the patient who had the disease to the disease itself, and disease could be studied in isolation, with the aid of inventions such as the microscope and special stains for examining slides and clinical instruments. The anatomy of the diseased body became increasingly important, while the person of the patient received less attention. Instead of learning by talking to patients, doctors were increasingly likely to learn by concentrating on their bodies, alive or dead. Much important medical examination now took place in the post-mortem room.

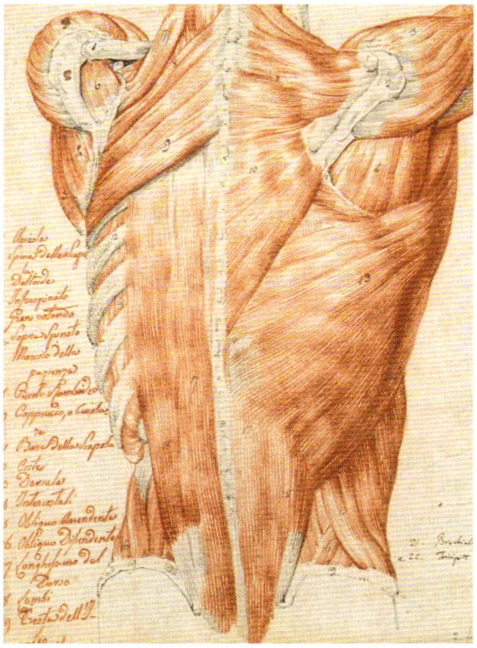

ABOVE As medical science developed, doctors concentrated ever more closely on the anatomy of the diseased body.

POST-MORTEM EXAMINATIONS

The story is complicated. Regular or routine dissection of corpses began in Italy in the thirteenth century, where it was sometimes done as part of a public demonstration undertaken in order to raise the status of medicine, and to establish it as a true body of learning suitable for university study, unlike the manual trade that many thought it to be. During the eighteenth century, dissection became part of the process of medical enquiry and important medical ideas emerged from post-mortem examinations. One such was that disease alters the body in ways that can be seen, described and used as a basis for research. These signs of disease could also help physicians better to understand disease in the living and so to improve their clinical skills. Post-mortem examinations allowed physicians to improve their skills in both diagnosis and prognosis by correlating the results with their patients' previous illness, comparing the lesions they found in death with the symptoms and signs they had observed when the patient was alive.

Examination of the dead body was developed by the Italian pathologist Giovanni Battista Morgagni *(1682–1771)* and was made more available to practising physicians by the work of Scot Matthew Baillie *(1761–1823)*, who published *The Morbid Anatomy of some of the Most Important Parts of the Human Body* in 1793. In 1801 the French physician Marie-François-Xavier Bichat *(1771–1802)* published his *General Anatomy, Applied to Physiology and Medicine,* which introduced the new concept of different types of body tissues (as opposed to body organs) as the basic units of the body. This became one of the foundations of medical science. In his book Bichat emphasized, 'You may take notes for twenty years … and all will be to you only a confusion of symptoms [and] incoherent phenomena. Open a few bodies, this obscurity will soon disappear.'

This theory of the anatomical localization of pathology, together with the correlation of clinical findings with structural changes in the body, was an outlook previously confined to surgeons. As a result the surgeons' approach to disease now became the most important. This became the basis of a new medicine and was enhanced by the development of the skills of clinical examination, by the physicians' increasing use of hands and by the new instruments invented for them.

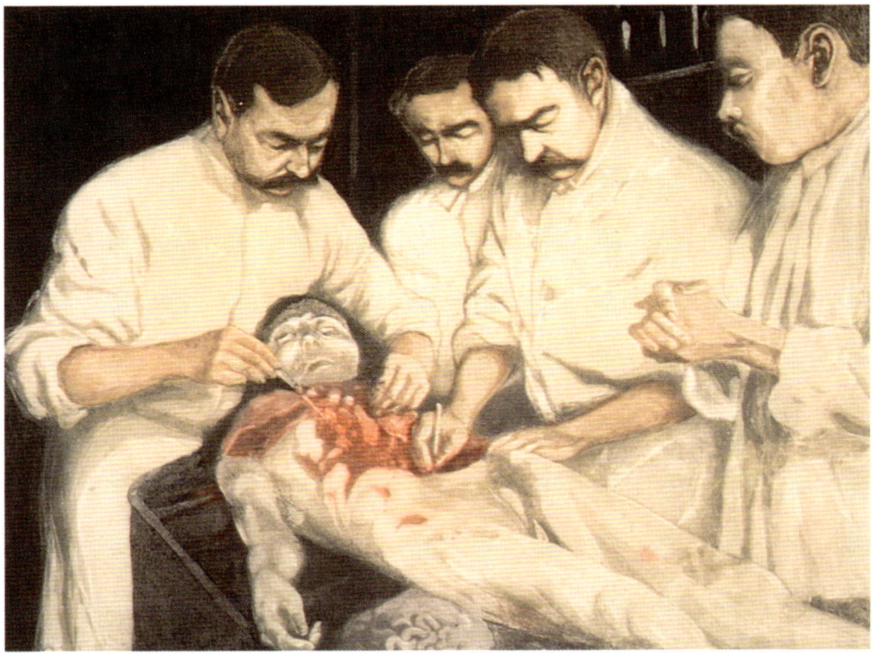

BELOW Post-mortem examinations enabled doctors to compare changes in the structure of the body with a patient's symptoms and signs of illness.

MEDICAL HARDWARE

Western medical science developed on the basis of clinical examination of the patient by the doctor. Previously direct examination had been purely external. From the beginning of the nineteenth century, the 'gaze', to use Foucault's term, began to turn inwards, aided by 'scientific' techniques and inventions.

THE STETHOSCOPE

The first clinical method to develop was the detection of pathology by the use of sound. This was first suggested by the Viennese physician Leopold Auenbrugger *(1722–1809)*. In 1761 he published his *Inventum novum (New invention)*, in which he described a method of examination he called 'percussion', producing sounds indicating the vitality of the internal organs. He believed that his method would revolutionize the diagnosis of chest disease. Like Morgagni, he believed that the key to medicine was the link between structural change and disease. He believed that this should be achieved by objective means, by physical examination of the living patient, but not by talking to him or her.

Auenbrugger's work did not catch on. It remained for a young French physician, René-Théophile-Hyacinthe Laënnec *(1781–1826)*, to change the scene. In 1819 he published *On Mediate Auscultation,* which described pathological lesions found in the chest at autopsy and showed how they correlated with disease detected in living patients. Laënnec developed an instrument that he named a 'stethoscope' to assist him in his examination of patients *(see box)*.

THE INVENTION OF THE STETHOSCOPE

Laënnec, rather than place his ear against the patient's chest, rolled paper into a cylinder as a listening device. He then improved the instrument in wood and named it the stethoscope (from the Greek words for 'chest' and 'to view'). This technique of examination was not excessively difficult to learn, was comfortable to use (as opposed to twisting the body into an awkward position in order to listen directly to the chest) and helped assuage the feelings of indelicacy that were associated with close physical contact between doctor and patient. Doctors rapidly adopted it and regarded it as a form of 'seeing' into the body, an extension of the 'gaze'. Since then almost every doctor has worn a stethoscope around his neck, if not in his ears.

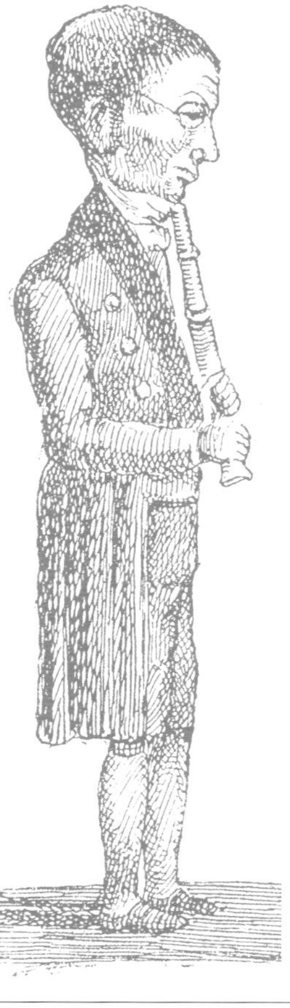

RIGHT Laënnec's first stethoscope was a tubular device with only one earpiece. The familiar binaural stethoscope followed in the 1850s.

EXTENSION OF THE 'GAZE'

The next important scientific invention for clinical examination was the ophthalmoscope. Until the early nineteenth century it was impossible to see into the blackness of the eye. Then the Czech scientist Jan Purkynje *(1787–1869)* discovered how to reflect light into the eye using a source of light and a lens, thus illuminating it. His work had little direct influence, but others then followed in the field, especially the German physician Hermann Helmholtz *(1821–1894)*, who invented an instrument that he called the ophthalmoscope. He published an account of his revolutionary invention in 1851.

The ophthalmoscope rapidly became popular with physicians, who gradually realized that the condition of the eye and what can be seen in it often reflects disease elsewhere in the body.

The next organ to be submitted to the new scientific 'gaze' was the larynx. The Italian Philipp Bozzini *(1773–1809)* made an instrument through which, using a light source and a series of tubes containing mirrors, it was possible to see into the body. The immense theoretical possibilities of this were recognized but not thought to be practical until they were developed further in Vienna. Eventually a Polish professor, Johann Czermak *(1828–1873)* designed the first laryngoscope, which made disorders of the larynx visible, and not simply audible as they had been previously, through hoarseness, cough, noisy breathing and so on.

By now the importance of being able to see into the body was being generally recognized. Sometimes moral considerations intervened – for example there was much understandable hostility

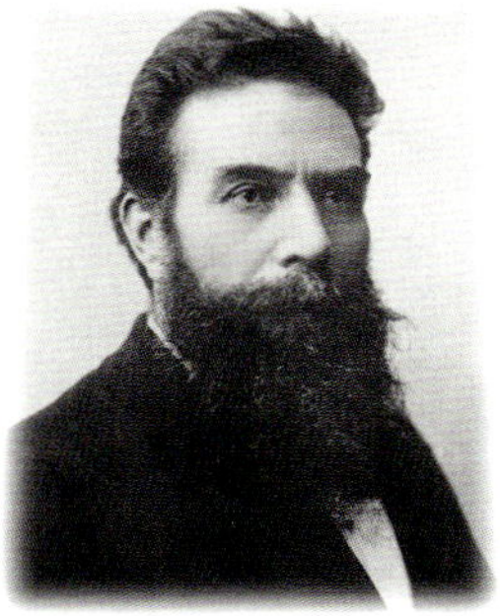

ABOVE Wilhelm Roentgen pictured in 1896, the year after he discovered X-rays.

to the vaginal speculum on the grounds that it offended female delicacy. Sometimes physicians objected to so much use of the eye because they were used to employing other methods.

Designs of instruments improved in the 1870s, when it became possible to have sources of light powered by electricity. In 1881 Thomas Edison invented the carbon-filament lamp, which greatly increased the brightness of artificial illumination. Another visual technique that emerged was photography, which began to be used to provide objective records of patients. This culminated in 1895 with the discovery of X-rays by the German physicist Wilhelm Roentgen *(1845–1923)*. At first this discovery met with little interest and even some ridicule, but the technique soon became popular and ever since X-rays have been one of the most powerful tools in the medical armamentarium. Refinements of the technique soon followed, including the fluoroscope and the use of bismuth to explore the gut on X-ray. During the twentieth century other visual techniques have been developed such as ultrasound, imaging and scanning. These methods are increasingly used in diagnosis, assessment and treatment and the instruments used are increasingly sophisticated and sensitive. For instance, it is now possible to look at every cell in the body and to operate instruments by remote control, often far inside the body, perhaps on a heart or blood vessel or foetus.

BELOW CAT scanning enables radiographers to see an X-ray image of a cross-section of the patient's body or head.

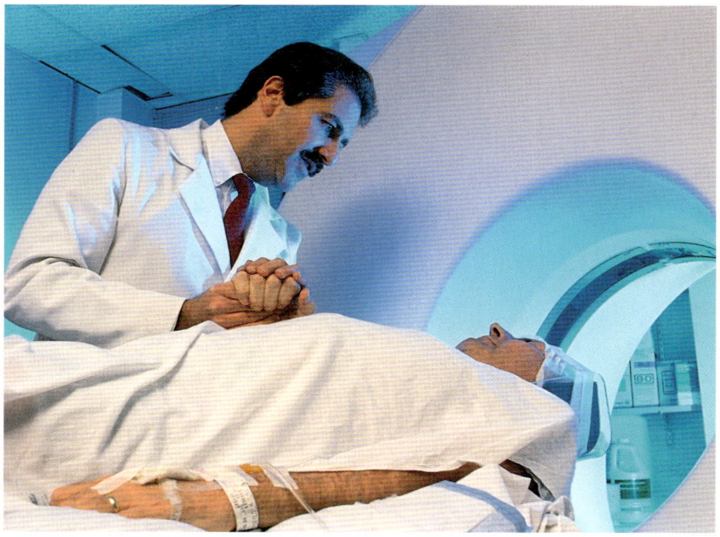

THE MICROSCOPE

The microscope has played an important part in medical science, and still does. Its application developed through several centuries with the improvement of lenses. One of the earliest experimenters with microscopes was the Dutchman Antoni van Leeuwenhoek *(1632–1723)*. In 1681 he discovered that protozoa and bacteria inhabited the human body, but he did not associate them with disease. One of the problems in using the microscope in medicine was that of optical defects caused by imperfections in the lenses, leading to the distortion of images, and spherical and chromatic aberrations. Initially these were so great that no one could be certain of the accuracy of what they saw. However, after the improvements in lenses introduced by the British microscopist Joseph Jackson Lister *(1786–1869*, father of Lord Lister), the microscope was used increasingly to study body fluids and diseases. Blood, urine, pus, phlegm and mother's milk were some of the fluids studied.

In 1843, Guy's Hospital in London established a department of microscopy and doctors began to take a serious interest in alterations in body tissues caused by disease. Gradually the idea developed that examination of post-mortem material with the naked eye alone was no longer sufficient.

Ideas about the basic structure of the human body also changed. The existence of cells had been known since the seventeenth century, but the new microscopes meant that knowledge of them could be greatly extended. In 1839 the German physiologist Theodor Schwann *(1810–1882)* showed that tissues were composed of cells, and in 1858 the German pathologist Rudolf Virchow *(1821–1902)* published his famous book *Cellular Pathology*. He insisted that new cells arose from other cells and not from undifferentiated fluid as had previously been thought. He also demonstrated that health depended on the orderly function of cells and that disease was caused by disruption of cellular function.

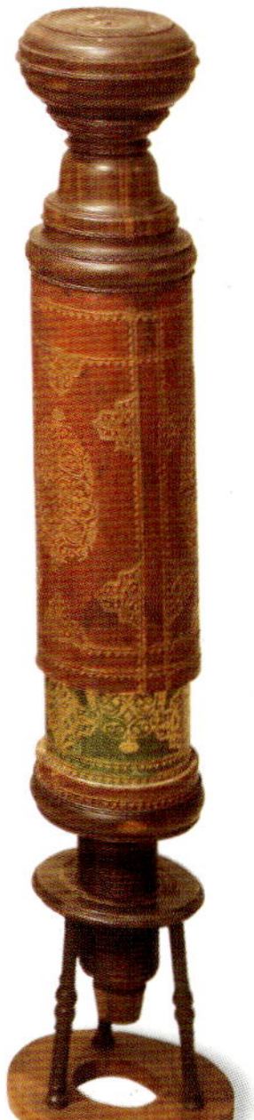

ABOVE Microscopes allowed doctors to study the tissues of the body in great detail. This example dates from the eighteenth century.

The adoption of the microscope as a tool of medicine led to the development of bacteriology (the study of bacteria), which became one of the most important laboratory supports of Western medicine.

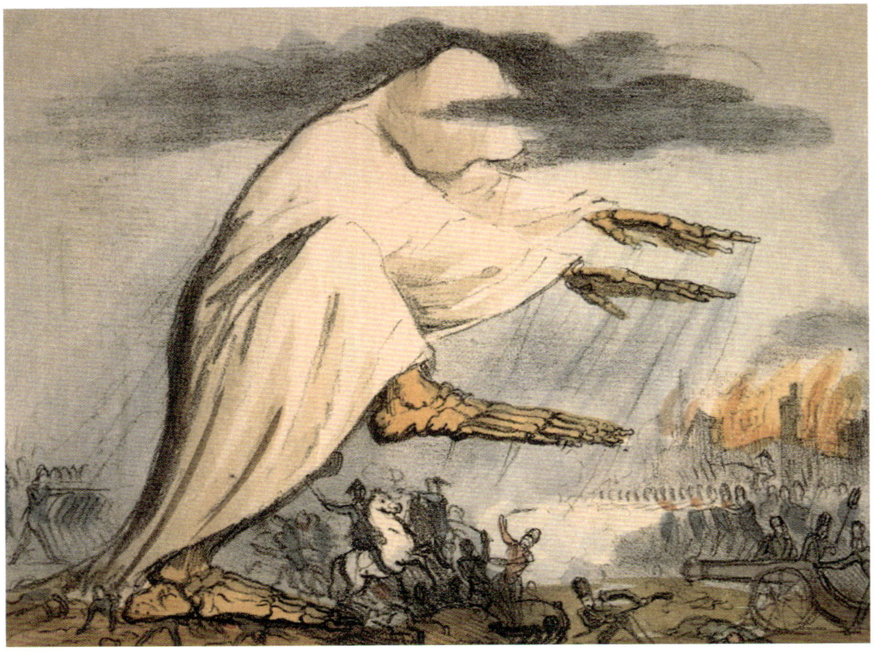

ABOVE A nineteenth-century cartoon depicting the inexorable advance of cholera. Robert Koch identified the bacillus responsible for the disease in 1883.

In 1840 the German pathologist Jakob Henle *(1809–1885)* published his essay 'On miasmata and contagia', in which he tried to show that tiny living creatures in the human body caused infectious diseases. The idea of 'germs' began to challenge the prevailing theory that diseases were caused by 'miasmata', or poisons in the atmosphere emanating from cesspits and rotting material. The two theories were prominent and the discussion about them was lively and contentious until the 1860s and the work of Frenchman Louis Pasteur *(1822–1895)* and British surgeon Joseph Lister *(1827–1912)* became known. Pasteur showed that putrefaction of organic matter did not occur in the absence of micro-organisms. Lister, worried by the appalling mortality rates from compound fractures (in which the broken bone penetrates the skin), devised methods of destroying bacteria in wounds during surgery. His method, a carbolic spray, was known as antisepsis. A few years later it was superseded by asepsis, which attempts to keep infection out altogether. This has been practised with increasing refinement ever since.

The German physician Robert Koch *(1843–1910)* took bacteriology further with his work first on anthrax, then on tuberculosis. He developed complex microscopical and chemical techniques and advanced the important sciences of culturing bacteria and staining microscope slides for examination. In 1882 he announced his finding of the tubercle bacillus. Bacteriology developed rapidly after Koch. During the 21 years between 1879 and 1900 the specific organisms of at least 21 serious diseases were discovered. These included gonorrhoea, typhoid, erysipelas, cholera, diphtheria, tetanus, pneumonia, meningitis, plague, syphilis and whooping-cough.

Ever since that time medical students have been taught the importance of Koch's postulates. It was long held that if they could not be demonstrated, the source of the illness could not be determined. However, it is impossible to adhere to these rules in the case of many diseases and the criteria are not now so strict.

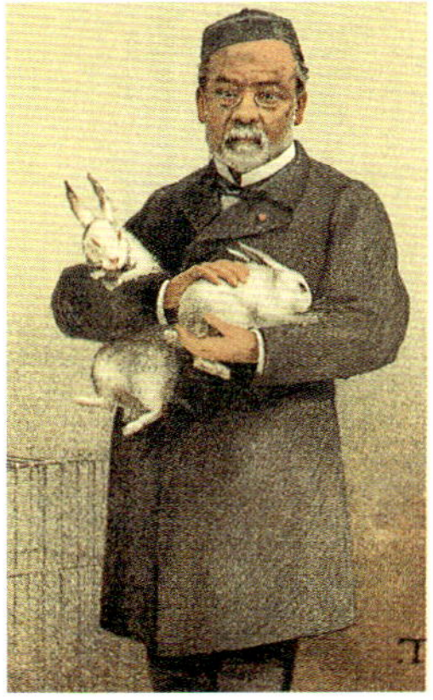

ABOVE Louis Pasteur dismissed the 'miasmatic' theory of disease. He argued that diseases were caused by germs and so effectively established bacteriology as a science.

KOCH'S POSTULATES

Robert Koch developed his ideas in what became known as 'Koch's postulates', which have been taught to medical students ever since. These were that the organism must be present constantly in diseased parts; that it must be able to be cultivated outside the body; and that it must be produced in a susceptible animal which had been inoculated with the cultivated micro-organism.

Koch's postulates are still valuable, especially as ideals, but many diseases do not conform to them, so they are no longer considered the essential basis of diagnosis that they once were.

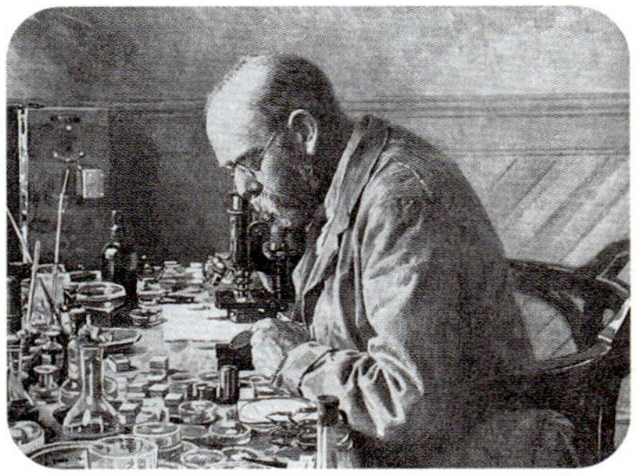

RIGHT Robert Koch's 1879 paper on 'The aetiology of traumatic infectious disease' established that bacteria were the cause, not the consequence, of infections.

MEASURING BODY FUNCTIONS

The basic sciences on which modern Western medicine is founded developed essentially during the first half of the nineteenth century. Microscopic anatomy or histology, physiology, pathology and pharmacy all progressed rapidly during this period and gradually came to be applied to medicine. During the eighteenth century and earlier, scientists had usually been either practising physicians or amateurs, often working in their own homes. Now there developed a new sort of scientist, full-time and professional, who worked in the field of medicine but did so in laboratories rather than at the patient's bedside.

The movement began in Germany, where the reformed universities provided a suitable environment for it. German universities were more important in the history of medicine at this period than were universities in the Anglo-Saxon world, where medicine was more individual and pragmatic. Germany was also more attuned to research and was less troubled by anti-vivisection and anti-dissection feelings or grave-robbing scandals, such as plagued Great Britain. Thus Germany came to lead the world in medicine in the second half of the nineteenth century.

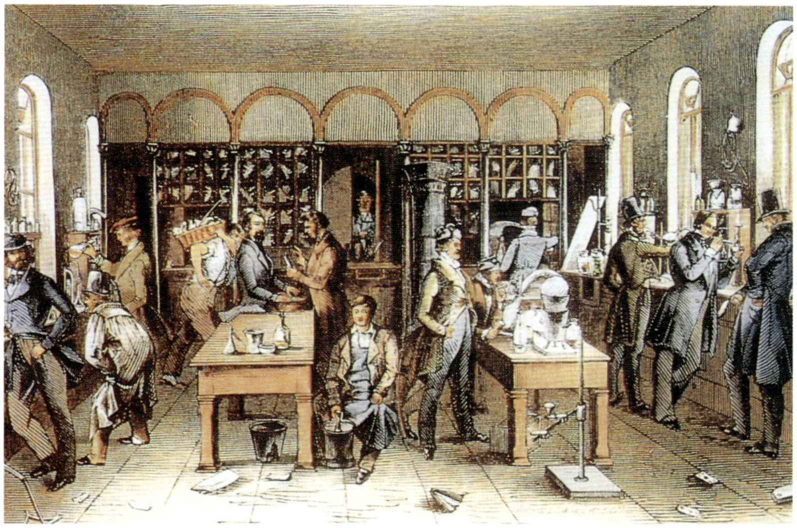

ABOVE German universities led the world in medical research in the nineteenth century. This engraving shows the chemist Justus von Liebig and colleagues in the Institute of Chemistry at the University of Giessen.

The development of the basic sciences had a profound influence on Western medicine. There was now an unprecedented corpus of knowledge concerning the structure and functions of the human body. Pathological signs could now be correlated with changes of structure. Deviations from the normal could be measured and assessed in a way that was previously impossible. New methods of treatment could be devised and predicted.

To the idea that illness was due to defects in body architecture was added the idea that measurements in relation to illness should be of changes in body *function,* such as temperature, breathing, heart beat and blood circulation. Unless changes in these functions were of very long standing in the patient, they did not change the structure of the body and so did not show at post-mortem dissection. This new study of function was the beginning of the medical science of physiology.

Instruments began to appear that could portray functions by measuring them numerically or transcribing them onto graphs, often on rotating drums covered with smoked paper and marked by an indicator arm. This transformed subjective monitoring of body function (such as of the nature of muscle contraction and the nature of the pulse) into objective data that could be seen by all. It became possible to construct many of the body functions as objective transcriptions that could be recorded, analysed and compared with those of the past or future.

The spirometer, which measured various aspects of breathing, began to rival the stethoscope. The sphygmomanometer measured blood pressure against a column of mercury and the sphygmograph recorded movements of the pulse onto paper and converted them into graph form. By the end of the nineteenth century there were machines that tracked the path of the electric currents of the heart. This developed into the electrocardiogram or ECG as a result of the work of the Dutch physiologist Willem Einthoven *(1860-1927)* in the early twentieth century, and this method of recording the cardiac cycle has subsequently became an essential part of the examination of the heart that is still used today.

Thus physiological functions were made 'scientific' and brought under the all-embracing 'gaze'. Medical diagnosis of patients' illnesses, along with methods of monitoring a patient's progress, became increasingly mechanical.

THE INVENTION OF THE THERMOMETER

One of the best known medical instruments is the thermometer. Attempts had been made to construct one for several centuries and one such had been invented by Galileo late in the sixteenth century, though he had not applied it to disease. There had been many technical hitches in developing it, but from the 1840s onwards the interest of physicians in such an instrument was roused. In 1868 the German physician Carl Wunderlich *(1815–1877)* published *On the Temperature in Disease* and thereby brought thermometry into prominence in medical diagnosis. Wunderlich was certainly the founder of modern clinical thermometry. He showed that the temperature of a healthy human being was constant apart from small diurnal swings, and that certain variations in temperature were characteristic of certain diseases.

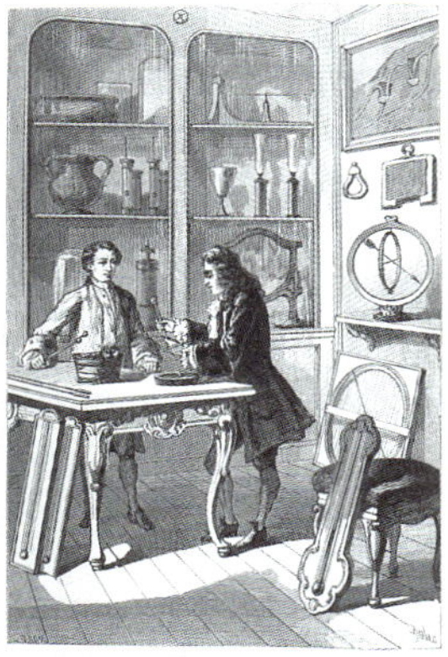

ABOVE **The French scientist Réné-Antoine Reaumur who devised a thermometric scale which made the boiling point of water 80° Reaumur.**

The early thermometers were difficult to use at the bedside because they were nearly a foot (30cm) long and took up to half an hour to register. According to Lauder Brunton, an English physician, doctors carried them under the arm 'as one might carry a gun'. Not long after Wunderlich wrote on the subject *(1868)*, the distinguished English physician from Leeds, Sir Clifford Allbutt, worked on reducing their size. The pocket thermometer was used in America during the Civil War, some time before it became customary to use them in Britain.

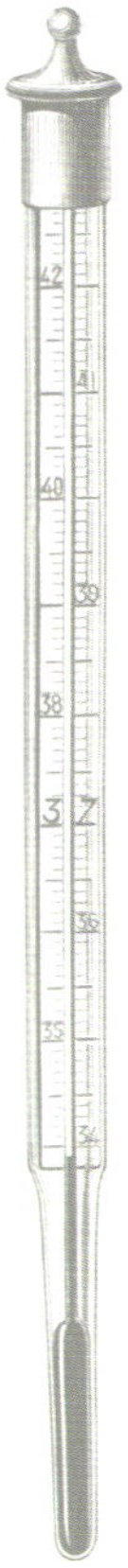

RIGHT **The short clinical thermometer was devised by Sir Clifford Allbutt in the 1860s.**

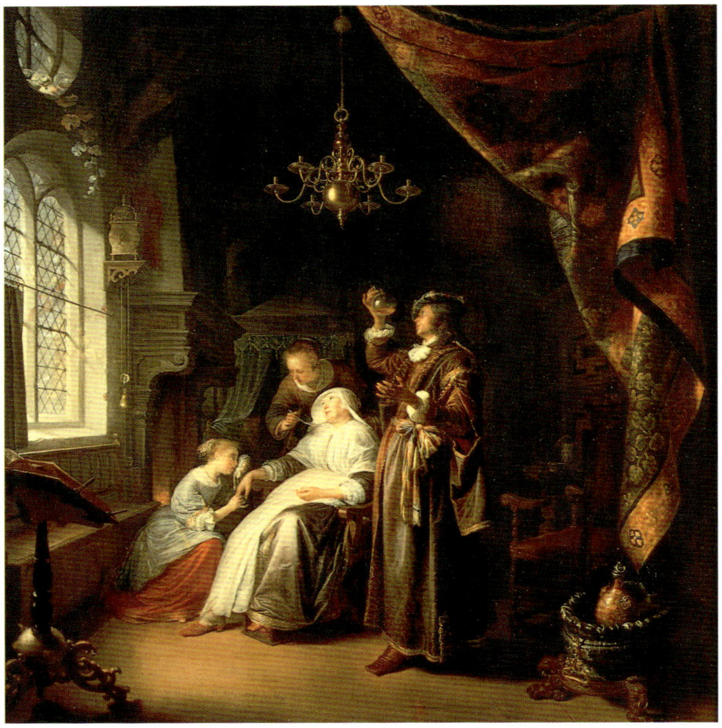

ABOVE **'The Dropsical Woman' by the Dutch painter Gerrit Dou *(1613–1675)*. In 1827 Richard Bright showed that dropsy was often associated with protein in the urine.**

LABORATORY MEDICINE

Many physicians were unsatisfied with correlating disease with structural changes in the body at post-mortem because such correlations could often not be found. Another line of thought developed. In 1848 a new medicine, called 'laboratory medicine', made its appearance in Paris under the leadership of Louis Pasteur (who was a chemist rather than a doctor), Claude Bernard *(1813–1878)* and the Société de Biologie. The various factions of the preceding half century had all been devoted to pathological anatomy, but laboratory medicine was different.

Chemistry had been used in medical diagnosis since the sixteenth century, a time when physicians attached great importance to visual examination of the urine. The Swiss doctor Paracelsus *(1493–1541)* recommended chemical analysis rather than mere visual inspection. During the eighteenth century, various chemical properties of urine in disease were discovered, especially in diabetes, but few physicians took a serious interest until Richard Bright *(1789–1858)*, in his *Reports of Medical Cases,* showed that 'dropsy', a common disease with accumulation of fluid in the tissues, was often accompanied by shrivelled kidneys and large amounts of albumin in the urine. From then on the use of chemistry to evaluate disease increased, though not without some opposition from doctors who believed that little could be gained from such examination because it was removed from the realities of health and disease. Other tests were devised for finding abnormal chemicals in the blood: protein, sugar, bacteria, products of infection and so on. Some of the tests could be done at the bedside, albeit often with cumbersome equipment, while others required a fully-equipped laboratory.

At the same time the microscope was being used to examine the blood and its cells. In 1877 William Gowers *(1845–1915)*, in his 'On the Numeration of the Blood-Corpuscles', showed how examination with the microscope could make certain tentative and difficult diagnoses certain. This was of enormous help to doctors, particularly in the everyday diagnosis of anaemia, which had hitherto been largely a question of guesswork. In anaemia the haemoglobin (red matter) in the blood is reduced, often because the red blood cells, which carry the haemoglobin, are themselves reduced or otherwise abnormal. This was a common condition in young women – probably partly because of their monthly loss of blood through menstruation. But hysteria was also common in young women. This was, roughly, the production of physical symptoms without physical disease, with the 'conversion' of psychiatric symptoms into physical manifestations, which were often similar to those of anaemia. Without adequate blood tests it was often difficult or impossible to distinguish between these two states.

TRANSATLANTIC DEVELOPMENTS

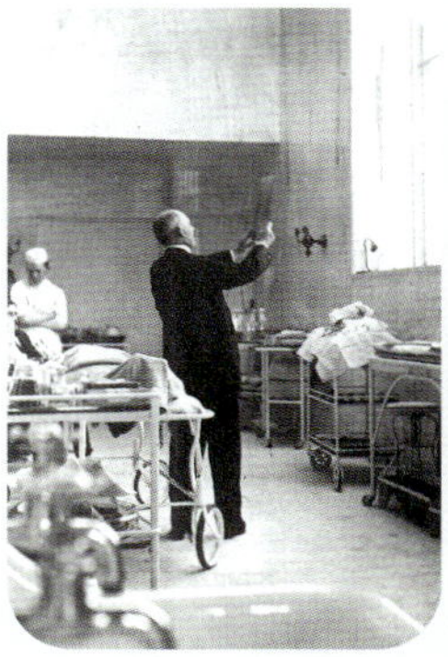

ABOVE William Halsted examining an X-ray at The Johns Hopkins Hospital where he was professor of surgery.

The German model of medical science, closely linking universities and hospitals, was copied in Johns Hopkins University, in Baltimore in the United States, which became and has remained a leader in the field. The American surgeon William Stewart Halsted *(1852–1922)*, who had studied in Germany, began to perform radical surgery there, which had a considerable influence on his colleagues and on the direction that medicine would take in the US. In Great Britain, on the other hand, medicine tended to remain less 'scientific' and was conducted more at the bedside, relying on 'clinical' experience and judgment rather than on 'scientific' tests and assessments. This was thought to be more agreeable for patients and the British boast was that 'On the Continent and in America they have the best science: in Britain, we have the best practice.'

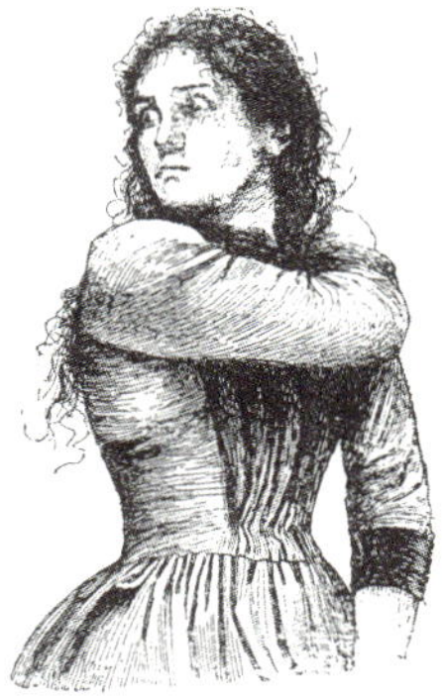

ABOVE In the nineteenth century hysteria was a common diagnosis to account for a wide range of female afflictions.

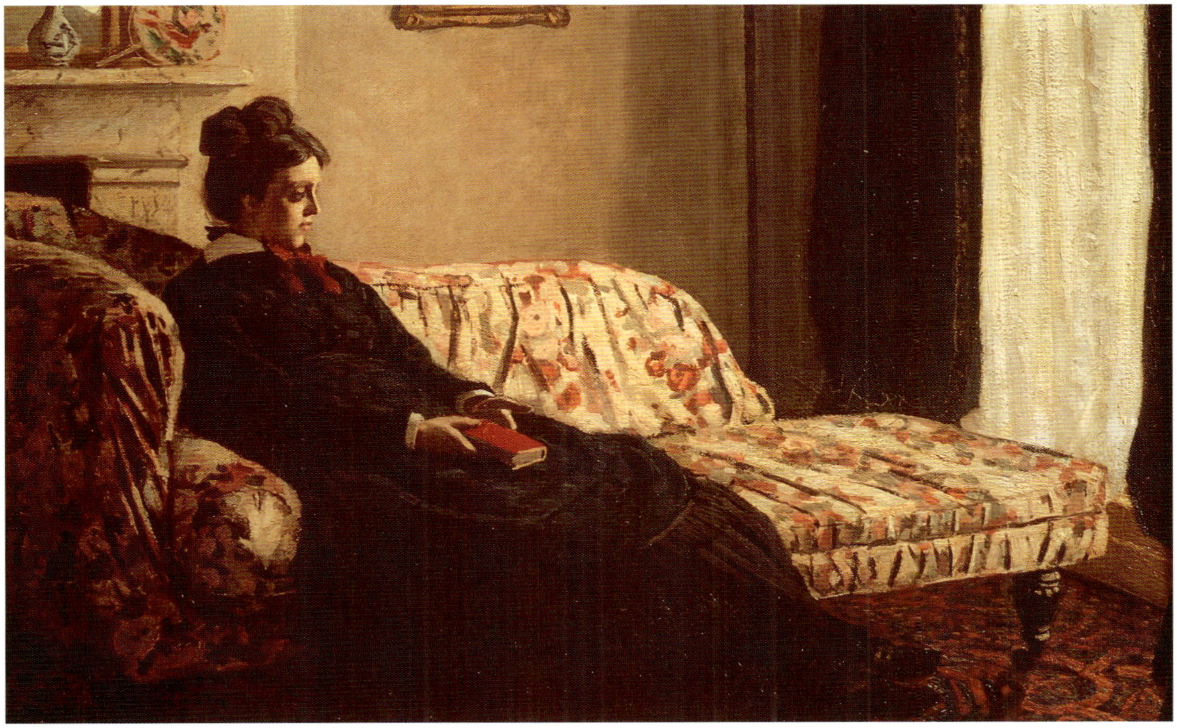

RIGHT Edouard Manet's pale subject (Mme Manet) may have been anaemic. Sir William Gowers' work in the 1870s enabled doctors to diagnose the illness with much greater precision.

These techniques were supplemented by other medical innovations, such as the alternative counting technique which utilized centrifugal force to pack the cells together, which then allowed clinicians to measure accurately the quantity of haemoglobin in the cells.

The discovery of bacteria as causal in disease led to the establishment of publicly-funded laboratories to identify widespread and epidemic infectious disease. Gradually there grew up a profession of those adept at laboratory techniques and doctors began to specialize in various forms of pathology, including bacteriology, chemical pathology and haematology. The work of these doctors was largely divorced from patients, and they spent most of their time working in laboratories.

SPECIALIZATION: AN INEVITABLE DEVELOPMENT

The development of specialists in the medical profession was slow and was initially tainted by association with quacks such as bonesetters and cataract-extractors. For this reason it was despised by the grand physicians and experienced as threatening by the burgeoning general practitioners. Originally, the early medical specialties, e.g., urology, ophthalmology and obstetrics, were not part of medicine at all, but were the province of lay practitioners and itinerant quacks. From the late eighteenth century onwards these fields were encroached on by upwardly mobile individuals who were in some important respects marginal to the medical profession. At the turn of the century *(6 January 1900)*, the British medical journal *The General Practitioner* observed of specialists, 'Their minds are narrowed, judgment biased and unbalanced by disproportionate knowledge of one subject.' In the end, it concluded, the patient would suffer, for unlike the patient's family doctor, the specialist 'knows nothing of the constitutional idiosyncrasies of the individual, which are essential to correct diagnosis and treatment.' This was a typical opinion of the medical profession.

Nevertheless, specialism developed inevitably as medical knowledge and medical science advanced beyond the scope of any individual. The first specialties were ophthalmology and gynaecology. The first specialist hospitals began to appear late in the eighteenth century. Between 1800 and 1890, 88 specialist hospitals were founded in London, 22 of them in the 1860s. They sustained hostility initially, even from within their own ranks. Even distinguished specialists, such as the paediatrician Abraham Jacobi *(1830–1919)*, complained that specialization tended to degrade the general practitioner, but these specialist hospitals, essentially a product of the development of medical science, were mostly set up by medical men who could not gain entry into the élite corps of physicians that formed the medical establishment. The trend for specialization has continued to the present day.

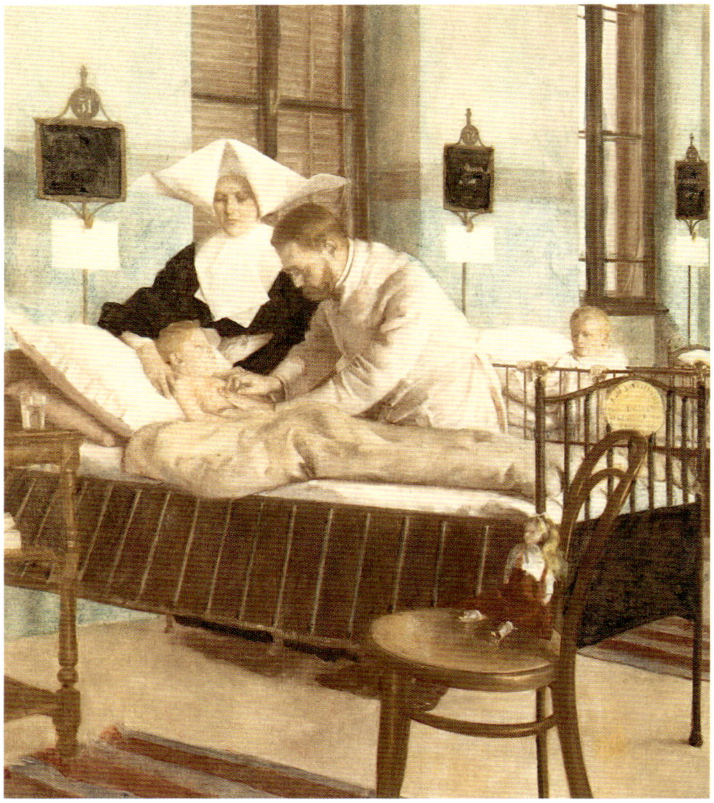

ABOVE A child is examined in a German hospital in 1892. The development of medical specialties was a significant feature of the nineteenth century, and the provision of specialist paediatric hospitals was well established in Europe by the middle of the century.

MEDICAL SOCIETIES AND JOURNALS.

The growth and development of medical science stimulated the establishment of publications dedicated to spreading information about new techniques and discoveries. So the nineteenth century was a period of proliferation of medical journals of all types. This trend has continued to the present time. New journals are constantly being founded as one specialty or subspecialty breaks away from its parent subject.

MEDICINE AND THE SOCIALLY DISADVANTAGED

The way in which medicine justifies social inequalities, such as those of social class, race and sex, shows how much it reflects the beliefs and prejudices of the day. For instance, today a single mother living in poor circumstances is likely to be diagnosed as suffering from depression, whereas the successful executive overworking in a bank or law firm is said to be suffering from 'stress'. Much nineteenth-century literature attempted to demonstrate the inferiority of non-white races. Negritude was sometimes regarded as a disease in itself, and was often identified as a source of disease on 'scientific' grounds. An example of this was *drapetomania,* a so-called disease which consisted of the strong desire of a slave to be free. There was much measuring of skulls, often of only a few selected specimens, to demonstrate that blacks and women had smaller skulls and so were inferior to white males. Another was the idea of Benjamin Rush *(1745-1813)* in 1792 that all negroes suffered from a mild form of congenital leprosy whose only symptom was blackness. Such ideas reinforced the *status quo* of society and enhanced the status of the medical profession. They were also part of the process of 'medicalization', in which medical theory and the medical profession gradually took over aspects of life in which they had hitherto played no part. Until this time, skin colour had never before been regarded as a medical matter.

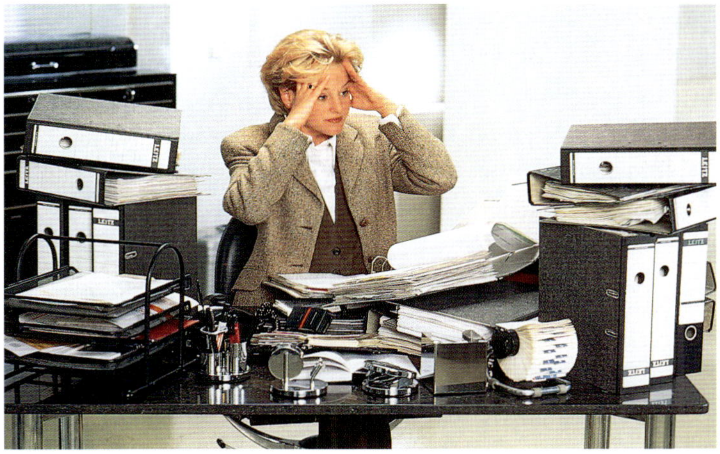

ABOVE Executive stress has become a commonplace diagnosis of the 1990s. 'Ordinary' people exhibiting the same symptoms may be diagnosed as depressed. Medicine thus reinforces stereotypes.

Commoner than the 'diseases' of blacks were those of women. As the power of religion declined and medicine became more authoritative and powerful, medical ideas came to embody, both explicitly and implicitly, current social ideas about women. These included ideas about their nature, role in society, abilities and limitations. Doctors thus gradually assumed a politicized role; they supported the established order and justified the control of women through medical authority. At the time middle-class women were regarded as pure, indolent and sickly. Working-class women were regarded as polluting and a potential hazard from infection. Much of the medical literature concerned middle-class women, who had the time and means to visit and support doctors. Popular literature also concerned the subject of female health but it revealed little, for doctors disapproved of popular health. Scientific medicine was essentially viewed as the preserve of the medical profession, with the patient simply adopting the role of passive recipient.

Medical 'scientific' theory stated first that women were ill because they were women, and second that they became ill if they tried to do anything beyond their conventional female roles, a Catch-22 situation. The 'illness' almost always related to the woman's reproductive system which, it was thought, limited their activities and ensured the need for the constant attendance of a medical practitioner. It was by its very nature pathological.

Puberty was viewed as a period of stress and crisis. Girls were to be treated as invalids during this period. Menstruation was also considered to be pathological. In 1862 Dr Edward Tilt, a London obstetrician, claimed in the British medical journal *The Lancet* that 'for thirty years the [uterus and ovaries] are thrown into a state of haemorrhagic and other orgasm every month.'

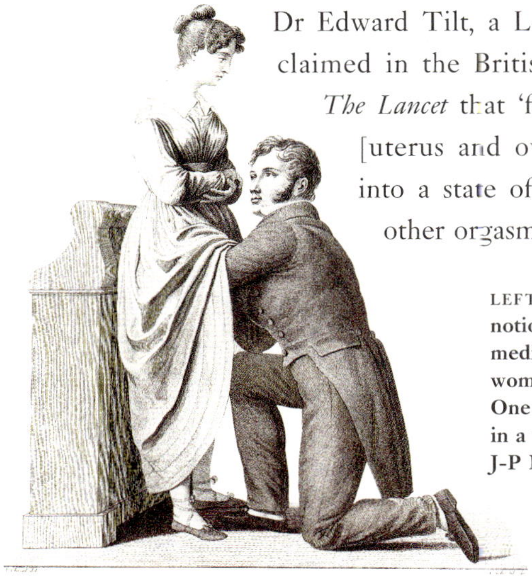

LEFT Nineteenth-century notions of decorum made medical examination of a woman's genitals a problem. One solution was illustrated in a textbook produced by J-P Maygrier in 1822.

Pregnancy was also regarded as an illness and was even thought to be a form of epilepsy. The expectant mother was treated as if she were sick and advised that she needed to stay in bed as much as possible during pregnancy. Care of the mother was moved away from traditional women midwives to become the preserve of male medical practitioners.

The menopause was also seen as pathological (i.e., a state that caused disease), in which 'the nervous force, no longer finding useful function, goes astray in every direction'. It was thought that the natural female physical functions of ovulation, gestation, labour, lactation and the menopause in turn dominated the entire organism of woman.

The process by which normal, biological or social human functions and variations were taken over by the medical profession as 'diseases' is called 'medicalization' *(see box)*.

BELOW In the past women have suffered from the effects of 'medicalization', whereby normal physical processes, such as childbirth or the menopause, have been categorized and treated as illnesses by the predominantly male medical profession.

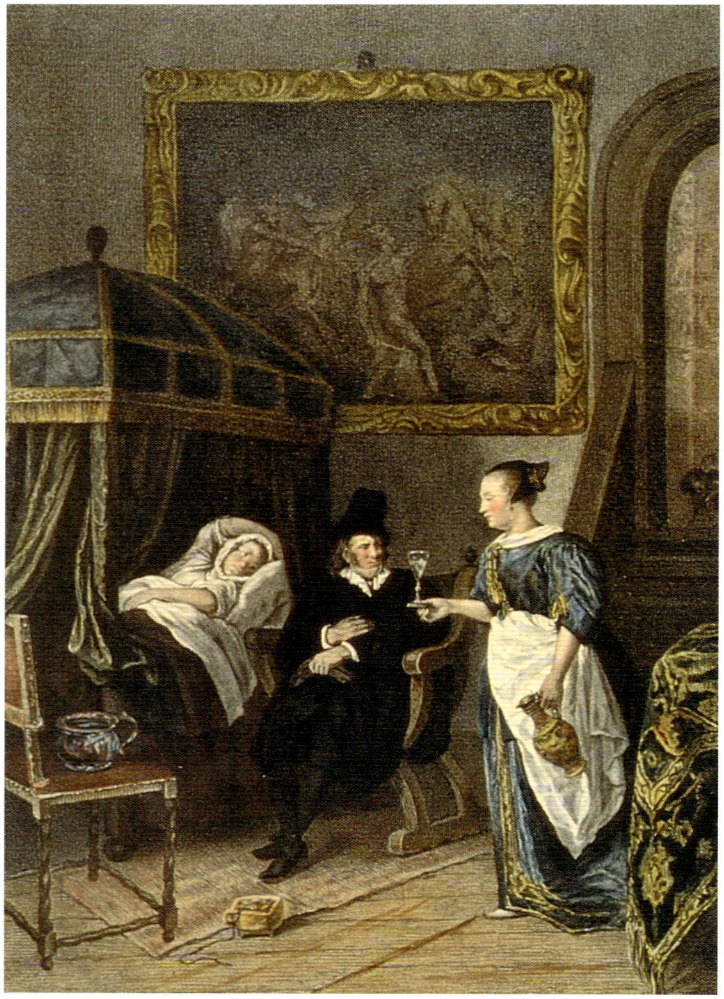

MEDICALIZATION

Western medical science was so successful and popular that it had little difficulty in extending its power to many aspects of daily life not previously regarded as its preserve. Variations in behaviour came to be regarded as 'diseases', to be treated by 'scientific' medicine. More and more areas of life accordingly became subject to medical definition and jurisdiction. During the process, problems were seen increasingly in medical terms and were defined in this way. New 'diseases' were discovered, constructed or invented by the medical profession. Medical treatments were advocated as solutions to those problems.

Anything labelled as an 'illness' or a 'disease' was deemed to require 'scientific' medical treatment. These included homosexuality, alcoholism, drug use, shoplifting, criminal tendencies, variations in sleep patterns, and some matters previously regarded as spiritual and religious, the province of the priest. Some of these new diseases exactly fitted common beliefs. For instance, the late nineteenth-century obsession with constipation was reflected in the disease labelled 'autointoxication', in which, it was believed, the contents of the large bowel poisoned the body. As a result, much attention was paid to laxatives and purgatives and, when surgery of the abdomen became possible towards the end of the century (with reliable anaesthetics and antisepsis or asepsis), operations to remove the colon became fashionable in both England and America.

More recent additions which have been similarly redefined by this process include, among many, contraception and fertility, normal pregnancy and childbirth, and conditions called 'multiple personality', 'post-traumatic stress disorder', 'attention deficit disorder' and 'false memory syndrome'.

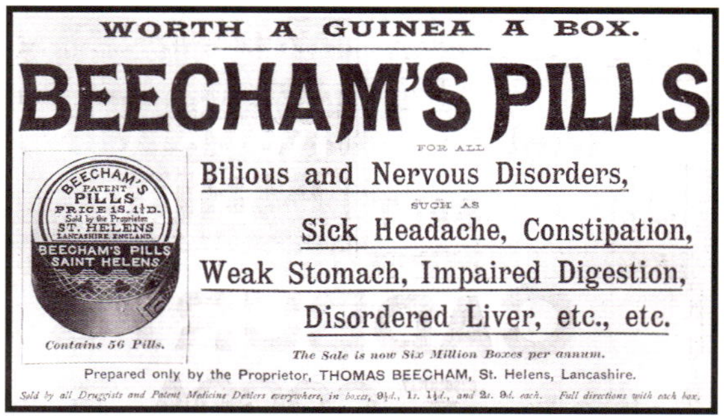

ABOVE In England, the Victorians were eager consumers of laxatives to ward off 'autointoxication'. Some even submitted to surgery to this end.

SCIENTIFIC MEDICINE IN THE TWENTIETH CENTURY

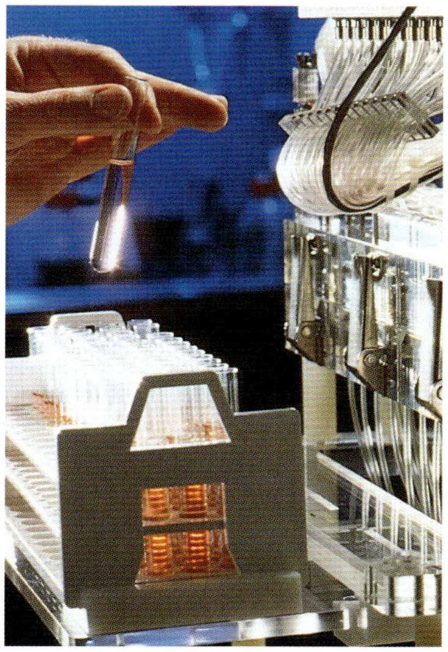

ABOVE **The adoption of control trials to evaluate the efficacy of new therapeutic drugs has resulted in some important medical breakthroughs in the twentieth century. The antibiotic streptomycin was validated in this way in the 1940s. However, a measure of caution is required; such trials are not infallible.**

Scientific medicine has made huge advances during the twentieth century. It is difficult to decide which have been the most important developments. Perhaps one should begin with the concept of controlled trials and their gradual adoption as a standard in research. This has been one of the big advances of the twentieth century. During the nineteenth century it was regarded as acceptable and 'scientific' to question a patient as he left the ward and mark him as a 'success' if he was grateful or trying to please the doctor. Many 'statistics' were published triumphantly to prove that certain treatments were valuable. Naturally, many of them were later shown to be useless or dangerous.

Then came the idea that patients who were being studied should be matched by 'controls' and compared with them. It was acknowledged to be important (though the precepts were often not followed) to plan the trial prospectively, not retrospectively, to compare like with like and, where possible, to study both groups in a 'double-blind' manner in which neither the patient nor the doctor was aware of who was being treated and who was part of the control group. Only by this method, properly carried out, is it possible to be certain about the results.

The first famous trial of this kind was carried out soon after World War II on the use of streptomycin in the treatment of tuberculosis. The results were spectacular in favour of the drug, but the double-blind controlled trial is not always an infallible method. Sometimes, even when huge efforts are made to perform all the procedures flawlessly, the results have been labelled 'the double-blind leading the double-blind'.

DIFFICULTIES WITH CONTROLLED TRIALS

It is often impossible to devise a double-blind controlled trial, or even a prospective one. Every attempt has to be made to match like with like, trying to make allowances for the influence of age, sex, class, race and so on. And whatever their validity, the results of scientific trials tend to be believed, rejected or shelved according to whether or not they suit the beliefs and prejudices of the profession and/or public. For instance, in the mid-twentieth century the Royal College of Physicians in London published the results of an elegant study into cigarette smoking and showed beyond reasonable doubt that it led to cancer. But it was not the conclusion that the public, and still less the tobacco industry, wished to hear; there was no political will to act on the data and it was only after many years that the unwelcome results were assimilated. Even today, in spite of a vast amount of supportive evidence, the conclusions are resisted by the tobacco industry and by some hardened tobacco addicts.

CLINICAL SCIENCE

By the end of the nineteenth century there was considerable interest in the sciences basic to medicine. They were developing particularly rapidly in Germany, where, unlike Britain and the United States, medical schools were attached to universities and were amenable to research. Increasingly, Americans went to German medical schools and research institutes. The United States, which had hitherto had mostly private medical schools, began to emulate European traditions by establishing basic science laboratories in its universities and medical schools.

Thus there developed the concept of clinical science carried out in clinical departments by men and women devoted to research and working with patients in a clinical setting. In this movement, Britain was far behind. There had been little difficulty in creating university departments in the basic sciences directed by full-time professors, but there had been no comparable academic development in the world of clinical practice.

In Germany, some clinical departments had their own laboratories and assistants, even though the professors often maintained large practices. One example was Bernard Naunyn *(1839–1925)*, a great German physician to whom clinic and laboratory were inseparable. At different periods in his life he was a professor of medicine in Berlin and several other German universities, where he headed clinical departments. As well as seeing many patients, he did much research into liver disease and diabetes mellitus. One of his assistants discovered the presence of ß-oxybutiric acid in the urine of patients in diabetic coma. Naunyn introduced the term 'acidosis'.

The United States was strongly influenced by what was happening in Germany. The American Medical Association, *(founded in 1886)* had a profound effect on the development of clinical research. From the beginning it encouraged clinical scientists. Salaried clinical scientists were appointed in the US early in the twentieth century at the Hospital of the Rockefeller Institute, the Johns Hopkins Hospital and some hospitals associated with the Harvard Medical School. Hitherto the United States had been lagging behind Europe in medical progress, but the development of these institutes and the appointment of medical scientists enabled it, with the aid of large amounts of money, to catch up with Europe and eventually to overtake it in medical knowledge and expertise. For most of the twentieth century the United States has led the world in most branches of clinical research and the country's clinical scientists have won many Nobel prizes.

Britain had to wait longer. In 1905 the famous Anglo-Canadian physician (Sir) William Osler *(1849–1919)* went from Johns Hopkins to Oxford as Professor of Medicine. He was dismayed at 'the medical educational desert' he found there and criticized it repeatedly. He founded the Association of Physicians of Great Britain and Ireland, but this differed from the United States in that it did not include basic scientists, pathologists, physiologists or bacteriologists, nor those in public health. Also, unlike the US, the meetings were closed, limited to physicians and their guests. So it was 'an intimate club of mainly academic physicians', which had little contact with individuals in other scientific disciplines. It therefore never had the same national impact on medical science as its American equivalents.

Nevertheless, by 1910 a number of outstanding British contributions to clinical research had been internationally recognized. Sir James Mackenzie *(1853–1925)* pioneered the polygraph and Sir Thomas Lewis *(1881–1945)* the electrocardiogram (ECG). Sir Archibald Garrod *(1857–1936)* of St

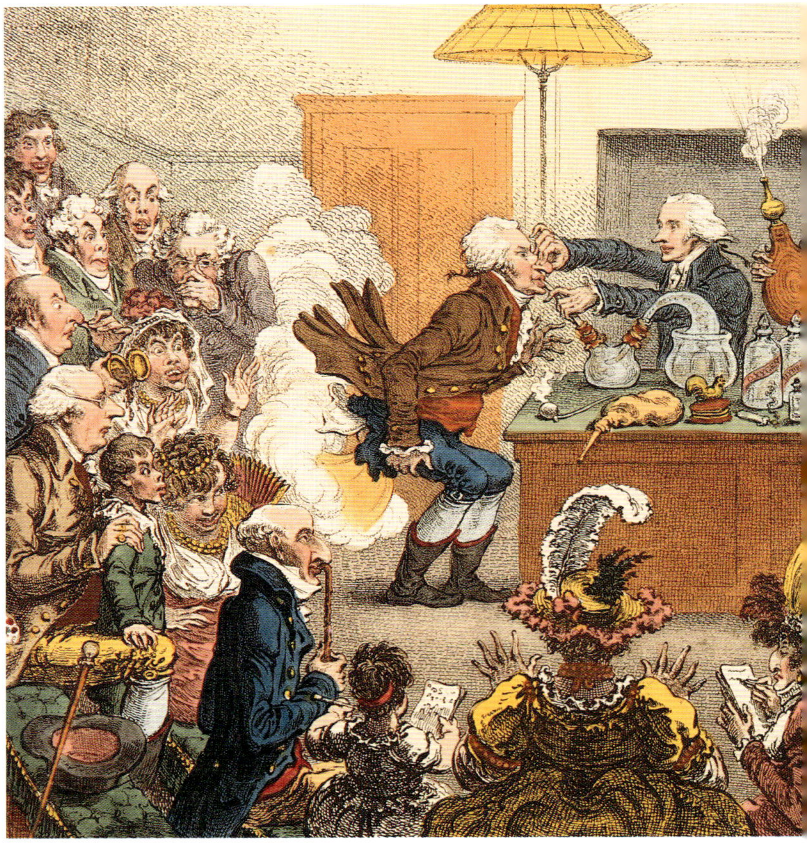

Bartholomew's Hospital in London had published *Inborn errors of Metabolism*. There was much research going on into the understanding of thyroid disease. Surgeons were improving their knowledge and inventing new operations. The British surgeon and physiologist Sir Victor Horsley *(1857–1916)* was making major contributions to the new specialty of neurosurgery.

In 1913 The Royal Commission on University Education in London under Lord Haldane *(1856–1928)* emphasized the importance of scientific research in clinical medicine but its findings were opposed by many and were shelved during World War I. Nevertheless, it laid the foundation for the establishment in British medical schools of modern academic departments in clinical subjects, where research would be emphasized. During the 1920s and 1930s such positions began to be created in British universities.

By 1925 there were five chairs of medicine among 12 medical schools in London, but their background tended to be in medical politics rather then academic medicine, and they had curious rules, such as that professors needed little or no experience of research and had to come from the same hospital. Thus some of them were inept and on the whole they were not as powerful or as able as their American counterparts.

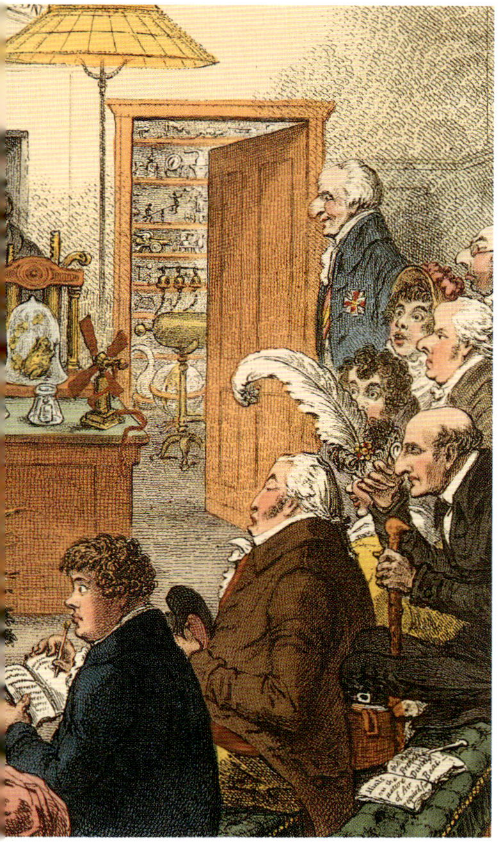

LEFT The brilliant English caricaturist James Gillray *(1757–1815)* applied his scurrilous and biting wit to the topic of scientific advance in this caricature from 1802 entitled 'New Discoveries in Pneumaticks! – or – an Experimental Lecture on the Powers of Air'.

BELOW The great American surgeon William Halsted *(1852–1922)* teaching in the theatre at Johns Hopkins University Hospital in Baltimore, where he was professor of surgery. Note that he is wearing rubber gloves; he pioneered their use in surgery.

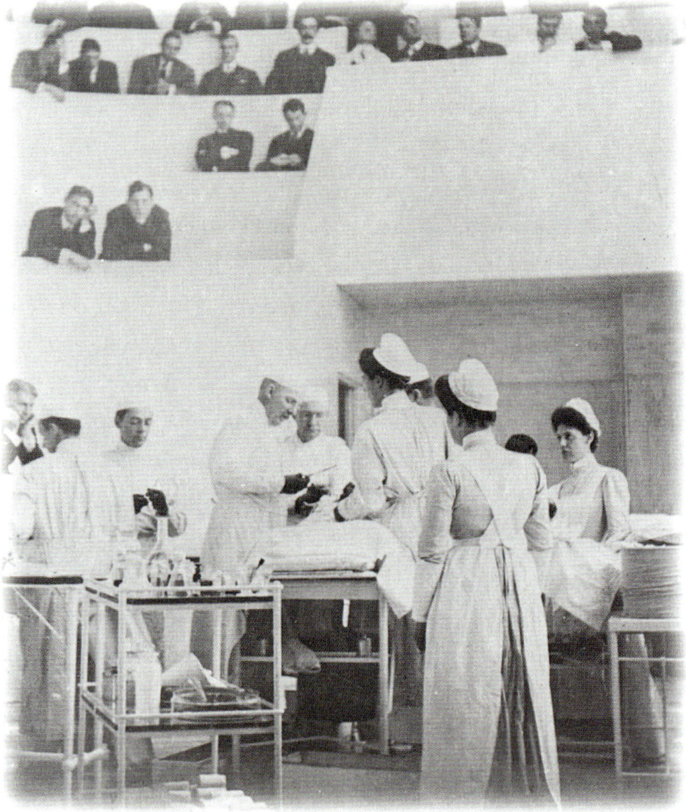

DISCOVERIES AND ADVANCES IN THE TWENTIETH CENTURY

The twentieth century has seen more discoveries and advances in medical science than all previous centuries put together, and medicine has become infinitely more powerful than it ever was before. Medical treatment in many fields has become immensely more effective. We have gained knowledge of matters and processes of illness that, at the beginning of the century, were unknown or mysterious. We can save lives, often easily, where before we could only watch victims die.

Two important areas of knowledge that began to develop early in the twentieth century concerned viruses and vitamins. Filterable viruses, organisms that could pass through all known filters, were discovered in the 1890s. Yellow fever was the first human disease proved to be caused by one of them. Many others followed, including smallpox, typhus, measles, poliomyelitis, rabies and viral meningitis. Because viruses are difficult and expensive to trace and study, a whole mythology has grown up round them in the public mind and there is a tendency to blame them for any unexplained disease.

It had been known for 200 years that sailors at sea remained healthy if given lemons, but scurvy, along with rickets, was common among Western children during the nineteenth century. The identification of vitamins as essential constituents of a healthy diet was an important advance in Western medical science. Many deficiency diseases were tropical, including beri-beri, pellagra and kwashiorkor (the last being a more complex deficiency disease), but once their causes were identified, if care was taken to see that children received an adequate diet, the conditions virtually disappeared. At least, knowledge existed of how to prevent them, even if it was not always put into effect. In the West, vitamins are the vehicle for a good deal of neurosis. Many people whose diets are perfectly adequate believe that unless they supplement these with expensive vitamins and supplements, they will become ill.

Another important early twentieth-century discovery in medical science was that of the main blood groups, A, B, AB and O. This made it possible to give blood transfusions with reasonable safety, which saves countless lives and facilitates advances in many branches of medicine, especially surgery.

Many diseases have been conquered or greatly relieved during the twentieth century through the development of medical science. One of the first and most important products of laboratory medical science was the discovery of insulin in the summer of 1921 by the Canadian physiologists (Sir) Frederick

Banting *(1891–1941)* and Charles Best *(1899–1978)*. It rapidly transformed diabetes from an invariably and often rapidly fatal disease into one that could be at least partially controlled. As a result, sufferers could expect many years of good life. Later in the century the treatment of diabetes changed again. Insulin is still used to treat it, but much of the management of the disease, especially in the older age-groups, consists in finding and maintaining a life-style that keeps the blood sugar within levels that are least likely to damage the blood vessels.

THE BENEFICIAL POWER OF DRUGS

Other diseases whose sufferers have benefited from modern medical science include leukaemia (especially in children, in whom it was usually rapidly fatal until the second half of the century), tuberculosis, pneumonia and other bacterial infections and many forms of cancer. Much of this has been brought about by drugs. Perhaps the most useful and spectacular of these were the antibiotics introduced between 1935 and 1945 and widely used ever since. The first were the sulphonamides, in 1935. Then penicillin became available, initially in very small quantities, during and after World War II, as a result of the research work of Alexander Fleming *(1881–1955)*, Howard Florey *(1898–1968)* and Ernst Chain *(1906–1979)*. It was followed by streptomycin and many more. Unfortunately antibiotics have been widely abused and used too frequently and for trivial complaints. As a result, strains of micro-organisms have developed that are resistant to antibiotics. For half a century the pharmaceutical industry coped with this situation, with immense profit, by producing a seemingly endless series of new antibiotics. Recently these have been running out and there is again great anxiety about the resurgence of infectious diseases. Another group of drugs that has become immensely important are the cytotoxic drugs, which are used in the treatment of cancer.

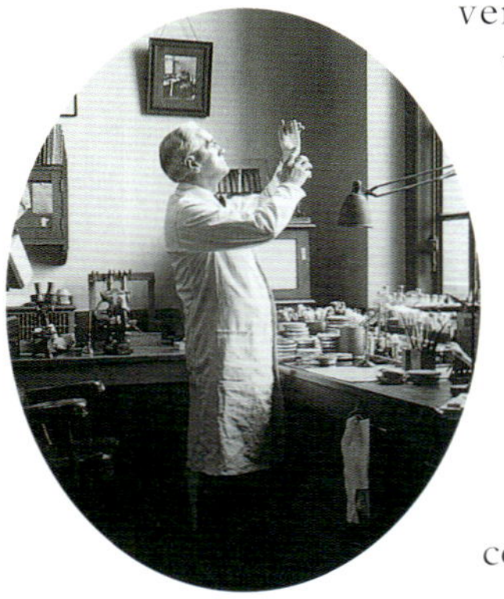

ABOVE **Sir Alexander Fleming, who discovered penicillin by chance in 1928.**

Many diseases can now be prevented altogether. Medical science has produced vaccines and immunization programmes which have largely eliminated many diseases that were previously prevalent and dangerous, including whooping cough, measles, diphtheria and poliomyelitis.

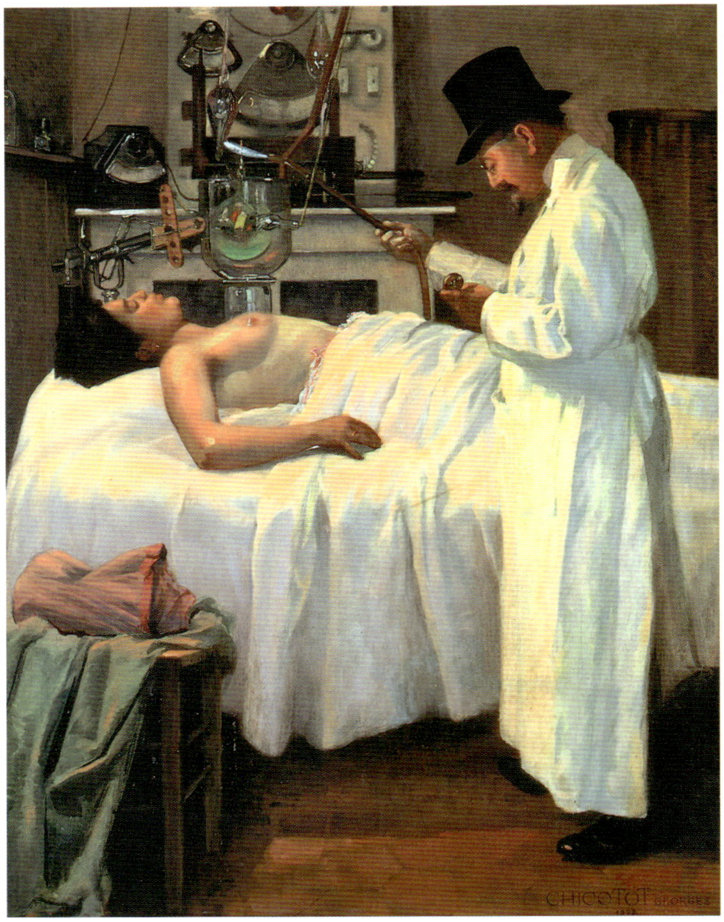

ABOVE **The use of radiotherapy to treat cancer dates back to the early years of the twentieth century. This painting by Georges Chicitot, dated 1908, is entitled 'The First Attempt to Treat Cancer with X-rays'.**

The twentieth century has been the century of therapeutic (as well as recreational) drugs. Many thousands have been developed by the pharmaceutical industry and some of these have been found to be invaluable. Drugs that alter mood and levels of consciousness have been significant among these. The barbiturates were introduced in 1903 and Evipan, the barbiturate anaesthetic, was introduced in 1932. These drugs had the disadvantage that they were addictive and were also used widely by suicidal people. In the middle of the century they began to be replaced by other drugs, notably the benzodiazepines, which included Valium and Librium. It was claimed that these were non-addictive, but this has proved not to be the case and addiction has become a serious, though often concealed, problem. Other important drugs have been the major tranquillizers, largely the phenothiazines, which have been widely used in psychiatry for major mental illnesses.

HIGH-TECHNOLOGY TOOLS

Technology is essential to medical science and this too has advanced enormously. Sophisticated apparatus for chemical tests have been followed by machines for kidney dialysis, controlling irregular heartbeat and many other purposes. During the second part of the century intensive care units for patients who are extremely ill have been set up and save many lives. Special care units have been developed to care for premature and ill newborn babies. Computers have revolutionized medical science and made many tasks feasible for the first time or simply much quicker than hitherto. Radiology has expanded with sophisticated radiotherapy, ultrasound, imaging techniques, scanning and so on. Techniques for studying and altering genes have also come into prominence.

Meanwhile surgery has advanced immeasurably compared with the plethora of fancy operations devised at the turn of the century. Plastic surgery developed markedly during the two World Wars, when it was increasingly helpful in the treatment of disfigured servicemen. Surgery in general has become less damaging and invasive and there are now techniques for doing minimal damage, for 'OK' ('orifice' and 'keyhole') surgery and, most recently, surgery performed under the 'eye' of a scan. Another branch of new surgery has been foetal surgery, in which the foetus is operated on inside the womb or removed from it temporarily and then replaced to continue gestating.

Foetuses are now screened for abnormality and, if thought to be damaged, are often aborted. Those prospective parents who have fertility difficulties now have a range of possible therapies to help them. Many of these treatments come under the heading 'IVF' or in-vitro-fertilization.

Preventive medicine has developed techniques of screening whole populations for disease rather than waiting for symptoms and signs to develop. This began with the mass X-ray units that screened for tuberculosis, but screening is now used in many other ways, most commonly screening for cancer. There is controversy about screening. Some people think that despite its apparent value, in fact it reveals many conditions that would never actually cause trouble, that all it does is create much anxiety, and that the number of false positive and false negative tests mean that the procedure is of little use.

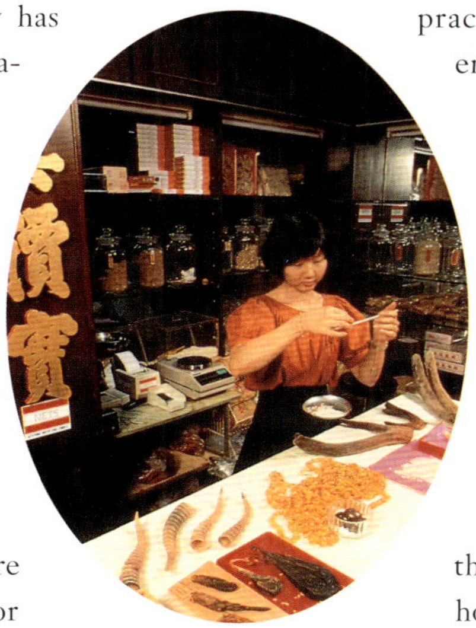

ABOVE Traditional Chinese medicine largely eschews the high-technology solutions preferred by Western medicine.

PSYCHIATRIC MEDICINE

An area of medicine that has not so far become truly 'scientific', and which is still an area of obscurity and ignorance, is psychiatry. The major tranquillizers (such as largactil and other phenothiazines) and lithium can control some schizophrenic patients, but many cannot tolerate them and their illnesses remain an unsolved problem. Lithium is of great help to some manic depressives, but not to all. Unfortunately, during the twentieth century psychiatry has extended its administrative power and organization more than its knowledge and practical effectiveness. Furthermore, there is an enormous lack of knowledge and expertise, as well as profound disagreements, about the interplay between body and mind.

This relates to the widespread public dissatisfaction with modern Western medicine. It may seem ironical that now, when medicine is more effective than ever before, it should attract so much discontent that many thousands of people are rejecting it, at least in part, in favour of other, complementary treatments. There are many reasons for this. One is that many modern treatments, however scientific they may be, are applied inappropriately or excessively. This is particularly true of drugs and surgery. The number of people damaged rather than helped by them (and sometimes damaged as well as helped) is enormous.

IATROGENIC DISEASE

In 1974 a Senate investigation reported that 2.4 million unnecessary operations were performed in the US per year and that they caused 11,900 deaths and cost about $3.9 billion. More deaths are caused annually by surgery in the US than the annual number of deaths during the wars in Korea and Vietnam. 'Iatrogenic disease', or disease caused by doctors, is thought to be rampant. Estimates for patients admitted to hospital because of poisoning by prescribed drugs have varied from 10 per cent to an astonishing 40 per cent. Our society has created a situation in which people tend to assume that there is 'a pill for every ill', and suffer as a result, often without realizing it.

THE RISE OF MEDICAL POWER

The process of medicalization is closely allied to the exercise of medical power. Medical power is the mainstay and objective of the medical profession, though not necessarily that of individual doctors. The growth of scientific medicine enabled the profession to grasp at the prospects of gaining and increasing its power over many aspects of human life where before it played no part. It did this regardless of whether or not by so doing it could actually help individuals or society, whether it had the technology to improve the situation, and whether or not it intended to try.

During the present century the medical profession has taken control of normal pregnancy and childbirth, sometimes making them abnormal, as well as contraception and abortion, without the intention of doing much about them. It has taken over 'drug addiction' and shaped it in ways that added to the prestige of doctors but did little to help the patients, and without admitting that no one knows how to treat drug addiction. This perpetuated and increased the drug problems of the Western world. It seems that doctors, have in one way or another taken control of most groups of people who are problematic to society.

It is not surprising that doctors are increasingly criticized for this process of medicalization, which is often seen as power-seeking rather than as the exercise of true medicine. Increasingly in recent years there has been criticism of the behaviour of doctors and doubt expressed about their motives, both individual and corporate. Many people also see medicalization as a system of social control imposed from above on a population, or even as a step towards totalitarianism. Some fear that, if they get the chance, doctors will seize the power to decide, for instance, who is and who is not fit to marry and have children, perhaps through the initial introduction of a compulsory premarital medical visit. Most disturbingly, during this century we have already seen doctors participating willingly in schemes such as the sterilization of the unfit, and the use of 'inferior' races for purposes of scientific research.

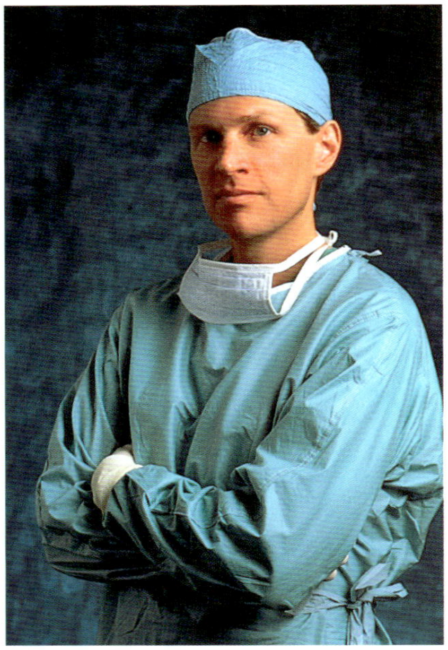

ABOVE **Critics argue that doctors have taken control of aspects of human life which should not concern them.**

Other writers have also feared the dangers of allowing medicine to take over matters of everyday life, particularly as there are ever more powerful drugs being pushed onto the market, and as ever more sophisticated surgical operations and other advanced forms of treatment become available. There are also dangers, many think, in medicalization, because it encourages people to allow experts to run their lives, thus undermining their personal autonomy and development. The radical American philosopher Ivan Illich *(1926-)*, a passionate critic of what he sees as our current culture of dependency and acceptance of institutional authority, propounds this view very strongly and claims he is convinced that 'the medical establishment has become a major threat to health'.

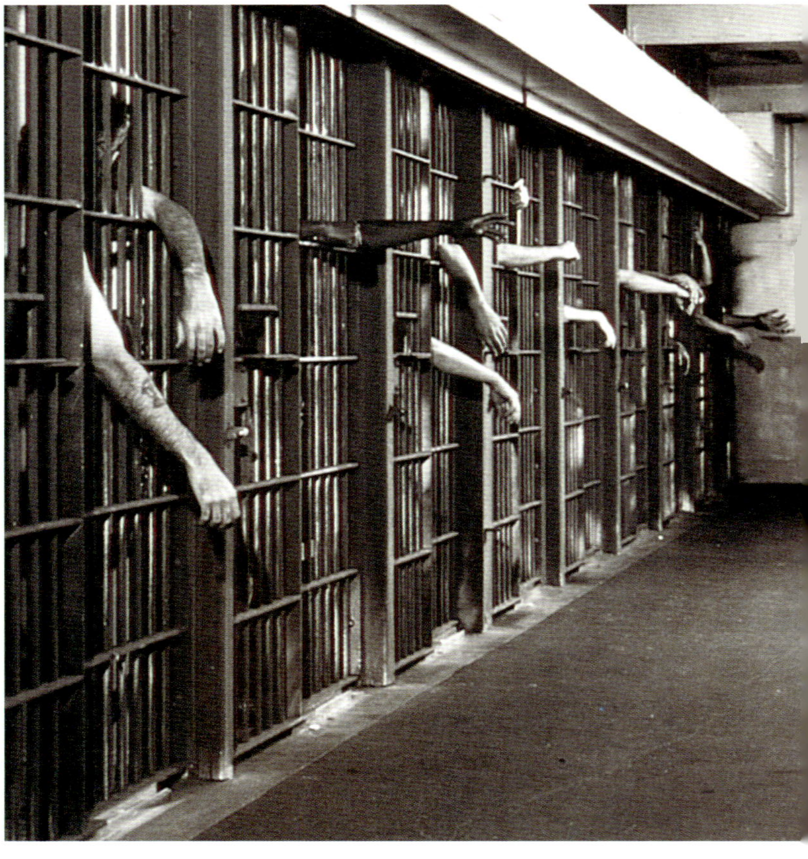

Some doctors have also used scientific medicine to impose moralistically biased views on society. For example, they have set themselves up as experts concerning drug-taking and have even invented a moral condemnation as a medical diagnosis, which they call 'drug abuse'. This diagnosis has been widely accepted, especially in official circles. Politicians tend to support the concept of medical power because it can be used in an authoritarian way to underpin the established order.

It would be wrong to think that the process of medicalization was simply instigated by doctors and imposed by them on an unwilling populace. It was, and is, also demanded by those who come under its sway. There is a tremendous public demand for medical services and it is impossible to say how far medicine will grow in response to that demand. One could argue that what doctors think and do merely reflects what the population demands that they think and do.

Certainly they seldom resist the demands of society, and they have willingly established a whole spectrum of disease in areas previously regarded as being none of their concern. The 'disease model' is widely used in analyzing and assessing social problems and these have added status to the medical profession even where they have not brought any significant progress towards greater understanding or power to solve the problems.

Many doctors have doubted the necessity for such widespread medical intervention and a few have challenged the medical power base, sometimes with disastrous results. Nevertheless, an increasing number are thoughtfully critical of the way in which they were trained and the relevance to the present day of the attitudes implicit in that training.

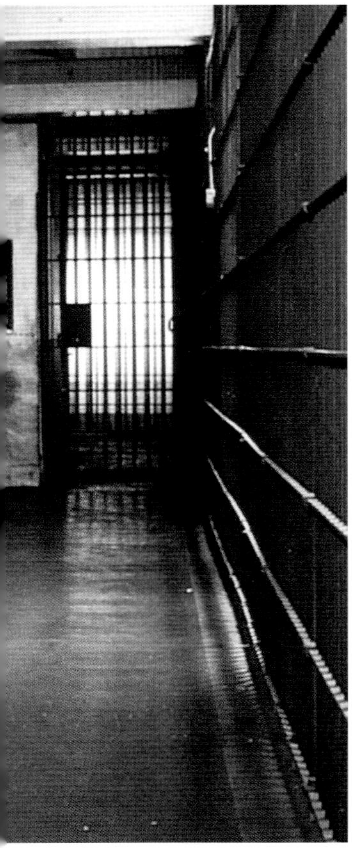

LEFT One of the consequences of the growing medicalization of our society is that people who are deemed anti-social or problematic are handed over to the care of doctors, as if they are suffering from a disease. Drug-takers are characterized as 'drug-abusers' in need of medical care. There is a danger when medical power runs unchecked; for instance, in the past doctors have used prisoners and 'inferior' races for scientific research.

Doctors have always had power and ideas about health and disease. They have known secrets, both about poisons and remedies, and about their individual patients. They have let it be thought that they know what they are doing even when they do not. They have probably always liked to 'medicalize' as a means of establishing themselves. They have used their power wisely, but they have sometimes abused it. They have great power over their patients, and its abuse is a serious danger to society, but ultimately they can be controlled only by those patients. Doctors and scientific medicine reflect society.

While judging a fiction contest recently in England, the author AS Byatt complained about the recurrent preoccupations which she encountered in many of the entries. She pointed out that British fiction is remarkably body-obsessed and the bodies with which it is obsessed are invariably sick or damaged.

We seemed to be in a world of human
bodies seen as objects of desire and violation,
a world in which most of the action was
penetration by the penis or the knife or the
needle, where everything dripped with
blood and other fluids.

AS BYATT

Fiction, like medicine, reflects the society in which it grows. Byatt also reflects the feelings of DH Lawrence:

When I went to the scientific doctor
I realised what lust there was in him to
wreak his so-called science on me
and reduce me to the level of a thing.
So I said: Good morning! and left him.

DH LAWRENCE, *THE SCIENTIFIC DOCTOR*

Many feel like this sometimes, but few would choose to die by refusing to have their acute appendix removed or would wish to deny life-saving antibiotics to a child suffering from the otherwise fatal tuberculous meningitis. Few would refuse a hip or knee replacement for an intolerably painful joint. Scientific medicine benefits us all. It is our own excesses and our follies that sometimes spoil its potential benefits.

CHAPTER THREE

HERBALISM

THE OLDEST TRADITION

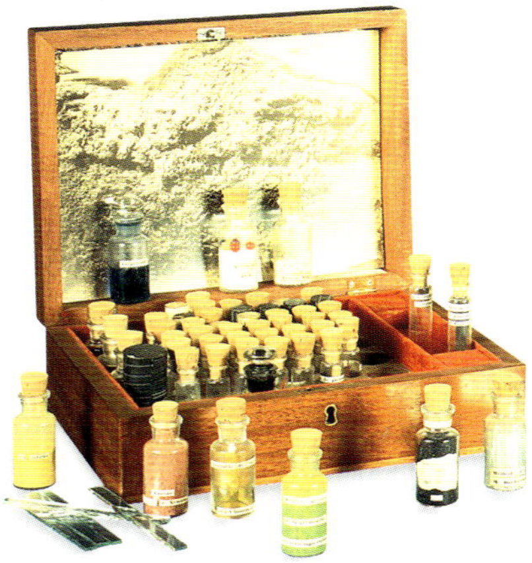

ABOVE Medical commercialism in the eighteenth century encouraged the sale of medicine chests, including herbal remedies, for use in the home.

NOWADAYS *the lore of herbs – offering a sense of an unbroken tradition – attracts not only the serious student, but also the curious and the dilettante as it reaches into many aspects of our lives. Consumer promotion of health and wellness, for example, encourages widespread popular interest in herbs, spices, elixirs, cordials, 'natural' perfumes and aromatherapy products. Furthermore, herbal lore continues to pull together and meld ideas from diverse cultures. The Western fascination with Chinese ginseng, for instance, embraces a mix of oriental exoticism, scientific information, and popular beliefs that the root is a powerful aphrodisiac as well as a tonic. Perhaps, too, the long recognized similarity of many ginseng roots to the human form remains mystical for some people, a mystique perhaps encouraged by often elegant commercial packaging.*

Written as recently as 1983 to a herbalist in rural Alabama, USA, the letter quoted opposite (with original spelling, grammar and syntax) reflects both continuity and change in the story of herbal medicines. Although the twentieth century has witnessed the decline or even total disappearance of herbal knowledge among most people in Western industrialized countries, renewed interest in herbs is evident today. This – part of the growth of alternative/complementary medicine and what is sometimes called the green movement – is fostered by many factors.

Aside from fears that the side effects of modern prescription medicines often make the cure worse than the disease, one significant factor in this renaissance is herbal lore. Although difficult to define, this is generally viewed as an accumulated body of ancient and modern knowledge about herbs, an eclectic mix of anecdote, tradition magic, myth and 'factual' information.

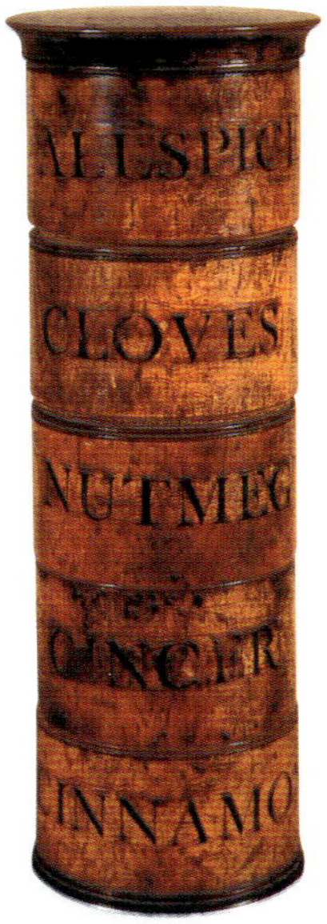

ABOVE A nineteenth-century spice container. Spices served as medicines as well as condiments in the Middle Ages.

LETTER TO A HERBALIST

I'm writing concerning the herbs, roots, weeds, etc. I read about you [a herbalist] in the Anniston Starr [Alabama]. I'm real interested about finding out about these. My mother has a weight problem which she can't loose weight no way she tries, she also had tyroid problems which now they've got them under control. But she still can't loose weight. I would very much appreciate you writing me back and giving me a list of [herbs]... How to fix them and your price list. I need information on what tree bark is it you can chew to stop the tooth ache, which plant to use to cure a stomach ache...The reason I'm writing to you for these is we don't have money to go to the doctor... please write us back we need your help desperately.

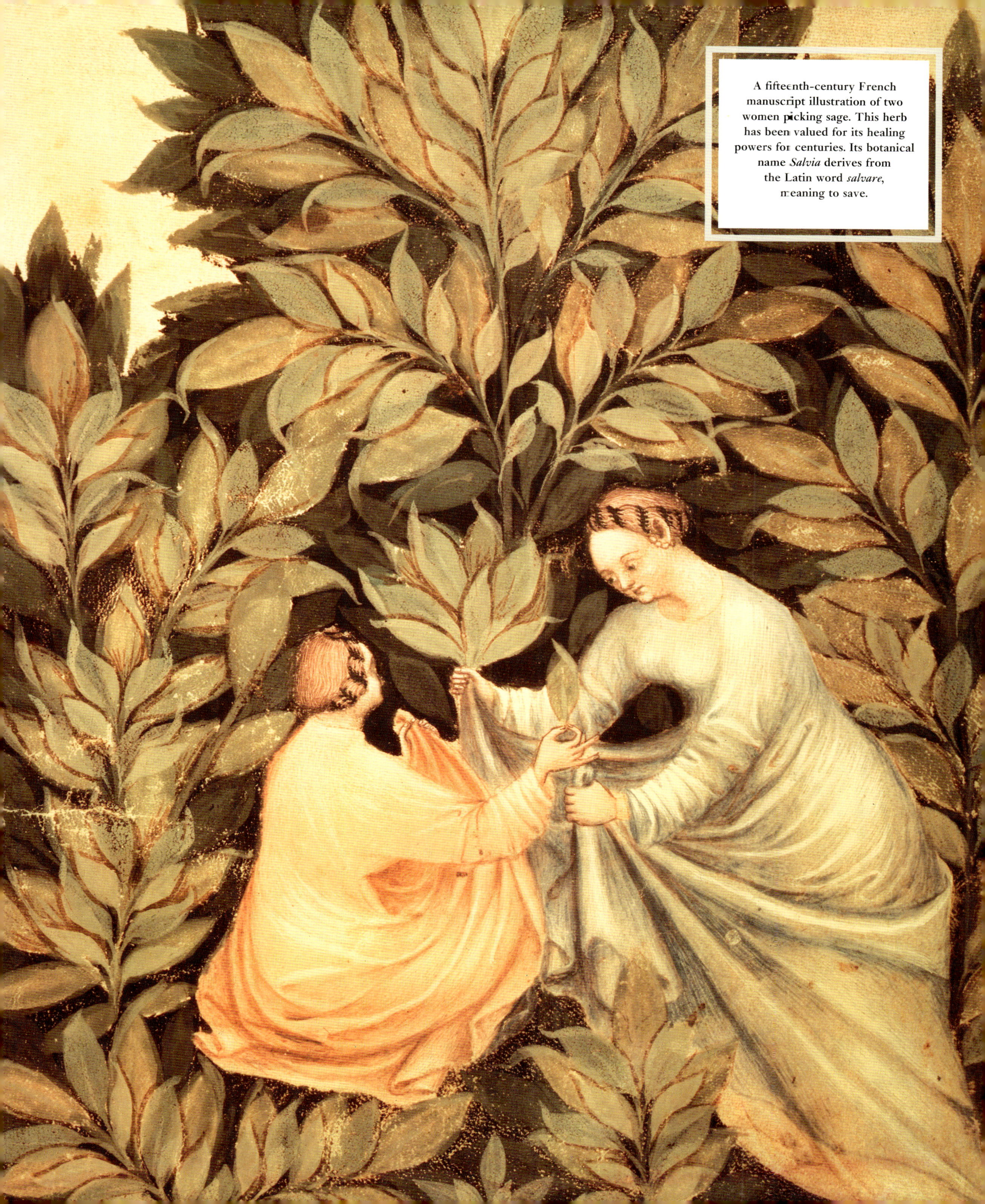

A fifteenth-century French manuscript illustration of two women picking sage. This herb has been valued for its healing powers for centuries. Its botanical name *Salvia* derives from the Latin word *salvare*, meaning to save.

Another 'exotic', one added recently to the Western herbal medicine market, is a new *(1996)* preparation of 'Cat's Claw' – an extract produced from a vine, *Uncaria tomentosa*, growing in the Peruvian rain forest. The bottle label bears the photograph of Lauro Hinostroza, a respected Peruvian curandero, along with the statement that he guarantees the purity of the product. In many ways, the new brand mirrors promotional material of the past, which tied the reputation of a herb with the experience of native North American people.

COMMONLY ASKED QUESTIONS

The past and present story of medicinal herbs – leaves, roots, bark, wood, or other parts of a plant – is intriguingly complex, a mix of empiricism, science, social and cultural forces. As the story unfolds, some commonly asked questions will be kept in mind. For instance, how effective are herbal medicines, either as simple herbs or in compounded preparations using more than one ingredient? Are herbs always safe? How widespread was, and is, herbal knowledge? Questions about efficacy are of special interest because many commentators, past and present, have criticized the usefulness of many, if not almost all, herbal medicines. However, if there is any justice to their view, why has knowledge of, if not necessarily belief in, many herbal practices – especially those that have not been mainstream – persisted over long periods of time?

Among various considerations relevant to answering these difficult questions, patients' viewpoints – confidences in and dislikes regarding herbs – are significant but sometimes overlooked. ('For colds, they'd give you senna – it was bitter and took me hours to get down,' said one Canadian recently). In fact, expectations about treatment depended on many factors such as whether it was part of long-standing family care or recommended by one of a diverse range of practitioners using herbs. Indeed, one of the more noteworthy features of the long history of herbal medicine is this diversity and range – from regular physicians, with their bookish tradition, to, say, illiterate herbalists noted for their empiricism. Some always ask, who is the real expert?

This chapter has as a central thread some key features of the Western herbal tradition. However, other cultural traditions are considered, not only to look at their particular features, but also to notice the melding of traditions, often with resulting change – syncretism, as anthropologists call it – for this, too, is a notable feature of the herbal story. Even traditional Chinese medicine, often viewed as resistant to change over the centuries, has undergone much adaptation, particularly in recent times.

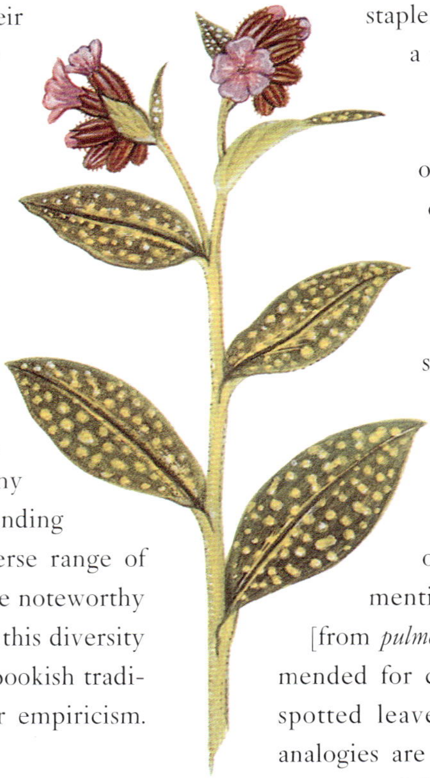

ABOVE The Doctrine of Signatures holds that a plant's appearance suggests its medicinal use. This is lungwort.

ORIGINS OF HERBAL MEDICINES

How did plants first come to be used for treating sickness? This takes us back to prehistory, to the time of unwritten records and to what is often disparagingly called 'primitive' medicine. It is widely considered that many treatments were introduced from accumulated observations arising from instinctive behaviour, from observations on the habits of animals, and from trial and error on humans. The latter could have been linked to trying out plants on the basis of their sensory properties (e.g., strong odour or taste), as has certainly been done much later, even by herbalists in the twentieth century. Perhaps, too, the familiarity occasioned by using plants for food and other non-medicinal uses led to significant observations. In the past, as in the present, many plants have served both as foods and as medicines. The corn silk fibres from the maize plant, for example, a staple food prepared in many ways, have long had a reputation as a diuretic.

Although the 'discovery' of medicinal uses is viewed as a triumph of observation, of empiricism untrammelled by theory, concepts and reasoning probably played a part. Many examples can be found in the later written record where analogy with other plants, or the application of a theory such as the Doctrine of Signatures, are relevant considerations. Although the Doctrine of Signatures has various shades of meaning, a basic idea is that the appearance (e.g., shape, colour) of a plant offers a clue to medicinal usage. A commonly mentioned example is the lungwort (*Pulmonaria* [from *pulmo*, Latin for lung] *officinalis*), which is recommended for chest ailments; with some imagination, the spotted leaves resemble a diseased lung. Comparable analogies are found in ancient Greek medical literature. Often cited is a plant – found growing in crevices of rocks and seemingly breaking them – administered for bladder stones. There is no reason to think that such ideas and manner of reasoning did not exist in prehistory, especially when we consider that ancient writings, such as those compiled by the Greek physicians Theophrastus *(c.370–288/5 BC)* and Dioscorides *(fl. c. AD 40–80)*, incorporated information from the oral tradition of medical folklore.

THE EFFECTIVENESS OF HERBS

What do we mean by the effectiveness of a herb? This is a relative term, for it can have different meanings for patient and for practitioner. Some commentators make a distinction between effectiveness (benefits under *ordinary* circumstances, which may be very variable) and efficacy (benefits under *ideal* circumstances). For the latter, many factors must be in place, aside, of course, from whether the treatment really is suitable for the problem. Medications have to be of good quality and administered in appropriate dosages. Moreover, in any assessment of the treatment, a placebo action has to be taken into account. Nowadays, this is generally defined as an action unanticipated by theory or known scientific data; placebo action is shaped by many factors, ranging from the relationship between practitioner and patient to a patient's confidence in the medication. Some describe placebo action as resulting from the power of suggestion, an idea that can be traced back to ninth-century writings.

Nowadays much debate exists over the usefulness of herbs in times past. Some see medicine in general as an 'unrelievedly deplorable story'. Well-known essayist Lewis Thomas, for instance, believed that medicine during century after century consisted of sheer guesswork and the crudest sort of empiricism. Others argue that very few historical drugs offered real benefit; any success is credited to the body's own ability to heal itself through immune defence mechanisms. Past critics of herbal therapy – from Galen *(AD 129–c.210)* in antiquity to eighteenth-century physicians such as William Cullen *(1710–1790)* – are often called upon to support negative opinions, though all such critics had their own extensive materia medica.

Contrarily, many commentators do not accept such negative views. They argue, despite the problems in identifying both ancient diseases and ancient remedies, that many herbal preparations were effective or, at least, gave ease or relieved symptoms (e.g., diarrhoea, general aches and pains and loss of appetite). Although this is not seen as 'curing' the underlying disease, the relief of symptoms – which, after all, is what much conventional therapy does today – contributes to an individual's well-being. Moreover, those with positive views about therapies often notice that herbalists consider that herbs are more effective in combination with medicines than when used on their own. The persistence of much herbal knowledge from antiquity to the present also favours effectiveness in the minds of many; however, this tends to overlook the role of theory and of cultural factors that have sustained many beliefs, magical and otherwise, about herbs throughout time. Some of the recipes of Graeco-Roman times that include magical components are not dissimilar from those recorded in the twentieth century.

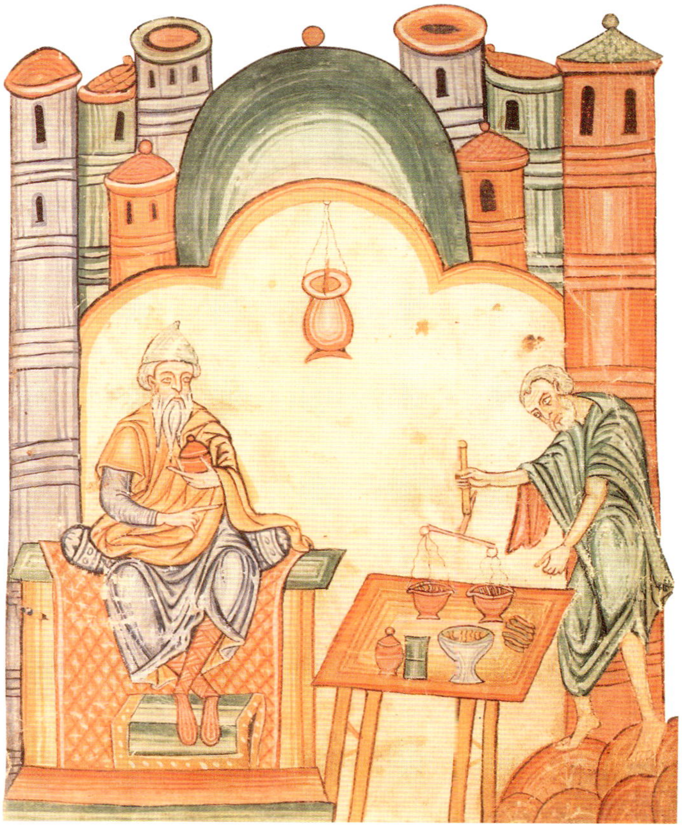

ABOVE Apothecary shops are common illustrations in medieval manuscripts. Evidently the apothecary was a source of specialist skills in the preparation of medicines in the Middle Ages.

MAKING CHOICES: HERBS

One of the most intriguing features of the story of medicinal herbs is the vast number recorded. Thousands of herbs have been known in most societies, though it is clear that only a core number have been or are still in common use. Perhaps 200 or so plants formed the basis of the ancient materia medica, and 70 or so the core of certain late medieval herbals. Estimates for today are very varied. It is commonly said that herbs are the basis of health care of 80 per cent of the world's population, though – as distinct from a few isolated constituents used in pure form – herbs have virtually no role in regular scientific medicine.

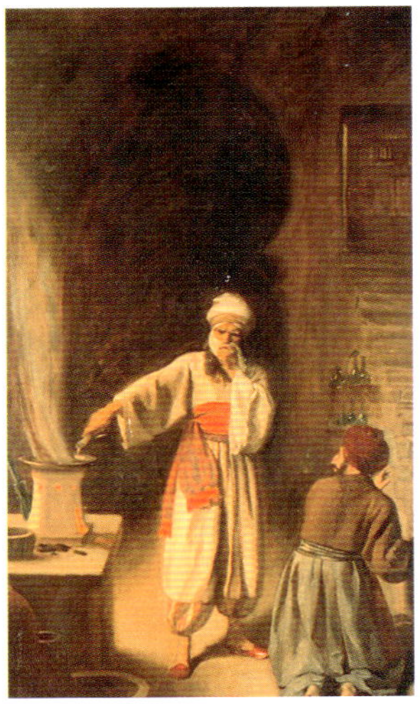

ABOVE **Rhazes, the Persian medical author. Arab medicine introduced new herbs to the West.**

Of interest, too, is the number of herbs that survive over long periods of time. A recent study of 257 drugs in more than 60 ancient Greek treatises, written mainly between 420 and 350 BC and linked with the name Hippocrates, claims that around 90 per cent are found in modern accounts of drugs; moreover, most of those used over time in Western medicine were known to the Graeco-Roman world. Many, too, can be traced back to the ancient Egyptian and Mesopotamian civilizations. Unfortunately, the information we have is only in the form of lists and recipes and uses. Knowing how ordinary folks in these times looked after themselves and what treatment they chose remains elusive. Did they rely on self care? When, if ever, did they call upon a medical practitioner?

HERBS IN ANCIENT EGYPT

Nakht, a common Egyptian weaver who died in the eleventh century BC, when aged between 14 and 18, suffered from schistosomiasis, tape worm (possibly associated with malnutrition), anthracosis of the lungs (presumably due to environmental pollution from cooking and heating), and pulmonary silicosis. Malaria was also a possibility. How stoic was he to his many ills? Were herbs used to purify the air in his sick room, if such a modern term is appropriate? Did he use powdered fleabane (*Inula* spp) as a dust to deal with the constant nuisance of fleas? How much of his health-care knowledge and that of his family can be found in the celebrated Ebers Papyrus, compiled around 1550 BC? We do not know for sure, though it seems likely that this ancient formulary of medicines covered much that was traditionally known in Egyptian society.

A particularly full account is given in the papyrus of the singularly attractive castor oil plant. However, as with information from other ancient sources, this tantalizes the modern reader as much as it informs. Laxative properties are noted, although not linked to the expressed oil (celebrated in our own time for this property). The account does imply usage to clean out the gastrointestinal system, an example, perhaps, of cleansing approaches – using castor oil or other laxatives – that have been commonplace in regular medicine until recent times. The papyrus does in fact mention the oil, but as an external application for certain skin conditions.

MAKING CHOICES: PRACTITIONERS

A patient's herbal treatment in times past often depended on their practitioner, who, in many circumstances, may have been the only one available for a consultation. Over time, a great diversity of practitioners – for instance, herb gatherers and herbalists, wise women, midwives, faith healers, druggists, quacks, botanical practitioners, regular practitioners – have all prescribed herbs. This is a conspicuous aspect of the story of medical herbalism. At times it has aroused much inter-practitioner rivalry and continues to do so, often due to different levels of education. In Graeco-Roman times, for instance, the erudite and learned Galen, who generally served the elite of society, contrasted sharply with most other 'physicians' in urban and rural communities.

At the same time there were 'laymen' with very extensive medical knowledge, like the Roman Celsus (*fl. c.* AD 25), author of the influential medical text *De medicina (On medicine)*, who practised on his own estates. Herbal knowledge has always been part of general culture. It is only since the nineteenth century that, increasingly, medical knowledge became the specialized expertise of the medical profession, which 'protected' it by the erection of many subtle boundaries. That is not to say that earlier physicians, with their experiences and skills – including forecasting the outcomes of illnesses (prognoses) – were not in demand. Indeed, there are grounds to suggest that the growing authority of the educated and learned physician, from, say, the twelfth century onward, owed much to public demand. On the other hand, there have always been some concerns over the bookishness and theories of physicians in general, compared with, for example, the accumulated wisdom of old women on which more will be said later in the chapter.

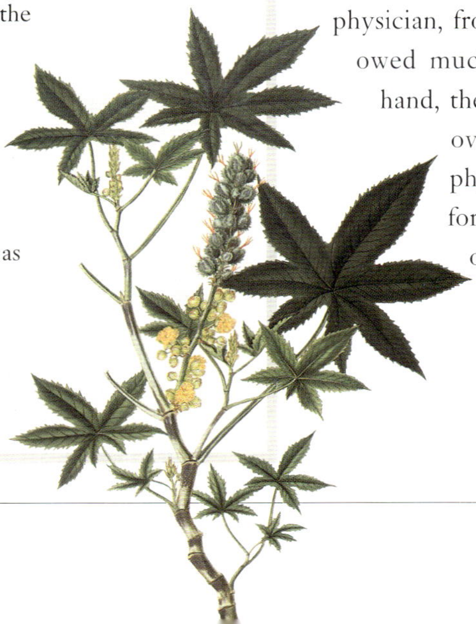

LEFT **The purgative properties of the castor oil plant were well known to the ancient Egyptians.**

TRENDS AND DEVELOPMENTS

GREEK MEDICINE: PERSISTING INFLUENCES

One of the most enduring concepts to persist in Western medicine, based on Greek foundations, was humoralism. This concept viewed (and, where humoralism still exists, still views) illness as arising from a disturbance in the natural balance of the body humours. The latter, based on body fluids, are phlegm, bile (yellow), blood, and 'black' bile or melancholy. Although evident in the Hippocratic corpus of writings that viewed health and disease as independent of supernatural factors, the persistence of humoralism in Western medicine stemmed largely from the encyclopedic writings of Galen. Health, the argument went, was restored by correcting an imbalance through treatment regimens in which food, drink, medicines and blood-letting were carefully orchestrated.

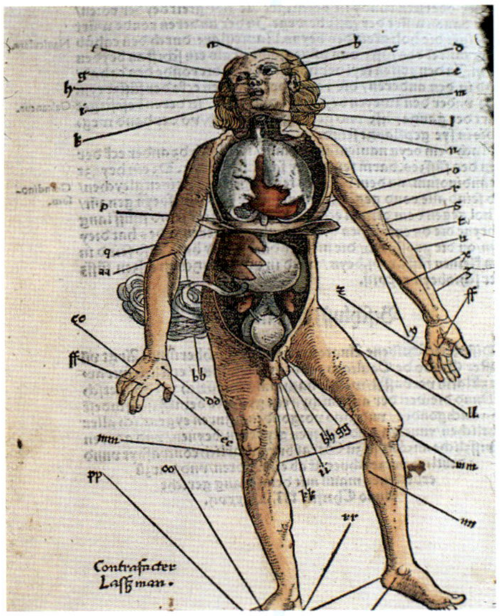

ABOVE **Blood-letting was one of the treatment regimens recommended by humoralist physicians who drew on the works of Galen for their authority.**

At the same time, one had to remember the place of outside factors such as bad air emanating from decaying matter or cesspits (miasma) and its effect on the body. The Galenic concept of non-naturals (food and drink, sleep and waking, air, evacuation and repletion, motion and rest, and passions and emotions) as determinants of health and disease also had long lasting influence.

The long-term influence of Galen (commonly called Galenism), which touched on more aspects of medicine than just humoralism, emerged with the passage of the so-called rational medicine of the Greeks into the Arab-Islamic world and then into the West. In the eighth century, Greek writings were translated into Arabic, and, later, in the eleventh century, a start was made on translating the Arabic into Latin. This transmission included writings on medicinal plants such as Dioscorides' *De materia medica (On medicines)*, compiled around AD 50 to 70; this pervasively influential work established an organized approach to the critical appraisal of herbs, including harvesting, preparation, storage, adulteration and how to test for it.

GALEN'S BEDSIDE MANNER

How ideas such as Galen's impacted on sick patients obviously affected the way patients viewed their medical conditions and their relationships with practitioners. Galen's patients, who generally knew much about medicine, faced a practitioner who, somewhat arrogantly, paraded his skills and expertise. Galen himself related an example of one-upmanship:

'At the door we met a servant carrying from the bedroom to the latrines a pot of which was full of excrement like bits of flesh or bloody discharge, a constant sign of liver disease. Without appearing to have seen anything I walked up to the patient with Glaucon [another physician] and felt his pulse wishing to find out if he was feverish or merely exhausted. The patient, who was a doctor, said that he was just getting back into bed after having passed a stool. The increased pulse rate is produced by the effort in getting up, he said. But while he was speaking I noted that in his pulse there was evidence of inflammation. Then, noticing on the window sill a pot containing syrup of hyssop I thought to myself, this doctor thinks he's got pleurisy because he feels the pain in the ribs which often occurs in inflammatory diseases of the liver. I postulated that, since he was getting pain, his respirations were rapid and shallow, and he was tormented by short spasms of coughing, he thought that he was suffering from pleurisy, and this was the reason why he was taking the syrup of hyssop. Realizing that fortune was now offering me a chance to raise myself in Glaucon's esteem, I placed my hand on the patient's lower ribs and on the right side, telling him that he was getting pain there. Both the patient, and Glaucon, thinking that palpation of the pulse alone had led me to diagnose the affected part, showed their admiration.'

The reputation of hyssop (presuming it to be *Hyssopus officinalis*) has continued into the present century for coughs and chest conditions, as an expectorant to bring up phlegm.

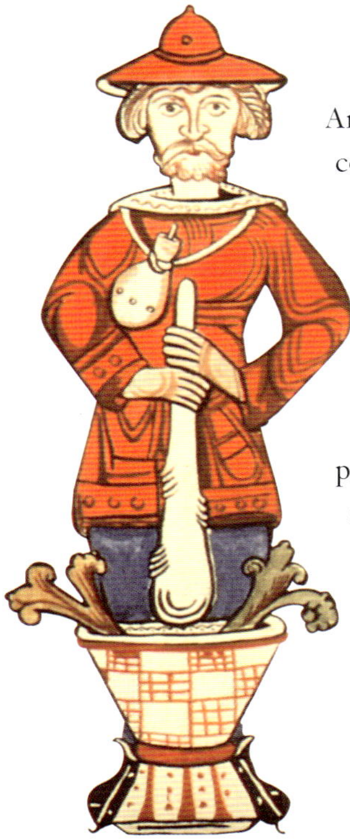

At the same time with the translations from Arabic into Latin, various ninth- to twelfth-century Arab contributions to therapy were passed on to the West. This included the addition of new drugs (a few from India and China) such as camphor, cassia fistula, senna, zeodary, nutmegs and possibly mace, tamarinds, manna and lemon, all of which ultimately gained a prominent place in herbal medicine; some new medical and cosmetic uses of plants already well known; an increase in the number of items in compounded medicines; and the use of sugar-based preparations such as electuaries, which used honey or syrup, and conserves.

These developments seem to have accentuated concerns over the quality of medicines, and some historians consider that this preoccupation contributed to the rise of pharmacy as a distinct occupation. Certainly, preparing medicines accurately could be very complex. The Galenic theory postulated that each herb (or other medicine) had two potential actions, either warming or cooling and either drying or moistening. Herbs were used, singly or more usually compounded together, to counterbalance the patient's disorder. To complicate matters, however, some herbs (e.g., cathartics) were considered to have specific therapeutic actions. All this led some Arabic authors to devise mathematical rules to determine the quantities of ingredients in a compounded medicine based on the qualities of each ingredient.

ABOVE In the Middle Ages the use of innumerable herbs in compounded medicines was common. Here an apothecary uses a pestle and mortar to mix and prepare ingredients.

While later writers took an interest in the complicated rules that developed, the effect was to foster a separation of what might be called academic medicine from conventional everyday practice.

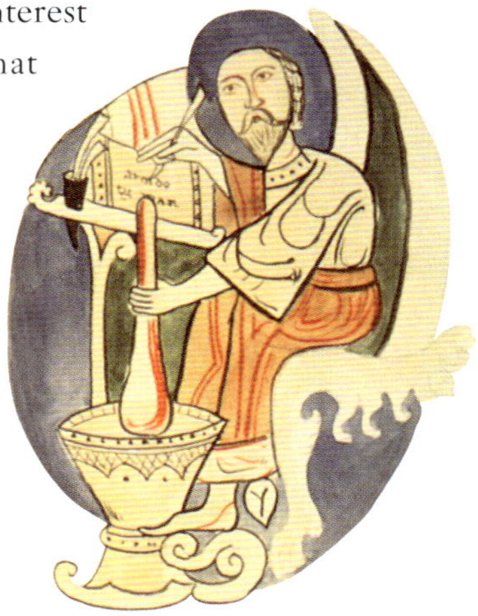

RIGHT The movement to specify rules governing the mixture of ingredients in compound medicines gave an impetus to the development of pharmacy.

Unquestionably, self-care remained the first line of treatment for most people. Over the years, physicians have often been ambivalent over self-care and complained that they have not been called soon enough to an illness in its early stages. Rhazes *(c.864–c.925)*, for instance, the celebrated Persian who wrote in Arabic, noted in his manuscript *A Treatise on the Small-Pox and Measles* (a work reflecting humoral doctrine) that, seemingly, he was not pleased with one of his patients.

> *A female patient, who was accustomed to drink camel's milk without my advice, and had become inflated by it, took some musk, without having been previously blooded or purged. Thereupon she fell into a continued fever, symptoms of the Small-Pox appeared, and after four days the pustules broke out. At the commencement of the disease she intrusted herself to me; so I immediately took care of her eyes, and strengthened them by a collyrium of cuhl rubbed up in rosewater. In consequence of this not a single pustule came out in her eyes, though they were very thick all around; so that the old women who were waiting upon her were astonished at her eyes being preserved. I made her take barley-water and the like for some time; and as her bowels were not relaxed, as is the case at the end of this disease, and she had still some remains of ardent fever, I conjectured this to be the effect of the residue of the humours that did not pass off by the bowels, as usual. I could not venture to bring this away all at once on account of her weakness; so I made her take the 'Aqua Fructuum' in the morning, and barley-water in the afternoon, for a fortnight, which occasioned two motions every day, and a complete purgation.*
>
> RHAZES, *A TREATISE ON THE SMALL-POX AND MEASLES*

The patient recovered completely after fifty days.

HERB LORE

The story of herbs in medieval times, no longer viewed as the dark ages, contributes much to herbal lore. Today, many people conjure up images of monks tending herbal gardens, and are familiar with Ellis Peters' celebrated mystery novels in which the main character, Brother Cadfael, tends a monastery herb garden in Shrewsbury, England, while investigating crimes. Some of today's herbal enthusiasts also delight in the famed verses about herbs in a monastic garden, written in the ninth century by Walahfrid Strabo. On sage he wrote:

There in the very front glows sage, sweetly scented,
It deserves to grow green for ever; enjoying perpetual youth;
For it is rich in virtue and good to mix in a potion,
Of proven use for many a human ailment.
But within itself is the germ of civil war;
For unless the new growth is cut away, it turns
Savagely on its parent and chokes to death
The older stems in bitter jealousy.

WALAHFRID STRABO, VERSES

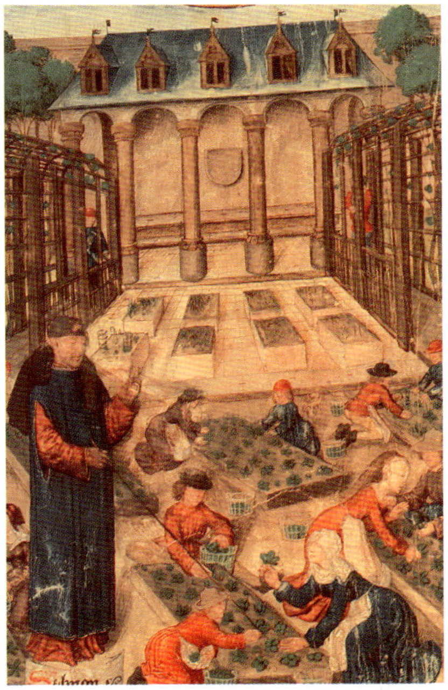

ABOVE 'The Garden of Medicinal Plants' – a fifteenth-century French painting. Medical botany was now well established.

One also finds, today, indulgence in modern 'medieval' feasts full of spices and sweetmeats, preserved and candied confections, such as once were prepared by the medieval apothecary. The Galenic hot qualities of spices made them important medicines as aids to over-indulgence and gastric upsets in general, as well as tonics. Apothecary shops are common illustrations in medieval manuscripts. Although the illustrations hardly offered medical information for the reader, they show that the apothecary was a source of specialist skills in the preparation of medicines. After pharmacy became an identifiable occupation in the Arab-Islamic world, a similar movement stirred in the West during the twelfth and thirteenth centuries. Ordinances, guilds and monopolies over certain goods began to support pharmacy as a specialist practice.

There is much reason to think that, in late medieval times, medical treatments contributed a great deal to the care and comfort of the sick, even though one can hardly overestimate the failures, especially in the many epidemics. The greatest scourge was the Black Death of 1346–47. Efforts to prevent and treat the disease were legion: flight, religious flagellation, careful living, specific attention to diet, the burning of aromatic herbs and the administration of a variety of herbs in part because of presumed anti-pestilential or cleansing properties. Many herbs were compounded into such famed preparations as Theriac and Mithridatium, which, with their dozens of ingredients, had a conspicuous life from classical times to the eighteenth century to treat cases of poisoning and as a cure-all for plague and other pestilential disorders. Amid the eighteenth-century reform of the materia medica, noted later, they faded from regular medicine, though some demand continued into the 1800s.

ARNAU OF VILANOVA'S WORDS OF GUIDANCE

The following passage from a lecture delivered in the last decade of the thirteenth century by the Catalan Arnau de Vilanova *(?1235-1311)* gives a good sense of attitudes to quality medicines, and the need for a physician to be careful over the choice and compounding of a suitable medicine.

'[Consider] suitability of that preparation, so that it be the strongest of its kind either absolutely or in relation to the illness for which it is prescribed: e.g., should figs (or ginger or dates) be given whole? Will this patient be better helped by figs from Persia or India or Damascus, or by Alexandrine or insular dates? There is great diversity found in things of the same kind, for example, ...plants that grow in the fields versus the same ones that grow in the mountains.

As for the medicine itself, the physicians should reflect on whether he can recognize it or not, and if he can he should ask to see it and judge it for himself. But if he is not acquainted with it, he should consider whether it has been described by the wise, and if so, when he has seen the plant, he should decide whether it corresponds to its description and [if so] choose it; while if it does not fit, he should not use it, but should choose instead something generally familiar and fitting the descriptions of the wise. And for students I give an example. You want to give eupatorium, but you are unfamiliar with it and the apothecary brings you wild salvia. If you want to avoid deception, be sure you know how the wise describe eupatorium... In the preparation [of a medicine] the physician must consider, in order, the cleansing, grinding, measurement, softening, and mixing [of its ingredients]. He should give instructions to his assistants, the apothecaries, about its mixing, telling them when [it is to be prepared], lest lacking his instructions they make it up later than they should.'

EARLY MODERN TIMES, 1500–1700

If anything, matters of quality and effectiveness of medicines became even more conspicuous in Renaissance times – generally viewed as the period following the introduction of printing in the middle of the fifteenth century until around the end of the sixteenth century. This was a time of critical appraisal of existing knowledge, a re-examination of ancient learning in the original Greek rather than Latin texts, and an appreciation of both first-hand observation and an ideal of improvement. Many printed herbals reflect the new mindset. Although naturalistic renderings of plants can be found in some early manuscripts, the primitive style of many medieval illustrations means that they were useless for plant identification. One sixteenth-century writer complained that important medicinal plants known to the ancients could no longer be recognized. However, the famed illustrations of Hans Weiditz in Otto Brunfels' *Herbarum vivae eicones (Herbal of living images) (1530)* moved illustrations toward showing plants in their natural state, and Leonhard Fuchs' works, *De historia stirpium (Inquiries on plants) (1542)* and *Neu Kreuterbuch (New Herbal) (1543),* underscored the value of combining figures with plant descriptions. William Turner's *A New Herball (1551),* the first herbal to be written in the English vernacular, offered careful descriptions of plants along with such warnings about errors as substitute plants that were being sold in apothecary shops for 'Venus heyre' *(Adiantum capillus-veneris).*

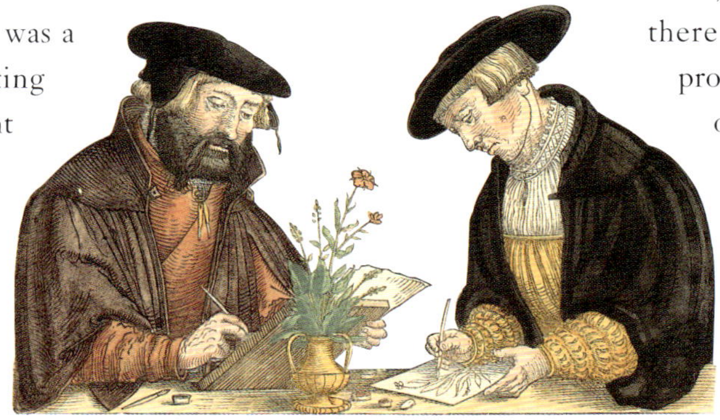

ABOVE **In the sixteenth century the standard of botanical illustration improved dramatically. Pictured here on the right is Albrecht Meyer who was the botanical artist for Leonhard Fuchs' *De historia stirpium.***

Sixteenth-century herbals paralleled a tremendous expansion of interest – commercial, botanical and medical – in plants, not only as a result of the desire to retrieve 'lost' drugs used in ancient Greek and Roman medicine, but also due to explorations in the New World. New botanical gardens such as at Pisa *(1543),* Padua *(1545)* and Leyden *(1587)* underlined the study of and teaching about medicinal plants, generally in the hope that therapy would be improved. Doctors in Padua in Italy, for instance, argued this would do away with the perpetration of errors and frauds in pharmacy, which was said to be causing the death of patients.

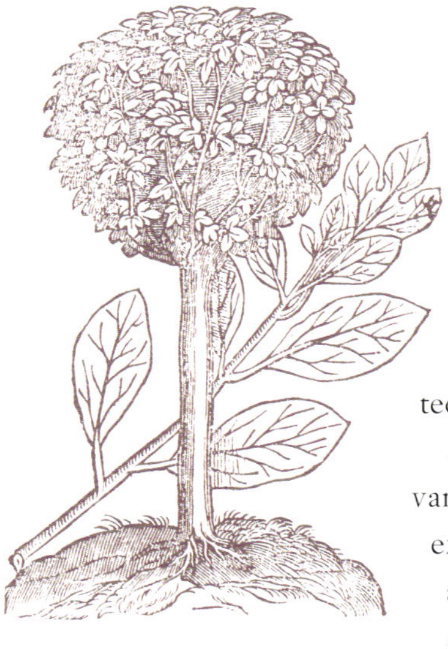

ABOVE **Sassafras as pictured in John Gerard's *Herball* (*1633* edition). The exploration of the Americas in the sixteenth century led to the importation into Europe of many New World medicinal plants like this.**

From the New World – the West Indies, Mexico, and south-eastern North America – there came medicinal plants and plant products: copaiba, balsam of Peru, balsam of Tolu, guaiacum, jalap, mechoacan, sarsaparilla, sassafras and tobacco, all well known prior to 1600. Unfortunately, it is not easy to estimate the popularity of these, though the scourge of syphilis drew much attention to guaiacum wood from the Caribbean. In 1517, it was stated that 3,000 Spaniards with syphilis had been cured by preparations of the wood. Such popularity did not survive the century, but the wood came to be used, like sassafras *(Sassafras albidum)* and sarsaparilla (*Smilax officinalis* and other species) – which also had some reputation in the treatment of syphilis – in conditions where blood purification was felt to be an asset. Another syphilis remedy of the time merits mention here as a rare introduction from China. China root *(Smilax china),* a botanical relative of North American sarsaparilla, reached Europe in the first half of the sixteenth century from Chinese traders via the Portuguese of Goa; although the root's reputation faded, like the others just mentioned, use of it persisted into the nineteenth century as a blood purifier.

Attitudes toward the new drugs depended on various factors. One was how they fitted into the existing Galenic theory, and agreement did not always exist on this. There were, too, differing attitudes toward exotics and indigenous remedies, an issue already noted. In one sense, this was highlighted by the title *(Joyfull Newes out of the New Founde Worlde, 1577)* of John Frampton's translation of the celebrated account of New World plants that had been written by Nicolas Monardes *(1493–1588).*

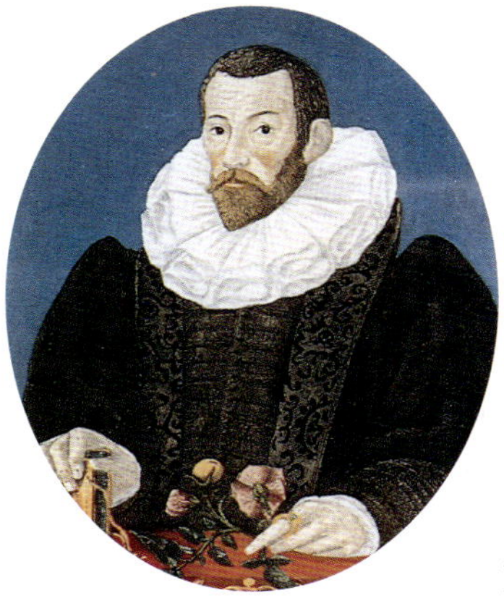

ABOVE John Gerard, who was herbalist to King James I and master of the Barber-Surgeons Company in 1607.

Monardes captures a sense of excitement of the times, if not the hard reality of the economics and politics that lay behind much exploration. On the other hand, attitudes toward 'exotic' plants from overseas were mixed. Timothie Bright's *A Treatise Wherein is Declared the Sufficiencie of English Medicines... (1580)* reflects how strongly many people felt that indigenous or local remedies were more effective for local diseases. Around the same time, another writer, John Gerard *(1545–1612)*, in his *Herball* of 1597, indicated the high estimation placed on imported goldenrod, as the following quotation testifies:

> *I have knowne the dry herbe which came from beyond the sea sold in Bucklers Bury in London for halfe a crowne an ounce. But since it was found in Hampstead wood, even as it were at our townes end, no man will give halfe a crowne for an hundred weight of it.*
>
> JOHN GERARD, *HERBALL (1597)*

Differences of opinion over exotics and indigenous remedies were not settled at the time, and have echoed ever since. 'Why send to Europe's bloody shores for plants which grow by our own doors?' was a question asked by Shakers – a religious sect and prominent herb growers in North America during the first half of the nineteenth century. Contrasts between the self-taught herbalist dedicated to using local and self-gathered remedies and the educated physician remains a contentious issue today.

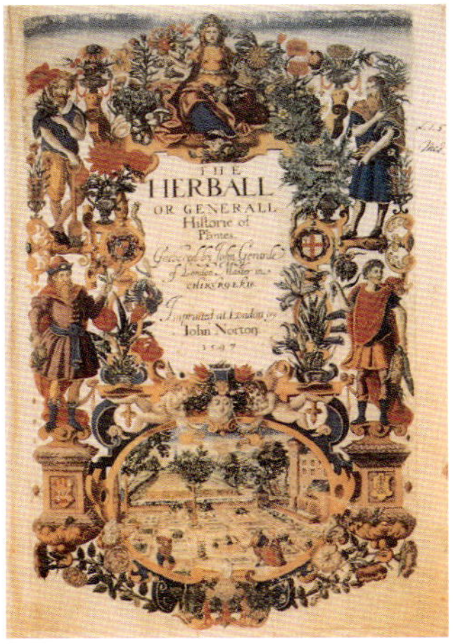

ABOVE The frontispiece to John Gerard's celebrated *Herball* of 1597. Gerard cultivated a garden in Holborn in London where he grew medicinal herbs. His influential book continues to remain popular to this day.

GERARD'S HERBALL

Within the English speaking world, John Gerard's *Herball (1597)* has made a significant contribution to herbal lore. Publications such as Marcus Woodward's *Leaves from Gerard's Herball Arranged for Garden Lovers (1931)* and modern reprints of the *Herball* continue to encourage popular interest in herbal writings of today. It is encyclopedic – more so the second edition of 1633, to which Thomas Johnson added over 800 plants to the 2,000 or so in the first edition. This 'coffee-table' book, with nearly 1,700 pages in the second edition, was commonly used in the seventeenth century and beyond by physicians and lay people alike. While the *Herball* has not enjoyed such a long publishing history as the celebrated herbal by Nicholas Culpeper *(1616–1654)*, still in print since 1653, Gerard's compilation has a sense of critical impartiality not found in Culpeper's book with its astrological content and anti-establishment stance. Gerard himself, in the spirit of the Renaissance, considered that the publication of the *Herball* was one way to preserve experiences, such as his gardening activities, along with medical information. As he wrote:

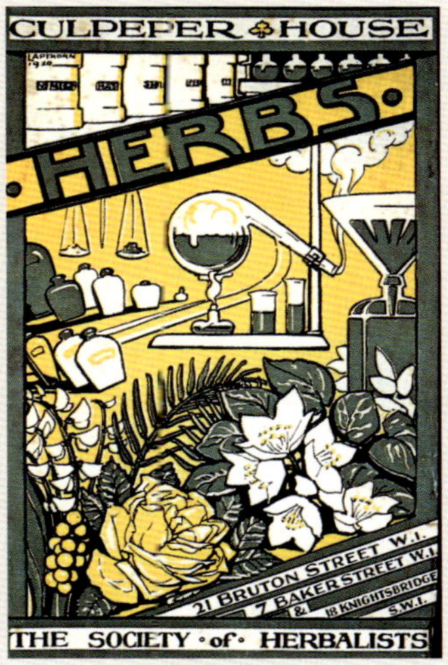

ABOVE Nicholas Culpeper's famous *Herbal* of 1653 has remained in print since its first publication. This 1930 advertisement is for Culpeper House, a popular herb shop in London.

> *But because gardens are privat, and many times finding an ignorant or negligent successor, come soone to ruine, there be [some] that have sollicited me, first by my pen, and after by the Presse to make my labours common, and to free them from the danger whereupon a garden is subject.*
>
> JOHN GERARD, *HERBALL (1597)*

WHY DID SO LITTLE LEAVE MEXICO?

Why did relatively few medicinal plants reach Europe from the New World or more strictly Mesoamerica? The question arises because of the richness of the medical flora as judged from such sources as the manuscript Aztec herbal (or Badianus Codex) written in 1552 by Martín de la Cruz, an Aztec physician, and Francisco Hernández's collection of over 3,000 Mexican plants assembled during the five years *(1572–1577)* he spent travelling there. Perhaps the explanation for limited transmission lies largely, as suggested by one historian, in the fact that little information was published in Europe. Certainly, Aztec theoretical concepts of a hot-cold classification of food and illness (soon admixed with those from Europe) were not far removed from European ideas at the time and offered no barriers to European interest. Nor is there evidence that local religious and magical aspects to the use of herbs was an inhibiting factor. When one looks at the richness of items available in the herb markets of Mexico today, it is clear that Europeans failed to explore a rich resource.

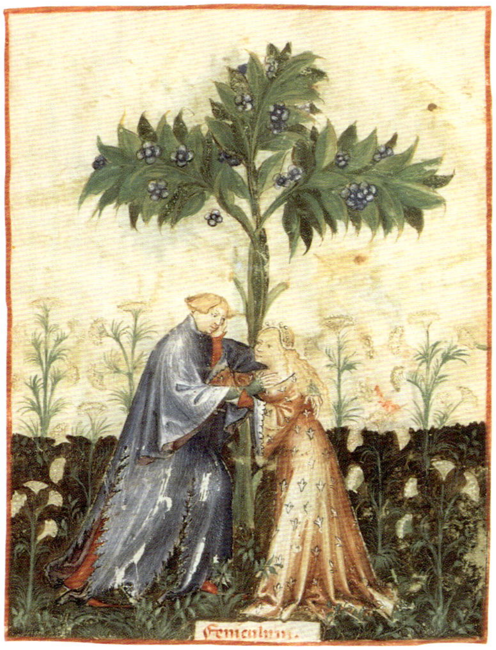

ABOVE An illustration of fennel from a fifteenth-century edition of the *Tacuinum sanitatis* or *Tables of Health*, a handbook based on an Arabic original. The herb was valued in medieval times as an aid to digestion and the flow of breast milk.

PREPARING HERBAL MEDICINES

The Swiss physician Paracelsus, or, more fully, Theophrastus Philippus Aureolus Bombastus von Hohenheim *(1493–1541)*, has been as widely discussed by historians as any other practitioner of the sixteenth century, yet he remains an enigmatic figure. Unconventional and with a difficult personality, much of his restless life was spent as a wandering physician and trenchant critic of Galenic medicine. Moreover, his own complex theory of disease with its emphasis on external causes – specific agents foreign to the body (e.g., from God, from stars or from minerals) – led

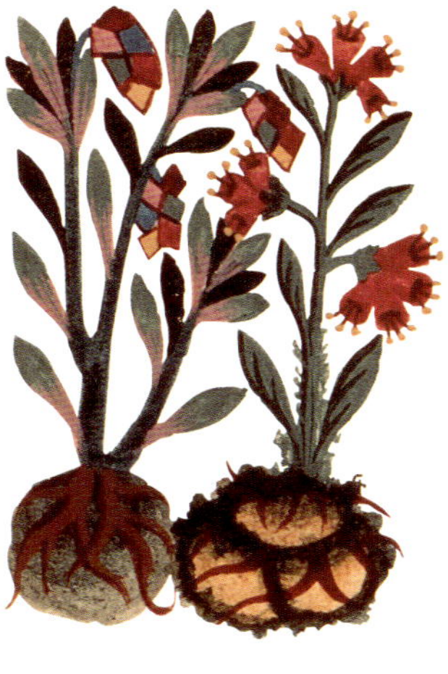

ABOVE European explorers undertook quite extensive research on the herbs of Mesoamerica in the sixteenth century, but despite their systematic efforts, few medicinal plants were actually introduced to Europe as a result.

THE LADY ALLINS WATER WITH SOME ADDITIONS

This is an example of an authentic herbal recipe from the end of the sixteenth century. Such recipes were not only prescribed by physicians, they were also in circulation as popular household remedies.

Take of:

- Cardus:
- Jesop:
- Scordum:
- Rew:
- Pimpernell:
- Turmentel:
- Scabuss:
- Peneroyal:
- Angelica:
- Egremony:
- Wormewood:
- Salandine:
- Wood sorril:
- Rosse a Solas:
- Dragon:
- Sage:
- Balme:
- Mungwort:
- Betaney:
- Hairewort:
- Hartstounge:
- Sentorie:
- Fumetorie:
- Buridge flowers:
- Buglous flowers:
- Marigold flowers:
- Roasmarie:
- Roots Liguors:
- Seader: Roots:
- Genson: Roots:
- Snack: Roots:

of each [root] an ounce & half

Of each of these herbs thire must be taken one Good hand full the Roasmary only excepted whereof you must take tow good hand fulls these herbes must be stript from their stalks. and shread without being washed at all in water and the roots must be cut into small peces and brussed a little then boath roots & herbs being mingled well together must be put to step for 24 howers in tow quarts of cannary wine and three quarts or white wine being close stopt yt no ayer get to it then Distill it in a could still with a gentle fire for towards the later end it will be very apt to burne. This quantaty is usually tow still fulls and will get something more then 4 quarts of water: which must be taken about 4 or 5 sponfull at a time being made bloud warme and sweetned with a little loafe sugar.

Paracelsus to argue for new, specific therapies. He did much to encourage the chemical search for the quintessences (what, today, we would call active constituents) of medicinal plants, as well as to popularize the use of chemical remedies. Although his immediate and considerable posthumous influence varied from place to place, his enduring legacy was a widespread questioning of many existing treaments and the stimulation of intense debates between Galenists and Paracelsians.

Paralleling Paracelsus' life-work and his interest in essences (and, to some degree, perhaps influenced by him), there was at this time a sharpening interest in distillation. This, which extends back to ancient times, was used to prepare an increased range of herbal remedies known as 'waters' and 'spirits'. In 1576 English surgeon George Baker wrote, 'We see plainly before our eyes, that the virtues of medicines by chimicall distillation are made more available, better and more efficacie than those medicines which are in use'. By the end of the century, countless recipes like that featured in the accompanying box (*see at left*) were in circulation not just among physicians and other practitioners, but as household recipes, at least in the upper social circles. The recipe, from a single handwritten sheet, is included here in its entirety, not only because of its intrinsic interest, but also because the erratic spelling is testimony to how mistakes were readily made in copying.

By the early eighteenth century, enthusiasm for distilled waters had declined markedly in professional medicine. John Quincy's popular *Compleat English Dispensatory* (e.g., *1719* edition) stated that many waters in the *London Pharmacopoeia* were 'good for nothing, or at least not worth distilling.' He added a condescending note that such preparations were, nevertheless, held 'in some esteem amongst nurses and ignorant people, and upon that account made, or pretended to be made and kept in the shops.' One has also to remember that some distilled items, such as rose water prepared by distilling water and rose petals, persisted in health care as well as in cosmetics and the kitchen. Not only have vast quantities of the water been incorporated in what has probably been one of the most widely-used skin preparations of all time, namely cold cream (often credited to Galen, hence also known as Galen's Cerate), but also it has been and is still widely used in cakes and desserts.

Spirits with their alcohol content were not criticized so harshly at the time. Cordials or cordial waters – generally distilled from spirits, herbs, spices and sugar – sometimes kept in handsome cordial chests, were commonly recommended as restoratives to refresh the spirits in swoonings and faintness, to strengthen the stomach, invigorate the heart, and such uses as to encourage sweating. Elixirs were still listed in pharmaceutical manuals in the early twentieth century and served as a legacy of cordials; some, too, are to be found today and, for many people, add to the mystique of herbal lore.

Distilled medicines straddled home and professional medicine, as did all aspects of herbal medicine. Self-sufficiency and self-care were, generally speaking, supported by the same medical knowledge, if not by the experience, possessed by well-educated physicians and other practitioners. The line between the medical knowledge of lay people and that of practitioners, as in earlier times, continued to be poorly delineated. On occasions, regular practitioners tried out recipes from a lay person, as did an English doctor called John Symcotts. In 1636 he had been attending a woman for a purpuric condition during pregnancy and noted: 'A beggar woman told the patient that she would recover if she took shepherd's purse in her broth. Hence I ordered her a broth of plantain, periwinkle, shepherd's purse, etc.' Symcott subsequently used this remedy in another case, so perhaps it was not just patronizing the first patient's wishes.

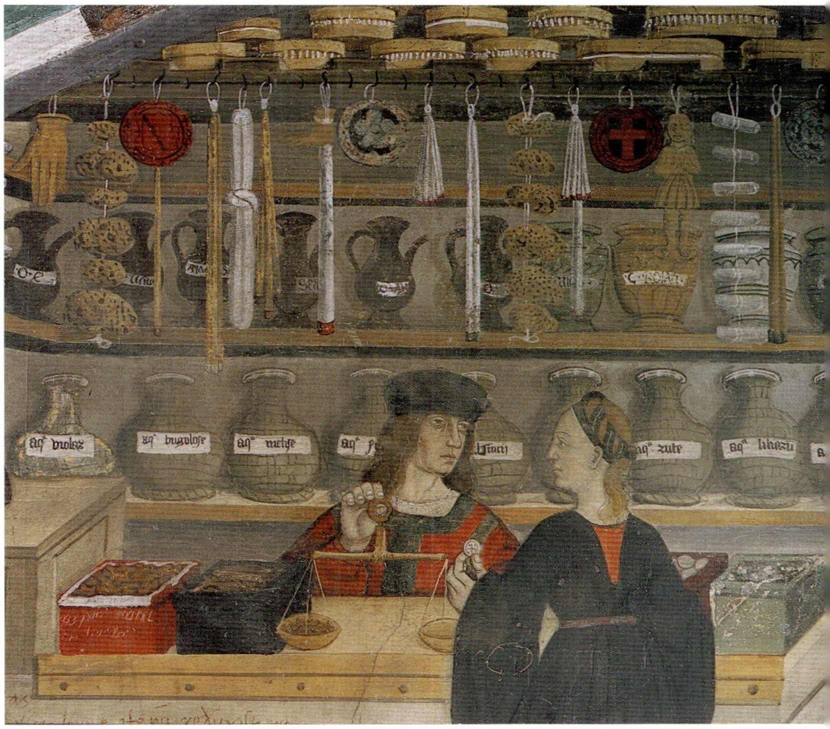

ABOVE This fifteenth-century Italian fresco from Issogne Castle in Val d'Aosta shows a patient buying a remedy from a prosperous-looking pharmacist. The rise of pharmacy as a specialist practice in the West had begun in the twelfth century. At a later date Paracelsus argued for reform in pharmaceutical practices.

Trying one medicine, then another, was routine for many people, though perhaps dissenting minister Richard Baxter *(1615–1691)* was not typical. He wrote that he had 'at several times the advice of no less than six and thirty physicians, by whose order I us'd drugs without number almost, which God thought not fit to make successful for a cure.' On one occasion he made up his own remedy of 'heath and sage, as being very drying and astringent without any acrimony: I boiled much of them in my beer instead of hops, and drank no other: When I had used it a month my eyes were cured, and all my tormenting tooth-aches and such other maladies.'

Resources for health care varied and there were medicines for the rich and for the poor. Elegant pomanders that hung around the necks of the wealthy were popular in the sixteenth and seventeenth centuries to hold aromatic substances purported to ward off disease, and as part of the long-standing way of dealing with bad air. Some pomanders opened into partitioned segments, each labelled for, say, ambergris, musk, lemon and rosemary. However, as English physician Thomas Moffet observed in 1655:

> *And the poorer sort [of people] may perfume their chambers with baies, rosemary, and broom it self. Make also a vaporous perfume in this sort. Take off mastick and frankincense, of each an ounce, citron pils, calamint roots, herb grass dried, and cloves of each three drams; make all into a gross powder, and boil it gently in a perfuming pot with spike-water and white wine.*
>
> THOMAS MOFFET, PHYSICIAN

Such aromatic fumigations (and others included pine rosin and 'tar') were also recommended at the time for burning on coals or in chafing dishes. One writer indicated that, at least in 1636, wormwood, rue and thyme were the cheapest herbs for strewing on floors – another way that was recommended to counteract the effects of bad air.

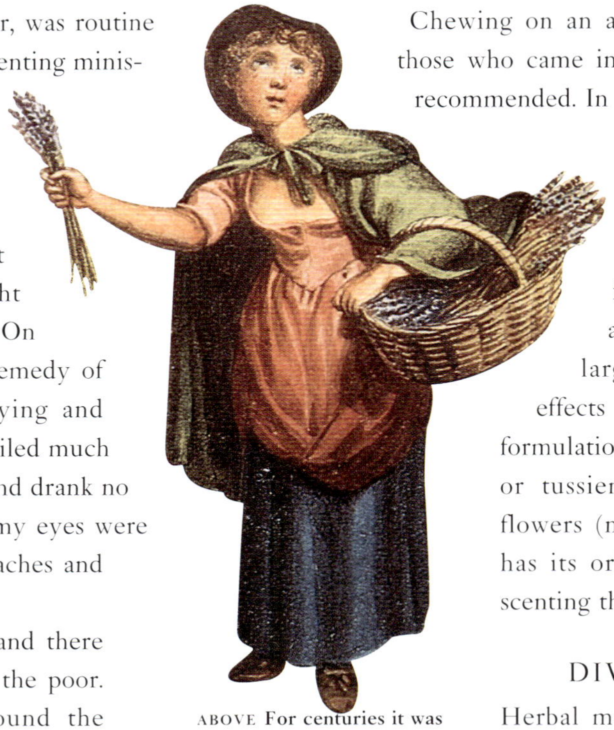

ABOVE For centuries it was believed that aromatic herbs were effective in warding off the effects of 'bad air'. This print of a lavender seller on the streets of London dates from 1806.

Chewing on an aromatic plant material, especially by those who came in close proximity to the sick, was also recommended. In 1664 the 'root called sedour' was noted for chewing 'in the company of such persons as are thought to be infected with the contagion' (meaning here the plague). Other botanicals mentioned from time to time for chewing were angelica and zeodary. It is clear that largely forgotten ideas of the harmful effects of bad air lie behind today's countless formulations of potpourri. Likewise, the nosegay or tussiemussie, a little bouquet of fragrant flowers (nowadays regaining some popularity), has its origins in the supposed desirability of scenting the air as much as in decoration.

DIVERSE PRACTITIONERS

Herbal medicine has long been practised by a wide range of practitioners. Because of the increased information arising from the printing revolution, a clear picture emerges of the diversity of unlicensed practitioners and of attitudes to them in the sixteenth and seventeenth centuries. Here we only have space to consider the role of women. Aside from their place in family care, a recurring topic in herbal lore is the role of 'old' or 'country' women (some midwives, many not) who, conventionally, are viewed as coming from humble circumstances. They are in contrast to experienced 'gentlewoman' whose practice, from privileged positions, often extended beyond their family to a community in general.

The knowledge of old women came variously from the oral tradition, experience and, perhaps, from the act of gathering and selling herbs. Some, however, were considered to have acquired their skills as a 'gift' or from such long-standing traditions as being a seventh daughter of a seventh daughter (though the latter concept more commonly applied to sons). Noted philosopher Thomas Hobbes *(1588–1679)* was one layperson who preferred to trust experienced old women rather than learned but inexperienced physicians. However, as more critical attitudes developed in the seventeenth century toward existing therapy, the value of experience without theory was often discounted, at least by physicians. Women and other lay practitioners were seen as employing 'old-fashioned', ineffective herbs. On the other hand, the eighteenth-century sentiments of

English physician and naturalist John Berkenhout (in his *Symptomatology, 1784)* continued to reflect some of the long-standing ambivalences with regard to the efficacy of regular therapy on the part of many:

> *I do not deny that many lives might be saved by the skilful administration of proper medicines; but a thousand indisputable facts convince me, that the present established practice of physic in England is infinitely destructive of the lives of his Majesty's subjects. I prefer the practice of old women, because they do not sport with edged tools: being unacquainted with the powerful articles of the* Materia Medica.
>
> JOHN BERKENHOUT, *SYMPTOMATOLOGY*

Not everyone was so comfortable, for there was always a lurking suspicion that countrywomen had a special knowledge of 'female' remedies, especially abortifacients, as well as of magic and witchery. The extent of the usage of abortifacients over time, as well as the effectiveness of many of them, is debatable, but some, such as pennyroyal and rue, remain very much part of herbal lore. Negative thoughts regarding the practices of 'old' women, especially with regard to their possible roles in abortion and in witchery, tend to overshadow the laudable activities of women with formal qualifications in times past, though they were relatively few in number. The situation has, of course, changed radically in the twentieth century. The old woman herbalist is now a rarity, at least in Western societies, while the increasing number of qualified women physicians generally have no knowledge of herbs.

THE EIGHTEENTH TO THE TWENTIETH CENTURIES

If we have a relatively clear picture of the diversity of practitioners around 1700, the eighteenth century raises many issues about 'Every Man His Own Physician'. Not only was self-care part and parcel of the Age of Enlightenment's faith in the diffusion of knowledge, but it was also part of a new medical commercialism. The latter ranged from a plethora of marketed medicines to the emergence of medicine chests for the home, stocked with herbs, chemicals and prepared medicines such as laudanum, derived from opium. The century, too, saw repeated calls for the reform of medicine and medicines, not only among physicians (at least academically-minded ones), but also influential laymen such as the founder of Methodism, John Wesley *(1703–1791)*. Wersley's popular, recipe-style *Primitive Physick (1747)*, with its emphasis on empiricism, is often viewed as a milestone in popular medicine, but its call for medical reform perhaps contributed to feelings that popular medical beliefs needed to be challenged and curtailed, as did excesses in the number of ingredients in many medicines.

There had, in fact, been a questioning of very complex medicinal preparations (polypharmacy) in the seventeenth century by critics of Galen, particularly through the posthumous influence of Paracelsus (see above) and such figures as Jean Baptiste van Helmont *(1579–1644)* and his posthumous work *Ortus medicinae (1648)*. Van Helmont criticized such common therapeutic measures as sweating, purging, blood-letting and vomiting, as well as the use of polypharmaceutical medicines. He described the latter as 'the confused hotch-potch mixtures in the shops, the betrayers of ignorance and uncertainty,' and added, 'the [Galenists] hope that if one thing help not, another will help: and so (through the preachment of Herbarists) they joyn many things together with each other.'

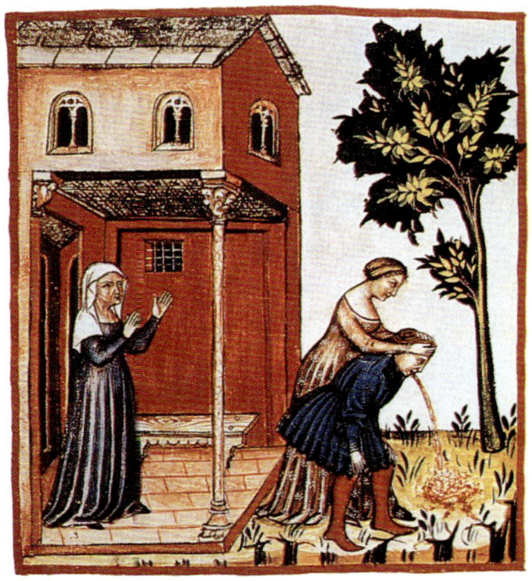

ABOVE The eighteenth century was a time of medicinal reform. Even earlier, writers like van Helmont had disputed the value of age-old Galenic remedies to induce vomiting or purging.

An English translation of van Helmont's work appeared in 1662 in the midst of growing squabbles in London between the supporters of chemical medicine and those who retained faith in the 'tried and tested', more herbally-oriented, Galenic therapy. Some 'chemical' physicians and 'chemists' were also concerned with bringing about social reform and, though they tended to take extreme positions, they contributed much to the atmosphere of change. Others were less overtly revolutionary such as physician Thomas Willis *(1621–1675)*. Well known in his own time, his *Pharmaceutice rationalis (Rational pharmacy) (1674)* encouraged critical attempts to improve therapy. Willis' work in applying new theories of physiology served as an impetus to simplify complex herbal medicines so as to minimize potential incompatibilities between ingredients.

THE MOVE TOWARDS SIMPLIFICATION

In the eighteenth century the movement toward simplification gathered momentum with considerable revisions of various pharmacopoeias. In 1774 British physician John Pringle *(1707–1782)*, writing to Albrecht von Haller about the new Edinburgh pharmacopoeia, gives a sense of the commitment to change:

'I do not think that we have yet thoroughly got the better of the prejudice that, by compounding many simple medicines together, we can answer several indications at once, and getting each particular, though it is the smallest dose, to equal the force of the whole simple in the largest.

You will find a list of simples, small in comparison with that of the other Pharmacopoeias and indeed of that of the last edition of their own Pharmacopoeia, but they seem to judge well in confining the number to that which was really useful and, being so, could with the better countenance insist on apothecaries keeping every individual simple fresh and good.'

Behind much eighteenth-century reform and simplification of pharmacopoeias was the application of developments in chemistry in order to find the 'real virtues of simples' and to standardize the composition of medicines. This was encouraged from a number of quarters. It was articulated by, for example, William Lewis in his successful *Experimental History of the Materia Medica (1761)*, where, like other writers of his time, he laid down a manifesto of sorts, 'to examine the several substances which are or have been in repute, with a view to ascertain, as far as possible, their real powers, and to establish this important part of medicine on a just foundation.'

A detailed study of the reform of medicines reveals that many herbs went out of favour, at least from professional if not home medicine. The compilers of the *Edinburgh Pharmacopoeia*, with revisions of the book every decade or so, reduced the list of 590 simples in 1735 to 222 in 1803. The *London Pharmacopoeia*, with fewer but more drastic revisions, rationalized the 1722 list of over 600 vegetable items to under 200 in 1809. In many cases the revision seems to have been done with confidence that the herbs were ineffective. In other cases it seems that they were pushed to one side as 'old-fashioned'. Some ask, did the passion for reform go too far? Obviously, such considerations have to be taken into account when assessing the historical usage of a plant and whether or not its record over time suggests efficacy.

BELOW 'The Apothecary's Shop' by Italian artist Pietro Longhi *(1702–1785)*. In the eighteenth century the use of herbs medically was considerably simplified.

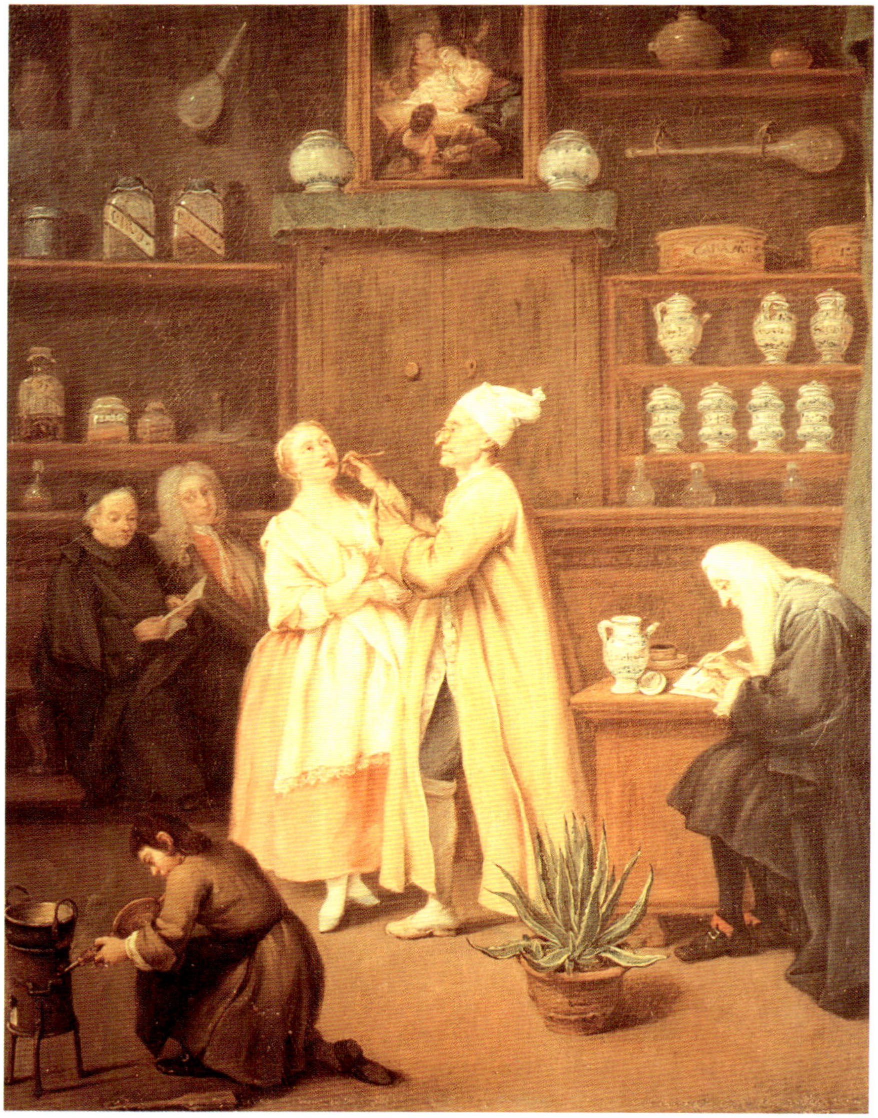

WILD AND TAME PLANTS

Herbalists commonly distinguish wild from cultivated plants. The latter, sometimes referred to rather charmingly as 'tame', are considered to make weaker medicines than plants harvested from the wild. Such folk knowledge reflects a long-standing recognition of a relationship that exists between the medicinal properties of a plant and the nature of the environment in which it grows.

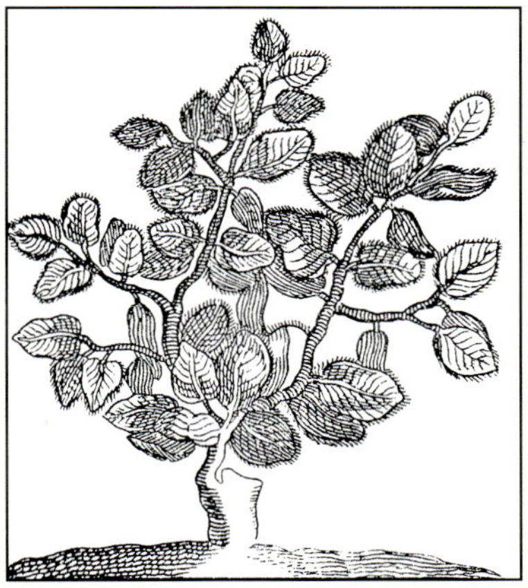

ABOVE A seventeenth-century engraving of the cinchona tree. An established remedy for malaria even then, when reliable supply from South America later became a problem, cultivated plantations were established in Asia.

Environment is important in the cultivation of medicinal plants, as has been appreciated for a long time, especially for plants cultivated as spices and perfume materials as well as medicines. In the nineteenth century, for example, it was found that commercial growing conditions for good quality lavender were better near Hitchin, Hertfordshire, in England, than near Mitcham in Surrey. In 1856 it was also noted that 'the ground for a plantation of lavender should not be surrounded by high hedges, [nor] in the immediate neighbourhood of any trees, which tend to retain too much moisture upon the plants, and thus cause the spring frost to cut off the flowers.'

Notwithstanding difficulties of finding the right conditions, the cultivation of herbs has often been promoted. This is not only for plants difficult to obtain in sufficient quantities, but also so as to help standardize quality. Various illustrations of this come from the nineteenth century with, for example, triumphant stories of overcoming problems of importation of cinchona bark of consistent quality (many species were used) from South America. Fragile seedlings were transported from there in order to establish cinchona plantations in India and the Far East, where the bark of the tree was much needed for the treatment of malaria.

Today, with a growing world market for herbs and great concerns over the perils of removing plants from their natural habitats and so potentially endangering species, cultivation is becoming an increasingly important issue.

NEW PLANTS

Reform and the elimination of items from the existing materia medica did not diminish the search for new medicines and attempts to improve existing ones. The celebrated cinchona bark, also known as Peruvian bark or the Bark (the source of quinine to be isolated in the nineteenth century), introduced from Peru in the seventeenth century, continued to preoccupy the minds of many. The tremendous difficulties in getting regular and authentic supplies led to various odysseys of plant exploration that remain an inspirational part of herbal lore. There was, for instance, the tragedy of Joseph de Jussieu, who, after almost 30 years of struggle in the jungles of South America searching for and documenting the sources of cinchona bark, had his specimens stolen as he was about the leave for Europe in 1761. Shortage of supply and uncertain origins of different commercial cinchona barks led to many searches for alternatives and for effective preparations of the bark especially since, as was said in 1772, 'many patients have an almost invincible aversion to it in powder form.' Ultimately, no alternative replaced the bark as a specific for the treatment of the feverish condition 'ague', which was generally malaria.

Part of the interest in the cinchona story is the legend that its introduction to the West emerged out of a local traditional remedy. Another example is the introduction of foxglove (*Digitalis purpurea*) by physician William Withering *(1741–1799)*. In 1785 he published *An Account of the Foxglove and some of its Medical Uses: with Practical Remarks on Dropsy, and other Diseases*. There, he indicates that he was encouraged to pursue studies after recognizing that foxglove was an active ingredient in a 'family receipt for the cure of dropsy... that had long been kept a secret by an old woman in Shropshire'. Later he heard about similar

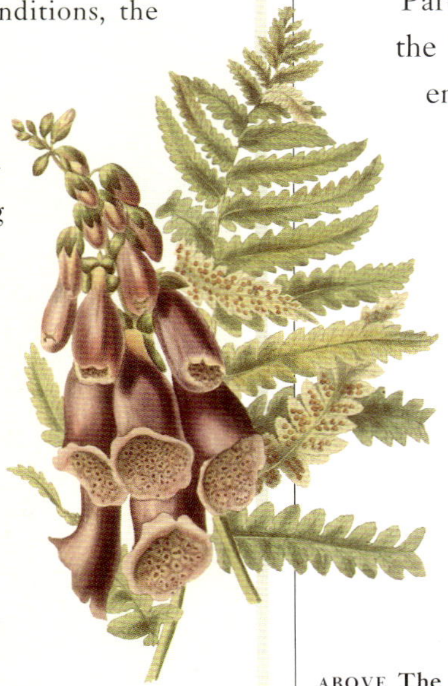

ABOVE The use of foxglove to treat dropsy was pioneered by William Withering in 1785. He drew on local traditional practices for his inspiration.

recipes as well as the success by another physician of 'an empirical exhibition of the root of the Foxglove, after some of the first physicians of the age had declared that they could do no more' for one of Withering's friends.

What is so striking about Withering's book is what we call the scientific approach in evaluating digitalis, including the establishment of appropriate dosage for treating dropsy. However, it is appropriate – in the light of many romantic accounts of the discovery of foxglove – to emphasize that Withering's work did not, in the hands of others, lead immediately to effective treatment of heart conditions. In fact, preparations of digitalis, after much inappropriate use in the nineteenth century, only became consistently useful following further pioneer studies published in the early twentieth century.

Another new dimension that was added to eighteenth-century plant therapy was the use of poisonous plants. In the 1760s Viennese physician Anton Störck *(1731–1803)* argued that the following plants, which until then had been little used in medicine, were valued remedies: hemlock (*Conium maculatum*), stramonium (*Datura stramonium*), henbane (*Hyoscyamus niger*), aconite (*Aconitum napellus*), colchicum (*Colchicum autumnale*), meadow anemone (*Anemone pulsatilla*), clematis (*Clematis alba*) and bastard dittany (*Dictamnus albus*). The initial reception of Störck's work was generally positive, and there was soon an acceptance that physiologically potent substances (i.e., poisons) could be an important part of a physician's armamentarium. Despite some influential critics, all the plants promoted by Störck continued to attract attention for some time. One incidental consequence of this innovation for the story of herbal medicine is that this development reinforced a prevailing feeling that the variety of herbs traditionally used by country women and other practitioners were old-fashioned.

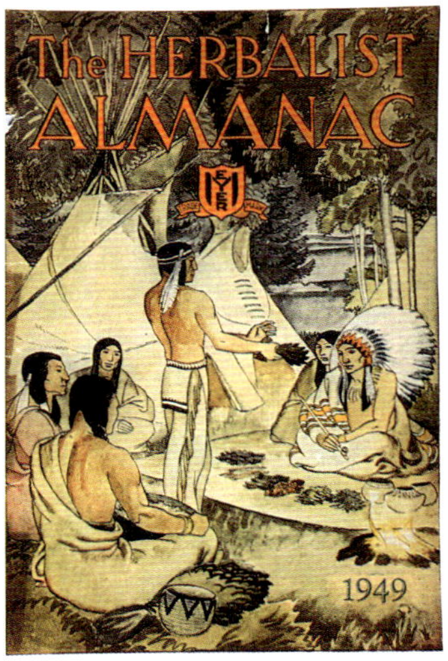

ABOVE Opinions differ as to the extent to which North American aboriginal medicine influenced that of the European settlers.

A further aspect of the new therapeutics in the eighteenth century that attracts the interest of historians is the contributions from the native people of North America. Did they contribute to the health care of the colonists, or did the latter rely almost entirely on medicines imported from Europe? The tantalizing nature of the questions is largely because, while many early accounts of aboriginal practices exist, most were written down in the nineteenth and twentieth centuries. As these are relatively modern records, it is difficult to know how much European information had, by then, been incorporated into aboriginal life. Conflicting interpretations exist among scholars about how much aboriginal medicine was transmitted to colonists. Some early scholars put forward negative opinions about the value of aboriginal herbal knowledge. James Mooney, for instance, in 1897, albeit at a time of much less knowledge of plants than exists nowadays, commented somewhat disparagingly on Cherokee knowledge:

> *Five plants, or 25 per cent of the whole number are correctly used; twelve or 60 per cent, are presumably either worthless or incorrectly used, and three plants, or 15 per cent, are so used that it is difficult to say whether they are of any benefit or not.*
>
> JAMES MOONEY

More recent writings offer differing views. Some believe that North American aboriginal people deserve great respect for adding much knowledge to the regular medicine brought over by the Europeans, while others consider that aboriginal materia medica beyond about ten plants had no major or substantial impact. Whatever the correct interpretation, it is fairly clear that aboriginal treatment influenced colonial home medicine or self-care more than it did regular medicine. Certainly, many significant observations can be found in eighteenth-century writings such as in Jane Colden's botanical notebook. Around 1750 she wrote about *Asclepias tuberosa*, 'the root of this Asclepias taken in powder is an excellent cure for the Colick, about halff a Spoonful at a time. This cure was learn'd from a Canada Indian, & is called in New England Canada Root.' Additionally, a mystique, some say a myth – which still exists – emerged about aboriginal knowledge of plants and medicine. In this connection we have noted 'Indian', or native American, associations emphasized in the advertising of or naming of medicines. A striking number of plants (not just those that are medicinal) have American aboriginal associations in their names, for example, Indian chickweed, Indian hemp, Indian pennyroyal, Indian pink, Indian plantain, Indian sage, squawroot, squawvine and wahoo.

CHINA: TRADITIONAL MEDICINE AND LINKS WITH THE WEST

At least two items, ginseng and rhubarb, of the eighteenth-century materia medica open up questions about another culture, China, and its traditional medicine. What is its character and its influence on Western herbal medicine? Chinese ginseng was brought to the notice of the West in the early eighteenth century by the Jesuit Father Jartoux. He stated that it was a remedy for various weaknesses and other symptoms. This encouraged interest in the North American ginseng, a related species that has never been considered as 'strong' as the *Panax ginseng* species from China. Although both ginsengs attracted interest in eighteenth-century Europe, there was no consensus of opinion about their value. William Woodville, for one, remarked in 1792, 'We know of no proofs of the efficacy of ginseng in Europe and from its sensible qualities we judge it to possess very little power as a medicine.' Nevertheless, the reputation of ginseng continues to intrigue the West.

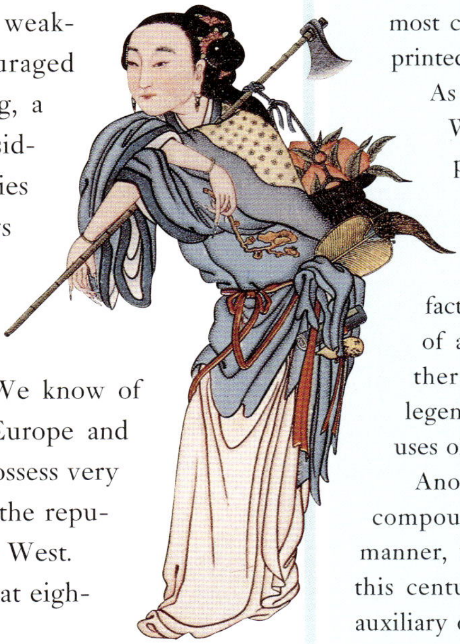

ABOVE China's traditional materia medica is extraordinarily rich.

Of Chinese rhubarb, it has been said that eighteenth-century Europe was swept by a veritable rhubarb mania. Although rhizomes of the plant were known in the West in Graeco-Roman times, its exact source, geographical and botanical, was unknown. A fascinating story exists of the search for origins, extending from the late fifteenth century until the second half of the nineteenth century. Only then was agreement reached that *Rheum officinalis* was the source of true Chinese rhubarb. All other *Rheum* species that had been found and studied up to then were considered far inferior therapeutically. It is not clear whether issues over exotic versus indigenous plants swayed opinion on occasions.

What issues arise from the stories of these two plants as well as a handful of others already mentioned (China root, camphor and ginger) – all entering Western medicine from China? One question, analogous to the one asked about Aztec materia medica, is why there has not been greater influence, in terms of more drugs being introduced? After all, we should bear in mind the richness of the Chinese materia medica with around 5,000 recorded plant species. Moreover, in recent times, many Asian plants have been introduced to Western horticulture without any knowledge of their traditional Chinese medical uses. We

CHINESE HERBAL MEDICINES

One of the striking features of traditional Chinese medicine is the complexity of the theory of herbal medicine; for example, to dispel cold, to counteract yin insufficiency, to stimulate qi and so on. Behind the theory is a long tradition of writings on medicines, which continue to serve as a fountain-head for traditional practice today. Perhaps the most celebrated, compiled by physician Li Shi-zhen, was printed posthumously in 1596.

As 'foreign' as traditional Chinese medicine is to most Westerners, it embraces concepts that have been part of the Western tradition and are still to be found today in alternative, if not in regular, medicine. Aside from the emphasis on restoring balance, noted in the text, one factor – common to the West and the East – is the use of a plant's sensory characteristics to determine its therapeutic properties. In fact, it is said that the legendary emperor Shen Nong learned the medicinal uses of herbs by tasting them.

Another noteworthy similarity is that widely used compounded medicines are formulated in a rational manner, with many analogies to Western medicines until this century. There is, for instance, a principal herb and auxiliary ones that promote the effectiveness of the principal and also counteract side-effects. A further component can be present to improve palatability. Many classical Chinese fomulae are sold as over-the-counter medicines, but obviously this does not allow tailoring of the formula to the individual needs of the patient, as would be done by a practitioner. Nor, of course, do commercial preparations involve the patient having to prepare them at home, say as a 'soup'. When, for example, a honeysuckle-forsythia remedy, perhaps containing nine herbs, is brought home from a Chinese pharmacy to treat 'flu, the ingredients are placed in a pan covered with cold water, brought to the boil, and then simmered for about five minutes. The 'juice' is drunk hot.

One well-known Chinese 'herbal' to have reached the West in recent years is the *Barefoot Doctor's Manual (1970)*. The work is designed to be used in rural areas by 'paramedics'. It is eclectic in so far as it contains the herbs and preparations used by formally educated practitioners, as well as those described as folk remedies. It shows that many traditional Chinese herbal medicines are used more on the basis of experience than on complex herbal theory.

ask the question, too, in the context of links between Asia and the West since ancient times. Aside from a maritime spice route, there was the famed Old Silk Road from China to the Middle East. Not only was this used in Graeco-Roman times for exporting Chinese silk to the West, but also for the import and export of many other products. Disagreement exists over the quantities of medicinals that were traded via these routes in ancient times. However, it seems clear that the enormous distance and consequent expense limited quantities and restricted items, notably aromatic spices, to all but the wealthy. In turn, this encouraged substitution and fraud.

If distances limited interest in and hence the use of Chinese herbs in the West, were other factors also relevant, such as differing theories of medicine? As was observed in connection with the introduction of New World drugs, acceptance of new drugs was partly related to them being rationalized on the basis of Western concepts of the time. However, although some students consider that differing concepts inhibited Western interest in Chinese herbs, those that reached the West came without Chinese theory. Moreover, while this theory is based on all things in nature – including humans – being in a sense one, and each possessed of the qualities of yin and yang in varying balanced proportions, such concepts are hardly remote from the notions of balance in the humoral system that has been an enduring influence on Western medicine. In both systems, when balance is lost, disease occurs. 'Rebalancing' was undertaken in a variety of ways. Chinese acupuncture, which has attracted interest in the West in recent years, has long been popular, although herbs have been the mainstay of treatment in China. The way the latter are used resonates, too, with the polypharmacy of Western medicine. Compounded prescriptions are the general pattern of prescribing and, even today, single herbs are rarely used by most traditional Chinese practitioners.

It is widely felt that traditional Chinese medicine has been resistant to change over the centuries; the first classic text, the *Yellow Emperor's Inner Canon*, compiled from earlier traditions in the first century BC or a little later, is still a working text, as are many ancient Chinese 'herbals'. However, although core concepts have been strikingly consistent, it is incorrect to suggest that Chinese medicine has been unchanging. The medical beliefs and practices that originated in China absorbed much from India, Tibet, Central and South-East Asia and, since the late nineteenth century, from the West. All traditional systems change over time. Likewise, key Chinese concepts were absorbed into various cultures.

ALTERNATIVE PRACTITIONERS

One noteworthy feature of nineteenth-century health care was the emergence of 'alternative' botanical practitioners. Although a great diversity of practitioners using herbs has always existed, and although many of them upset regular practitioners, there is little sense of an alternative *movement* in conflict with regular practice until the 1800s. Then, groups of practitioners promoted the use of herbs in ways different from regular medicine.

One of the more noticeable groups were practitioners of homeopathy. Widely adopted on both sides of the Atlantic, homeopathy was founded by the German Samuel Hahnemann *(1753–1843)* and is best known for using infinitesimally small doses of medicines. For the most part, homeopathy employed, and continues to do so, the range of herbs once used within the framework of herbal medicine in general. The majority of physicians in English-speaking countries were vigorously opposed to it. American physician Oliver Wendell Holmes' attack on homeopathy in 1842, 'Homeopathy and its Kindred Delusions', continues to be revered.

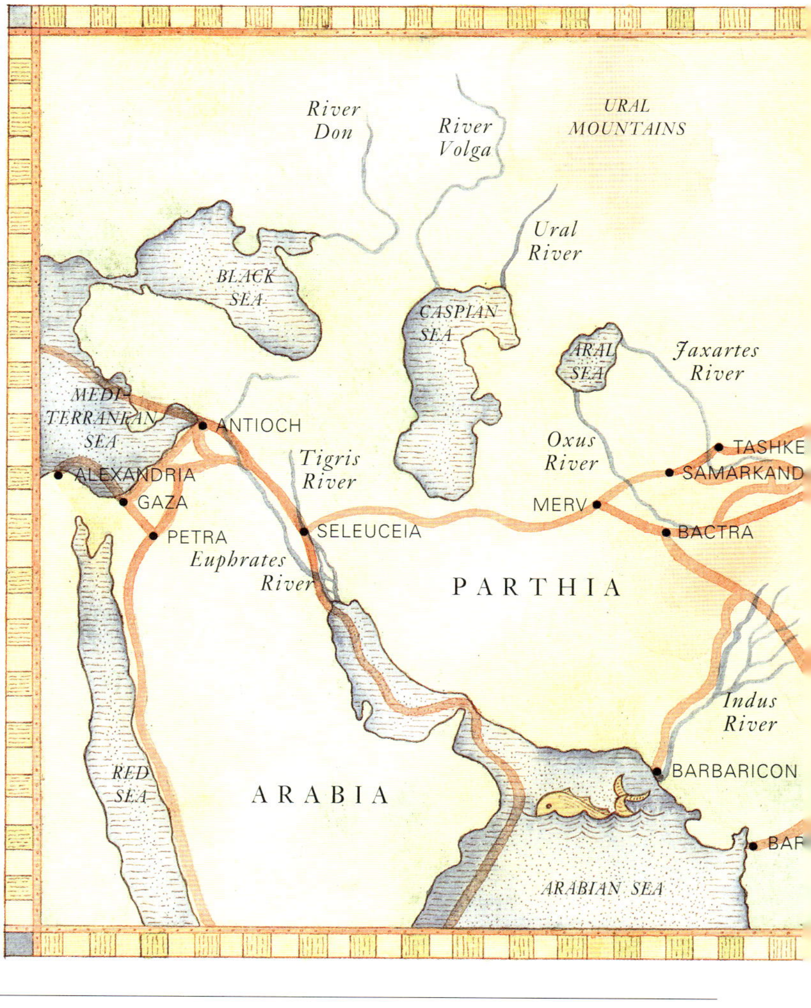

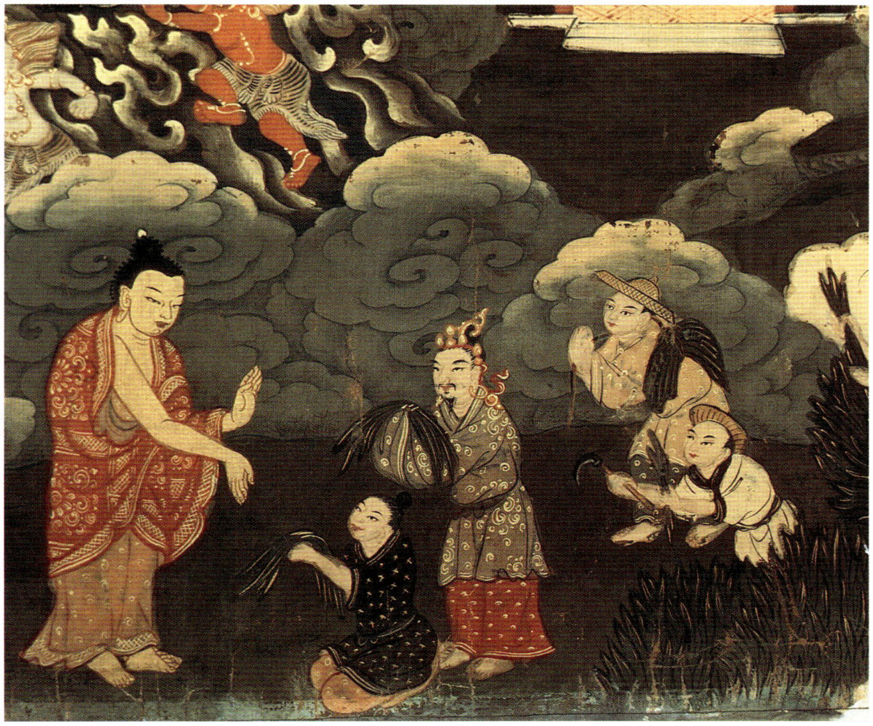

FLOWER REMEDIES

Homeopathy is practised in different ways, from the 'classical' to the 'unconventional'. Additionally, related treatments have emerged. Recently, Bach remedies (flower remedies), named after the British physician Edward Bach *(1880–1936)*, have become increasingly popular. They are recommended primarily for helping with emotional aspects of illness. Moreover, it is not surprising that certain Bach remedies are among many recommendations for the herbal treatments of today's ubiquitous problem of stress.

Bach developed his remedies from a belief that the dew formed on flowers became impregnated with the flower's healing 'energies'. The collection of dew was obviously tedious and laborious, and instead Bach made preparations in sunlight by floating freshly picked flowers (e.g., crab apple, honeysuckle, wild rose) on water. Significant differences exist between Bach and regular homeopathic remedies. One is that the former, while being prepared according to carefully laid-out guidelines, are not 'potentized'; in other words, additional 'energy' is not conveyed to the remedy during its preparation, as is the case with homeopathic medicines. The underlying concepts also offer sharp contrasts. Unlike homeopathic theory, Bach argued that the flower energy prevented mental attitudes becoming physical ailments. 'Disease is in essence the result of conflict between the Soul and the Mind,' he said.

It is tempting to see the uses of the Bach remedies – recommended, for example, for apprehension, indecision and loneliness – as having some kinship with the 'language of flowers'. This, commonly, has more to do with love and morals, but it also speaks to emotional states and well-being. Symbolism and emotions are very much part of the culture of flowers, as they are of herbal medicines in general.

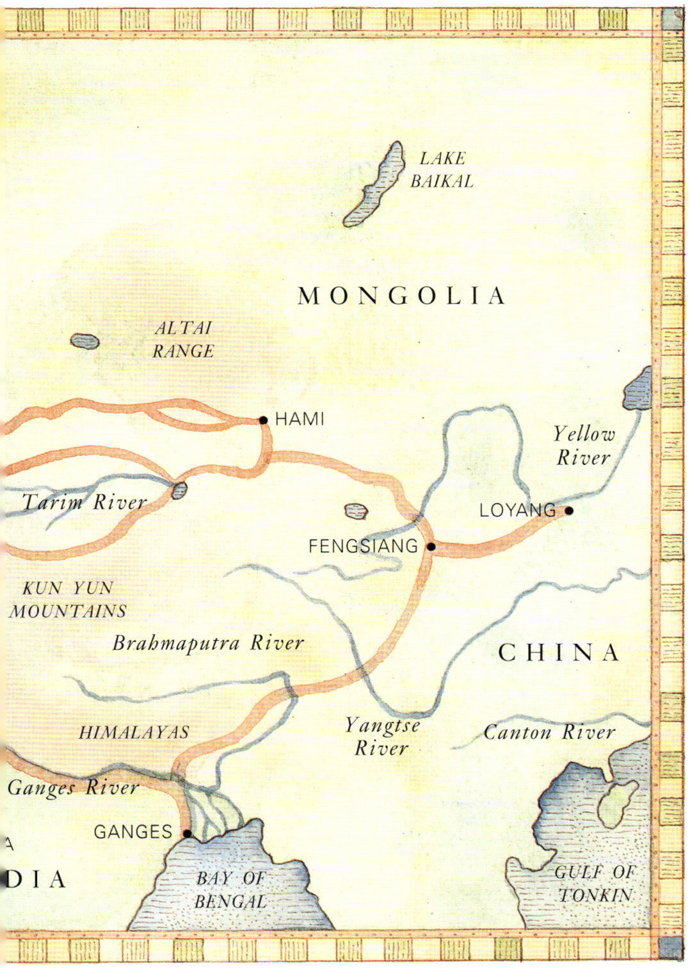

ABOVE An eighteenth-century Tibetan painting showing the Buddha being offered herbs. Tibetan medicine was strongly influenced by Buddhism.

LEFT The map shows the route of the Silk Roads from Loyang in China to India, and to Antioch, Petra and Alexandria in the Middle East. As well as silk, spices and medicinal products were also traded along these routes in Graeco-Roman times.

BELOW Edward Bach believed that his flower remedies were infused with healing 'energies' absorbed from a variety of flowers.

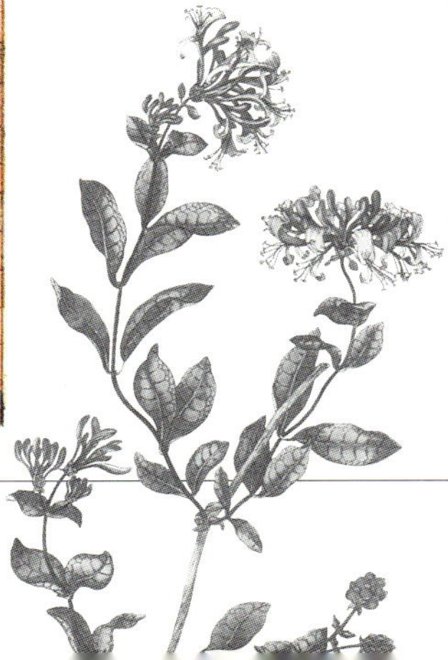

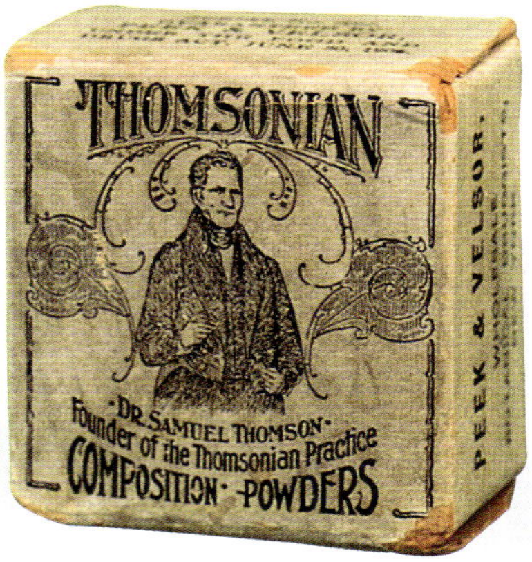

ABOVE A box of Thomsonian Composition Powders. Thomsonian medicine rejected medical orthodoxy in favour of medicinal herbs.

An example of a more limited movement, although not without influence on the alternative herbal movement of today, is Thomsonian medicine established in the United States by Samuel Thomson *(1769–1843)*. In line with many who have expressed disquiet with professional medicine, Thomson said that he learned about herbs from an old woman; then, after personal success in curing his own ailments, he promoted a medical system that achieved lay popularity partly through its relatively simple treatment concept of balancing excess body heat or cold. Thomson opposed the so-called 'heroic' administration of large doses of calomel and the letting of considerable quantities of blood that characterized much regular medical treatment at the time. Of the nearly 70 medicinal herbs he recommended for treating illness, lobelia and cayenne pepper are considered the core ones.

Thomsonianism, which has been called a people's health movement, began to change in the 1830s because some of its practitioners strived for more 'scientific respectability'. Splinter groups, each of which has its own fascinating story, emerged. Thomsonian teachings were spread initially to Great Britain by AI Coffin. Like Thomson, Coffin's appeal was a popular one, which engendered the ire of physicians. One wrote to the editor of the *Pharmaceutical Journal* on 5 August 1849:

> *I want you to have from me a short article on 'Coffinism.' Not on coffins, but on 'Dr. Coffin.' Sometime ago, a patient died in my neighbour-hood from the enormous doses of lobelia inflata [given] under Coffin's recomd. He is a quack...*
>
> LETTER TO THE *PHARMACEUTICAL JOURNAL (1849)*

Certainly, Thomson's favoured lobelia led to, apparently verified, deaths from overdosage.

Along with the 'alternative' herbal practitioners, many other herbalists practised within the framework of the Western tradition as reflected in the writings of Gerard, Culpeper, Wesley and other popular medical authors. In 1810, G. Swain, in the mountains of North Carolina, offered thoughts on his development as a herbal practitioner:

> *I found myself under the necessity of keeping a few simples for cases of emergency, and for the want of advice of a physician I was compelled to consult such books as Domestic Medicine, Family Physician, Primitive Physick and what not. Although I ever detested the idea of a plowman invading the office and assuming the character of a physician, yet necessity has no law and a man will commit sacrilege to save life!*
>
> G. SWAIN, 1810

IMPROVING MEDICINES

Concerns about the quality of herbs and herbal preparations received even more attention in the nineteenth century, with concerted efforts to apply new scientific knowledge, especially from chemistry, to the subject. A significant development – in line with the efforts, since the time of Paracelsus, to isolate 'essences' – was the early nineteenth-century extraction of a particular class of plant constituents, alkaloids. This started to have an impact in the early 1820s with morphine and quinine; at least 42 alkaloids were isolated between 1817 and 1898. Since then, thousands have been investigated. Relatively few, however, have found and retained a place in medical practice. Some are relatively recent, such as alkaloids from the Madagascar periwinkle, which are being used for treating certain kinds of leukaemia.

Aside from new, pure constituents, many improvements occurred in the preparation of pills, infusions, tinctures, extracts and so on. To give one

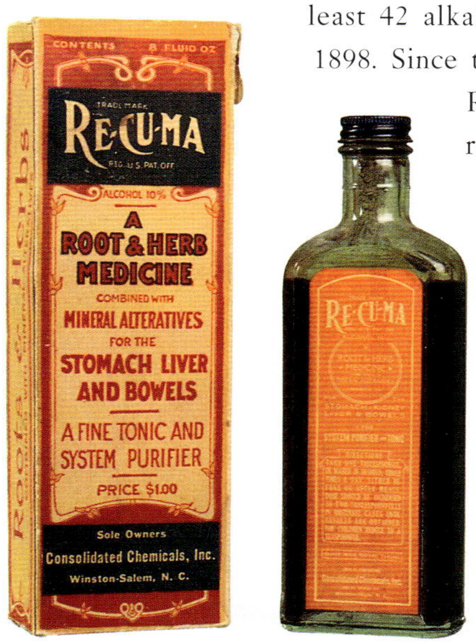

LEFT Like many commercially marketed herbal tonics, Re-cu-ma was highly alcoholic in content.

example, consider the nineteenth-century development in the preparation of extracts. This arose out of concerns over decomposition of constituents arising from excess heat and oxidation, when the initial liquid extract was concentrated, especially when preparing dry extracts. The advance that helped to alleviate the problem was the introduction in 1819 of *in vacuo* evaporation by English chemist John Barry, who wrote:

> *It has not failed to be a matter of regret with medical men that many of the pharmaceutical extracts, although prepared from materials of the same quality, vary considerably in their efficacy, in consequence of having suffered partial destruction in the process of inspissation [evaporation].*
>
> JOHN BARRY, CHEMIST

Barry's new technique did much to overcome heat destruction and oxidation. The new approach was immediately accepted, and technical problems were subsequently improved.

Another significant trend in quality control focused on the crude herb itself. This paralleled the expanding commerce of drugs in the nineteenth century and the development of a new scientific discipline, pharmacognosy – the scientific study of crude drugs. The latter investigated botanical and geographical origins, developed standards for identifying powdered herbs with the microscope, as well as chemical and other tests that detected adulteration, especially of powdered drugs, say, with earth or excessive moisture. However, by the time these and other considerations became routine in quality control, the use of herbal medicines was waning in the face of a growing number of chemical remedies available on the market from around 1900, ranging from aspirin to barbiturates. By around the 1950s, few herbs were used in regular medicine and, as a result, quality control of the herb market lessened.

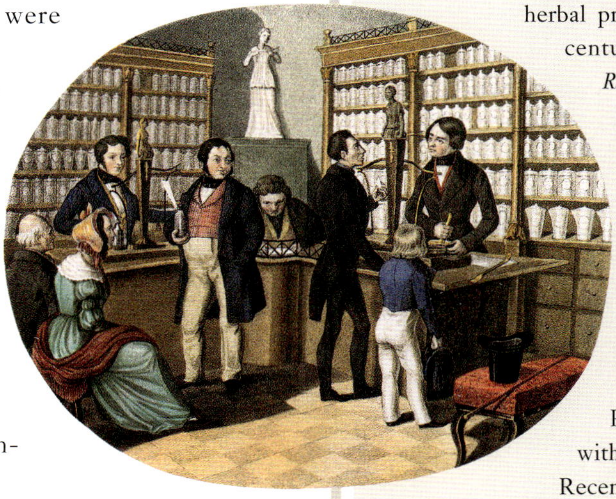

ABOVE An engraving of a German pharmacy in 1838. Both professionalism and commerce in pharmacy were growing at this time.

HERBS AND MODERN PHARMACEUTICALS

Apart from simple teas (aqueous extracts, perhaps sweetened with honey), the preparation of palatable herbal medicines can be complex. Such topics as compounding multi-ingredient medicines and the isolation of active principles with minimal decomposition are discussed in the main text.

Toward the end of the 1800s the production of medicines in the pharmacy and, commonly, small manufacturing companies, was changing. Certain companies, later to become household names (e.g., Burroughs Wellcome, Squibb and Parke, Davis) had research commitments to quality control and to mass-produce new single dosage forms (for instance, capsules, hypodermic injections and tablets). In 1923 Parke, Davis, for example, made clear that its ten preparations of the heart medicine digitalis were all standardized by a biological test developed in the company's laboratory.

Since the 1920s, however, paralleling the growing power of pharmaceutical companies in shaping health care, the spectrum of available products changed; traditional herbal extracts continued to decline with the appearance of new synthetics and major new classes of drugs such as hormones and vitamin supplements and antibiotics. While new herbal products have been introduced in this century, some, such as reserpine from *Rauwolfia serpentina* were swamped by synthetics. The move away from herbal extracts was not accepted by all practitioners. Their argument that whole plant preparations were often safer and more pleasant for patients than isolated active principles often supports the case for the reintroduction of herbal medicines today. Regrettably, these are often marketed without adequate quality control.

Recent books with titles such as *The Design of Drugs to Macromolecular Targets (1992)* reflect the current mainline research approach to find new drugs: the design of synthetic molecules based on knowledge of drug receptors in the body. Searching for pharmacologically active natural products was put on the back burner some years ago by almost all major pharmaceutical research centres. However, signs exist that this is changing; new, exciting chapters in the story of herbs as scientific pharmaceuticals may be forthcoming.

HERBALISM PAST AND PRESENT

Our account of herbal medicine has revealed continual concerns over the quality and effectiveness of medicines. Constant changes in the practice of medical herbalism have taken place within regular medicine and self-care, along with a growth in alternative forms of herbalism. Yet there is little evidence that even the most vigorous critics of particular herbal treatments questioned the overall value of herbal therapy per se. Often it was single herbs and particular preparations that were challenged. Of course, the modern cynic will say, 'That's all they had.'

Questions about effectiveness are difficult to answer and occasion much debate nowadays. There is a tendency to use today's standards of clinical trials as well as current expectations in assessing past therapies; certainly, they are commonly dismissed in the absence of double-blind clinical trials. Yet there is a responsibility to examine past treatments on their own grounds, so to speak, and to consider, where necessary, the magical or religious practices as well as other treatments (e.g., diet) that accompanied the administration of a herb. A close look at all the issues at play in the past shows that a patient's choice of herbs and of practitioner was a key characteristic. Generally, a sick person could readily take charge of his or her treatment, always a significant issue, particularly in chronic conditions.

We must recognize, too, that we do not have the same experience with herbs that people had in the past; we do not know how useful one composition was when compared with a similar one; and few now have the experience of tailoring herbal therapy to individual needs, rather than a particular disease, including the important matter of dosage. It is noteworthy that many herbalists today echo concerns expressed in John Ayrton Paris' popular textbook, *Pharmacologia* (e.g., *1840* edition), over the extensive reform that had been underway in the eighteenth century and later:

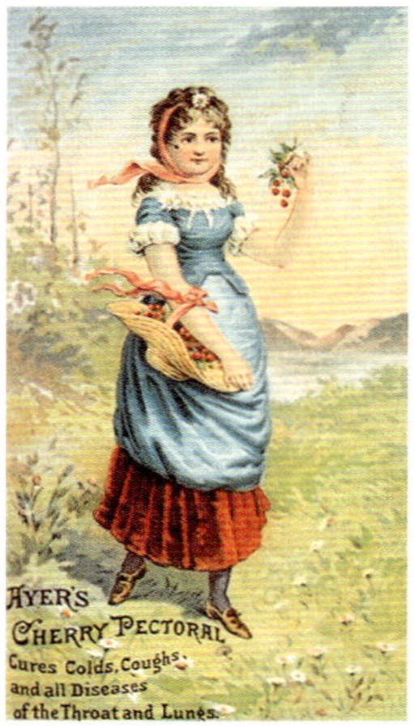

ABOVE An advertisement for Ayers Cherry Pectoral (*c.1900*). Despite its extravagant claims to 'cure all diseases of the throat and lungs', the effectiveness of such proprietary remedies is questionable.

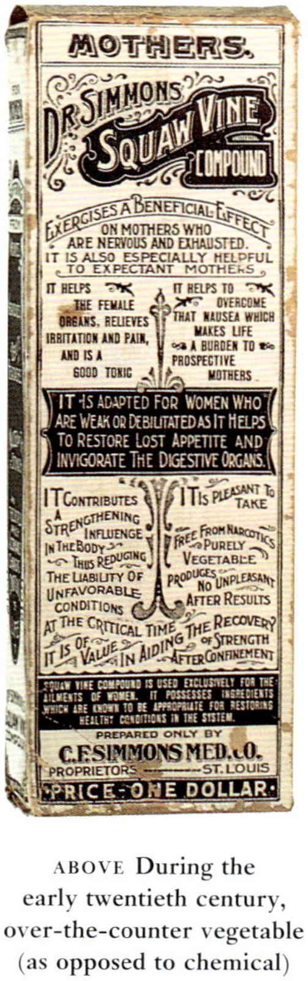

ABOVE During the early twentieth century, over-the-counter vegetable (as opposed to chemical) remedies were promoted.

I would remark that modern pharmacopoeias are shorn so much of old and approved receipts on account of their being extraordinary compounds, as to be almost useless in some cases…
I was informed by the late Dr. Harrison that, in the Horncastle Dispensary, of which he was for several years the physician, he never employed any other remedy for curing the malaria of Lincolnshire than equal parts of Bistorta (astringent) and Calamus Aromaticus (bitter and astringent) neither of which plants, separately, ever produced the least benefit in such cases. Bezelius attempted to form a compound of this description by adding to the bark of the Ash, some Tormentil Root and Ginger; and he [was successful].
Too much importance cannot be assigned to the art that thus enables the physician to adapt and graduate a powerful remedy to each particular case, by a prompt and accurate prescription… If he prescribes upon truly scientific principles he will rarely in the course of his practice compose two formulae that shall, in every respect, be perfectly similar, for the plain reason that he will never meet with two cases exactly alike. Now let me ask what constitutes the essential difference between the true physician and his counterfeit – between the philosopher and the empiric? Simply this – that the latter exhibits the same medicine in every disease, however widely each may differ from the other in its symptoms and character; while the former examines, in the spirit of philosophic analysis, all the existing peculiarities of his patient, and of his discord...and [then] adapts with a sound discretion and with a correct judgement of his [medicinal] agents, such means as may be best calculated to control and correct [the patient's] morbid condition.

JOHN AYRTON PARIS, *PHARMACOLOGIA*

Paris also emphasized that compounded plant remedies possess pharmacological activity not found in the individual plants; indeed, sometimes they possessed unexpected activity.

We see, then, a complicated scene of herbal medicine in the past. Improvements occurred, to be sure, but the many cross-currents of conflicting information paint a complex picture. The current herbal medicine scene in Western societies, generally viewed as alternative to regular medicine, is no less complex, with its eclectic approaches. One of these approaches can be called rational herbalism (the phytomedicines of Germany are generally placed in this category). Although this is loosely defined, it is largely a continuation of part of the regular Western medical tradition since the time of Paracelsus, namely, acceptance of a plant and its activity on the basis of science alone. Indeed, the emphasis on 'science' makes rational herbalism a favoured approach by government and licensing bodies in both developed and developing countries. Some promoters of rational herbalism have training in pharmacognosy, which, as mentioned earlier, once dealt with the identification and quality control of crude drugs. Herbs, then, tend to be approached almost exclusively via constituents rather than as part of therapeutics; in consequence, rational herbalism tends to dismiss such questions as, do herbal tonics and stimulants have a place in current treatment solely on the basis of their long history and widespread acceptance within popular culture?

Rational herbalism contrasts with the eclecticism that can be found in many modern writings. Such eclecticism mixes major systems of world healing – for instance, traditional Chinese medicine, traditional European medicine and Ayurvedic medicine from India. This herbal 'renaissance', as it is often called, or new herbal eclectism, can embrace many other cultures and concepts. These include 'traditional native American medicine,' as well as ancient concepts of alchemy and modern ideas of flows of energy in the body. Such mixing of various cultural traditions and concepts is largely untested and many believe that insufficient experience exists at the moment to assess its validity.

Another form of herbal practice is 'nutritional.' Its proponents rationalize the current use of herbs, at least in part, by their 'natural' nutrients. Nowadays, innumerable herbalists combine nutrition, prevention and treatment. The inherent contradictions that arise from mixing theories is sidestepped by arguments that empirical observations are of greater significance. Such a cavalier approach to theory troubles many. This is especially so among those who fail to consider the possibility that an alternative medical theory, however weak as a theory, may embrace sound observations. The negative feelings that many people harbour in relation to modern herbalism serves as fertile ground for specific criticisms, especially that many herbal medicines are unsafe.

BELOW One of the characteristics of the current herbal renaissance is its eclecticism – it draws inspiration from many cultures, China among them. Pictured here is the second-century Taoist physician Hua Tuo. He is thought to have used herbs as narcotics for surgery.

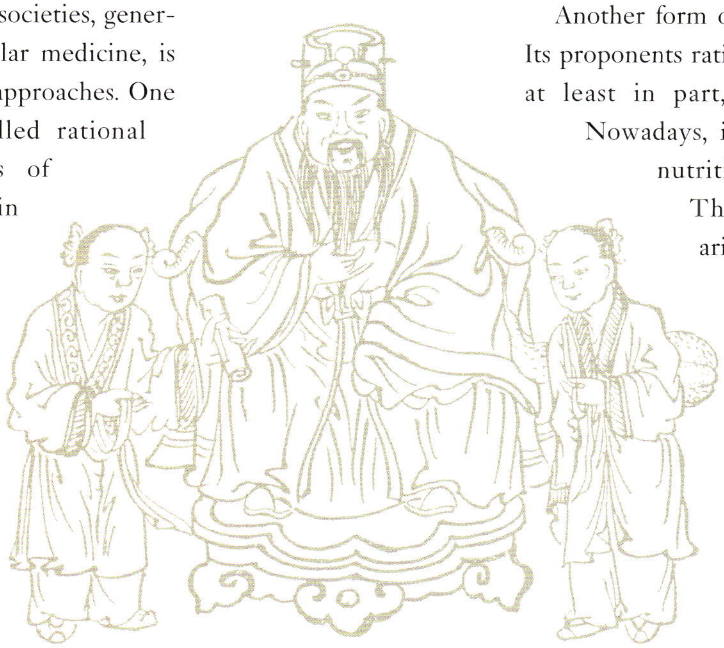

BELOW The Ayurvedic tradition of medicine from India draws on an extensive materia medica, including hundreds of herbs.

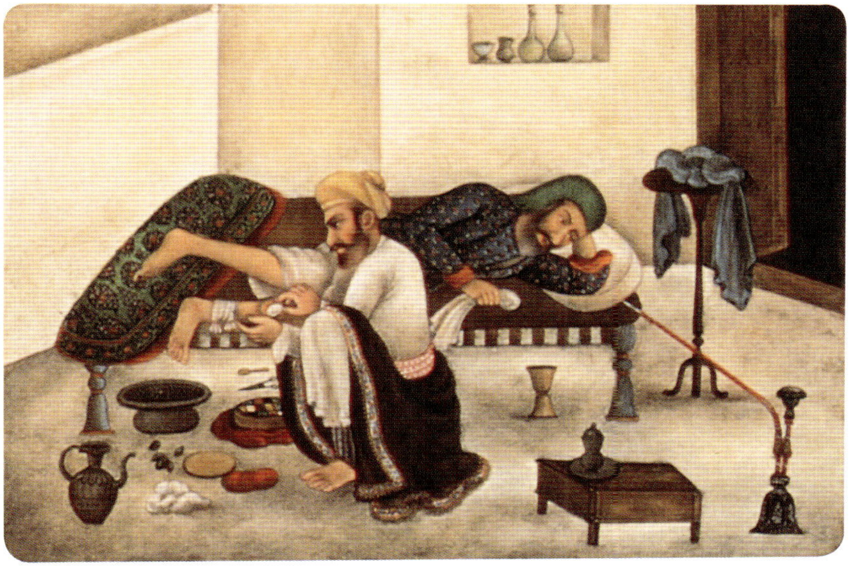

SAFETY ISSUES

It is no secret that health hazards from using herbal remedies can range from acute toxicity to insidious, long-term effects. In recent years, medical and scientific literature has frequently drawn attention to actual and potential liver damage as a result of using herbs. Two well-known remedies, comfrey and sassafras, fall into this category. However, potential harm attends the use of many other herbal therapies if they are not used appropriately. The question arises, is there sufficient information and adequate controls available to protect individuals? Most people, unless they believe in total personal freedom (or they live where substantial controls exist, as in Germany), answer this with a No. They argue that more quality control is needed, whether it be by practitioners or governments.

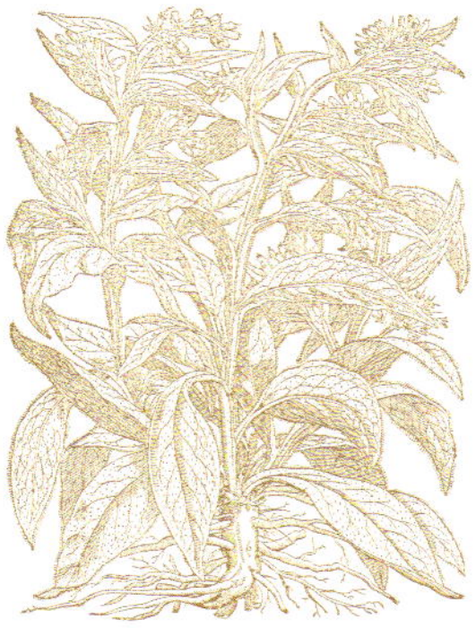

ABOVE Consumption of herbs is not hazard-free. Excessive use of comfrey may cause liver damage.

There is also a need for more general knowledge among users, not only on specific herbs, but also on topics that encourage critical questions. One example is the potential problems that can arise from using common names for herbs, for such names can refer to more than one plant. A recent herbal states that, for a gentian root tonic, 'feel free to substitute Sampson's snakeroot if it is available.' This suggests that Sampson's snakeroot refers only to Gentian species, whereas, in places, it can refer to *Psoralea* spp., *Aristolochia serpentaria*, and *Echinacea angustifolia*. Obviously, very different medicines may be made from these plants. The use of common names is of particular relevance to the recent growth of interest in herbal teas, for there is a growing tendency to use herbs regularly as beverages, rather than, as in the past, medicines. Although problems sometimes arise from the quality of commercial teas and of certain ingredients if taken in large amounts, most health concerns exist over teas brewed from single herbs gathered from the field or purchased from stores.

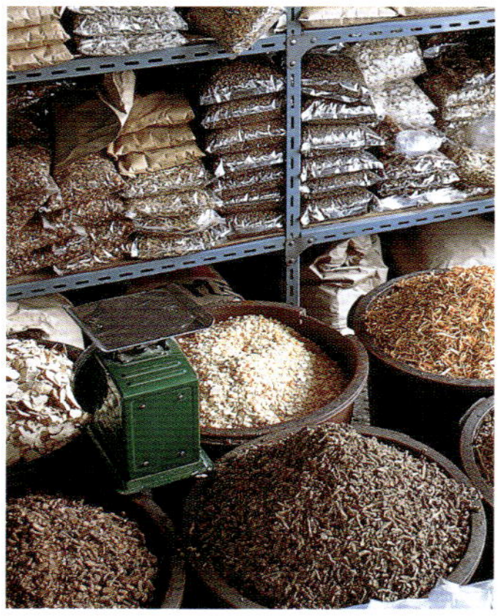

ABOVE Stocks of prepared herbs and traditional medicines awaiting sale in a Chinese market.

One issue runs throughout the story of herbs, namely the relationship that exists between professional medicine and self-care. This chapter has tried to indicate that herbal usage by regular physicians, by families in the home, or by the diverse range of other practitioners had much common ground until the nineteenth century. Then, and into the twentieth century, considerations such as the changing nature of medical practice, the emergence of the pharmaceutical industry, and the increase in commercial practices which were reshaping much of self-care undermined the position of herbal practice as the cornerstone of regular medical therapy. Nowadays, with the Western world's renewed interest in herbal medicine, relationships between regular and herbal medicine need attention. Policies about such relationships in our future schemes of health care are needed. Input is wanted from many people who have knowledge and appreciation of the use of herbs as medicines.

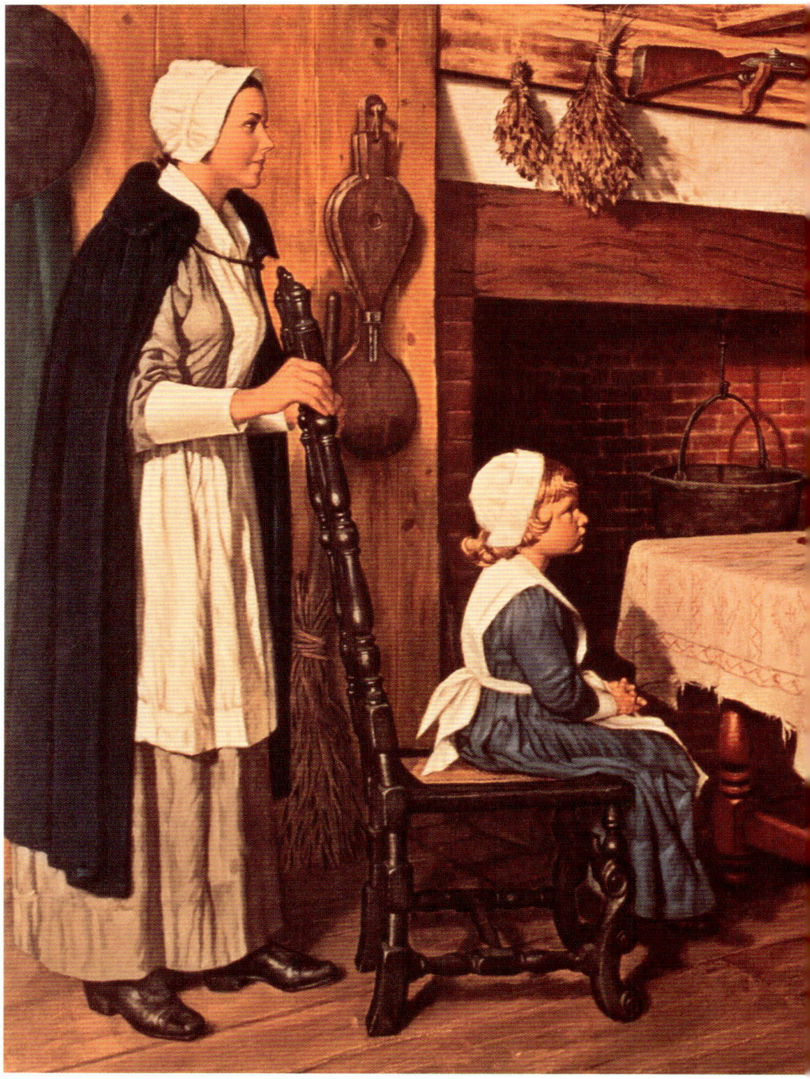

Relationships between scientific and herbal medicine are also important wherever herbal medicine remains a central part of medical care, as it does throughout much of the non-Western world. Strong traditions of herbal practices still exist in Central America as well as in China, Tibet and India, and other non-Western cultures. There are many calls to study these traditions scientifically, in the hope of finding new drugs for regular medicine. In turn, this raises many issues, ranging from ownership of intellectual property rights to traditional herbal knowledge to the repercussions on a local culture brought about by the exploitation of its herbal resources.

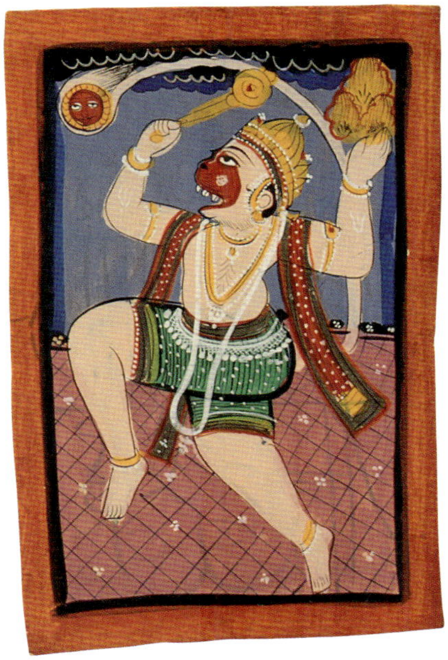

ABOVE The Hindu monkey-god Hanuman of the Sanskrit epic *Ramayana* carrying the 'Mountain of Healing Herbs'.

It may turn out that newly discovered medicines are too expensive for local people, while they may also lose a precious resource in consequence of inadequate conservation measures.

Another issue arising from today's shrinking globe deserves further comment. Are herbal practices, especially those recently introduced from, say, China, Peru or any other country, as effective in the West, where they are commonly administered in ways different from those in the countries of origin? After all, Western patients do not have the sense of a long history and testimonials that may well have supported a treatment in, say, China.

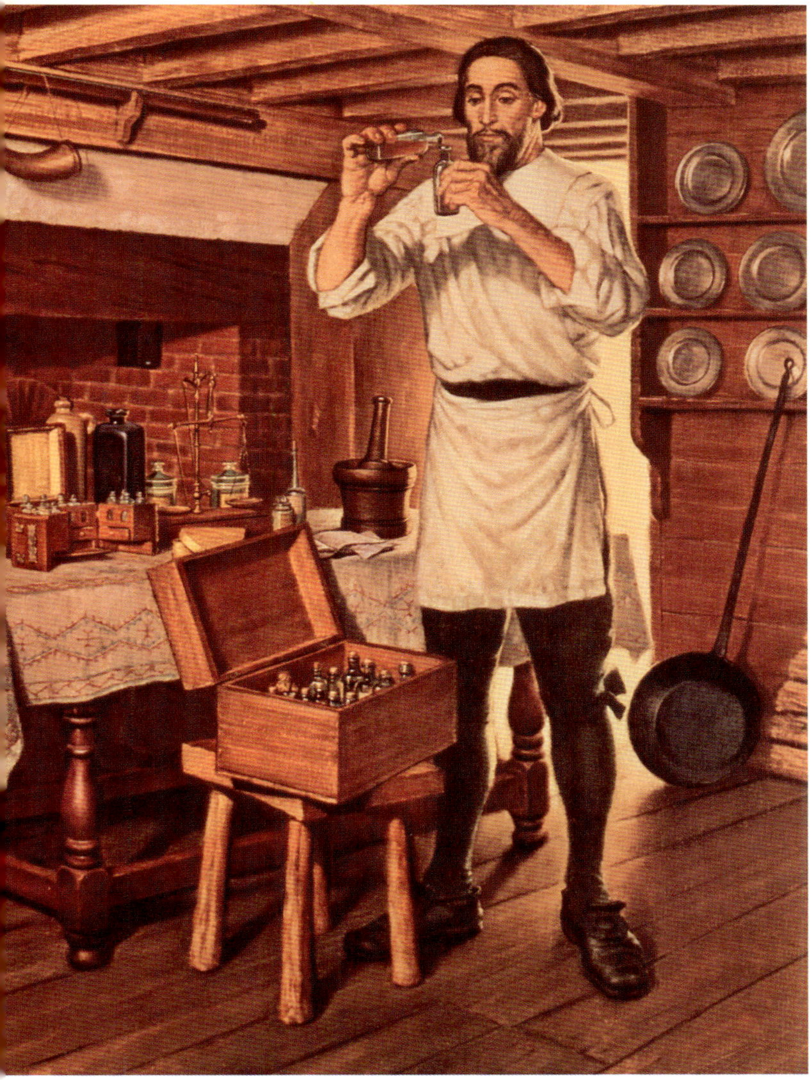

LEFT Nineteenth-century self-help: 'Governor John Winthrop Performing Apothecary Services in his Home' by Robert Thom.

There is no easy or single answer to this concern. In some cases the pharmacological activity of constituents – assuming the preparation and dosage is adequate – may be far more significant than cultural factors. In other cases, this is apparently not so. On the other side of the coin, there is the question, to what extent can traditions in, for instance, China, Tibet and India, supported as they are by respect for ancient authorities, accommodate the influences of Western scientific medicine?

Unquestionably, everyone interested in medical herbal lore has more than a lifetime's work in exploring, in many cultures, persistent and changing elements, fashions, myths and other factors relevant to effective treatment. There are, too, the new politics that surround investigations of herbs within traditional cultures, the need to conserve medicinal plants and much, much more. Such explorations hold the promise of finding significant health-care knowledge and of helping many people, perhaps even the writer of the rather despairing letter that opened this chapter.

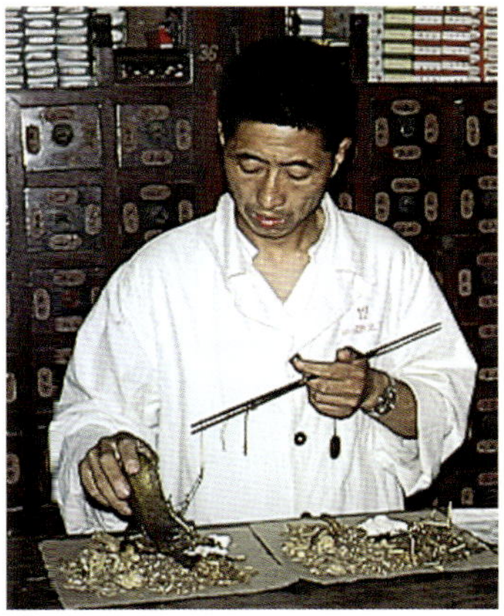

ABOVE What does the future hold for the herbal traditions of both the East and the West?

CHAPTER FOUR

THE BODY IN BALANCE

MEDICINE & DYNAMIC EQUILIBRIUM

IN 1794, *Britain sent its first official embassy, led by Lord Macartney, to the court of the Chinese Emperor, QuianLung. Every member of this mission, from Lord Macartney to his valet, was encouraged to study the manners and manufactures of the mysterious Chinese people. As it happened, the first occasion for such observation was a medical one: John Barrow, a member of the initial landing party in China, immediately fell ill from the effects of gorging on an unfamiliar Chinese fruit. Instructed by the Imperial Court to offer the foreigners every courtesy, the Chinese authorities immediately sent a respected physician to attend the stricken man. However, despite Barrow's prompt recovery under Chinese treatment, this pioneering cross-cultural medical encounter cannot be counted as an unqualified success.*

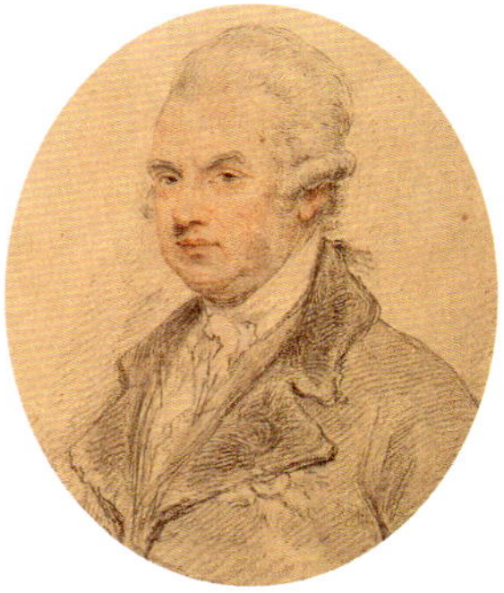

ABOVE Lord Macartney led the first British diplomatic mission to China in 1794.

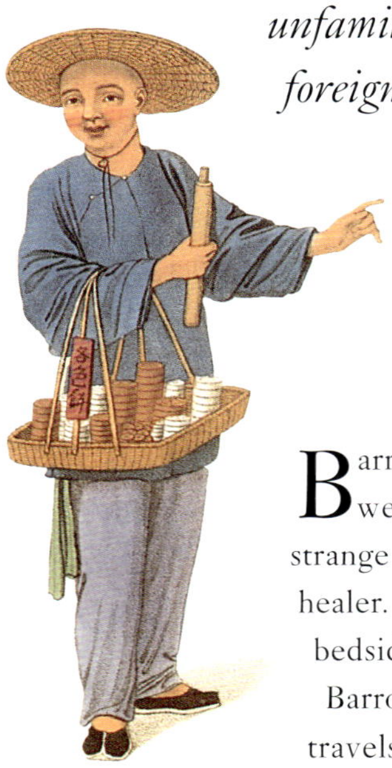

ABOVE This illustration of a Chinese apothecary dates from 1799, just a few years after Macartney's mission first arrived in the country.

Barrow and his countrymen were shocked by the strange behaviour of the Asian healer. He came to the patient's bedside and, in the words of Barrow's own account of his travels in China published in 1804, '[w]ith a countenance as grave and a solemnity as settled, as was ever exhibited in a consultation over a doubtful case in London or Edinburgh, fixed his eyes upon the ceiling, while he held my hand, beginning at the wrist, and proceeding towards the bending of the elbow, pressing… with one finger, and then… with another… This performance continued about ten minutes in solemn silence…'[1] Not only did the healer take Barrow's pulse at multiple points on the wrists, but he never asked the patient any questions, and arrived at his diagnosis entirely from examining the body. Ironically, the Westerners, accustomed by the norms of eighteenth-century European medicine to telling their doctors what ailed them, were incredulous of a diagnosis achieved without their personal assistance. Nor was the Chinese response to European medical practice more favourable. After a lengthy consultation with the embassy's Scottish physician, one high-ranking Chinese courtier remarked that the doctor's ideas of illness 'were so extraordinary that it appeared … as if [they] had come from an inhabitant of another planet.'[2]

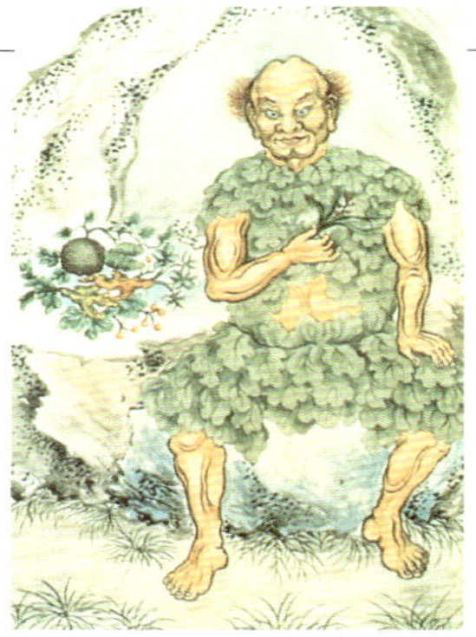

ABOVE The legendary emperor Shen Nong, the Divine Farmer, who is revered in China as the discoverer of herbal medicines. Scholars of the Han dynasty *(206 BC–AD 220)* recorded the herbal knowledge ascribed to him in a text entitled *Shen Nong Bencao Jing*. This watercolour was painted in Shanghai in 1920.

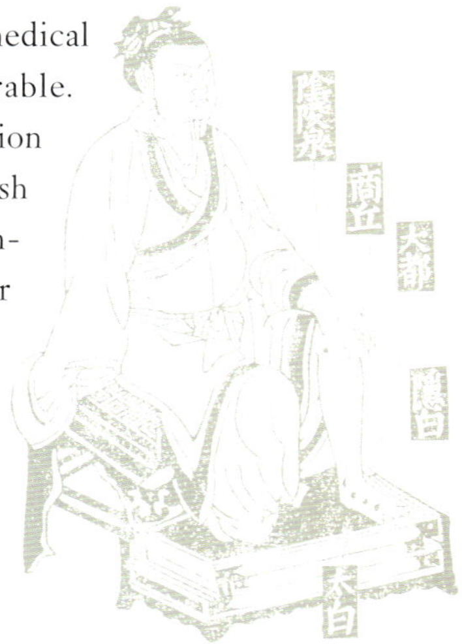

RIGHT A drawing from an ancient text on acupuncture by Wang Wei-I showing the lower course of the Thai-Yin acutract.

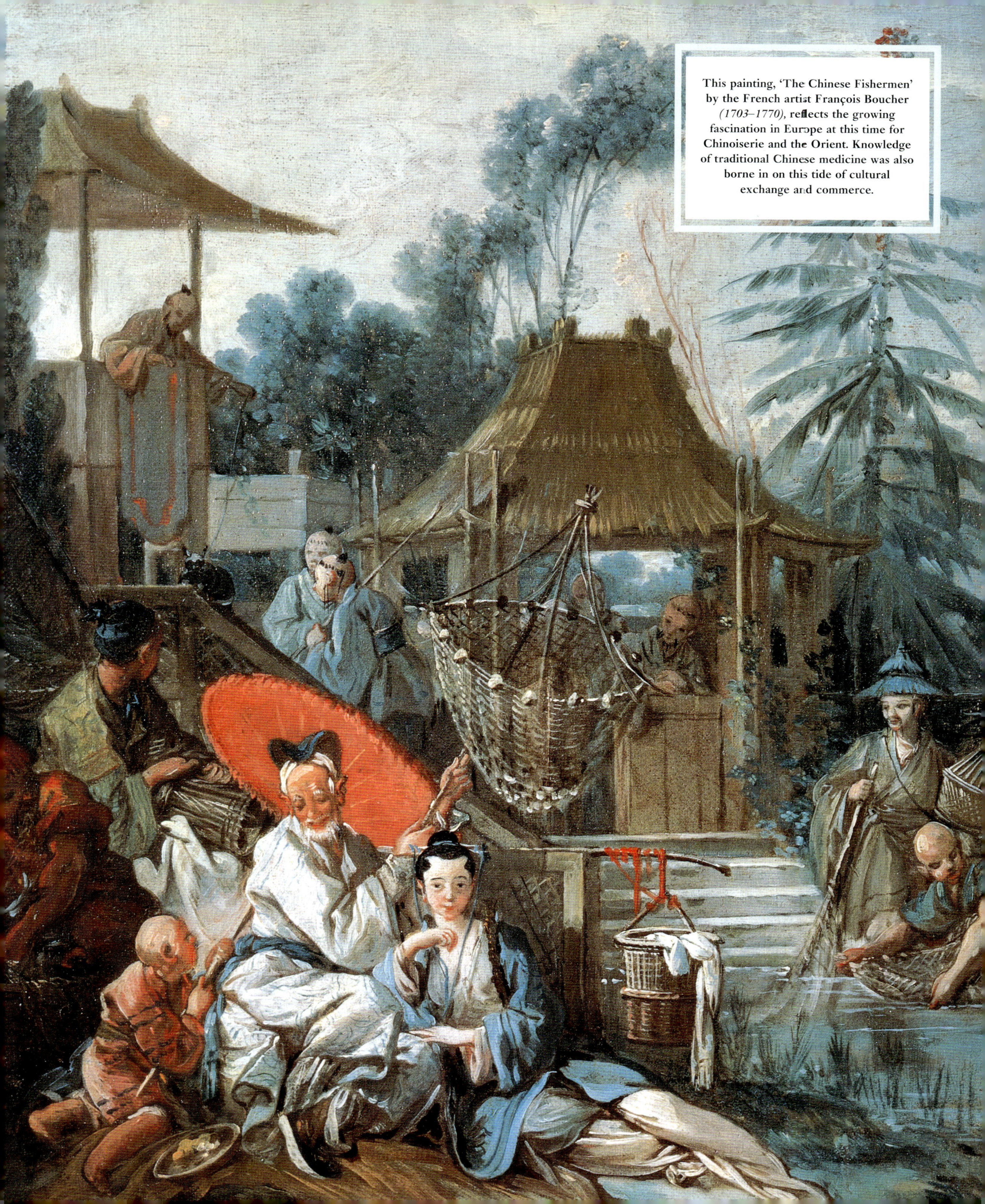

This painting, 'The Chinese Fishermen' by the French artist François Boucher *(1703–1770)*, reflects the growing fascination in Europe at this time for Chinoiserie and the Orient. Knowledge of traditional Chinese medicine was also borne in on this tide of cultural exchange and commerce.

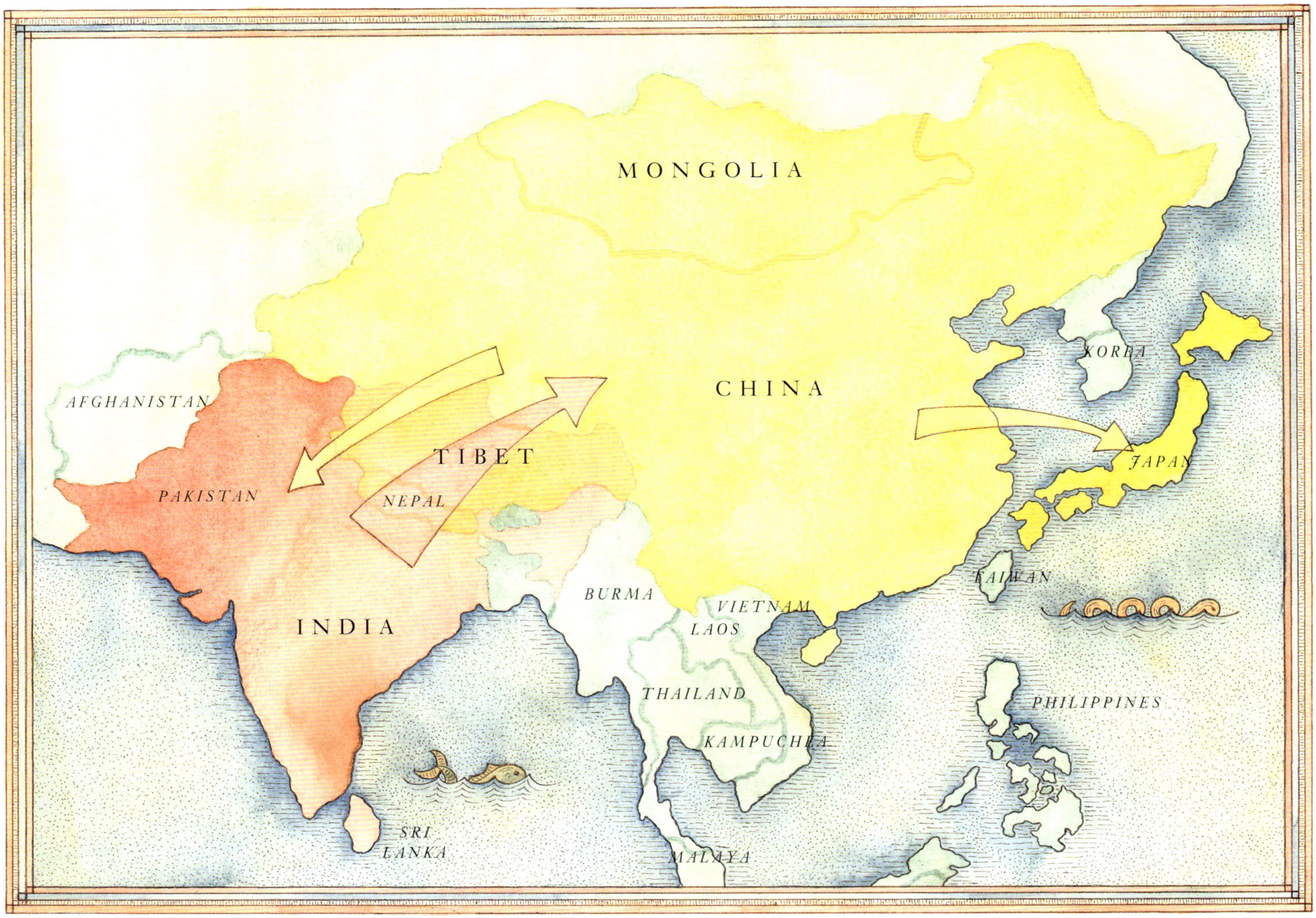

ABOVE The healing traditions of the Indian sub-continent (Ayurveda, Siddha and Unani) and China exerted reciprocal influence on one another, and on medical practices in Japan, Nepal and Tibet.

At first, the medical practices of India and East Asia may look as strange to contemporary Westerners as they did to those first British observers in China two centuries ago. Certainly, the average European or North American does not expect to be prescribed a herbal concoction for allergies or angina, or needle-pricks for menstrual cramps. Such a patient might be even more surprised to be told that her cramps were due to an excess of yang energy. The strikingly different medical and surgical techniques used in Asian medicine are based on ideas about the body, health and disease that initially seem alien and utterly unlike anything predicted by Western medical science. But, in fact, the concepts underlying Ayurveda, acupuncture and other Asian medical practices are closely related to the medical traditions of the West.

KEY TO MAP

- CHINA — *Chinese medicine*
- INDIA — *Ayurveda*
- INDIA – PAKISTAN — *Unani medicine*
- TIBET & NEPAL — *Tibetan medicine*
- JAPAN — *Japanese medicine*
- TAMIL NADU — *Siddha medicine*

SHARED TRADITIONS OF THE BODY

Classical Western medicine, traditional Chinese medicine and Ayurveda share the belief that the human body is a microcosm of the universe. Like their European counterparts, Indian and Chinese medical thinkers believed that the body was composed of the same materials as the cosmos; moreover, they linked each organ system to a particular elemental substance. For example, ancient Chinese astrology focused on five planets: Mars, Jupiter, Saturn, Venus and Mercury. Chinese thinkers consider the natural world to consist of five elements (or, to express it more accurately, five types of processes, each of which is represented by an archetypal substance) – metal, wood, water, fire and earth.

Unsurprisingly, given the belief that the human body reflects the universe in miniature, Chinese medicine recognizes five viscera – the heart, the liver, the spleen, the lungs and the kidneys. Each of these vital organs is linked to one of the five elemental substances – fire, wood, earth, metal and water, respectively. Their affinity with these substances signifies a connection between the organs and the processes of which their linked element is emblematic. Thus, each organ also acquires a set of other attributes associated with that element; these include specific odours, tastes, colours, sensation, emotions, seasons and even compass directions. In short, each of the sensible aspects of the natural environment had a representative within the body, in one of its five viscera. Like the Chinese, classical and medieval European doctors associated the different elements with specific body parts, and in Ayurvedic texts, the five great Hindu elements are inseparably joined with aspects of the body and objects of the senses.

These close theoretical connections between the body and the external world naturally affected the ways in which Chinese and Indian (as well as early Western) healers understood sickness and health. Practitioners in each of these medical systems consider disease to be a state of imbalance within the body, caused by imbalances, interactions or disharmony between individuals and their environment. Consequently, the aim of medical treatment was to preserve or restore the healthy equilibrium both internally and externally. This was no simple task; it demanded constant vigilance in monitoring activity levels and diet as well as the effects of the weather, the changing seasons and aging. Moreover, in Chinese and Indian medicine, changing states *either* of body or of mind could affect the healthy balanced state – an excessive emotion might cause a bodily illness or be caused by one.

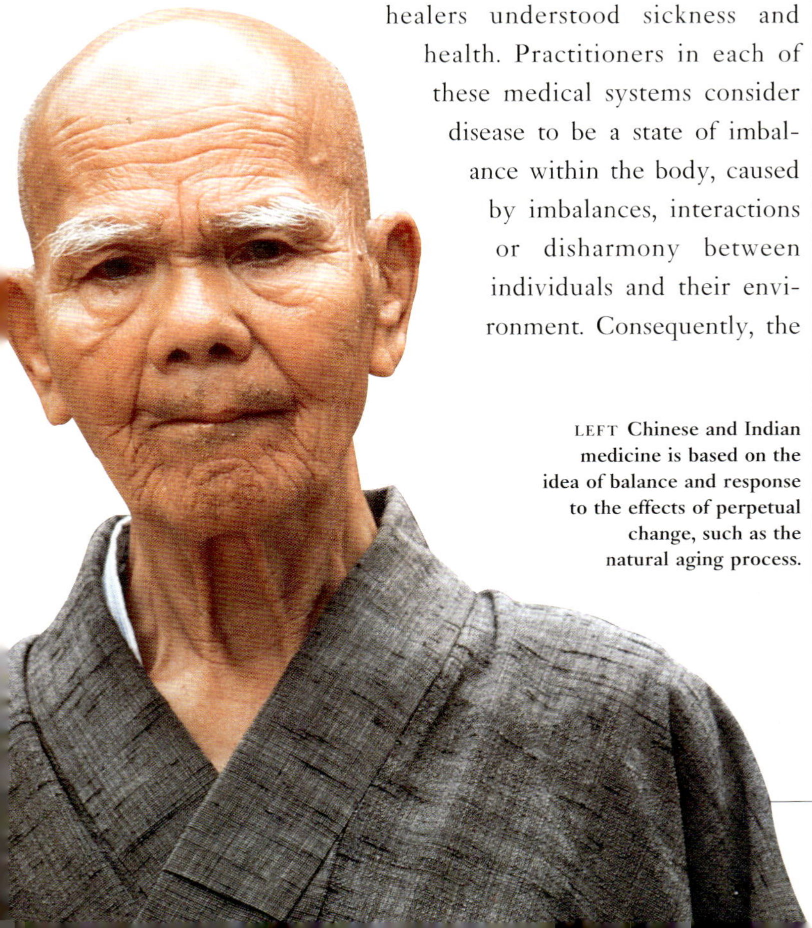

LEFT Chinese and Indian medicine is based on the idea of balance and response to the effects of perpetual change, such as the natural aging process.

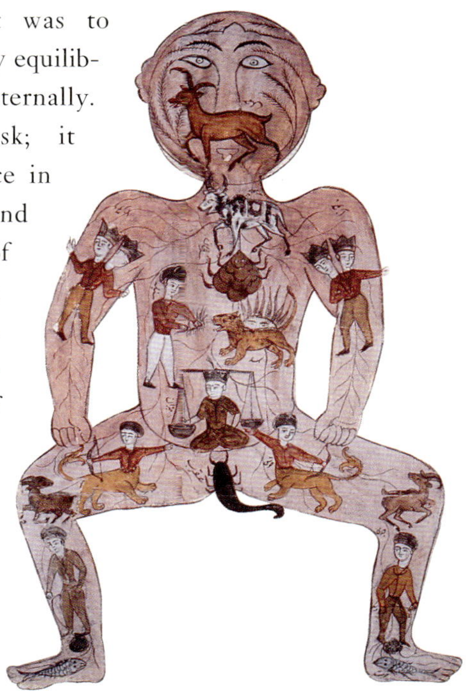

ABOVE The belief that the body reflects the universe in miniature informs Chinese and Ayurvedic medicine; it also recalls the astrological tradition of the West.

Like the most materialistic practitioners of Western medicine, although for significantly different reasons, Asian healers and medical practitioners treat consciousness as an organ of the body rather than a separate entity residing within it. The canonical texts of the Ayurvedic literature concur that while the mind creates the body, it is also dependent upon it. As one Western commentator observed, in Indian medical thought 'the soul can (with great difficulty) be extracted from the body, but then so (with much greater ease) may a heart or a tongue.'[3]

In early Western medicine, these interactions between body and mind, and body and environment, were thought to be mediated by the humours – blood, black and yellow bile and phlegm. These fluids were produced by the different organs and circulated through the body. Their production could be stimulated or retarded by physical or mental exertion or by diet, but it was also affected by the changing seasons and by the aspect of the planets with which each was associated. Only when the balance between these humours was appropriate, not only to the climate and season, but also to the subject's age employment and general character, would that person be healthy. In Indian and Chinese medicine, a similar doctrine obtains; the relationship between organs within the body and between the body and the natural world is understood to take place through the medium of fluids imbued with unique properties and actions affecting the physical and mental state of the body.

INDIAN MEDICINE AND THE ENERGETIC BODY

As with so much of India's culture, its indigenous medical practices are rooted in the ancient liturgical texts called the *Veda* – 'the knowledge'.[4] These ancient texts, themselves shaped by the even older Dravidian culture of the Indus valley, took their current form in the second millennium BC. They describe the origins of the universe, the natural world, the human race and the social order. Perhaps more importantly, the Vedas set out the principles upon which Hindu religious, moral and social life is based. In the process, they paint a fragmented but fascinating picture of an understanding of health and the body based on religious and magical principles, but also upon direct and careful observation of natural events. Thus, in the *Rig Veda (c.1500 BC)* and the *Atharva Veda (c.1000 BC)*, mysterious internal diseases like fevers are assigned supernatural causes, but are described in some detail; sufferers are advised to pray for relief and give offerings to angered demons or to benevolent deities, but they are also prescribed plant medicines. Meanwhile, the visible and clearly mundane causes of external ailments, like wounds and skin rashes, are acknowledged. The Vedic texts also list several internal organs, and mention various surgical interventions.

The first group of specifically therapeutic writings emerged at the end of the first millennium BC, and explicitly declare themselves to be based on the Vedic tradition. However, they also clearly draw on the learning of heterodox groups like the Buddhists and Jains and on the writings of individual ascetics. Although these communities had different goals and principles, they shared the aim of integrating the Vedic principles into daily life, rather than allowing them to become isolated as mechanically performed rituals. Unsurprisingly, the medical practices which emerged from this more austere and contemplative milieu stress moderation, both in life-style and in medical treatments, as the most powerful aid to health.

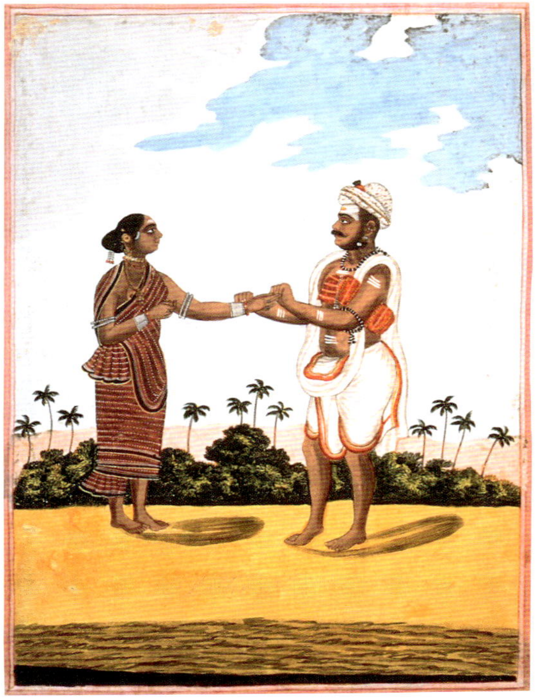

ABOVE An Indian doctor taking the pulse of a woman patient. Pulse-taking is one of the most important diagnostic tools in Ayurvedic medicine.

RIGHT An undated Sanskrit manuscript dealing with the teaching of physicians.

BELOW The attainment of Samadhi, from an early ninteenth-century volume showing Hatha-yoga postures or asanas.

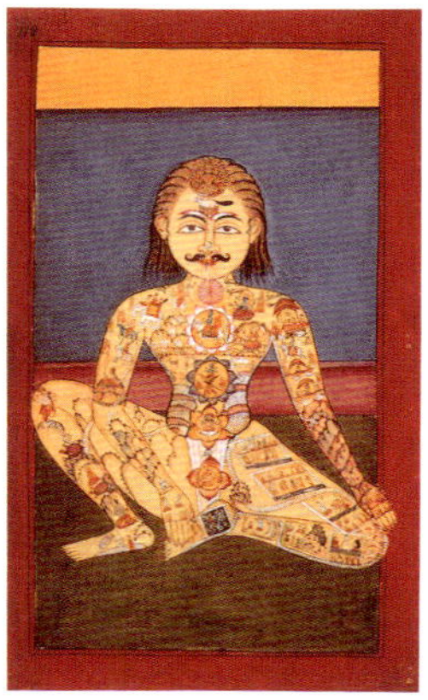

Two of the basic texts of Ayurvedic medicine, the *Caraka Samhitā* and the *Suśruta Samhitā*, were almost certainly written at this time, although the earliest definite reference to these compendia dates from the late fifth century. At that time, commentators described copies of the *Caraka* and *Suśruta Samhitās*, transcribed from Sanskrit originals by travelling Chinese monks. These texts refer internally to the fact that their contents had been altered and supplemented by authors subsequent to the eponymous (and divinely inspired) Caraka and Suśruta. Thus, from their inception, the central texts of Ayurvedic medicine were clearly organic constituents of the culture in which they were produced. The *Caraka* and *Suśruta Samhitās* achieved their modern forms by the end of the first millennium AD, but interpretations of their contents have continued to evolve and change, even after the texts themselves were fixed. The former concentrates on medical and the latter on surgical remedies, but both also describe the body and offer guidelines for healthy living. One of the most crucial of these guiding principles is based on the idea of desire as both the force which sparked the creation of the

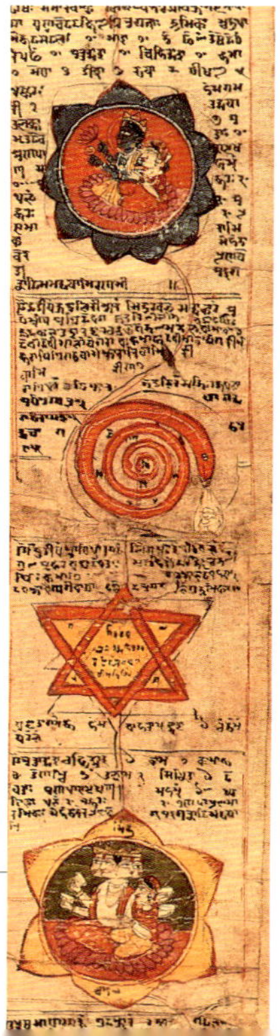

THE PHILOSOPHICAL ROOTS OF AYURVEDIC THEORY

Ayurvedic medical solutions often appear to be simply pragmatic, based on careful empirical observations. However, Ayurvedic texts and scholars draw heavily on theology and philosophy (darshana) to explain and justify their therapeutic choices. Thus the Vedas, and their ancient commentaries, the Upanishads (written between 1000–500 BC), are integrated as sources of authority. Over time, certain dominant schools of philosophical thought have also left clear imprints on the structure and theoretical basis of Ayurveda. Threading through the entire system of Ayurvedic medicine are the ideas drawn from the *sāṅkhya darshana.*

The sāṅkhya (or samkhya) system of philosophy, named for its basic text, which is the *Sāṅkhya Karika* of Isvarakrishna (c.200), is structured around the separation of spirit from its enslavement by matter. Its adherents sought *moksha* (liberation) of the spirit, or 'subtle body', from gross matter. This 'subtle body' was described as a material constituent of all living beings, albeit minuscule in physical terms. Like the kernel of a seed, the 'subtle body' was believed to accompany the *atman*, the individual soul, through the cycle of birth, death and rebirth, through change and disintegration, and the sorrow that inevitably results from attachment to worldly things which are subject to change and decay. The 'subtle body' was the enduring record of karmic actions and reservoir of accumulated karmic energy, whether good or bad.

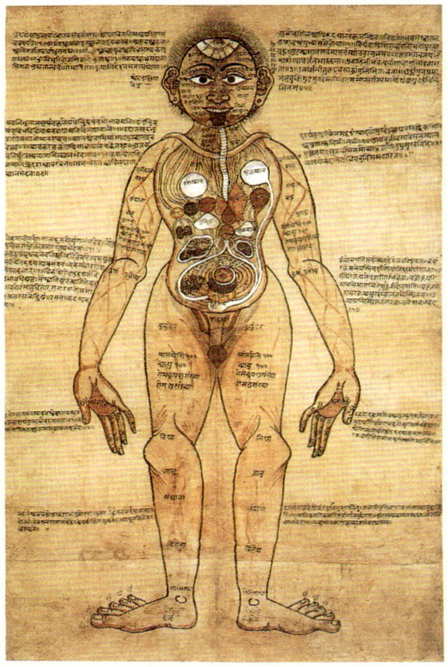

ABOVE A rare illustration of Indian ideas of anatomy, taken from a Nepalese medical manuscript.

Sāṅkhya also draws a distinction between consciousness and the physical or material. Although the former is incapable of action or effect by itself, in proximity with matter, consciousness provided the motivation and direction. Consciousness, in the sāṅkhya system, is the cause of activity (and thus even of life itself). The material being, by contrast, has the potential for activity – the potential to produce effects – but is without consciousness. Thus, in this complicated system, consciousness depends on the material to produce effects which will allow it eventually to be emancipated from materiality! The two most obvious results of this system for medical thought are that karma could be called upon as an explanation for inexplicable and tragic illness; and that the mind and the body, could not be treated as separate entities.

Sāṅkhya philosophy divides all disorder or pain into three categories: intrinsic, extrinsic and divine. In Ayurveda, these become endogenous, exogenous and Karmic. However, sāṅkhya's most substantial contribution to later Ayurvedic thought probably came from its doctrine of the intrinsic properties of substances – equilibrium *(sattva)*, activity *(rajas)* and inertia *(tamas)* are material attributes and present in all matter. Their distinct physical traits allowed these intrinsic properties to be used in medical diagnoses: sattva is cool and light, calm, pure and virtuous; rajas is active and hot, passionate, and happy or sorrowful; tamas is heavy and dull, stupid or lethargic, and dark and evil. Clearly, a predominance of one property over the others would have ramifications for treatment of the individual. The intrinsic properties were also assigned colours – white, red and grey/black, respectively – and in the body were represented in semen, blood and fat. They were also strongly associated with bodily functions and the organs which performed those functions.

In yoga, (based on the *Yoga Sutra* of Patanjali, written in the 2nd century BC), the cosmology of the sāṅkhya school was further elucidated. Sattva, the subjective consciousness, develops into the mind and the ten senses, five of cognition (the five Western senses) and five of action: speech (communication), hands (creative action), feet (locomotion), genitals (reproduction) and anus (excretion). Tamas evolved into the five objects of the senses (sounds, tactile objects, visible forms, tastes and odour). By being available to the senses and thus the consciousness, these phenomena in turn *produce* the five great elements: earth, water, air, fire and space. The elements each represent a stage in the purification of the material, in its slow and painstaking evolution from gross matter to pure spirit, able once more to achieve reunification with the universal soul or energy. They are also, with the immaterial self, the fundamental constituents of the physical body. Rajas as an intrinsic material trait is more or less self-explanatory; it is the range of interactions between sattva and tamas. The meditative exercises developed in yoga were intended to use innate qualities of the conscious body to free the spirit, the atman, from the constraint of its material cage – a cage built by the oppressive attachment of the material, desiring mind to the physical world.[5]

universe from undifferentiated spirit and that which will destroy it. In the microcosm of the human body, passion and desire disturb the healthy equilibrium; if desire is satisfied in moderation, the temporary disturbance it causes can be constructive; but if desire becomes immoderate, unsatisfied, or is immoderately satiated, its feverish heat can destroy health.

AYURVEDIC MODELS OF THE BODY

The body in Ayurvedic medicine is represented by two somewhat different models. One, easily recognizable to the average Westerner, describes the body as a system composed of ducts and tubes, valves and burners. This is similar to the hydraulic model which became popular in Europe as the workings of the circulatory system came to be known in the seventeenth century. It is the product of centuries of careful, empirical observations, and serves to answer most of the 'how' and 'what' questions in medicine: 'How do the humours flow around the body?', and 'What makes the body warm?'

The other way of understanding the body in Indian medical thought, especially in a Tamil variant of Ayurveda called Siddha medicine, portrays it as an alchemical laboratory. The healthy body takes in gross matter and, through the many stages and metabolic processes of digestion and circulation, purifies it. This process releases (to the body) the component of spirit or energy which exists in every natural object, and which is identical with the life-force. This metaphor for the body also has a Western parallel – although a more ancient one than the circulatory system – and, as we will see, a Chinese analogue. It explains the functions of bodily processes, and seems to have arisen as a way to address medical 'why' and more complex 'how' questions: 'Why do humans eat and excrete?', 'Why do people fall ill?', 'How does the weather affect health?' Of course, each of these visions of the body places a strong emphasis on balanced and healthy interactions with the environment.

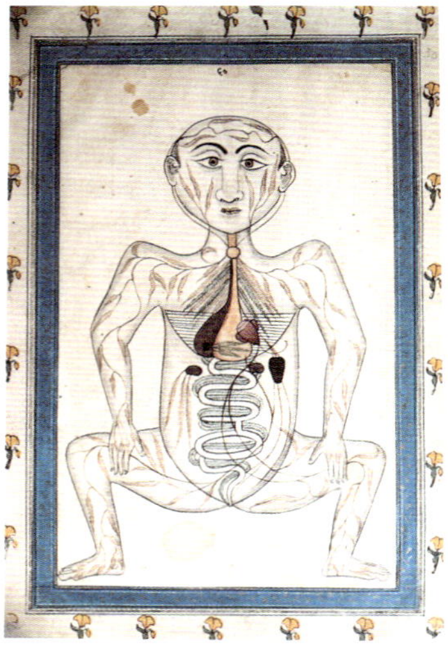

ABOVE Ayurvedic models of the body picture it both as a system of tubes, valves and burners, and as a type of alchemical laboratory.

The classical medical texts of Ayurveda use both of these models, usually together, to explain the physical phenomena of health, illness and death. In both constructions, the body consists of seven bodily tissues – *dhātu* in Sanskrit. The dhātus bind the spirit and the mind to the physical body, strengthening and supporting them. In order of refinement, the dhātus are *rasa* (plasma or bodily juices), blood, flesh, fat, bone, marrow and *'sukra* (the male and female reproductive fluids). Rasa is the most unrefined of the tissues, and is derived directly from food. It in turn nourishes – or is refined into – blood, which becomes flesh, and so on. Each substance is purified and integrated into its more subtle essence.

Around these stable elements circulate Ayurveda's equivalent of

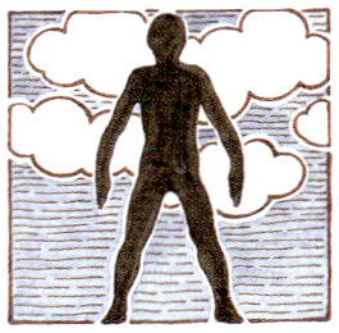

ABOVE Vāta corresponds to wind or breath and represents the element of air. It energizes and mobilizes the body.

BELOW A scene from the Govinda Gita showing Krishna, the hero of the Hindu epic, the *Mahabharata.*

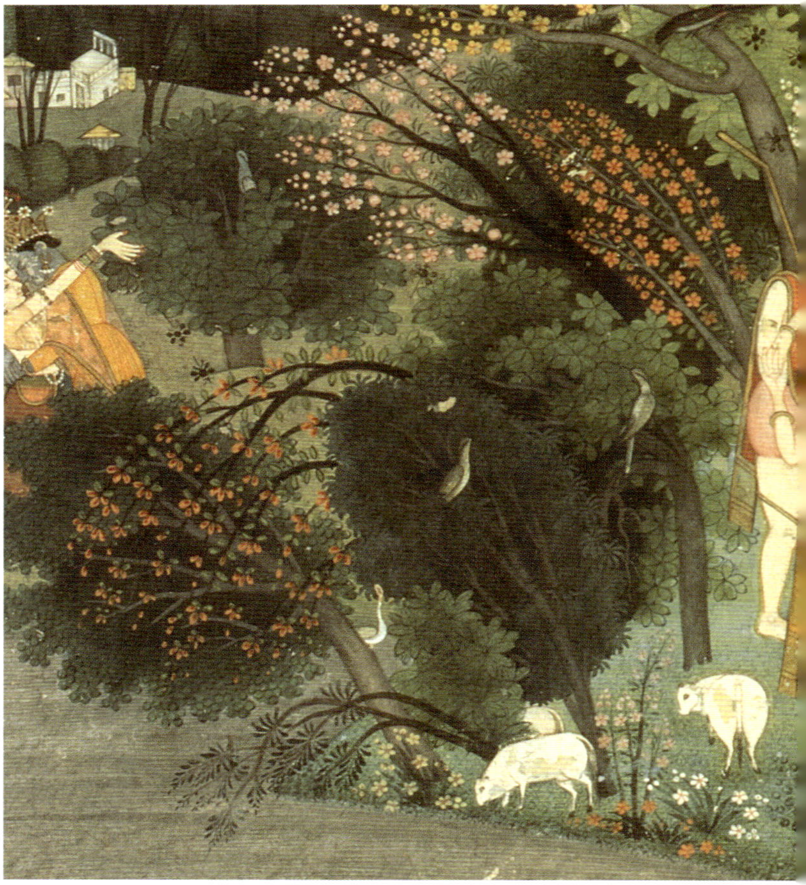

the Western humours (*doṣa* in Sanskrit). The three doṣas are called vāta, pitta and kapha; they correspond to wind or breath, bile and phlegm, but these physical substances, the vehicles which carry the doṣas around the body, are only part of the story. Simultaneously, the doṣas represent the active elements – air (paired with space), fire (paired with water) and water (paired with earth) – in the alchemical model, and thus are linked to the attributes and affinities of those elements. The doṣas have one further association, which unites their alchemical and their hydraulic roles: they are the less stable, more impure forms of the vital essences, *agni, prāṇa* and *ojas.* These three essences are the forms in which the elements of air, fire and water exist in living beings. Agni is the medium through which mind and body communicate with each other and the environment; prāṇa is the power which forces the body to act as a functional unit; and ojas forms the actual linkage between the body's disparate units, enabling agni and prāṇa to have their effects.

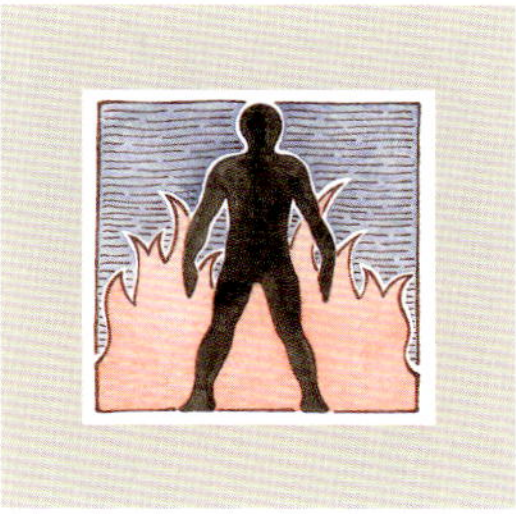

ABOVE Pitta corresponds to bile and represents the element of fire. Pitta influences vision, digestion and the generation of heat.

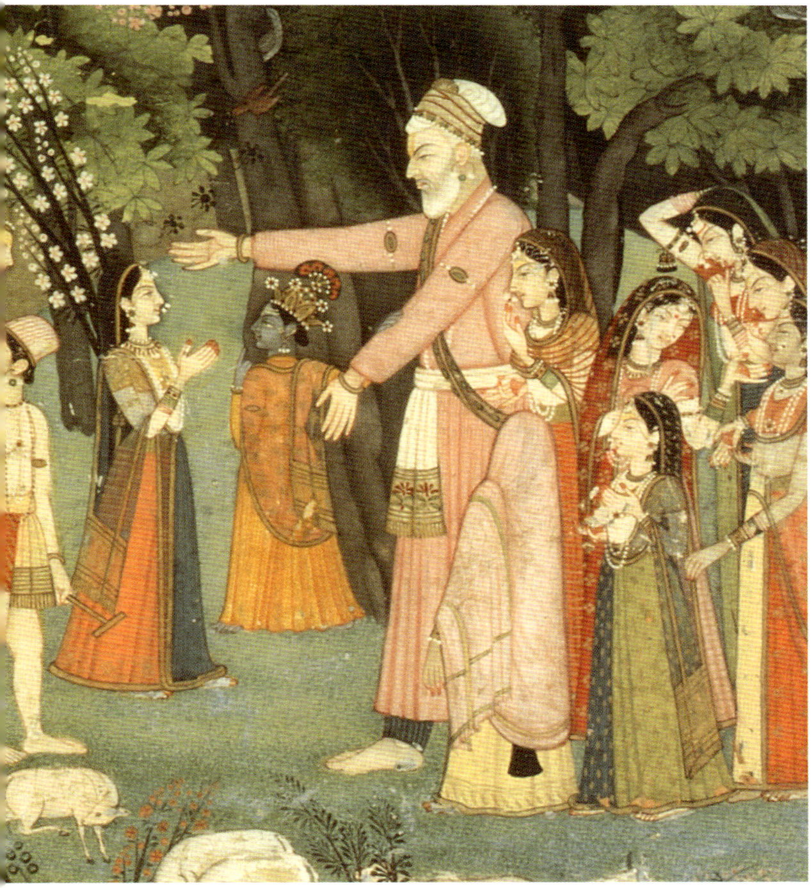

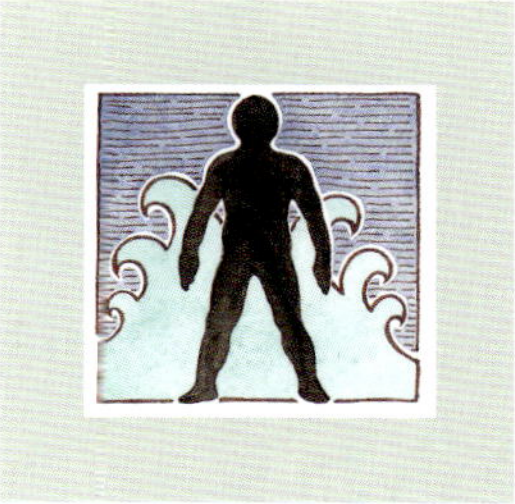

ABOVE Kapha corresponds to phlegm and represents the element of water. Kapha maintains the stability of the body and promotes smooth working of the joints. Strength is related to kapha.

Given this complicated network of associations and functions, it is unsurprising to discover that the doṣas' role in the body is also complex. In health, they permeate the body, with each doṣa dominating one region of the body – the large intestine, the navel and the chest, respectively. If any or all of them are deficient or in excess, they bring disease; yet the doṣas are vital to the preservation of life. They are the substances which shape and motivate the elements in living beings. The vāta enables the body to move, energizes it and is responsible for the action of urges; the pitta plays a role in digestion, vision and heating the body; and the kapha stabilizes, relaxes and unites the body. All substances in the natural world are composed of some combination of the five elements and are classified by the element which is predominant; living things are classified by their predominant doṣa.

The body has one other fluid constituent, ojas, which differs from prāṇa and tejas in that it is discussed in terms of physical traits. Ojas is at the pinnacle of the physical components of the body – it is the essence of *'sukra* – but its immaterial component remains central to its nature.

> *'It is said, however, that the ultimate power in all the body tissues, right up to seed, is ojas. Although it is based in the heart, it permeates, maintaining the continuity of the body. It is unctuous,...pure, and slightly reddish yellow. When it goes, one is lost; when it stays, one survives. It is that from which the various states present in the body arise. The things that make ojas decrease are: anger, hunger, worry, grief, fatigue and the like...But when the ojas increases, one's body feels well, properly nourished, and strong.*
>
> VAGBHATA, *HEART OF MEDICINE*

This combination of material and immaterial characteristics suggests that the most appropriate translation for ojas might be 'energy', or even 'vital energy'.

VITALITY IN MOTION: CHINESE IDEAS OF THE BODY

The rationale underlying Chinese medical thought, and the connections made between cosmology (theories of the universe) and the natural world – including the human body – are similar in many respects to those found in Ayurveda. As in Ayurveda, medical thought is rooted in a more ancient narrative of the creation of the universe and of the natural world. This story, like that of the Vedas, combines an over-arching belief in the unity of nature with a group of ordering categories – into one of which all natural objects must fall – which are defined through a set of material traits and characteristics.

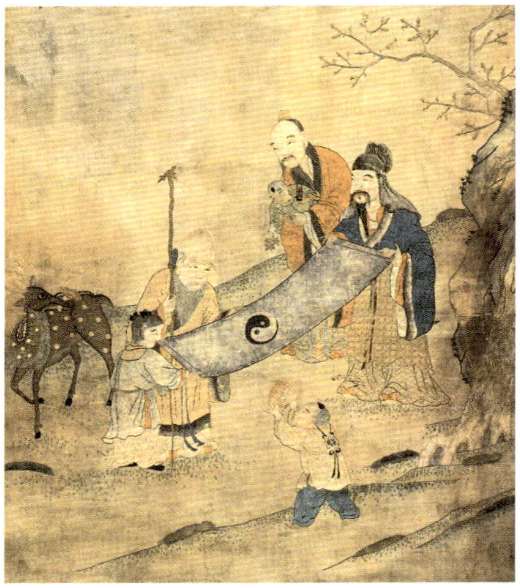

ABOVE This seventeenth-century Chinese painting shows people studying the T'ai Chi symbol which represents the opposed but complementary categories of yin and yang. Yin and yang are imagined as two faces of a mountain, one sunny, the other in shade.

The first recorded traces of the system which Westerners know through the names of its components, *yin* and *yang*, are found in the *Shih-ching*, a group of traditional songs composed in the first millennium BC. These verses draw lines of correspondence or association between sets of opposing states of being, characteristics and physical phenomena. Thus, the opposed characteristics of feminine and masculine are joined respectively to similarly opposed physical phenomena like dark and light, wet and dry, cold and warm. All of the first terms were associated with the category yin, and all the latter with its opposite term, yang.[6] Yet within each predominantly yin or yang object, characteristics associated with its opposite occur; in Chinese thought, nothing is pure yin or pure yang *(see tables on opposite page)*.

The earliest surviving medical text, the *Huangdi Neijing* (or *Yellow Emperor's Inner Canon*), written c.200 BC, draws heavily on this system of yinyang correspondence, and on the Five Element theory which counterpoints it. Like the Ayurvedic texts, the *Neijing* depicts the human body as a microcosm of the universe. This vision of the body also reflected in minute detail the state and culture within which it was written. The body was conceived as a tiny country, with a ruler, 11 other state officials, ministers and assistants working in harmony to run the transport and communication systems *(see box above)*.

Within the body, these functions of transport and communication took place via twelve waterways *(jing)* – reflecting the twelve great Chinese rivers – and ever-smaller sub-channels called *luo* and *sun*, as well as vessels called *mai*, located in vital regions of the body. Through each of these channels flowed a

THE TWELVE STATE OFFICIALS

XIN *('heart-mind')* The ruler; in charge of the 'heart-mind' or centre; also responsible for propitiating the *shen* (spirits)

FEI *('lungs')* Official responsible for internal links and monitoring conditions.

GAN *('liver')* Military decision-maker and strategist.

DAN *('gall bladder')* Minister in charge of justice and verdicts.

CHANZHONG *('central altar')* Directs official messengers and creates/authorizes the feeling of joy.

PI-WEI *('spleen-stomach')* Two officials responsible for taste and storing food.

DACHANG *('large intestine')* Official responsible for transport and transformation (of food).

XIAOCHANG *('small intestine')* Officer responsible for disposing of excess.

SHEN *('kidneys')* The body's enforcer and motivator, as well as the storer of power and controller of capacity.

SANJIAO *('triple-burner')* Opens sluices and manages watercourses – keeps the transport system in order.

PANGGUANG *('bladder')* Official concerned with regions in which fluids are stored and altered[7]

fluid substance called *qi (see page 105)*; *mai* also contained blood. All along the channels were points or depots called *xue,* where the flow of qi was accessible to outside (medical) influence. These channels connected the organs to each other in various ways, and also allowed each internal organ to communicate with a surface organ on the body: heart to tongue, liver to eyes, spleen to mouth, lungs to nose, kidney to ear – an idea that was eventually to become essential to the diagnosis of illness. When these channels and the internal world surrounding them were well-regulated, then it was believed the body thrived; when they failed, however, so did the body's health.

As with the Ayurvedic sense organs, each Chinese organ was associated with one of the archetypal substances, and with all of its linked qualities and affinities *(see table overleaf).* Beyond this model of the body, the *Huangdi Neijing* offers descriptions of diseases and therapies, with comparatively little theory. Great praise is given to preventive medicine, underlining the Chinese tradition that a good doctor 'cures' patients before they are ill. Another important medical text, the *Nanjing (Classic of Difficult Issues),* thought to date from the first or second century BC, consolidates the theoretical components of the *Neijing* and unites theory with practice and diagnostics.

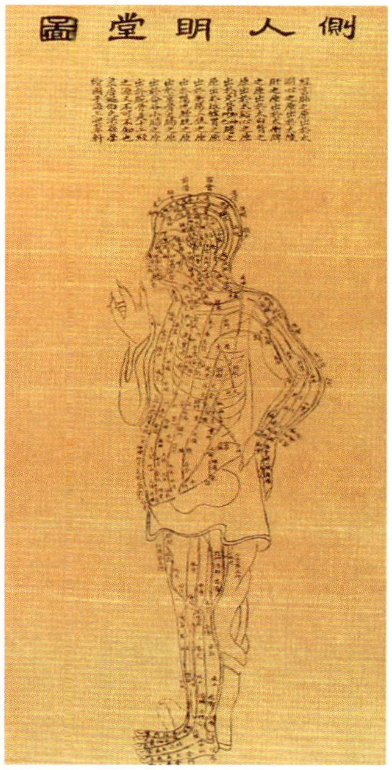

ABOVE An acupuncture chart reprinted in 1906 from an original that is thought to date from the Song Dynasty *(960–1279).*

YANG

GENERAL Masculine, heavens

QUALITIES Light, hot, dry

IN THE BODY
The upper parts and back, the outer parts (e.g., hair, skin), the shallower organs; the hollow organs are all relatively more yang

ORGANS
Yang organs are those which receive, break down and absorb that part of food that will become Fundamental Substances; they also transport and excrete the rest

CHARACTERISTIC ILLNESS
Fire Pernicious Influence. Here, the climactic condition of heat has invaded a body imbalanced by excess yang energy. Symptoms include sudden fevers and hot rashes – typical Western diagnosis might be a bacterial infection, like Streptococcus

YANG THERAPIES
Acupuncture and moxibustion, because they move from exterior to interior

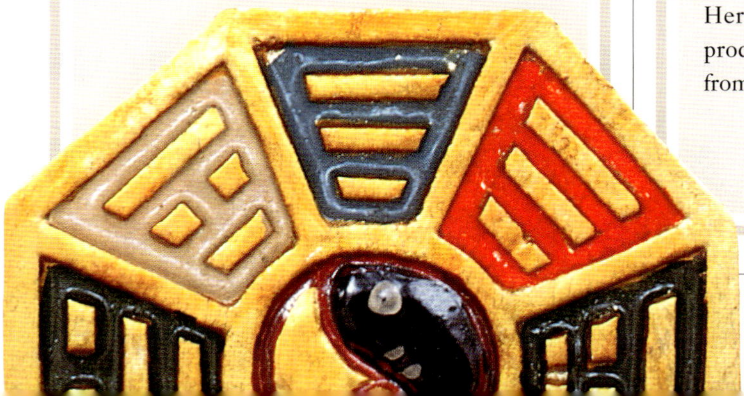

YIN

GENERAL Feminine, earth

QUALITIES Dark, cold, wet

IN THE BODY
The lower parts and front, the inner parts and deeper organs, and the solid organs are relatively more yin

ORGANS
Yin organs are those which produce, regulate, transform and store the Fundamental Substances: *qi* (essence or energy producing movement), blood, *jing* (essence or energy producing organic development), *shen* (spirit, material consciousness), fluids (bodily juices)

CHARACTERISTIC ILLNESS
Dampness Pernicious Influence. Here, the climactic condition of dampness has invaded a body imbalanced by excess yin energy. Symptoms include heavy mucoid secretion and discharges, oozing skin – typical Western diagnosis might include herpes zoster, other viral infections

YIN THERAPIES
Herbal treatments, as their effects are produced through digestion (and thus move from interior to exterior)

BELOW A stone rubbing from a Beijing temple that illustrates the concept that the body is a country in miniature with a ruler (the 'heart-mind') and other bodily officials regulating its functioning.

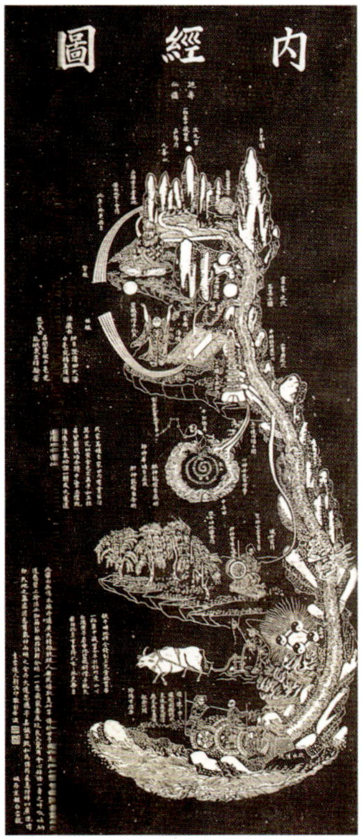

THE FIVE PHASES AND THEIR ASSOCIATED QUALITIES AND ELEMENTS[8]

QUALITY/ OBJECT	ELEMENT/PHASE				
	Wood	**Fire**	**Earth**	**Metal**	**Water**
direction	east	south	centre	west	north
colour	blue-green	red	yellow	white	black
climate	windy	hot	damp	dry	cold
human sound	shouting	laughing	singing	weeping	groaning
emotion	anger	joy	pensiveness	grief	fear
taste	sour	bitter	sweet	pungent	salty
yin organ	liver	heart	spleen	lungs	kidney
yang organ	gall bladder	small intestine	stomach	large intestine	bladder
orifice	eyes	tongue	mouth	nose	ears
tissue	tendons	blood vessels	flesh	skin	bones
smell	goatish	burning	fragrant	rank	rotten

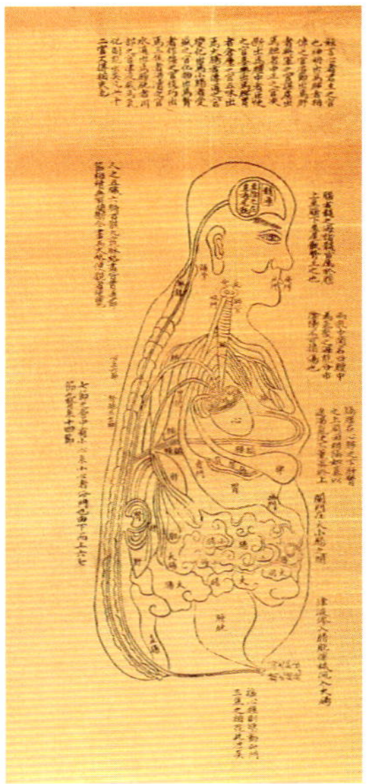

ABOVE A traditional depiction of the Chinese model of human internal anatomy, taken from a 1906 copy of an eighteenth-century original.

BELOW The T'ai Chi symbol of yin and yang is emblematic of continual change and renewal.

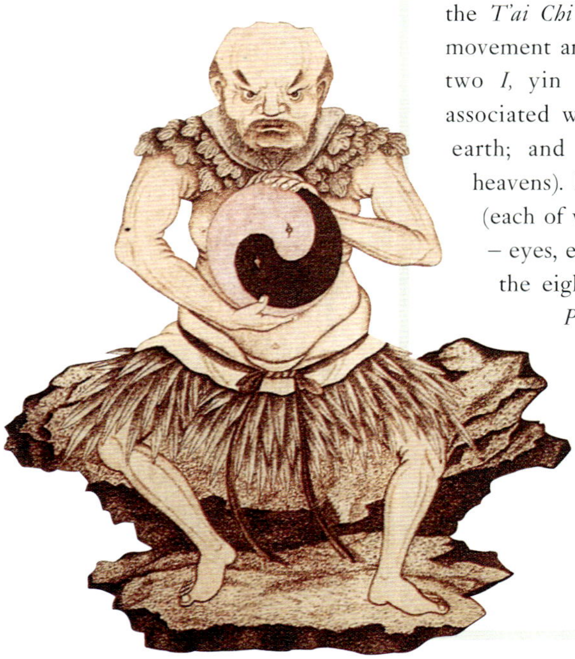

THE PHILOSOPHICAL COSMOLOGY OF CHINESE MEDICINE

Chinese medicine is organized by two central theories, drawn from speculations about the creation of the universe, and from direct observation of the natural world. The Doctrine of the Two Principles relates that the *Wu-Chi* created the *T'ai Chi* (infinite void); the differentiation of movement and stasis in the *T'ai Chi* generated the two *I*, yin and yang (which are respectively associated with the feminine, darkness, and the earth; and the masculine, lightness, and the heavens). From the two *I* came the four *hsiang* (each of which is associated with a sense organ – eyes, ears, nose, mouth), and from the *hsiang*, the eight diagrams (or *Pa-Kua*); each of the *Pa-Kua* represents a point of the compass and a primal substance: ether, water/vapour, fire, thunder, wind, water/liquid elements, mountains, earth).

The second central doctrine is that of the Five Elements or Processes: metal, wood, water, fire, earth. The elements correspond both to planets and to organs; thus the heart, liver, spleen, lungs, and kidneys are respectively paired with the elemental processes symbolized by fire, wood, earth, metal, water; and the planets, Mars, Jupiter, Saturn, Venus, Mercury.

The organs are also linked to the attribute of the Five Elemental Processes: the five colours, tastes, climates, directions, odours, emotions, animals, numbers, fruits, sounds, and grains. Thus, to take one example as a general illustration, the element wood is emblematic of the active process of growth, and is the product of activity – of growth. It is associated with the Spring, and with two organs, the liver and the gall bladder, which were considered to be active regulators of the rest of the body. The liver caused the circulation of qi and blood – in other words stimulated activity. The gall bladder as well played an active role, storing and dispensing the digestive fluids produced by its yin partner, the liver.

CHINESE IDEAS OF ANATOMY

The remarkable model of the body set forth in the *Neijing* became more abstract in the *Nanjing* and subsequent medical writings, while the different fluid and solid substances of the body also received more detailed attention. The duties which in the *Neijing* were assigned to 'officials' developed into a set of 'organs'. Chinese medicine has traditionally been concerned with the functional rather than the physical body – in other words, instead of concerning themselves with anatomy, Chinese doctors focused on physiology. Thus, although they share names with the Western anatomical organs, the 'organs' in Chinese anatomy are actually groups of closely related physiological functions.

These texts also lay out the principle fluid components of the body – the Fundamental Substances. Like their analogues in Ayurvedic medicine, these follow a hierarchy from more to less material. The juices of the body, ranging from sweat to saliva to the gastric juices, are directly extracted from food. They nourish the body, and act as lubricants. Blood, too, is derived from food, but it is composed of the most refined fluids in combination with purified food. It is a more potent source of nutrition, and circulates around the body for that purpose. Jing, qi, and shen – collectively known as the *San Bao* or 'three gems' – are altogether more complex substances. Jing is the essence, or the natural energy or strength that the body derives from food; in the Taoist tradition it is associated with semen.[9] Jing, and the qi into which it is refined, act together to allow the body to grow and develop, and give it the capacity to act. Shen, which in the Neijing's microcosm were natural spirits whose propitiation was the chief duty of the Xin official, in this system represents the individual's consciousness. It is the substance which enables awareness, and it is unique to human life. The traditional formula for expressing the relationship that these substances have to one another is strongly reminiscent of Ayurvedic ideas: 'Refine the jing to transform the qi, refine the qi to transform the shen, refine the shen and return to the void.'[10] However, although without shen the body dies, it plays a comparatively small role in medical practice. Qi and jing are more accessible to human and medical intervention.

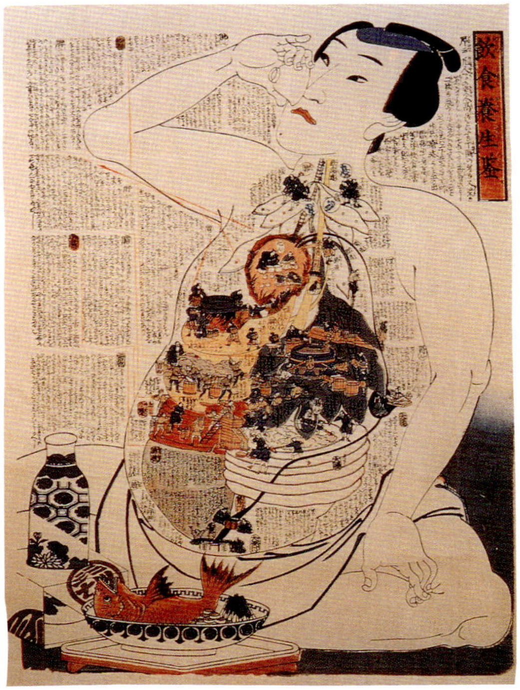

ABOVE Traditional Japanese medicine is largely based on Chinese practices which started to be studied in Japan from around the sixth or seventh centuries AD. This woodcut print from Japan (c.1850) illustrates how overindulgence can lead to various kinds of skin afflictions.

As in Ayurvedic medicine, the subtle and complex fluids – and in particular, qi – act as the mediators between body, mind and environment. By about 200 BC, qi had assumed primary importance in the Chinese search for health and longevity; the scholar Zhuang Zi *(c.369–286 BC)* wrote, 'Man's life is due to the conglomeration of the qi, and when it disperses, death occurs, so it is said that one qi pervades the universe...'[11] The free circulatory movement of qi is considered essential to the maintenance of a healthy balance between the different organs, and all of the qualities and attributes which they represent. Ojas (spirit or energy) is the closest analogue of qi in Indian medicine, while the aether or pneuma of the ancient Greeks also resembles qi in many respects.

Qi has many forms and natures, both in linguistic and in philosophical terms. The word itself can refer to the literal breath, and wind in the meteorological sense, as well as this vital energetic fluid. Moreover, as a primary component of numerous compound words, qi takes on still more connotations. Among the most important of these compound words are *yiqi, yuan-qi,* and *zheng qi.* The first term signifies the single and unified qi (here, think of qi as combining the meanings of spirit/energy/force), which permeates all things – in other words, the *dao.* Each person is born with a certain amount of this unitary qi, called yuan-qi (inherited/original qi); it serves to unify and protect the body's different elements so that it becomes strong enough to repel external forces. Zheng-qi is the most important form of qi in medical terms; it means the 'proper breath' and refers to the form of qi which circulates around the body, nourishing and protecting the organs and tissues. This form of qi is particularly susceptible to human interventions – exercise, diet, medicine and even change of climate.

'PATIENT, HEAL THYSELF': TAPPING THE VITAL ENERGIES

The conception of the body which underpins Indian and Chinese medicine is fundamentally one of a fluid entity, unified but permeable to environmental forces. In Ayurvedic medicine, the body is, either through perception or through digestion, interacting with not only the physical environment it encounters, but also with the social structure, changing mental states, and even the accumulated karma of the soul which inhabits it (and which, during its tenure in the body, takes the form of ojas). All of these can either strengthen or weaken the body, because all are endowed with vital energy, and affect the consciousness through the senses or the emotions.

The Chinese body lacks the historical dimension – the interaction between karmic energy and physical matter – but is equally entwined with internal and external environments. Thus, the medical practices of both these systems aim to augment, redirect or restore the body's health-giving interactions with its mental, physical and cultural surroundings. In other words, therapies in South and East Asia have been practically and theoretically designed to tap the vital healing energy and to restore its component substances, whether physical humours or subtle fluids like qi or ojas, to a proper state of dynamic balance.

The basic aims of Ayurvedic medicine are expressed within the two syllables of its name. As the *Caraka Samhitā* explains, 'It is called "ayurveda" because it tells us *[vedayati]* which substances, qualities and actions are life-enhancing *[ayusya]* and which are not.' Among the 'life-enhancing' practices advocated in Ayurvedic medical texts from as early as the sixteenth century is yoga (which evolved from meditative and alchemical practices contemporaneously with, but separately from Ayurveda). The *Su'sruta Samhitā* includes several chapters on the subject of meditative exercise, and among the few images found in the Indian medical canon are pictures of different yogic postures. Yoga emerged from the Siddha medical tradition; this variant of Ayurvedic medicine envisions medicine almost exclusively in terms of nurturing, manipulating and balancing the body's innate vital energies. Unsurprisingly, it is also the branch of Indian medicine most strongly influenced by the alchemical model of the body. In this respect, Siddha philosophy closely resembles the early Taoist beliefs upon which traditional Chinese medicine is based.

Like Ayurveda, Chinese medicine uses a combination of physical movements and introspective thought, called *Dao Yin* within the medical tradition, as a part of its preventative medicine and healing arts. The idea behind both yoga and *Dao Yin* (now often subsumed under the broader term *qigong* or 'qi-exercises') is to combine the powers of the mind and the body to distill qi/ojas, and to purify the very substance of the body. In the *Yoga Sutra* of the yogi Patanjali, meditative exercise was a way to enhance mental focus and force. The goal of such concentration was religious: by withdrawing completely from the material, one could reunite one's atman with the divine universe. The essential aspect of this practice for medical purposes was that yoga required the regulation of all body parts, and the withdrawal of attention from internal and external stimuli.

In the process of guiding the atman on its journey towards *brahman* (the universal one), the yogi also gained access to the flow of energy through the body, and was able to transform the humours, and especially the 'sukra, into ojas. This additional energy lengthened the yogi's lifespan, and consequently the amount of time available for reaching enlightenment *(moksha)*. In Chinese culture, as well, one goal of meditative exercise was to increase the lifespan. The philosopher Zhuang Zi gently mocked his own contemporaries' mad pursuit of longevity through *Dao Yin*, describing their actions as, 'Breath[ing] in and then out in many different ways, spitting out the old and taking in the new, strolling like a bear and stretching like a bird, and all just to achieve long life. This is what such practitioners of the *dao yin* ... enjoy.'

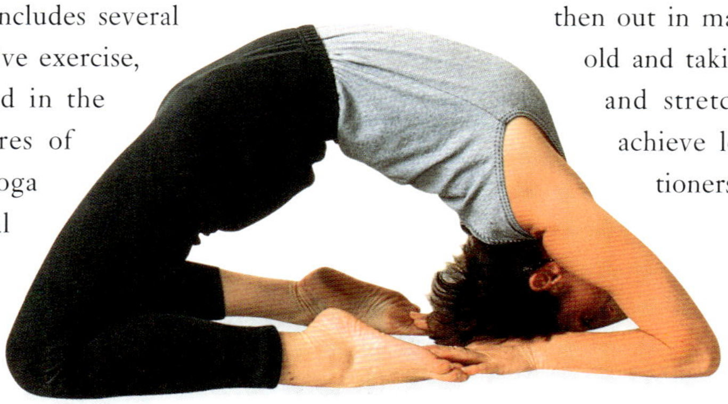

LEFT Yoga is one of the 'life-enhancing' practices that is recommended by Ayurvedic practitioners. It derives from the Siddha tradition of southern India.

Both yoga and Dao Yin use breathing exercises in combination with fasting – in fact, one Chinese technique, called tortoise breathing, reputedly allowed adepts to survive for months only on water. Similar stories abound about Indian yogis. Ge Hong (*AD 284–364*), a noted Chinese physician and alchemist, wrote in a collection entitled *Bao Pu Zi*:

> *If one cannot obtain herbs, one can still live to several hundred years of age if one practises respiration and fully grasps its principles… Those who fully grasp the principles of cultivating health, unremittingly practise respiration, perform Dao-Yin exercises morning and evening to promote and stimulate blood and defensive energy… can indeed be free from illness.*[12]
>
> GE HONG, *BAO PU ZI*

However, Ayurvedic and Chinese physicians realized that few people would have the necessary personal discipline required to achieve such levels of vitality through the practice of meditative exercise alone. Even the enthusiastic Ge Hong knew that most people would inevitably rely on medical therapies and a proper diet to prevent and treat illness. Over the course of the first millennium AD, Dao Yin exercises were modified and then fully integrated into the medical canon. Of the resulting combination, Ge Hong wrote that 'Although medicinal preparations are the basis of longevity, their benefits will be greatly enhanced if one is able to combine them with respiration techniques.' He and his successors believed that qi, guided by the mind and enhanced by therapeutic measures, could attack and cure bodily illness. As with yoga, the role of Dao Yin in this task was to increase the sufferer's capacity to gather and guide qi, and focus the mental energies. The different movements of the therapeutic qi-gong exercises assisted the Dao Yin practitioner to focus on a particular body part, and encouraged the qi to flow in the proper direction.

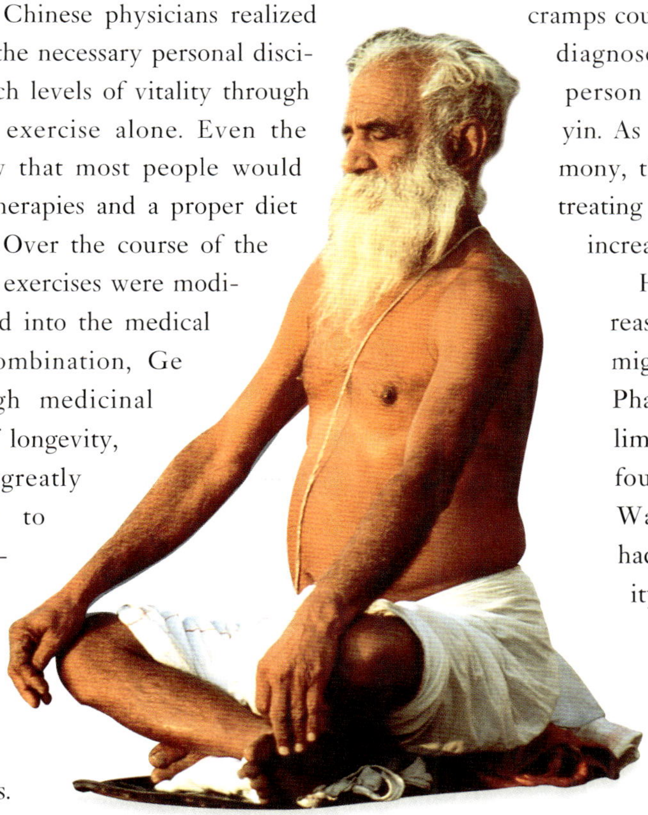

ABOVE Yoga draws on the notion that control over the mind can be aided by physical exercises. These can help the devotee achieve a state of spiritual enlightenment and liberation from the body.

DIAGNOSIS IN ENERGY MEDICINE

Yin, yang and the Five Phases in Chinese medicine, and the Five Elements and three doṣas in Ayurveda play a central role in the diagnosis and treatment of disease in both medical systems. The systems of correspondence constructed around these theories provides a set of physical, apparent clues to the hidden underlying characteristic condition of each patient. Thus, a woman with perpetually cold hands and feet, pallor, a pale tongue and terrible menstrual cramps could be readily diagnosed as a person with excess yin. As one of the primary forms of bodily disharmony, the physician might feel comfortable simply treating the woman with remedies chosen in order to increase her natural yang energy.

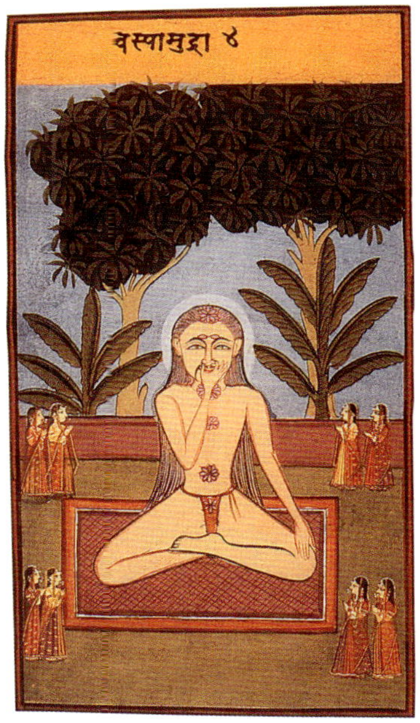

ABOVE The yoga position Vaspamudra from a nineteenth-century album that illustrates and explains a variety of postures.

However, to gain more insight into the reason for her imbalance, the careful physician might try to determine for which of the Five Phases she had the greatest affinity – her cold limbs would suggest Water, and if she had a foul, chemical odour, the association with Water would be confirmed. However, if she had a fragrant odour, it would suggest an affinity with Earth. The physician might also look for a failure in one of the organs. To do so, the practitioner would consider the relationship between the visible surface organs and their connected pairs of internal organs, as well as the Five Phases associations between organs and, say, colours. Chinese diagnostics involve the use of all of the senses, as well as detailed questioning of the patient; in combination with careful observation of each individual's demeanour, the patient's history should reveal any social and environmental factors relevant to disease.

Ayurvedic medicine relies heavily on the theories surrounding the three doṣas (which are, of course, aspects of the active elements) to organize the rich information provided by a patient's symptoms. Diagnosis aims to uncover the general state of the patient – how body, mind and environment are interacting. Thus an Ayurvedic doctor is trained to diagnose according to *darśana, sparśana* and *praśna:* visual inspection (including inspection of the aura which is produced by the body's ojas); palpation and other techniques involving physical contact – especially pulse diagnosis; and aural interrogation – questioning the patient and listening to the sounds of the body.

By the sixteenth century, Ayurvedic texts asserted the importance of interrogating the 'eight bases': the sensory viscera – eyes, tongue, voice and skin; the excreta – faeces and urine; the pulse; and the general appearance of the patient. It is in the last category that considerations of emotional and social states most clearly fit, but an Ayurvedic doctor would see traces of these traits in each of the other bases as well. Through these means, the physician would isolate the region of the body which was afflicted, the dhātu (tissue) affected, and the doṣa whose settled and unnatural presence in that tissue was causing disease. The same symptom, for example swelling, might indicate any of the three doṣas, depending on its location, temperature, colour, texture and the sensations reported by the patient. Thus, physicians would turn back to the classical Sanskrit texts, which set forth verse after verse explaining the particular correspondences between the humours, different symptoms, the diseases which those symptoms might indicate and various forms of treatment. Prognosis, again based on theories of doṣa correspondences, was set forth in other texts. By analyzing disease in terms of the relationships between the qualities, the substances and their actions, Ayurvedic doctors added structure to their empirical experience of disease. However, the complexity of those relationships preserved the diagnostic flexibility essential to dealing with individual patients.

The crucial role of the circulating subtle fluids in Ayurvedic and Chinese medicine is certainly visible in their diagnostic techniques. In particular, both cultures came to depend heavily upon the pulse as a way to read the internal workings of the body. In Chinese medicine, the pulse of each organ can be read at the wrist, while Indian doctors used the pulse to gather information about the movements of the *tridoṣa.*

However, the best way to assess the importance of these substances is to examine their place in the therapeutic armoury of each tradition. As we have seen, both systems developed styles of meditative exercise designed to enhance the production of their respective vital energies, qi and ojas. Both Chinese medicine and Ayurveda have breathtakingly extensive pharmacopoeia; remedies in each tradition are designed to strengthen the body's subtle fluids. Finally, both medical systems have external applications which aim to stimulate and modulate the motion of these essences. Indeed, one of the therapies in question, acupuncture, is among the most familiar aspects of Asian medicine to Westerners.

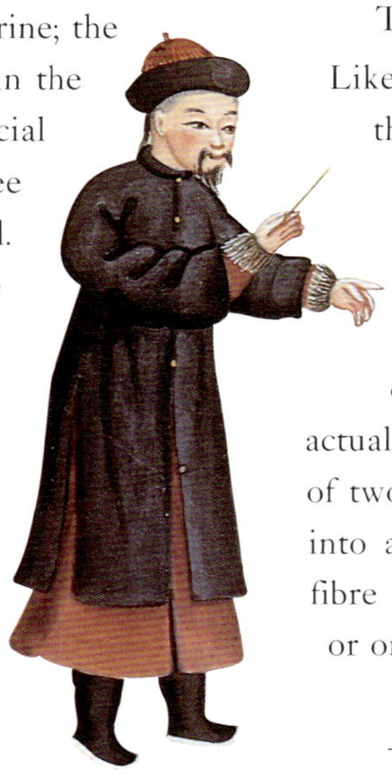

ABOVE AND BELOW Perhaps the most familiar symbol of traditional Chinese medicine to Western eyes – an acupuncturist with his needle approaches a patient.

THE BASIS OF ACUPUNCTURE

Like all Chinese therapies, acupuncture is based on the system of channels and organs described in the *Neijing.* Because these interconnected channels approach the body's surface at specific, empirically recognizable points, the flow of qi through the organs and around the body can not only be monitored with diagnostic techniques but actually altered and re-routed. This can be done by one of two external means: either a needle can be inserted into a specific point, or a small amount of vegetable fibre (moxa, dried mugwort) can be burned just above or on the surface of such a point.

The first traces of acupuncture are millennia old – stone needles have been found by archaeologists at prehistoric sites. Centuries of acupuncture practice have resulted in a rich surface map of the body, with hundreds of known points whose association with the internal organs and functions are well-established. Various points also have known associations with the treatment of specific symptoms and diseases. Acupuncture points are called *xue,* and have been found everywhere on the body; however, certain areas of the body's surface, such as specific points on the hands, feet and legs, are considered too dangerous to treat with the needle. In China, acupuncture is typically used in conjunction with the technique of moxibustion. Moxibustion involves the burning of pellets of vegetable fibre on or just above the surface of acupuncture points.

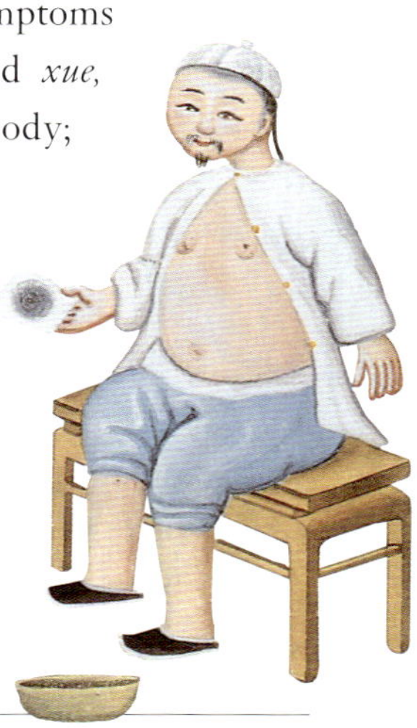

Although ancient, acupuncture is also an evolving technique. In the twentieth century, it has been modified to incorporate the use of electricity, and a new application for the needle has been found: acupuncture can produce powerful anaesthesia, with no side effects and with the patient remaining fully aware. In Japan, too, the twentieth century has seen the emergence of a new way to manipulate the acupuncture points and channels. Known as *shiatsu,* it combines the manual stimulation of acu-points with the techniques of massage and meditation to relax the body and treat chronic pain. Shiatsu practitioners claim Dao yin and anma (a type of massage which originated in ancient China, but was transmitted to Japan before AD 950) as sources for their therapeutic technique. However, they also call upon Western anatomical and physiological data to explain the effects which shiatsu produces. Anatomical knowledge of the body is integrated with the classical Chinese map of the body. Shiatsu practitioners use traditional Chinese diagnostic techniques – emphasizing touch-diagnosis – to assess patients, but select therapeutic points according to this innovative cross-cultural model of the body. Thus, instead of trying to alter the movement of circulating qi directly, shiatsu uses manual pressure to correct and re-align the body's tangible structures and rhythms. In addition, although most of the points manipulated in shiatsu are either traditional acupuncture points or lie along the acu-channels, they can be elsewhere.

Ayurveda's external applications are far less familiar to modern Westerners, although eighteenth- and nineteenth-century patients would recognize them immediately. Collectively known as *pañcakarma,* they include enemas, purgation and therapeutic vomiting. These treatments are considered to benefit illnesses caused by vāta, pitta and kapha imbalances, respectively. These Ayurvedic treatments differ from the external applications of Chinese medicine in that they do not attempt to affect the ojas directly, but rather to create the conditions in which ojas is created and held in balance. They are described as allowing and encouraging the fluid doṣas, prone to flooding, to return to their appropriate areas of the body, and then to be reduced to more healthful levels. Pañcakarma follows a prescribed pattern; in preparation, the body is covered with oil and warmed to the point of sweating – this step makes the doṣas more fluid. The second phase is designed to excite the humours, to prepare them to leave the body. The enema, purge or emetic is administered, to remove the excess doṣa, and to purify the body. Finally, the body is calmed, and the doṣas are considered to have returned to balance.[13]

ANIMAL, VEGETABLE AND MINERAL

Both Chinese and Indian medicine have enormous and incredibly various pharmacopoeia, drawing upon the animal and mineral kingdoms, as well as the more usual herbal sources. The types of animal substances used range from cow urine and dung to pulverized bull's testes to honey and tiger bones. This wide range stems from the fact that different medical principles underpin different categories of animal-based drugs. For example, the cow is sacred to Hindus, and every product derived from it is consequently considered not just pure but inherently beneficial by Ayurvedic medicine. The principle behind the use of tiger-bone or rhinoceros horn in Chinese medicine is that of magical correspondence: in other words, the strength associated with the tiger is supposed to be passed on to the person who consumes tiger bone. Today, some traditional Chinese healers are working to find alternatives for these substances, use of which is now illegal, to protect the endangered species from which they are derived. The substances they have discovered may have greater chemical and medical effects, but they have not yet gained the confidence of the consumer.

In fact, rhinoceros horn and tiger-bone have no pharmacological activity. They only achieve therapeutic results from the belief of patients and physicians in the power attributed to them. However, other substances which entered the materia medica by this means have proved more valuable. For example, bull's testes and the ovaries of other animals contain the hormones which stimulate the libido; even though both types of organ were probably first used because of the animal's status as a symbol of virility or fertility, the drug derived from them is active, and must have produced positive results in patients.

The third category of materia medica consists of the mineral medicine. The minerals range from salt and sulphur, to gold, lead and silver, clay, glass and mercury. Precious minerals were used in much the same way as the more exotic animal substances; their rarity and costliness were considered to confer upon them specially beneficial qualities. They were also considered to be more pure than other material substances, and thus to be endowed with more of the vital energies. Gold in particular was favoured because of its incorruptibility. Indian, Chinese and Western healers all relied upon powerful and poisonous mineral drugs – especially mercury – to treat some of the most dangerous and intransigent diseases. All were aware of the hazards of such drugs, but saw no other therapeutic alternative.

CROSSING THE BOUNDARIES OF CULTURE: WESTERN RESPONSES TO EASTERN MEDICINE

In the early years of the East India trade, and until as late as the first half of the eighteenth century, Europeans openly acknowledged the similarities between Western medicine and its Indian and East Asian counterparts. The stumbling early translations of Ayurvedic and Chinese medical texts emphasized features like the humours, which resembled classical doctrine, and the traditions of pulse diagnosis, which were portrayed as foreshadowing the European discovery of the circulation of the blood. In this phase of East-West relations, Europeans in India, China and Japan actively sought out the expert knowledge of those cultures, buying and translating classical texts and sending the resulting material back to the metropolitan centres of Europe. Most of these curious travellers were Catholic priests, usually specially trained Jesuit missionaries.

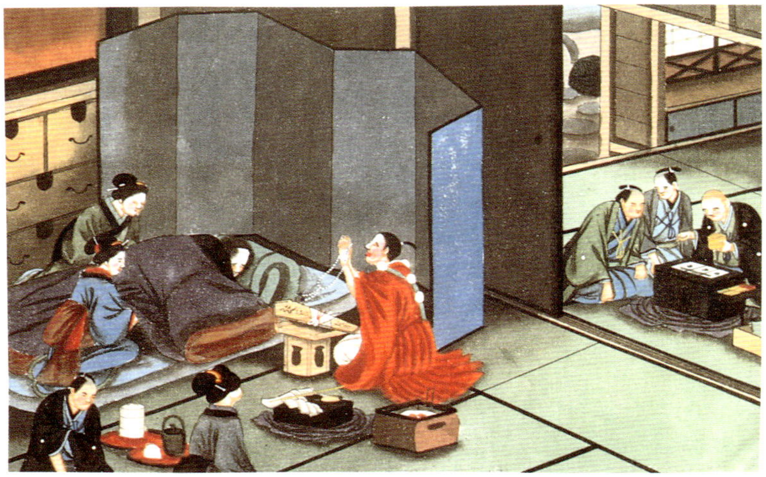

ABOVE European knowledge of Japanese medical practices initially came about principally through the work and publications of Wilhelm Ten Rhyne and Engelbert Kaempfer.

The other major group of Europeans in Asia were traders, agents of the East India Companies of Great Britain, France and the Netherlands, and in the Manchu north of China, Russia. In the years between 1670 and 1800, a vast and various collection of information about these unknown and exotic countries accumulated in Europe. Fact and fantasy were often mixed, and the problem of translation in relation to technical subjects – like medicine – made telling the two apart even more difficult. Descriptions of acupuncture, for example, were sent back to Europe both by the priests in China and by the physicians at the Dutch trading post in Japan. The former described Chinese medical theory with some sympathy, but their descriptions of acupuncture were wildly inaccurate. In 1685, one European, drawing his information from these Jesuit sources, described acupuncture as, 'that perforation of all parts of the body which they do even of the very brain itself, transfixed from one side of the head to the other with a metal bodkin a cubit in length or longer…'[14]

The European physicians in Japan certainly gave more accurate physical descriptions of acupuncture, and were quite positive about the needle's potential to heal. However, they almost entirely neglected the theories underlying acupuncture practice. Given that their information about Chinese medicine was gathered orally, in Portuguese – generally a second or third language for these northern Europeans – from Japanese interpreters who spoke only a smattering of that language themselves, and often only slightly better Chinese, this lacuna is perhaps forgivable!

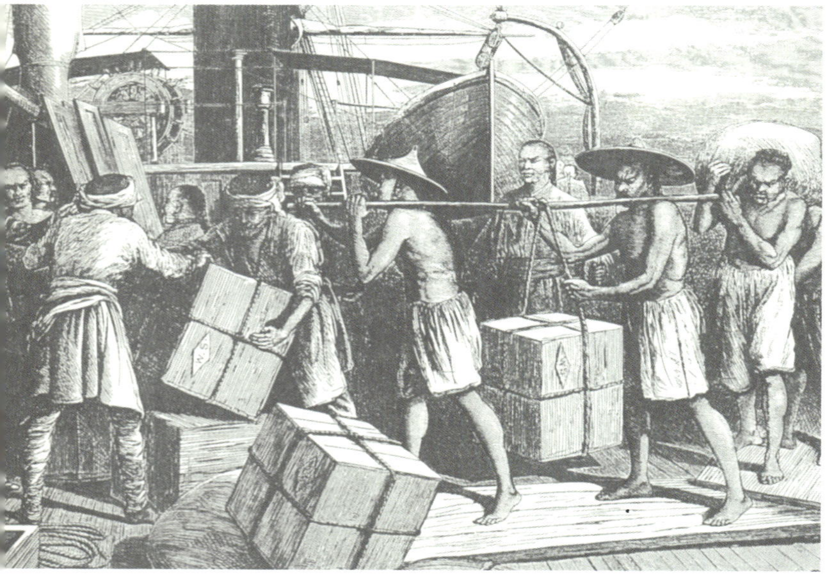

LEFT When diplomatic and trade relations between East and West were established in the eighteenth and nineteenth centuries, a conduit for the exchange of medical knowledge also became available.

LEARNING ABOUT CHINESE MEDICINE: THE PRIESTS AND THE DOCTORS

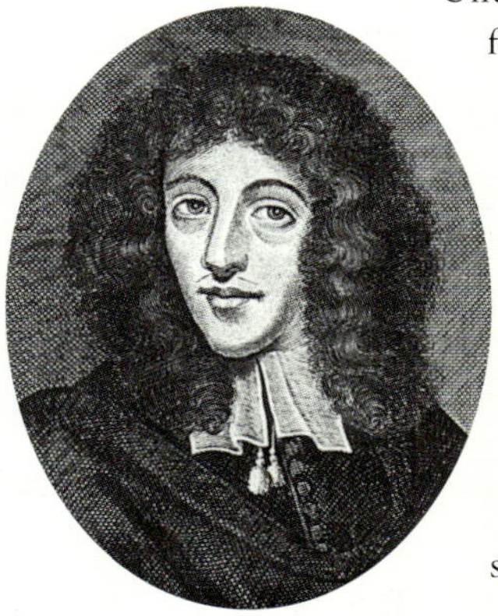

ABOVE **An engraving of Wilhelm Ten Rhyne at the age of 34. He was a physician at the Dutch trading colony of Deshima, and his account of acupuncture introduced Europe to the practice.**

Until the 1850s, Westerners were forbidden to learn Chinese. Only one group was exempt from this rule: those who would settle forever in China, live by her laws, and swear never to return to their native countries. This restriction, intended to protect China from internal strife and external influences, ensured that for several centuries, almost the only Westerners who spoke Chinese were priests, sent by the Catholic Church to convert the great Empire to Catholicism. Japan, too, had been a target for Catholic missions, but the internal strife feared by the Chinese had actually broken out in Japan. Japanese Christians were persecuted and their priests were either executed or driven out; by 1641, Japan was closed to all foreigners save the tiny and closely guarded Dutch trading colony on Deshima. To further limit potential contacts between the Dutch and the Japanese citizenry, the foreigners were allowed to bring medical personnel with them.

Despite their scant numbers, the priests in China and the doctors in Japan made discoveries about traditional Chinese medicine (which formed the basis of Japanese practice as well). The Jesuits, and in particular a Pole named Michael Boym *(d.1659)*, sent back detailed descriptions of Chinese diagnostics, Five Element theory, and the doctrine of yinyang. He even included maps of the acupuncture points, but interpreted them as points where the pulse might be taken. In Japan, Wilhelm Ten Rhyne *(1647–1700)* and Engelbert Kaempfer *(1651–1716)* provided Europe with its entire fund of knowledge about acupuncture, as well as the first maps of the acupuncture channels *(jing)*. Both men were medically trained and aware of the new scientific developments in Europe; it was perhaps this knowledge which made them sceptical of the medical theories surrounding the practice of needling. Nonetheless, they encouraged Europeans to experiment with the foreign technique, and described the needles and the illnesses for which they were used in great detail.

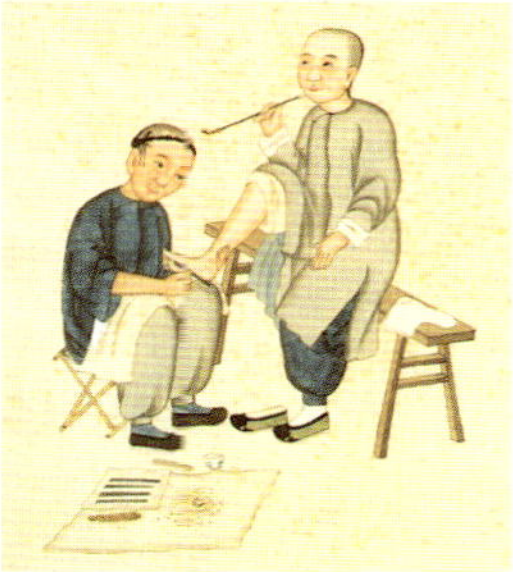

ABOVE **An early nineteenth-century watercolour of a Chinese chiropodist by Zhou Pei Qun.**

Why did these men, all of them fully occupied with other tasks, take the time to study the medical practices of another culture – even risking, in the case of Ten Rhyne and Kaempfer, their own jobs and their informant's lives? Both groups had what might be called ulterior motives. The Jesuit mission in China had committed itself to conversion from the top down. This was a reasonable, but expensive strategy, and in order to keep the Vatican interested, the Jesuits had to portray China as the supreme prize, and its occupants as worthy of the cost and effort devoted to the mission. At a time when medicine and science were beginning their long ascent in status, the Jesuits needed to portray the Chinese as excelling in those fields. So they went looking for evidence that this was indeed the case, and found it in sophisticated Chinese theories of the pulse.

Ten Rhyne and Kaempfer, too, had pragmatic as well as idealistic goals to fulfil through their research into the manners and medicine of the Japanese. Both men sent their work back to Europe to be published, and Kaempfer in particular planned to base his subsequent career around his Japanese experiences. Their knowledge of acupuncture was stock-in-trade, as well as the fruit of genuine intellectual curiosity.

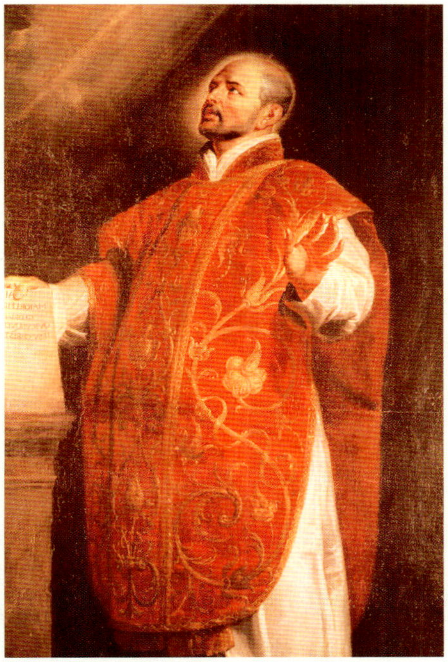

LEFT **St Ignatius de Loyola *(?1491–1556)*, the founder in 1540 of the Society of Jesus – a portrait by Peter Paul Rubens. Jesuit missionaries in the Far East were introduced to traditional Chinese medicine.**

LEARNING ABOUT INDIAN MEDICINE: SOLDIERS, TRADERS AND MISSIONARIES

In India, interactions between Europeans and the various indigenous peoples took place on a larger scale and with much greater freedom than in either China or Japan. From their colony in Goa in the early sixteenth century, the Portuguese avidly sought information about Indian drugs and herbal medicines. In the seventeenth and eighteenth centuries, the Dutch and British East India Companies, despairing of their ability to supply their soldiers, sailors and traders with sufficient Western drugs, also sought Indian alternatives. Both groups did extensive research on the botany of the Indian sub-continent, with a particular focus on finding and studying medicinal plants.

Early British traders actively sought out Ayurvedic practitioners to question them about local remedies and regimens. In the process, they discovered that the Western Galenic system had strong similarities with Indian medical thought. Meanwhile, Indian practitioners expressed great interest in Western surgical techniques – due to cleanliness taboos and the poor status of surgery in India, the techniques described in the *Su'sruta Samhitā* were no longer practised. However, this early atmosphere of co-operation and collegiality could not survive the combined onslaught of increasing numbers of Europeans (including doctors), new standards of medical practice, and the rise of scientific medicine, with its emphasis on anatomy and chemistry. The British government was weaned from its pre-1860 policy of encouraging (as a cost-saving measure) the use of native drugs and medicines, and laws designed to protect and promote Western medicine were enacted in the 1910s.

Given the decline of surgery in India, it is ironic that the most successful medical export from India to Europe was a surgical operation. The technique was designed to restore the nose. Intriguingly, the British learned of it from a brickmaker, who in turn seems to have gained his knowledge from family traditions. The operation began with the creation of a flat pattern of the appropriate size and shape to replace the missing nose. This pattern was then placed on the centre of the forehead, and cut out of the skin beneath it, leaving a slender connecting strip of skin intact to preserve circulation. After roughening or cutting the cheeks at the edge of the open sinus, the raw edges were joined and sutured. The 'nose' was bandaged and shaped, and reeds were inserted into the air passages. When the nose had almost healed, it was trimmed and reshaped.

SCIENCE AND WESTERN MEDICINE

Meanwhile, back in Europe, the sciences which inform modern medicine were emerging at a rapid rate; after Harvey's discovery of the circulation, and with the rise of anatomy, elite doctors in European medicine were gaining confidence in the idea of 'medical science' – a collection of objective, rather than subjective experiences of the body. As the Macartney mission's response to the physician-centred process of Chinese pulse-diagnosis showed, this idea was slow to filter out of the medical books and reach the general population. However, even as many European medical practitioners continued to doubt the value of new anatomical knowledge, Westerners posted in Asia began to make anatomical accuracy a criterion for judging non-Western medical systems. Chinese and Ayurvedic medical knowledge (and several thousand years of distilled experience and observation) were in general disregarded because the medical theories underpinning them did not depict the physical body as it was understood by Western anatomists.

Nonetheless, the rise of Western medical science did not completely eliminate East-to-West transmission of medical knowledge. Moxibustion and acupuncture, first described in Europe in the late seventeenth century, enjoyed several waves of European popularity in the eighteenth and nineteenth centuries, respectively. Moxibustion, which bore a close resemblance to the traditional Western technique of actual cautery (using extreme heat to stimulate or eliminate diseased tissues), was accepted fairly readily, although it was stripped of its underlying theory. Moxa was milder than its European counterpart, and had strong and vocal support among a

BELOW **Moxibustion – here being practised in Japan – enjoyed brief spells of popularity in Europe during the eighteenth and nineteenth centuries.**

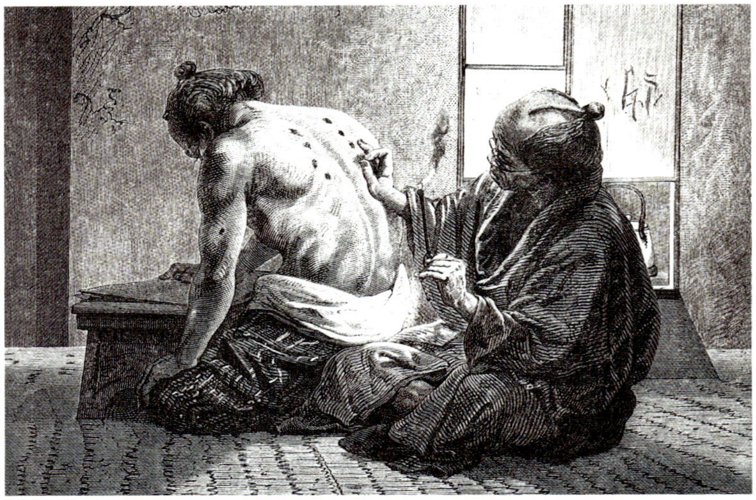

well-travelled and well-read elite. Acupuncture, on the other hand, had no European analogue. After the publication of Wilhelm Ten Rhyne's medical treatise on the technique in 1683, acupuncture was discussed, but not practised, by an elite group of European physicians. The cures Ten Rhyne claimed for the needle were considered incredible, and the Chinese anatomy upon which acupuncture was based was portrayed as 'curious', even ludicrous. Subsequent first-hand reports of acupuncture were ignored by the few doctors and surgeons who could purchase access to them. Medical compendia and dictionaries were more readily available, and many of them referred to acupuncture; however, they consistently described it as an Asian mode of blood-letting. Since European medicine was already richly endowed with different methods of bleeding, an alien alternative attracted little attention and no professional support in the century following its European debut.

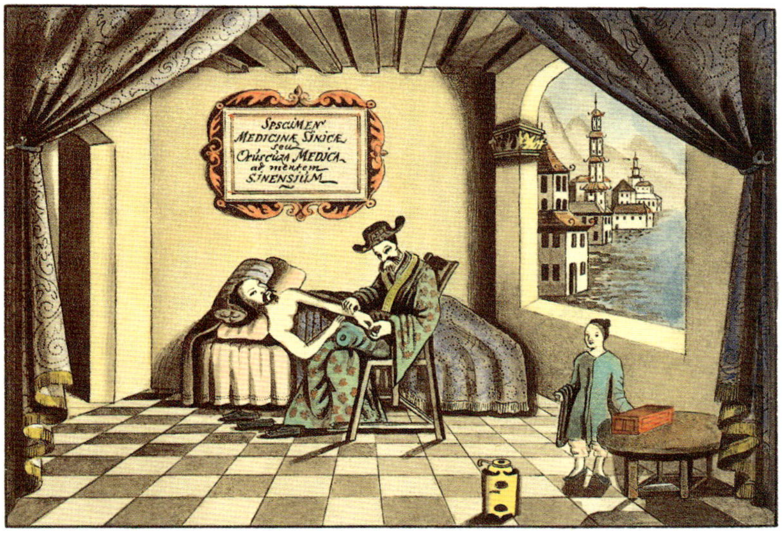

ABOVE This image is the frontispiece of Andreas Cleyer's 1682 work on Chinese medicine *Specimen medicinae sinicae*. Note the brazier and needles.

By the end of the eighteenth century, however, the picture had changed radically; a form of acupuncture was being used in the great hospitals of Paris, especially in those specializing in rheumatism, gout, sciatica and other chronic and nervous afflictions. More importantly, acupuncture had come to the attention of the first generation of medical experimentalists. The French medical press described the empirical success of acupuncture and reported experiments on its mode of action. These reports rapidly circulated around Europe, accompanied by the eye-witness accounts of foreign medical students in Paris.

By the second decade of the nineteenth century, the British press had succumbed to the forces of curiosity and rising interest, and reports on the successes of this exotic medical import began to appear with increasing frequency. For twenty years, references to acupuncture peppered medical periodicals. Private doctors and public hospitals throughout Europe experimented with the technique, and sought an explanation for its curious effects. Laymen also played a part in promoting acupuncture-use. In Britain, for example, one gout-sufferer who had been cured by the needle named his favourite racehorse 'Acupuncture' and promoted the technique in his local area.

This rapid surge of interest in acupuncture, however, died away nearly as quickly as it arose. Its status was tarnished by the appearance of several dubious medical practices also involving needles, such as the painful technique known as Baunscheidtism, as well as by the swift decline in China's reputation after their defeat by Great Britain in the Opium Wars. But the most important factor in the disappearance of acupuncture was the changing standards of proof and authority in European medicine. The continued use of a treatment which could not be understood and explained by conventional scientific methods was becoming unacceptable in medical circles.

By mid-century, acupuncture had receded almost to invisibility in the West. Acupuncture was still used by individual practitioners and in some hospitals, and both patients and practitioners witnessed its beneficial effects in ailments like sciatica, rheumatism, gout, tetanus and muscular injury, and the use of the needle continued to spread, albeit slowly, through informal networks. However, although acupuncture gradually re-emerged in the medical press, it never regained its early visibility in this medium. Changes in the structure and status of the medical profession, and in the construction of therapeutic authority within Western medicine as a whole, made acupuncture indigestible to orthodox medicine.

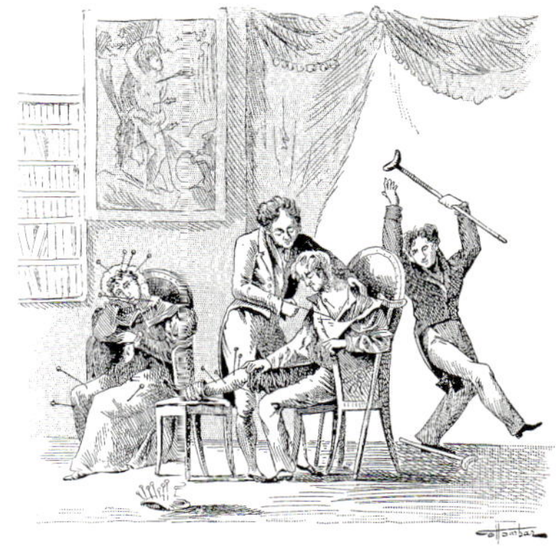

ABOVE A rather sardonic view of 'the marvellous effects of acupuncture' from an early nineteenth-century French source.

ENERGY MEDICINE IN THE WEST

MESMERISM

Given the general lack of interest in and often outright hostility to Chinese and Indian medical theories which prevailed at the end of the eighteenth century, it is perhaps ironic that this period also saw the rise of mesmerism in Europe. Mesmerism was based on an idea about the vital energy of the body remarkably similar to those underlying the Chinese practice of qigong. In 1775, Swiss physician Anton Mesmer *(1734–1815)* claimed to have discovered a genuine natural substance, which he called 'animal magnetism'. It was a 'subtle fluid' in both the classical and the Newtonian senses – Mesmer himself likened it to gravity and aether as well as the newly discovered 'galvanic fluid', electricity.

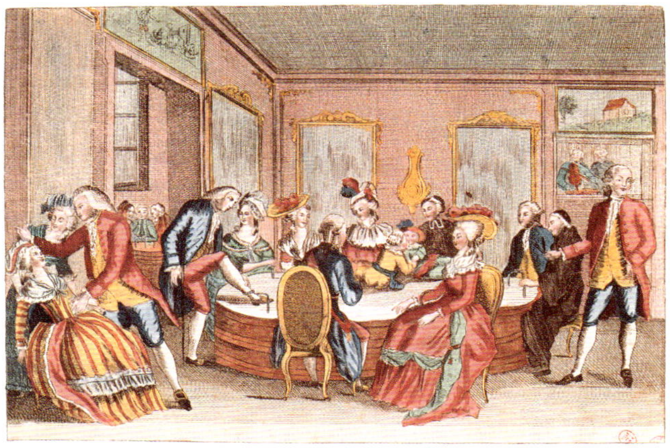

ABOVE Anton Mesmer's concept of animal magnetism finds a parallel in Indian and Chinese theories of vital energy. For a while, his salon was immensely fashionable.

By 1784, Mesmer confidently answered the question 'What is magnetism?' with the statement that, 'It is the property which bodies have of being susceptible to the action of a universally distributed fluid, a fluid which surrounds all that exists and which serves to maintain the equilibrium of all the vital functions.' He might almost have been quoting from classical Chinese or Ayurvedic descriptions of their respective vital energies. The possibility that such a substance might exist in the human body first occurred to him in response to an older work which suggested that the human body, like the seas, might feel the gravitational pull of the planets – in other words, that human tissues were subject to 'tides'. Indeed, Mesmer also defined animal magnetism as 'the property of the animal body that renders it sensitive to the action of heavenly bodies and of the earth.'

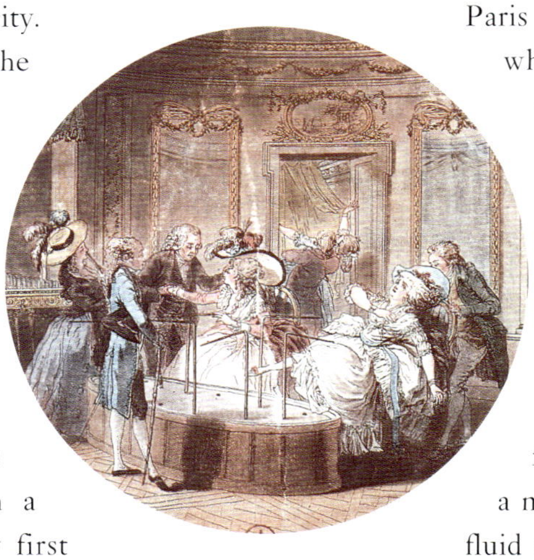

ABOVE Mesmer is seen, centre left, with patients who are holding metal handles protruding from a tub filled with water and magnetic metal objects. Two of the ladies appear to be experiencing a mesmeric 'crisis' or trance.

Mesmer was convinced that the presence and proper action of the magnetic fluid, like those of qi and ojas, ensured health. Conversely, a sick person might be cured of nervous conditions by the stimulation of his or her mesmeric fluid, or by a dose of the substance transferred to them by an individual super-endowed with animal magnetism by reason of moral and physical superiority. Mesmer himself was such a person naturally, but less fortunate individuals could build up their reservoirs of animal magnetism through efforts of will. Alternatively, a sick individual could benefit from the pooled (or stored) magnetic energy of a group of normal people. After an initial rebuff in Vienna, Mesmer set out in earnest to popularize his discovery. In 1778, he moved to Paris and began by offering treatments to those who attended his clinic-salon in Paris. He called his new, quasi-masonic establishment 'The Society of Harmony', and gave it the motto, 'All things in due weight and measure.' Clearly, Mesmer sought scientific credibility as avidly as popular acceptance! His salon was dominated by an enormous 'tub' filled with water and magnetic material – mainly metal bars and iron filings– which Mesmer considered to be a mesmeric magnet, charged with the collected fluid of his own and his patients' animal magnetism. From the periphery of this tank projected metal handles. His patients would grasp these during treatment, and Mesmer would will the tub's stored energy into his patients' bodies, triggering the mesmeric 'crisis', or trance.

Supported by a wave of interest in the new discovery of electricity, for a time Mesmer's technique produced good results; patients proclaimed the success of his cures, and the scientific establishment looked on bemusedly. Most of Mesmer's

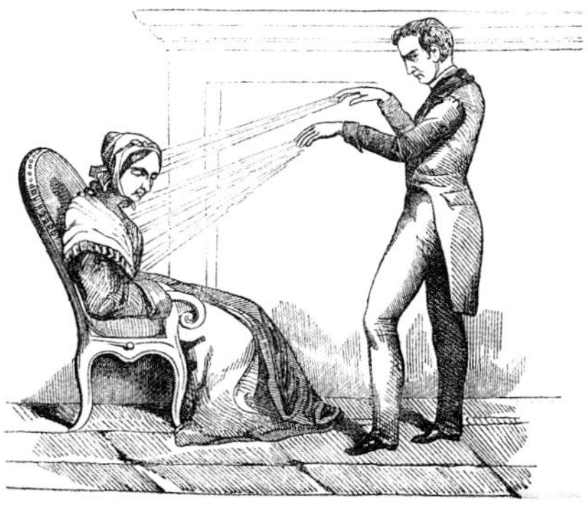

ABOVE Mesmerism upset orthodox opinion because it seemed to pose a threat to the virtue of its female disciples.

successful cases were among middle- and upper-class women, whose attendance at his clinic was due as much to fashion and politics as to medical complaints. These patients, surrounded by acquaintances and fellow sufferers, were fixed by the intense gaze, and sometimes stroked by the wand of Dr Mesmer. If a 'crisis' was produced, the individual might faint, cry out – perhaps with pleasure, perhaps in pain – or even fall into a fit. It was this peculiar, unpredictable and highly personal interaction between a male physician and predominately female patients, combined with a taint of political radicalism, that got Mesmer in trouble.

The medical profession, which had snubbed him in 1781, began a formal investigation of his technique and the new fluid for which he claimed so much. Despite the reaction which Mesmer could produce in his clients – and which he was able to train others to produce as well – no physical substance was found to exist. His discovery was publicly discredited by the findings of a Royal Commission in 1784. It did not, however, decline in popularity for lack of experimental proof. Rather, mesmerism was undermined in orthodox medical circles because it existed in an atmosphere of sexual tension and titillation. Mesmer was not disgraced by the collapse of his theory in the face of science; he was driven out of Paris by the unstated assumption that his therapeutic invention threatened the virtue of his predominantly female patients.

The technique itself, stripped of its claims to a material basis and often trading under the untainted name of hypnotism, continued to be applied in the private spaces of the patient's home or the doctor's surgery. In fact, mesmerism was exported to India by a surgeon named Esdaile, who used it to produce anaesthesia during surgical operations. Today, Mesmer is regarded as a founder of psychotherapeutic hypnotism. Although modern hypnotism has given up its claim to an imponderable fluid as an aid to healing, the analogy between hypnotism and the comparatively new practice of qigong healing (in which an expert skilled in qi-manipulation uses his or her own qi to direct that of a patient) has been remarked upon by practitioners of both therapeutic disciplines.[15]

HOMEOPATHY

Like Ayurvedic medicine and acupuncture, homeopathic medicine is based on a sense that the body interacts in complex ways with its natural environment, and on an assumption that the body has the innate power to heal itself. Homeopathy, however, is a thoroughly Western invention. In 1796, disgusted by the harsh and dangerous practices of orthodox medicine, a German physician named Samuel Hahnemann *(1755–1843)* laid the groundwork for a new medical science, which he called homeopathy. This science was based on two principles and a number of observations. The first principle was that *'similia similibus curentur'*, or 'like cures like'; the second was the 'Doctrine of Infinitessimals', or the smallest possible dose. Hahnemann based the first principle on his own observation that certain medicinal substances produced in the healthy body exactly the symptoms which they relieved in the sick one. However, it is also a form of the ancient notion of correspondence (which also shaped Chinese and Ayurvedic herbalism).

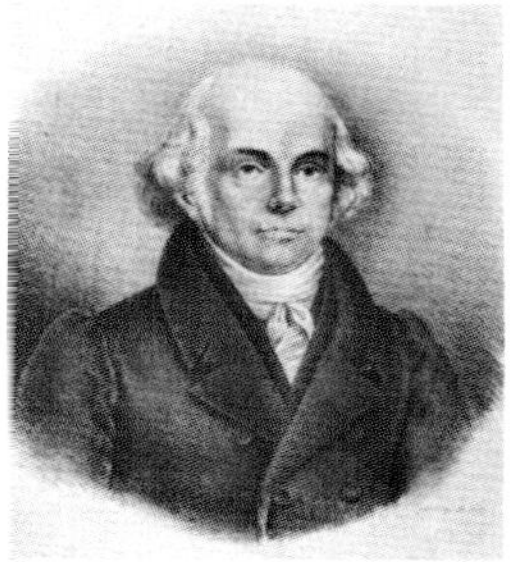

ABOVE Born at Meissen in Germany, Samuel Hahnemann was the founder of the practice of homeopathy.

In the case of homeopathy, the administration of drugs was intended to assist the body's natural tendency to restore itself to balance, by triggering or hastening the excretion of disease-causing material. Once the source of imbalance was removed, the body would heal itself – therefore a drug that cut short the cycle of suffering could only be beneficial. Although Hahnemann and his followers did not give this tendency a physical form – like ojas, qi or aether – they were calling on the same basic concept: that within all living bodies resided an inherent healing power. As Hahnemann wrote in *The Organon of the Healing Art*:

> *In the healthy condition of man, the spiritual vital force, the* dynamis *that rules the spiritual body, rules with unbounded sway, and retains all parts of the organism in admirable, harmonious vital operation ... The material organization, without the vital force, is capable of no sensation, and performs all the functions of life solely by means of the immaterial being (the vital force) which animates the material organism...*
>
> SAMUEL HAHNEMANN, *THE ORGANON OF THE HEALING ART*

TREATING LIKE WITH LIKE

Hahnemann believed that the homeopathic method of treating like with like was superior to the orthodox method of treating with opposites, largely because the artificial disease produced would overwhelm the weaker natural disease, and drive the body towards its natural denouement. 'By giving a remedy which resembles the disease the instinctive vital force is compelled to increase its vital energy until it becomes stronger than the disease which, in turn, is vanquished.' Historically, this idea of the self-regulating 'instinctive' vitality underpinned Western medicine's frequent use of drugs to produce vomiting or purging. Other techniques intended to harness the body's own restorative efforts involved making the patient sweat (based on the observation that the positive resolution of a life-threatening fever was frequently signalled by profuse perspiration) and in the technique of blood-letting.

The second homeopathic principle, Hahnemann's novel idea, and the most controversial aspect of homeopathy both in the nineteenth century and today, was called the 'Doctrine of Infinitessimals'. The smaller the dose of a medicine, the more effective it was likely to be in producing its effects, and the less likely it was to disrupt further the ailing patient's already delicate balance of health. He based this principle on the observation that prescribing large doses of 'Similars' strongly aggravated the symptoms of disease, while smaller doses still produced cures. The source of this counter-intuitive behaviour, he reasoned, was the efficacy of homeopathic drugs in stimulating the vital force. Over time, he came to believe that the process of dilution itself made the crude substance of each drug purer, and consequently more potent – rather than diluting the active material, he believed he was refining it.

Although the principles of homeopathy were comparatively straightforward, putting them into practice was far from simple. To treat a disease successfully according to the homeopathic method, Hahnemann claimed that:

We only require to know, on the one hand, the diseases of the human frame accurately in their essential characteristics and their accidental complications, and, on the other hand, the pure effect of drugs; that is, the essential characteristics of the specific artificial disease they usually excite, together with the accidental symptoms caused by difference of dose, etc. and by choosing a remedy for a given natural disease that is capable of producing a very similar artificial disease we shall be able to cure the most obstinate diseases.

SAMUEL HAHNEMANN, OP. CIT.

Despite Hahnemann's sanguine tone, homeopathic practice clearly demanded no small burden of prior knowledge, especially as few drugs had been tested on healthy individuals. Moreover, the experiments he prescribed to discover the 'pure effect of drugs' required that each proposed medical substance be tested alone. This protocol essentially prohibited the use of compound drugs. Homeopaths made a virtue of this necessity, by claiming that the simplicity of their medicines made them all the more natural and readily assimilated by the body.

From the mid-nineteenth century to the second decade of the twentieth, the popularity of homeopathy soared; homeopathic journals, medical societies and universities were established in Europe and North America, as well as in India. The middle and upper classes flocked to this mild medicine, accepting it as a reprieve from the violent purges, poisonous mineral compounds and drastic blood-letting of medical orthodoxy. Homeopathy also appealed to the romantic ideals of the day, fulfilling the desire of the middle classes to return to an Arcadian nature and simplicity lost in the turmoil of the Industrial Revolution. However, faced by this stiff competition, orthodox practitioners began to moderate their therapeutic measures. With the advent of anaesthesia, regular medicine, too, could claim to be mild, and the continued rise of science as a basis for medical authority gave them a theoretical edge. The regulars could put forward more compelling explanations for disease, even though they still often

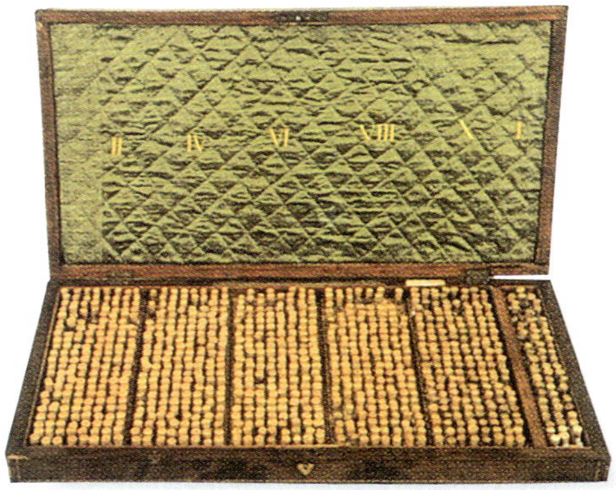

ABOVE **Hahnemann's own medicine box. He angered the apothecaries of his day because he dispensed his own preparations.**

lacked effective therapies for them. Moreover, scientific tests of homeopathic remedies apparently proved them to contain no 'active' ingredients. As governments began to regulate the medical profession, orthodox institutions were able to restrict the claims of their homeopathic competitors. Homeopathy entered a steep decline, from which it is only now recovering.[16]

EASTERN INFLUENCE ON WESTERN PRACTICE TODAY

Western doctors and scientists today are aware of the ancient and still vital systems of medical thought and expertise that originated in India and China. Perhaps more importantly, Asian medical practices are becoming a part of the popular culture of medicine in Europe and North America. The consumers as well as the practitioners of medicine are increasingly interested in these non-Western models of health and health care. Like acupuncture, mesmerism and homeopathy in the nineteenth century, Chinese and Ayurvedic therapies today are seen as potential alternatives to Western medical orthodoxy.

The allure of Asian medicine is, of course, linked to the 'exotic' philosophies and cultures underlying it, but its immediate appeal to consumers stems from its emphasis on the particular and subjective experience of the patient. Arising from long traditions of subjective – but nonetheless rigorous and painstakingly recorded – exploration of consciousness and the mind-body, both Chinese and Ayurvedic medicine have developed techniques to read and assess the experiential account of illness. Both traditions value this account, told from the patient's perspective, as a diagnostic and therapeutic tool. In contrast, the Western medical tradition is marked by a heavy reliance on the observer's account of the disease; authority is given to objectivity and objectivity tends to be equated with truth.

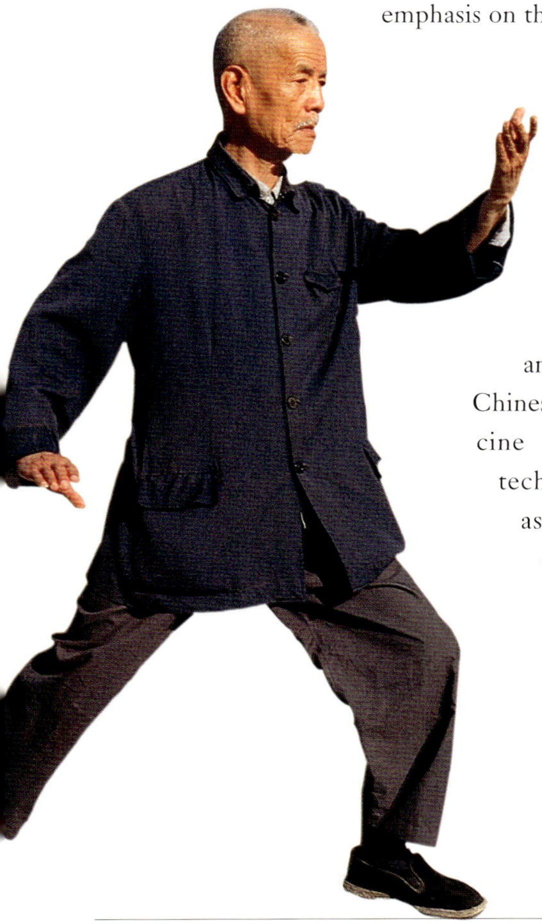

LEFT Eastern techniques of health care are receiving an increasingly enthusiastic reception in the West. T'ai-chi Ch'uan is one of a number of disciplines that have been taken up in recent years by Westerners.

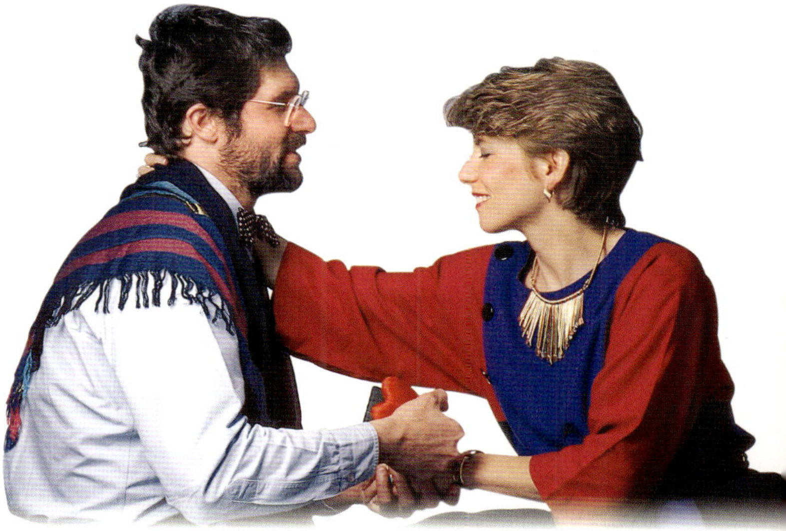

ABOVE A doctor comforting a patient with AIDS. Orthodox Western medicine finds its traditional orthodoxies challenged by diseases like this.

However, in the face of consumer demand and competition from medical alternatives, and struggling to cope with diseases like AIDS and the chronic ailments of old age, Western medical science is finally re-awakening to the clinical worth of subjective experience. In 1841, a Briton in China wrote to his medical colleagues posted in all the exotic possessions of the British Empire. He strongly encouraged them to study the local medical practices, observing that:

> *Every nation and tribe has what we may call its national therapeutics and nosology. It has some conceptions of disease peculiar to itself, some modes of treatment not observed elsewhere. In principle and extent, they may be very humble, in detail united with error and mistake, but I think we should have to search a long time before we found one that would not afford one fact for our information, or one hint to awaken our curiosity.*
>
> GT TRADESCANT LAY *(1841)*

Perhaps today, more than 150 years later, the Western medical community, practitioners and patients alike, will be able to benefit from his sound and sensible advice.

CHAPTER FIVE

SURGERY AND MANIPULATION

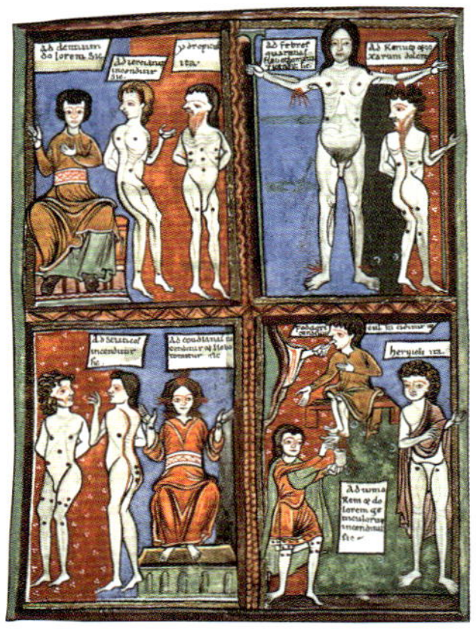

ABOVE These twelfth-century vignettes show cauterization points.

THE WORD 'SURGERY' *comes from the Greek* cheirourgein, *made up of* 'cheir' – *hand, and* 'ergo' – *to work. Literally, therefore, the term means 'to work with the hand'. Surgery is defined as those manual procedures used in the management of injuries and disease; in the words of the* Oxford English Dictionary *definition, it is 'the art or practice of treating injuries, deformities and other disorders by manual operation or other appliances'. Man has always been subject to violence – contusions, fractures, dislocations, impalements, eviscerations – and the earliest surgeons in the days before history was recorded were no doubt those men and women who showed particular interest and skill in dealing with such injuries.*

Long before written records existed, we have to rely on the only available evidence, ancient skeletons, to learn something of the diseases which affected primitive man and of the earliest surgical endeavours. Archaeologists have provided evidence of arthritis, bone infections, tumours and of dental disease from the earliest times. Fractures, of course, are obvious and splints of wood and of bark have been found in ancient Egyptian excavations. However, remarkably and inexplicably, the earliest major surgery of which we have undoubted evidence is trephination of the skull, which dates back to at least 5,000 BC in the Stone Age period. Not only did primitive surgeons, using no more than crude flint or stone instruments, actually bore holes through the skulls of patients, but there is undoubtedly evidence that a proportion of their patients survived. We know this because about half of the skulls excavated show evidence of healing around the edges of the bone defect. Moreover, this operation was performed in widely different areas of the world. Trephined skulls have been found in Western Europe, including England, as well as in North Africa, Asia, the East Indies and New Zealand. In North America, evidence has been found of the operation from Alaska in the north, down through the continent to Peru in South America.

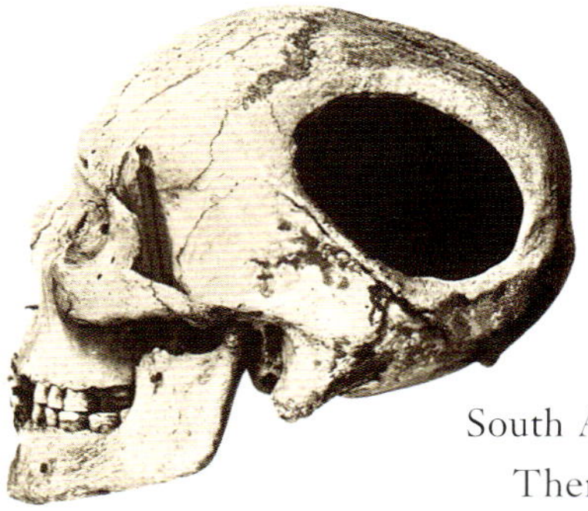

ABOVE Trephined skulls such as this provide the first concrete evidence of surgery in ancient times. Possibly the operation had a magical, rather than therapeutic, purpose.

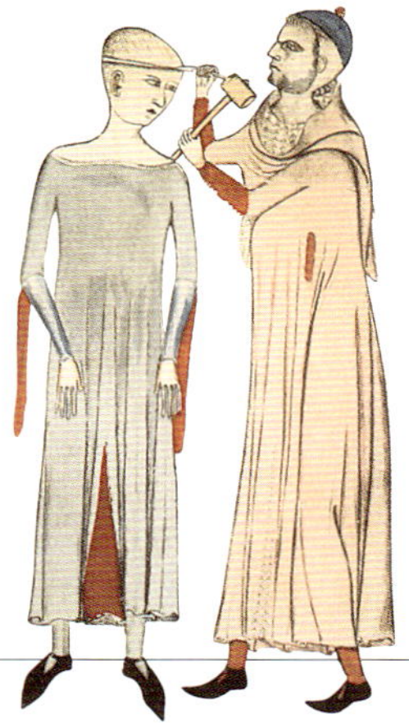

There are many unanswered questions. Did this operation, which is today regarded as a sophisticated procedure to be done by expert neurosurgeons, arise spontaneously in numerous centres throughout the world, or did knowledge of the operation spread gradually from place to place? Why was the operation performed? In many cases, it was undoubtedly carried out because of trauma to the skull. In many other examples, however, there is no evidence of skull injury and also evidence that the operation was repeated at intervals of time. We can only guess that it might have been performed on patients suffering from mental illness, intractable headaches or epilepsy to let out the demon which possessed the patient (a belief still common in some primitive races).

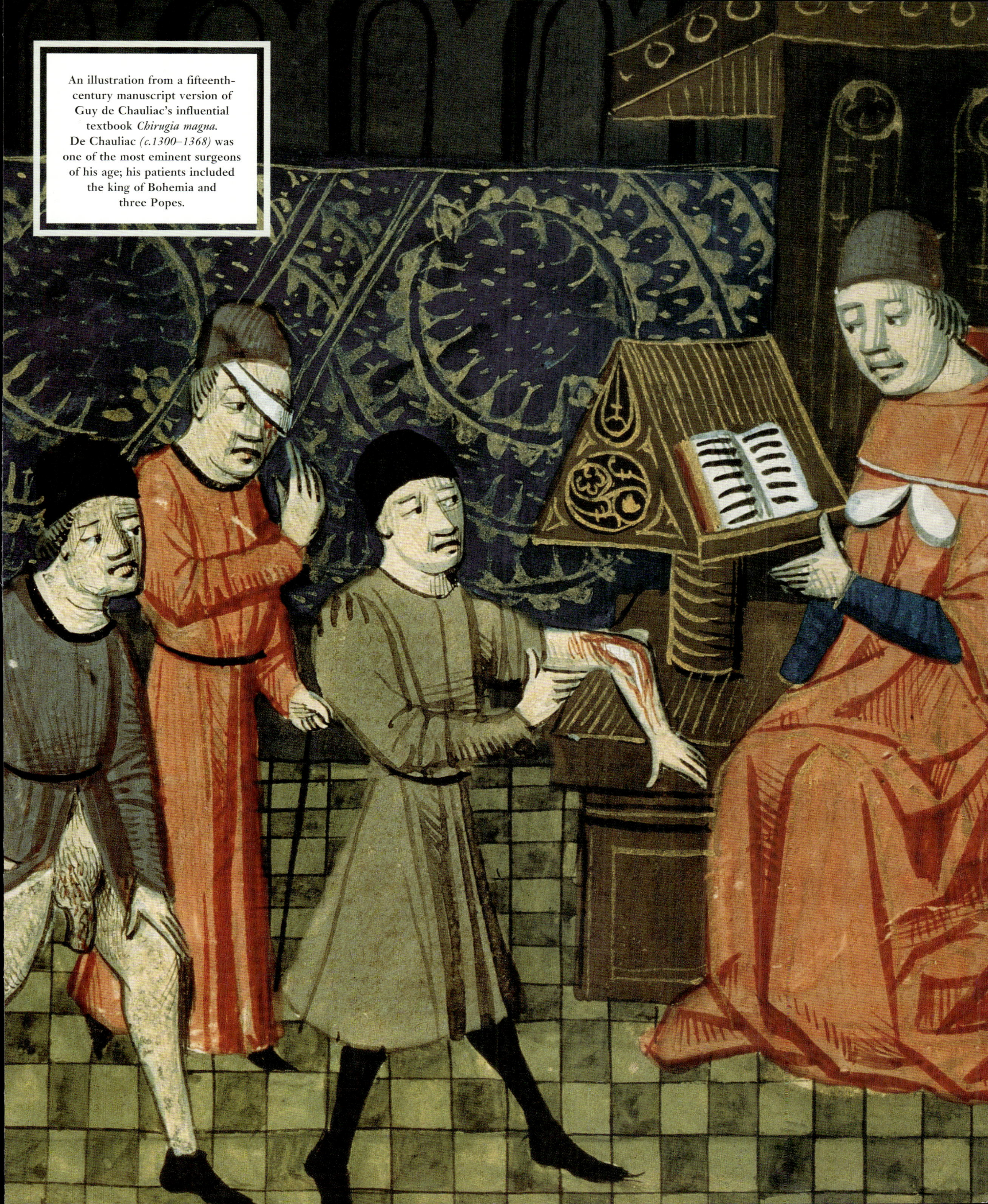

An illustration from a fifteenth-century manuscript version of Guy de Chauliac's influential textbook *Chirugia magna*. De Chauliac *(c.1300–1368)* was one of the most eminent surgeons of his age; his patients included the king of Bohemia and three Popes.

THE ANCIENT MIDDLE EAST

The first written records, which came from ancient Babylon and Egypt, interestingly enough contain the earliest references to medical care, and report what were obviously active interventional surgical procedures.

Writing was invented in Mesopotamia, the valley between the rivers Tigris and Euphrates, in the time of the Sumerians, who founded the city of Ur about 3000 BC. The script comprised wedge-shaped (cuneiform) signs inscribed with a stylus on soft clay, which was then baked. Successively, the Sumerians were conquered by Sargon of Akkad at about 2500 BC, who was soon to be overcome, in turn, by the Assyrians.

The medicine of Mesopotamia was primarily medico-religious. Practitioners were priests and, after 2000 BC, they were ruled by the strict laws included in the code of Hammurabi. This code, carved on a black stone about 8 ft (2.4m) high, which was discovered at Shush in Iran in 1901, can be seen today in the Louvre Museum in Paris. At its top, we see the emperor Hammurabi of Babylon receiving the laws from the sun god Shamash. His code laid down rewards for success and severe punishment for failure on the part of the surgeon – it was obviously a dangerous profession in those days! It is evident from these writings that surgical conditions such as wounds, fractures and abscesses were treated by these early surgeons.

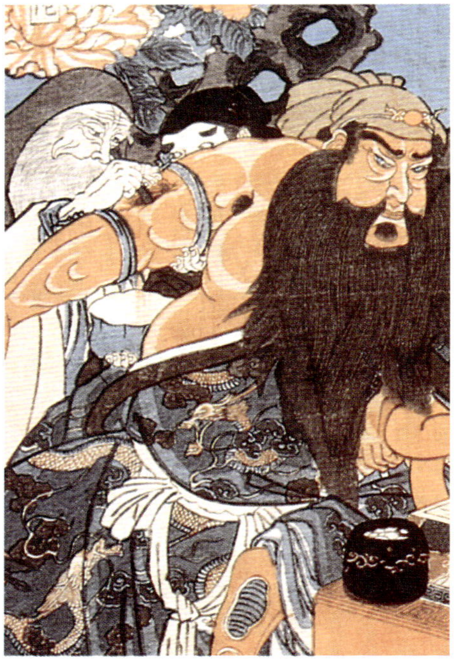

ABOVE The Chinese surgeon Hua Tuo operating on the arm of warlord General Kuan Yun.

The civilization of ancient Egypt dates from around 3000 BC. With it came the development of the pictorial writing of hieroglyphics and the discovery that writing material could be prepared from the papyrus reed. In 1862, Edwin Smith, an American Egyptologist, discovered a papyrus of immense interest, the world's earliest surgical text. Dated at around 1600 BC, it contains material probably derived from even more ancient times. It comprises 48 case reports, which commence with the top of the head and which proceed systematically downwards – nose, face, ears, neck and chest, and then mysteriously stops in mid-sentence at the spine. Having described the physical signs of the patient, the surgeon then goes on to decide on the outlook of the case; if the prognosis is good or if there is a possible chance of success, treatment is then advised. If hopeless, then the patient should be left to his inevitable fate.

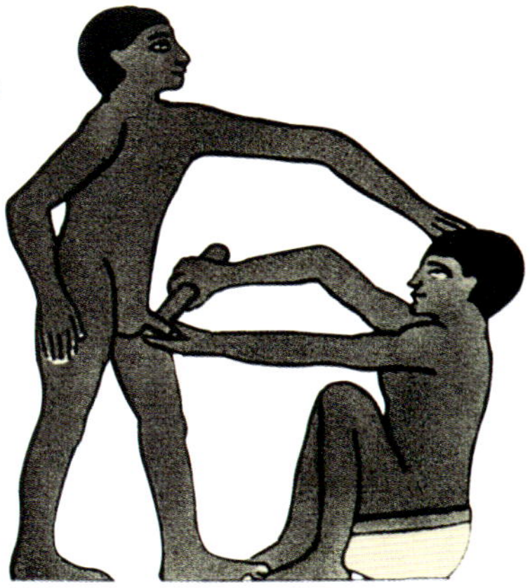

ABOVE A depiction of circumcision in ancient Egypt, from a carved relief c.2500 BC. This was probably a religious ritual.

From these writings it appears that the only surgical conditions treated, just as our evidence from Babylon suggests, were wounds, fractures and abscesses. The only exception is that circumcision was performed, presumably by priests, as part of a religious ceremony among the nobility. This is documented as a carved stone relief, dated about 2500 BC. Presumably the Jews of ancient Egypt learned this custom, which was then incorporated into Mosaic law.

From the earliest days of Egyptian civilization, belief in reincarnation meant that members of the royal family and nobility had their bodies preserved. Initially this was merely done by drying the corpse in the sand, but over the centuries more and more sophisticated techniques of embalming were developed. As a result of our examination of these preserved bodies, a great deal has been learned of diseases of ancient Egypt. These include congenital deformities such as club foot, dental caries, arthritis and fractures. Some of these show treatment by quite sophisticated splinting.

CHINA

Chinese civilization dates back to perhaps 2000 BC. Priests of the Shang Dynasty, around 1500 BC, left texts scratched on bone which refer to maladies of the eyes, teeth, throat, nose, legs, abdomen, kidney and bladder and mention epidemics which may have been malaria, cholera and the plague. However, ancestor worship and the Confucian philosophy forbade the mutilation of the body of a dead person, and Chinese physicians were opposed to any invasion of the human body. This meant that surgical intervention was frowned upon, dissections of corpses were not performed; even up to modern times there was no true anatomical research, and knowledge of the human body was mostly theoretical. There was indeed only one ancient surgeon of note, Hua Tuo *(?AD 190–265)*, who is pictured operating on the arm of General Kuan Yun. He offered trephination of the skull to Prince Tsao Tsao, who was suffering from severe headaches. The Prince suspected that his surgeon wished to murder him and ordered his execution. Hua Tuo might have indeed been a foreigner who entered China from India and was therefore acquainted with the Indian art of surgery.

INDIA

About 1500 BC, the Aryans invaded India from Central Asia, bringing with them the Sanskrit language. The earliest writings on Indian medicine are to be found in the Vedas, or books of knowledge, which were believed to be of divine origin. Here we read of 'sages' who would carry bags of healing herbs, care for the injured, remove spears and arrows from the wounded and who employed a plant, named after the god Soma, which would relieve pain. They also cauterized wounds and snake bites and may even have developed a catheter to relieve retention of urine that was purported to 'open the flow of urine again like a dam before a lake'.

The two earliest Indian medical authors were Caraka and Suśruta. Whether these were two actual historical personages or names to which collected works of medical literature are attributed will probably never be found out. This collection of writings, of which many copies and versions exist, contain much of surgical interest. Works were translated into Arabic around AD 800 and often quoted in the writings of Rhazes.

Suśruta describes 20 sharp and 101 blunt surgical instruments, stresses that individuals who wish to study medicine and surgery should be born of good family, desire to learn and possess strength, energy of action, contentment, character, self-control, a good retentive memory, intellect, courage, purity of mind and body, and a simple and clear comprehension; qualities which we would certainly look for in today's medical students. A disciple was expected to study for at least six years. It is quite evident that Hindu surgery at this time reached a high state of excellence. For example, there is a detailed description of the operation of couching for a cataract. In this procedure, the opaque lens of the eye is mobilized and pushed downwards into the lower part of the eye to allow the restoration of vision.

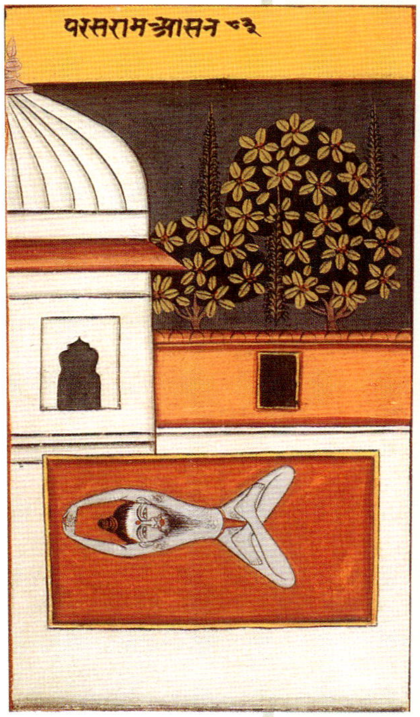

ABOVE **The *Suśruta Samhitā*, one of the most important Indian medical texts, devotes considerable attention to yoga. This is a nineteenth-century illustration of the *Parasaram* posture.**

COUCHING FOR CATARACT

This detailed description of an eye operation quoted below appears in the earliest Indian medical texts.

'In the morning in a bright place, the temperature being moderate, let the physician sit on a bench as high as his knee opposite the patient. The latter, having washed and eaten and been tied, sits on the ground. After he has warmed the patient's eye with the breath of his mouth, rubbed it with his thumb and detected the uncleanness which has formed in the pupil, he orders the patient to look down at his nose. Then, while the patient's head is held firmly, he takes the lancet between his forefinger, middle finger and thumb and introduces it into the eye towards the pupil, on the side, half a finger's breadth from the black of the eye and a quarter of a finger's breadth from the outer corner of the eye. He moves it back and forth and upward. Let him operate on the left eye with the right hand or on the right with the left. If he had probed correctly, there is a sound, and a drop of water comes out painlessly. Speaking words of courage to the patient, let him moisten the eye with women's milk, then scratch the pupil with the tip of the lancet without hurting... if the patient can see objects, the doctor should draw the lancet out slowly, lay cotton soaked in fat on the wound, and let the patient lie still with bandaged eyes'.

SUŚRUTA SAMHITĀ

Suśruta also describes what must have been the earliest plastic surgery procedure, the restoration of an amputated nose by means of a skin graft. Removal of the nose was a punishment for adultery in those days, so there was no shortage of patients for this operation. Interestingly, it evidently remained in practice in India among itinerant surgeons for hundreds of years. A newspaper account of this in 1840 prompted Joseph Carpue of London to perform a very similar operation, using a forehead flap of skin, with success.

Today, much emphasis is placed on surgical training using models for improving technique. It is interesting that the writings of Suśruta include advice on how surgeons should practise the art of suturing (or stitching) on animal skins or strips of cotton, improve their bandaging on life-sized dolls, practise surgical incisions on watermelons or cucumbers and practise the ligature of blood vessels and of blood-letting on lotus stems and the veins of dead animals.

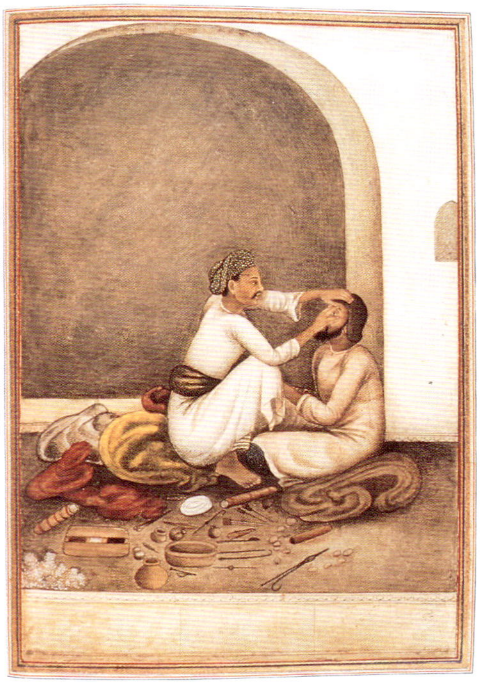

ABOVE This painting dating from 1825 shows an Indian oculist treating a patient with the surgical instruments of his trade laid out next to him.

ANCIENT GREECE AND ROME

Much of our modern medical traditions and many of today's medical terms derived from Ancient Greece. The Greek culture absorbed knowledge from Mesopotamia via Asia Minor and also from Egypt. By the 6th century BC, medical schools were flourishing on the island of Kos and on the adjacent peninsula of Cnidos (now in modern Turkey). One of the teachers of Kos was the man who is commonly regarded as the 'Father of Medicine', Hippocrates. He was born on Kos in about 460 BC, the son of a physician. He undoubtedly existed and is mentioned by his younger contemporary, Plato. However, the Hippocratic collection of writings, about 60 works, are now regarded as being the product of a number of authors, writing over a period of several hundred years and often expressing contradictory views. Hippocratic writings are characterized by being factual; they contain descriptions of careful observations of actual patients, eschew any elaborate theories of disease and base treatment principally on rest, diet and a few simple medications.

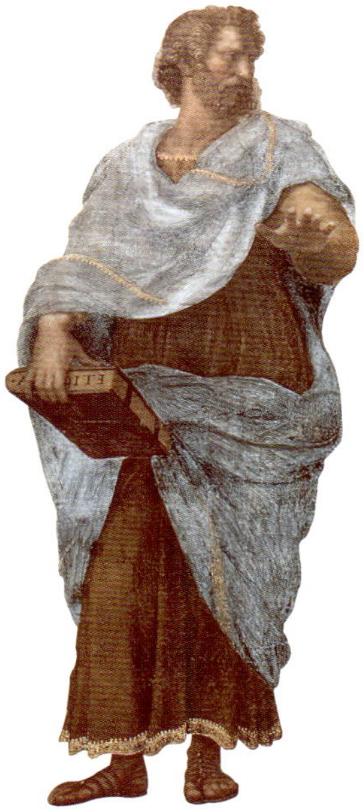

ABOVE The Greek philosopher Plato *(c.427–347 BC)*, who was a contemporary of Hippocrates. Plato's ideas formed the mind of his pupil Aristotle.

From the surgical point of view, the Hippocratic writings give us descriptions of the treatment of wounds, fractures and dislocations and also describe elective operations for a number of surgical conditions. In the treatise entitled *On Wounds of the Head,* there is detailed description of trephination (the removal of circular sections of the skull) for treatment of fractures of the skull, even noting, 'while trephining, often remove the instrument and dip it in cold water. If you do not do this, the trephine, becoming heated by the circular motion and heating and drying the bone, may burn it and cause an unduly large piece of the bone round the sawing to come away'. The trephine was either held between the palms of the hands and rotated by the action of rubbing them together, or was rotated by a cross-piece and thong. In the volume *On the Articulations,* we find a description of the method of reducing dislocation of the shoulder which is still used today, and, indeed, is termed the Hippocratic Method:

The patient must lie on the ground upon his back while the person who is to effect the reduction is seated on the ground upon the side of the dislocation; then the operator seizing with his hand the affected arm, is to pull it, while with his heel in the armpit he pushes in the contrary direction.... but a round ball of a suitable size must be placed in the hollow of the armpit, for without something of the kind the heel cannot reach to the head of the humerus.

ON THE ARTICULATIONS

DESPERATE REMEDIES

In the book *On Haemorrhoids*, the description of their surgical treatment fills one with admiration for the courage of the patients in Ancient Greece. 'Having laid him on his back, and placed a pillow below the breech, force out the anus as much as possible with the fingers and make the irons red-hot, and burn the pile until it be dried up, and so that no part may be left behind…' Another method of curing haemorrhoids states, 'You must prepare a cautery, an iron that exactly fits is to be adapted to it; then the tube being introduced into the anus, the iron, red-hot, is to be passed down it and frequently drawn out so that the part may bear the more heat and no sore may result from the heating, and the dried veins may heal up'. One notes, however, that should the patient not consent to surgical treatment, various prescriptions are advised for local application!

Among the many Greek immigrant surgeons must be mentioned Soranus of Ephesus *(AD 98–138)*, who studied in Alexandria and flourished under the Roman emperor Hadrian. As well as writing on fractures and skull injuries, Soranus can be regarded as one of the founders of obstetrics. He introduced the Roman birth-stool, which had supports for the back and arms and a crescent-shaped aperture. Soranus also described the necessity of emptying the bladder before delivery of the baby and performed packing of the uterus for haemorrhage. However, the most famous of the physicians of this period, and indeed perhaps of all time, was Galen *(AD ?131–201)* of Pergamum, whose writings were regarded as having almost biblical authority for the next 15 centuries. After training in Alexandria, Galen became surgeon to the gladiators in AD 158 and in the next five years developed an extensive practice in traumatic surgery. He then moved to Rome, where he spent the remainder of his life and became physician to the emperor Marcus Aurelius. He dissected and experimented extensively on animals (human dissection was not permitted) and wrote vast numbers of books – on anatomy, physiology, pathology, therapeutics and, indeed, on every branch of medicine known at the time. He produced no specific surgical text, but his writings on surgery are scattered through his books. He described operations for varicose veins, reconstruction of cleft lip, removal of polyps from the nose and suture of the intestine after penetrating injuries of the abdomen.

Although there was much good in Galen's writings, the whole corpus of his knowledge was regarded as sacred by later generations. Galen's writings remained almost unchallenged until the sixteenth century, when men learned once more to observe nature. The dissections of Vesalius *(1514–1564)* swept away many of Galen's false anatomical concepts and William Harvey *(1578–1657)*, using experimental observations, proved the true nature of the circulation of the blood.

Tradition states that Romulus and Remus founded Rome in 753 BC. By 201 BC, Rome had defeated Hannibal, annexed Carthage on the North African coast and was dominating the Mediterranean. Roman surgery was strongly influenced by Greece. Upper class Romans considered medicine in general, and surgery in particular, beneath the notice of a cultured individual and most practitioners were imported from Greece. However, it was a Roman nobleman, Celsus *(25 BC–AD 50)*, who has left us an encyclopaedic survey of medicine at that time. Although Celsus was almost forgotten for some centuries, he was the first classical medical writer to be printed *(AD 1478)* and his writings were highly valued during the Renaissance. He describes the surgery of injuries, fractures and dislocations, diseases of the nose, ear and eye, of hernia, bladder stone, varicose veins and fistula.

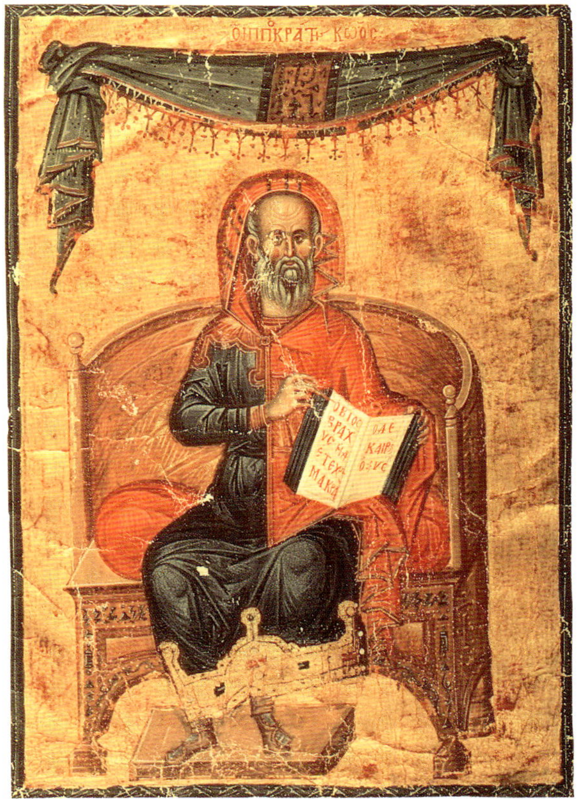

ABOVE Hippocrates. In his hand is a book with his most famous aphorism: The life so short, the art so long to learn.

BYZANTIUM, ISLAM AND THE MIDDLE AGES

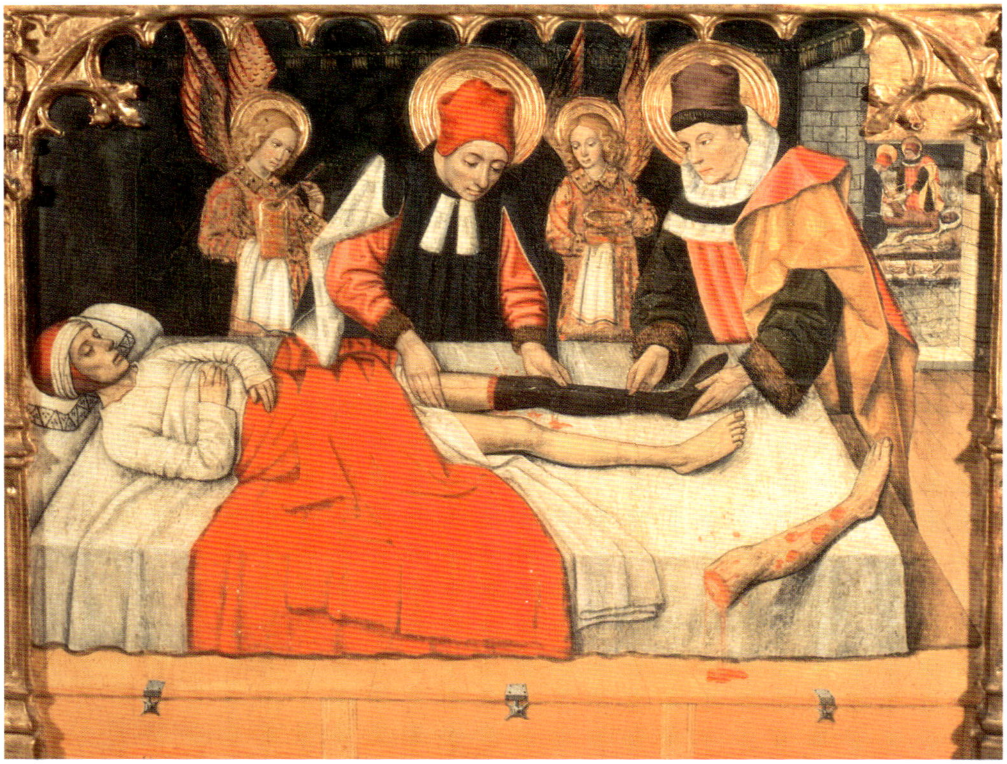

ABOVE St Cosmas and St Damian graft the leg of a Moor onto a white patient. This painting is by the Spanish artist Jaime Huguet *(c.1448–1492).*

The period of observation and experiment closed with the death of Galen, whose life coincided with the greatest period of the Roman Empire. After him, the Empire gradually disintegrated and medical authors became the mere compilers of the works of their predecessors. In AD 395, the Roman Empire was divided into a Western and Eastern division. In the West, Rome fell to the invading Goths in 476. Western Europe was plunged into the long centuries of the 'Dark Ages', characterized by widespread ignorance and lack of social progress. In the East, however, the Byzantine Empire persisted and flourished until the capture of Constantinople by the Turks in 1453.

The Byzantine Empire saw the rise of the cult of healing saints, the most famous among them being the physician brothers, Cosmas and Damian. They practised in Aleppo, in modern Syria, but were martyred for their faith in the fourth century AD. Visitors to their tomb reported miraculous cures and the brothers later became the patron saints of medicine. The most famous legend associated with them relates that a man with a gangrenous leg prayed at the church of St Cosmas and Damian in Rome. There a miraculous operation took place; the man's gangrenous leg was removed and the leg of a blackamoor who had recently died was grafted onto the stump. When the patient awoke in the morning he had two sound legs – one white and one black. The story of this extraordinary graft, (which preceded modern transplantation by many centuries!), was the subject of hundreds of paintings, some by the great masters.

Little of importance was added to either medicine or surgery during this time. However, a number of encyclopaedic writers produced extensive collections of the works of earlier Greek and Roman physicians and surgeons. These works, later translated into Arabic, formed the basis of the medical knowledge of Islam, from where it was to be returned in Latin translation to medieval Europe. The degree of surgical sophistication revealed in these documents is of great interest. For example, Oribasius *(AD 325–403)*, a native of Pergamum, the birth place of Galen, provides a treatise devoted to the treatment of fractures by mechanical appliances, including screw traction and elaborate multiple-pulley systems. Aetius of Amida *(AD 502–575)*, physician to Justinian I, gives the first description of ligature (tying) of the artery above an aneurysm – a pathological dilatation of the vessel.

Perhaps the most famous of these encyclopaedists was Paul of Aegina *(AD 625–690)*. He proposed that his writings should be a compendium of Greek and Roman medicine and succeeded in his aim. Little is known of Paul, except that he studied and practised in Alexandria. The sixth volume of his works is entirely devoted to surgery. He gives an excellent description of the operation of tracheotomy (cutting into the windpipe), in which he mentions the importance of correct positioning of the patient and the safe site for opening the windpipe. He also describes amputation of the breast for cancer, trephination of the skull and the surgical treatment of a hernia. Compared with earlier Greek writers, however, the surgery described by Paul shows certain regressive tendencies which would dominate therapy throughout the Middle Ages. Bleeding, cupping and the extensive use of the cauterizing iron for all sorts of conditions were going to dominate surgical treatment throughout the Middle Ages. Indeed, because the translation of these works from the Greeks and Romans were to be taken as literal truths which could not be questioned, little advance would be made in surgical progress for many hundreds of years.

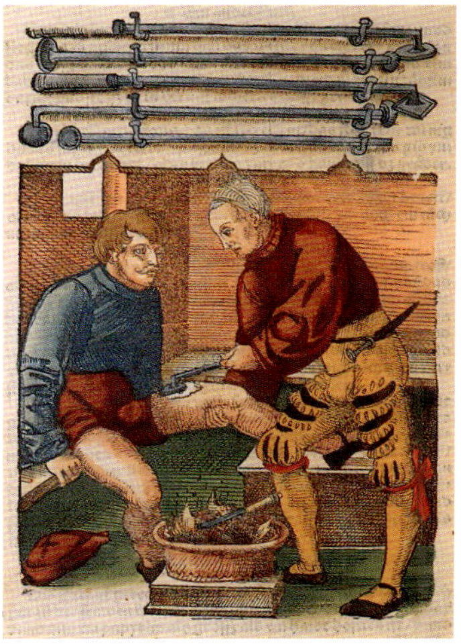

ABOVE A medieval patient enduring the agony of the use of a cauterizing iron to stop his bleeding.

ISLAM

The teaching of Mohammed *(AD 570–632)* united the peoples of the Arabian peninsula. Over the next century the Islamic empire spread eastwards to the Indus, and along the coast of Northern Africa to the Pyrenees in the west. Around AD 750 this large empire fell apart, into the Eastern Caliphate, with Baghdad as its capital, and the Western Caliphate, with its seat of government at Cordoba in Spain. Much of Byzantium came under Muslim rule, and although the Arabs were at first indifferent to the learning of infidels, they gradually came to appreciate it. The medical writings that had been rendered into Persian and Syrian were now translated into Arabic, so that Greek and Roman medicine were spread far and wide in the Arab world, particularly to important cultural centres in Cairo, Baghdad and Damascus in the east, and Cordoba, Seville and Toledo in the west. Arabic scientists and physicians published important works. Through Latin translations, many of them were produced in Toledo, where, in the twelfth century, a translation institute was founded, and these works became available in Western Europe. However, Arabic medicine contributed little further to the treasures of Greece and Rome; surgery, in particular, remained at a standstill. Prohibition of dissection meant that there were no advances in anatomical knowledge, haemorrhage was greatly feared, and much faith was placed in the use of the cautery.

ALBUCASIS' COLLECTION

Only one of the many medical books written in Arabic treated surgery as a separate subject. This was the *Collection* of Albucasis *(936–1013)*. The author was born and practised in Cordoba and wrote an extensive work which covered all branches of medicine. The last of its 30 volumes is devoted to surgery. In his introduction, Albucasis complains that surgery had almost completely disappeared as a specialty in Spain. Proficient surgeons could no longer be found as a result of the absence of anatomical knowledge. He gives several examples of surgical incompetence:

> *I have seen an ignorant physician incise over a scrofulous tumour of the neck of a woman, open the cervical arteries and provoke such haemorrhage that the patient died in his hands. I have seen another doctor undertake the extraction of a stone in a very old man. The stone was huge; in performing the extraction he removed a portion of the bladder wall. The patient died in three days.*
>
> ALBUCASIS, *COLLECTION*

The text of the book is taken largely from Paul of Aegina with few additions. Surgery is to be avoided wherever possible and the cautery preferred to the knife. Bleeding, cupping and the use of leeches are important means of treatment. An interesting finding in Albucasis's chapters on the treatment of fractures is a good description of fracture of the penis. He recommends splinting it by means of a goose neck, which is pushed over the member.

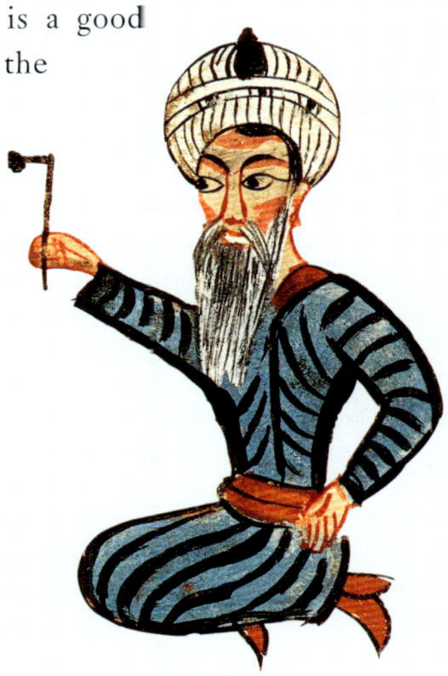

RIGHT A thirteenth-century Arabic doctor preparing a medicine. In all probability this physician would have read some, if not all, of Albucasis' 30-volume work on medicine, the *Collection*.

THE MIDDLE AGES

The Dark Ages of the Western world followed the fall of Rome. The sick and dying might find comfort in religious establishments, where they could be looked after by monks and nuns, but edicts in the twelfth century forbade clerics from shedding blood, which meant that the educated classes were prohibited from performing any type of surgery. The practice of surgery therefore rested in the hands of a few people: barbers, wandering charlatans and a small number of competent practitioners, who alone kept the glimmering light of surgery alive.

The first reawakening of Western European medicine was in Salerno, near Naples. Indeed, it was reputed that as early as the ninth century a hospital existed there. From its beginning, the School of Salerno was a lay organization and not under ecclesiastic control. By 1240, regulations were laid down concerning medical education, which included the length and content of the medical curriculum, the form of the examinations and a mandatory post-graduate year. The school had the sole right to approve for practice all physicians and surgeons in the area. Women as well as men were included, not only as students but as professors. The first revival in anatomy took place at this school, and although there was not the opportunity for human dissection, animals, especially the pig, were dissected.

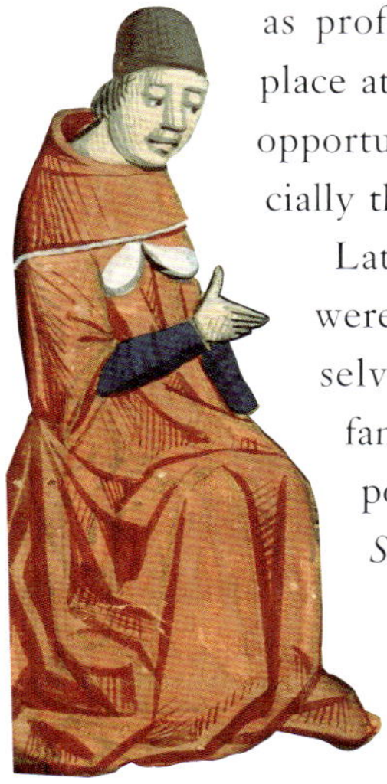

ABOVE Guy de Chauliac's famous book on surgery was a standard text for more than 200 years.

Latin translations of the Arab encyclopaedias were available, but the Salernian doctors themselves published their own texts, the most famous of these, the *Regimen Sanitatis,* being a popular guide for healthy living. In 1170 the *Surgery of Roger* (Ruggiero Frugardi) was published, the first independent surgical text to appear in the Western world. This was sequenced from head to foot and even described the repair of an injured intestine, by stitching it over a wooden tube.

From Salerno, the teaching of surgery spread to Bologna and then, in the thirteenth century, the French school of surgery became influential, with the formation of the Confraternity of St Cosmas and Damian founded in Paris. The great French teachers of the time included Lanfranc *(?–1315),* who originally practised in Milan, Henri de Mondeville *(1260–1329)* and Guy de Chauliac *(1300–1368).* Guy de Chauliac studied in Toulouse, Montpellier and Paris and studied anatomy in Bologna. He practised in Avignon and his fame is based on his book *Grande Chirurgie,* which was written towards the end of his career and which was an immediate success. The text was lucid and systematic although essentially conservative and with little personal contributions from the author. Indeed, he states in the introduction, 'I have added nothing of my own, except perchance some little of that which the smallness of my mind has judged profitable'. The book went through many editions and translations and indeed served as the principal textbook of surgery for the next two centuries until finally becoming superseded by the works of Ambroise Paré in the middle of the sixteenth century. The first volume of the book is on anatomy, which Guy considered indispensable to the surgeon, and he stressed the importance of human dissection.

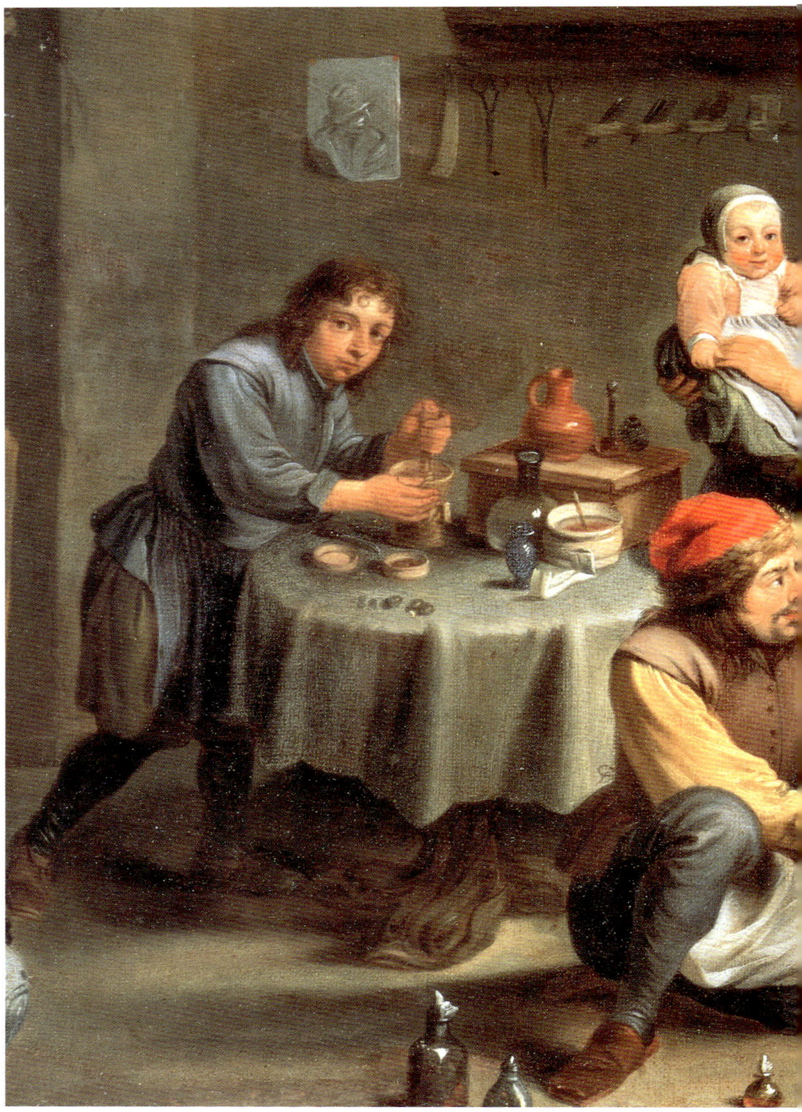

ABOVE For centuries the practice of surgery rested in the hands of often poorly educated barber-surgeons. One such is pictured by David Teniers *(1610–1690).*

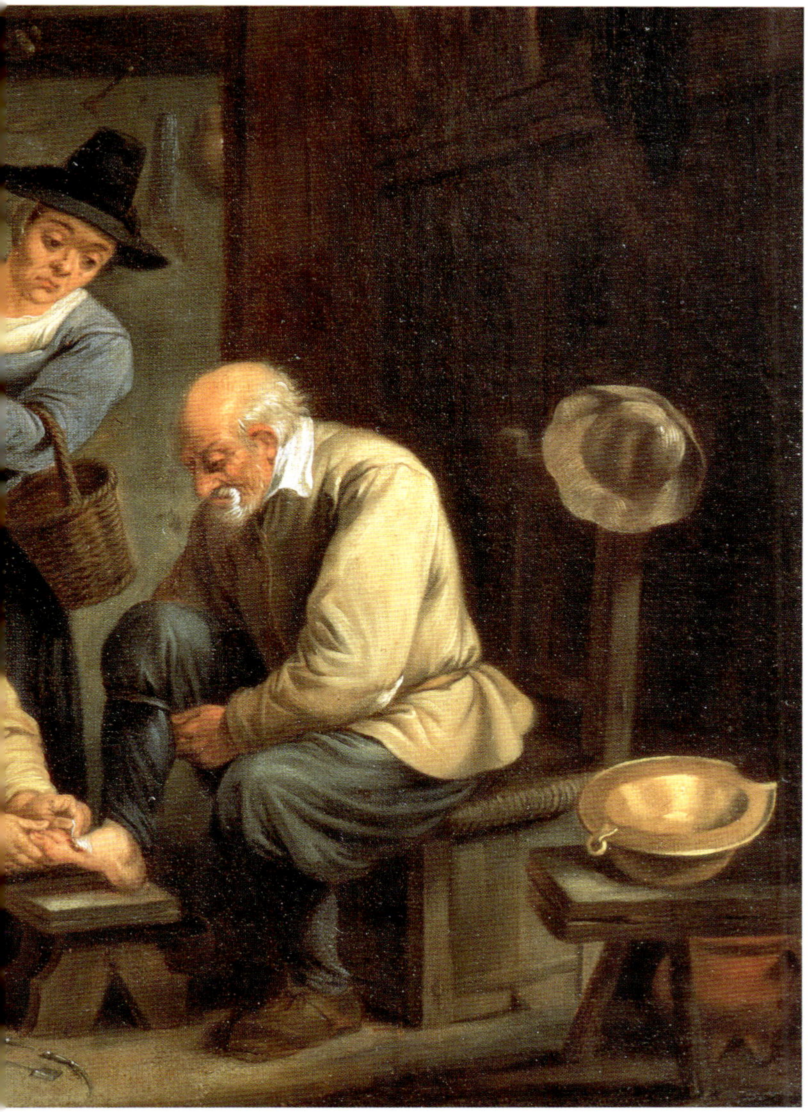

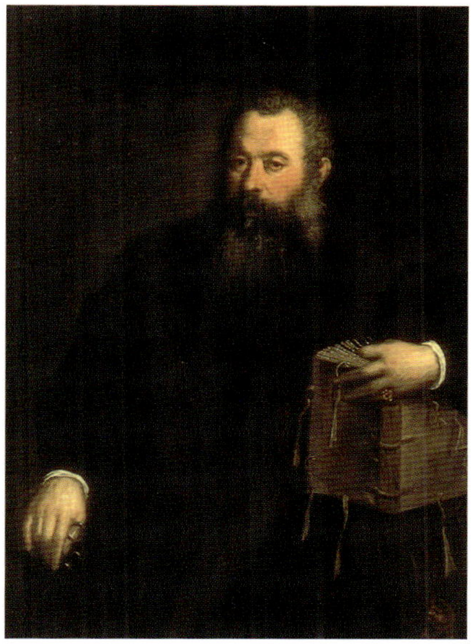

LEFT This portrait of Andreas Vesalius is by the great Venetian painter Titian *(c.1487–1576)*. Vesalius' work on anatomy corrected many of the errors that had been made by Galen. It must be judged one of the most influential of all medical books.

BELOW The draughtsman that Vesalius chose to illustrate the seven books of *De humani corporis fabrica* was the German Stephen Calcar. His drawings of the dissected body were beautifully precise.

THE RENAISSANCE IN EUROPE

The conquest of Constantinople by the Turks in 1453 saw an influx of Byzantine scholars into the West, especially into Italy, bringing with them the classical writings of Plato, Hippocrates and others. In medicine, the stubborn adherence to the excessive influence of Galen was replaced by physicians, surgeons and anatomists who based their views on facts and scientific observation. Indeed, new translations of the standard authors, for example by Thomas Linacre *(1460–1524)*, who was personal physician to both Kings Henry VII and Henry VIII of England and the first President of the Royal College of Physicians in England, demonstrated that many of the established tenets, held with almost religious fervour for hundreds of years, were based on poorly translated, second-hand versions of the classical authors, including Galen himself.

The technique of printing which used movable type, invented by Johannes Gutenberg *(1400–1468)* of Mainz, allowed books to be produced cheaply and in large numbers. It soon became obvious that further progress, particularly in surgery, could only be made by a detailed study of human anatomy. The papal ban on human dissection became less and less strict and was finally lifted by the early sixteenth century. Pioneers of human dissection included Mundinus *(?1270–1326)* of Bologna and Jacob Sylvius *(1478–1555)* in Paris. However, the man who dominated the scene and who made an enormous contribution to surgical progress was Andreas Vesalius *(1514–1564)* of Louvain. His public dissections during his seven years in Padua drew enormous crowds of students. His efforts were crowned by the publication of his *Fabric of the Human Body* in 1543, the outstanding illustrations in which can be used for teaching even today. Vesalius corrected many of the anatomical misconceptions of Galen. In surgery, therefore, the scene was now set for a true revival in learning.

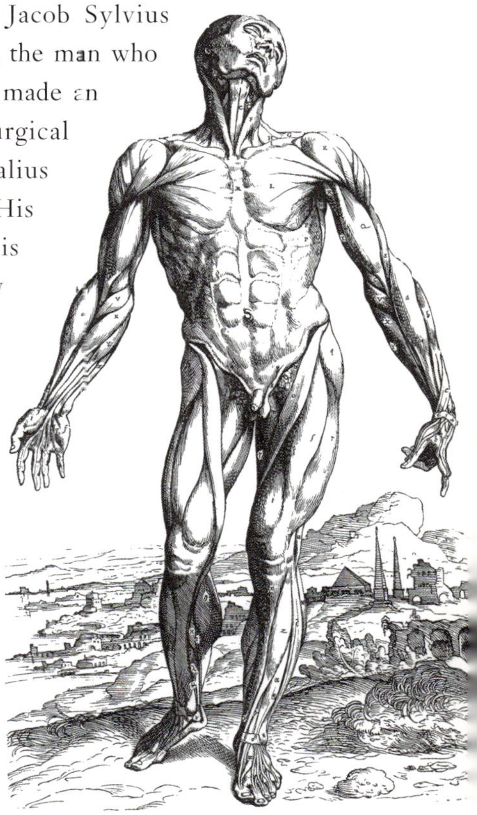

THE SURGERY OF TRAUMA AND OF WARFARE

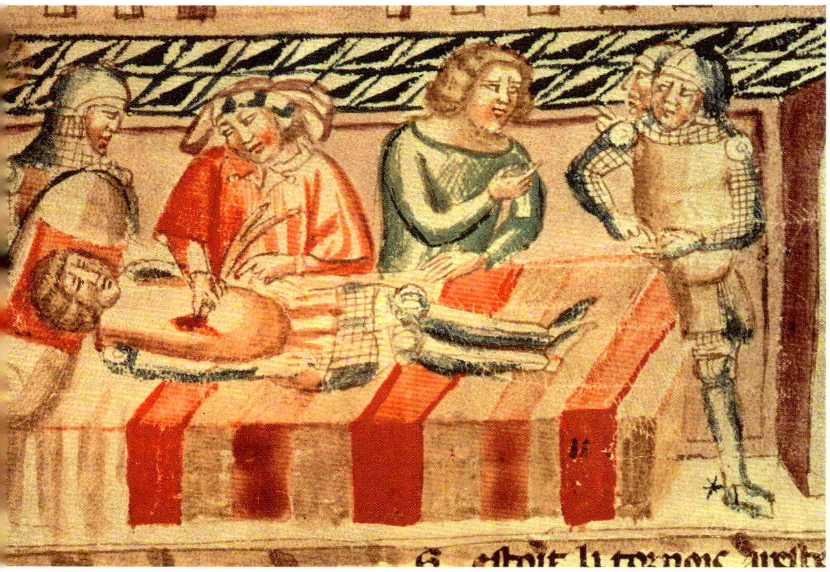

ABOVE Warfare and surgery go hand in hand. This medieval illustration of the siege of Troy shows care of a wounded soldier.

Throughout human existence, man has been an aggressive animal and much of the trauma people experience is inflicted by one member of the species on another. The very earliest evidence we have of this is seen in a cave painting in the Pyrenees dated from some 30,000 years ago, which seems to show arrows being shot at a man (or could it be a woman?). Until the invention of gunpowder in the fifteenth century, war wounds were inflicted mainly by knives, swords, spears, arrows and cudgels. These produced lacerating injuries which might kill the victim by penetration of a vital organ or by haemorrhage. However, if the victim survived the immediate injury, he or she was very likely to survive the injury itself. This was because these lacerated wounds produced little tissue destruction and thus allowed the natural powers of the body's healing to cure the victim. So surgeons became skilled at dressing and bandaging their victim's wounds and splinting their fractures. The various ointments they used, although probably usually ineffective, at least did little harm. Haemorrhage might be treated by pressure on the wound, cautery or by ligaturing the bleeding artery, a device introduced by Alexandrian surgeons around 250 BC and described by the Roman writer Celsus in the first century AD. The medieval surgical textbooks often carried an illustration of a 'wound man' which showed the various injuries the surgeons of the Middle Ages might be called upon to treat.

The introduction of firearms completely changed this picture. The gross tissue destruction produced by the musket ball and cannon provided a wonderful medium for the growth of bacteria, especially anaerobic microbes, those that thrive in the absence of oxygen and which grow on dead tissues, especially the organisms that produce tetanus and gas gangrene. Thus dreadful wound infection and gangrene of a type not previously seen was encountered by surgeons treating these war wounds. Now this, of course, was centuries before our knowledge of the bacterial causation of wound infection and it was not unreasonable for military surgeons to conclude that these awful complications were due to the poisonous nature of the gunpowder itself. The solution was obviously to destroy the poison and this was done by means of a red-hot cautery or by the use of boiling oil poured into the wound. The great popularity of the latter was undoubtedly due to the writings of the Italian surgeon Giovanni da Vigo *(1460–1525)*, whose surgical treatise entitled *A Compendious Practice of the Art of Surgery* was first published in Rome in 1514. It went through more than 40 editions in many languages and greatly influenced the surgeons of his time.

Of course, we now know that this practice had the opposite effect to the one desired; the red-hot cautery and the boiling oil simply destroyed more tissue then the missile itself and aggravated an already serious situation, as well as inflicting untold torture upon the poor soldier victim.

Now we come to one of those great landmarks that punctuate surgical history; a surgeon who, through his example and writings, greatly influenced progress in the management of wounds. Ambroise Paré *(1510–1590)* was born in the little town of Laval in France, the son of a barber. At the age of 22 he came to Paris as an apprentice to a barber-surgeon and then moved to the great Hôtel Dieu as resident surgeon. In that immense medieval hospital, the only one in Paris at that time, he gained great experience. At the age of 26 he commenced his career there as a military surgeon. In those days, there was no organized medical care for the humble private soldiers of armies in the field.

Surgeons were attached to individual generals and other important personages, and might, if they wished, give what aid they could to the common soldiers in their spare time. Otherwise, these poor fellows had to rely on the rough help of their companions or of a motley crowd of horse-doctors, farriers, quacks and mountebanks, or of the female camp followers. Paré was appointed surgeon to the Duke of Montejan, who was Colonel-General of the French infantry. In his first of many campaigns, in Turin in 1537, he made the fundamental observations that he described so brilliantly in his important book *The Apologie and Treatise.* He recounts how, when he had run out of boiling oil, the established treatment for firearms wounds, he applied instead 'a digestive made of egg yolk, rose oil and turpentine'. In the morning Paré was amazed that patients treated with the digestive medication felt little pain in their wounds, while the others were in great pain. 'Then I resolved never again to so cruelly burn the poor wounded by gunshot.'

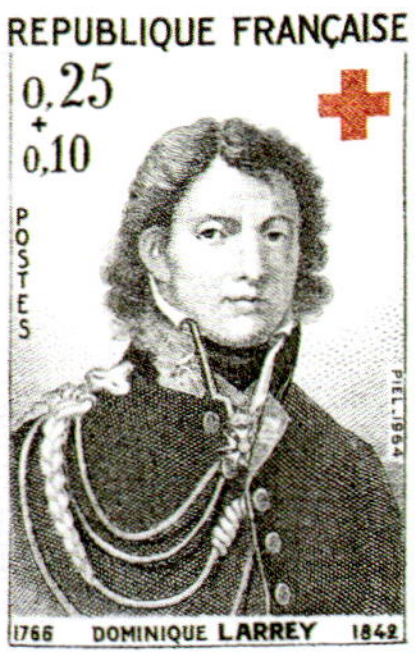

ABOVE The French military surgeon Baron Dominique-Jean Larrey.

BELOW Ambroise Paré revolutionized the treatment of battlefield wounds. He abandoned the use of cautery in favour of ligature of the blood vessels.

Paré also went on to show that bleeding after amputations should be arrested, not by the terrible method of the indiscriminate use of the red-hot cautery, but by simple tying of the blood vessels. A prolific writer, who used contemporary French rather than Latin, Paré had the widest and most beneficial influences on surgical craft in the sixteenth century. In his very first campaign he ended his description of the treatment of a gunshot wound of the ankle with his most famous phrase, which perhaps should be the prayer of every surgeon: 'I dressed the wound and God healed him.'

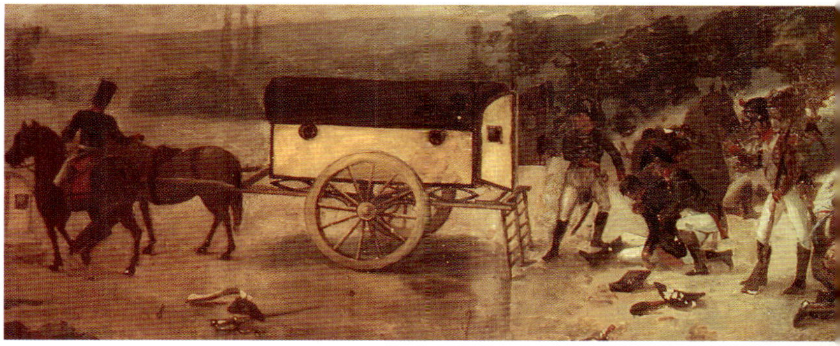

ABOVE In the 1790s Larrey pioneered the use of horsedrawn *ambulances volantes,* or 'flying ambulances' such as this, for rapid removal of the wounded from the field of battle to the nearest dressing station.

For more than two and a half centuries after the death of Paré, little advance was made in the treatment of wounds in general and of war wounds in particular. Infection was the main problem, and without knowledge of the bacterial nature of this complication, little could be done to prevent it. Amputation, performed as soon as possible after wounding and, without the boon of anaesthesia, carried out as rapidly as possible, remained the best remedy for a major limb injury. Dominique-Jean Larrey *(1766–1842)*, one of the greatest of military surgeons, with his vast experience in the Napoleonic wars, greatly improved the organization of military surgeons and introduced rapid evacuation of the wounded from the battlefield to the dressing station with his specially designed 'flying ambulance'. His work provided the foundation for the present day concept of the importance of rapid removal of the wounded out of battle to surgical care.

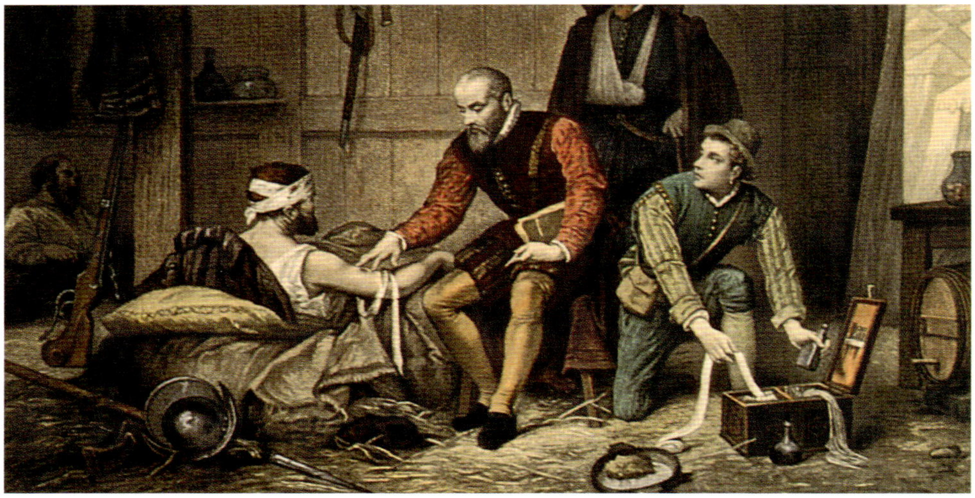

The introduction of ether in 1846 as an anaesthetic agent by William Morton *(1819–1868)*, a dentist in Boston, and of chloroform by Sir James Young Simpson *(1811–1870)* in Edinburgh the following year, assuaged the agonies of the surgeon's knife, but the ravages of wound sepsis remained. Thus, in the American Civil War, the first major conflict in which anaesthetics were available, operations for missile wounds were performed painlessly, but still with the high mortality rate familiar from past centuries.

LISTER AND ANTISEPSIS

Now we come to perhaps the most important contribution to the management of wounds; not just those of trauma, but also wounds produced by the surgeon in the course of operative procedures – the work of Joseph Lister *(1827–1912)*. Lister was appointed Professor of Surgery in Glasgow in 1860. At this time, like so many surgeons before him, he was puzzled by the observation that a closed fracture, no matter how severe, would heal without infection. In contrast, a compound fracture, which might only be complicated by a minor puncture wound, would usually become infected and the victim was lucky to get away with his life, let alone his limb. In some way, the exposure of the fracture to air seemed to be lethal. In 1865, Thomas Anderson, Professor of Chemistry at the University of Glasgow, told Lister of the work of Louis Pasteur *(1822–1895)*, which proved conclusively that putrefaction of milk, wine, urine and meat was due to bacteria and not merely to exposure to air. At once it became obvious to Lister that it was not the air itself, but the bacteria that it carried into the wound, which resulted in the suppuration, pus and gangrene which plagued the surgical wards of those days.

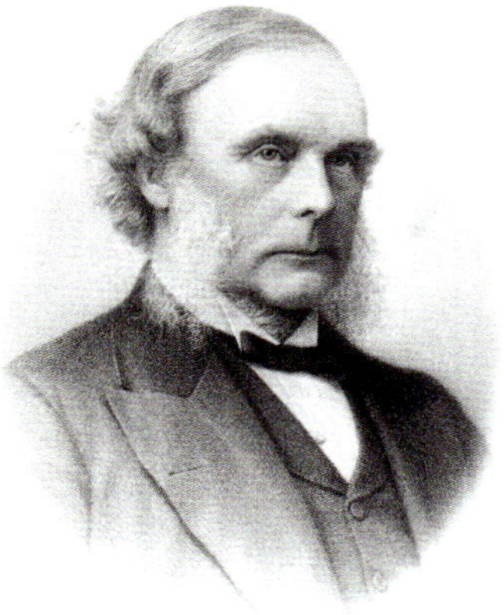

ABOVE **Sir Joseph Lister, the British surgeon who established the principle of antiseptic surgery in 1865.**

Pasteur had shown that heat could kill microbes, but as it was impossible to apply heat to the wound without burning the patient, some chemical substance had to be found. After a number of experiments, Lister read that carbolic acid had been used with excellent results as a means of purifying the stinking sewage at Carlisle, England. Lister's first sample was a sticky, smelly fluid almost insoluble in water, but soluble in oil. A purer preparation was soon obtained and was soluble in 20 parts of water. This was used in Lister's historic operation on the fractured leg of James Greenlees *(see box)*.

A NEW ERA OF ANTISEPSIS

On 12 August 1865, an operation was performed that was to mark the watershed between the two eras of surgery, the primitive and the modern. The patient was a boy named James Greenlees, aged 11 years, admitted to the Royal Infirmary, Glasgow, with a compound fracture of the left leg caused by the wheel of an empty cart running over the limb. The treatment, carried out by Joseph Lister in a small ward at the Infirmary, consisted of careful application of carbolic acid to all parts of the wound, which was then dressed with lint soaked in the same fluid and the leg was then carefully splinted. Under the dressing, the blood and carbolic acid formed a protective crust, beneath which, miracle of miracles, the wound healed soundly. The dressings were continued and, six weeks after his accident, young James walked out of the hospital and into surgical history.

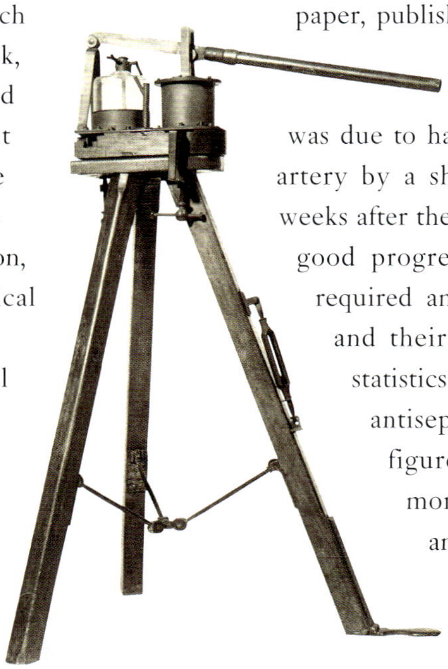

ABOVE **This is the carbolic spray equipment developed by Joseph Lister to kill germs in the operating theatre. The development of antiseptic surgery put paid to the notion of 'laudable pus'. Wound infection was shown to be harmful.**

Lister delayed publication of his remarkable results until a total of 11 patients had been treated by antiseptic method. His paper, published in the British medical journal *The Lancet* in 1867, noted that of the 11 cases of compound fracture there was only one death, which was due to haemorrhage as a result of the perforation of the artery by a sharp fragment of the fractured femur several weeks after the injury, when the patient appeared to be making good progress. One other case developed infection and required amputation of the leg; the other nine recovered and their limbs were saved. The improvement in the statistics on Lister's own wards after the adoption of this antiseptic technique is shown by his own published figures. Before antisepsis, he noted a 46 per cent mortality in 35 amputations. Subsequently, when amputations were carried out using the antiseptic method, 40 operations were performed with only six deaths, a 15 per cent mortality.

Enormous new vistas of surgery now lay open as surgeons could confidently make an incision through intact skin without incurring an extreme risk of wound infection. It was Lister who showed that such operations, for example to straighten out deformed limbs or surgery on tuberculous joints, could be performed safely.

THE TWO WORLD WARS

It is said that the only thing to benefit from war is surgery. Certainly, the next important advance in wound treatment took place in the horror of World War I. In the early days of 1914, surgeons were horrified at the terrible injuries which high velocity missiles produced on human flesh and bone. The massive tissue destruction, combined with teeming bacteria from the fertile fields of Flanders, produced dreadful infection and could not be combated by Listerian antisepsis. Gas gangrene occurred with an incidence never seen before or since, and tetanus complicated 8.8 per 1,000 wounds.

The scenes in the advanced surgical units (called Casualty Clearing Stations) seemed to revert to the days of Ambroise Paré, but the front-line British and French surgeons had solved the problem by 1915. The solution was to excise all dead tissue, remove all foreign material and leave the wound open, lightly packed with gauze. This meant that healthy, well-oxygenated tissues would have the maximum chance of overcoming infection. Then, five days later, the wound could be sutured, a technique termed 'delayed primary suture'. This has become the standard method of treating war wounds in every campaign since then.

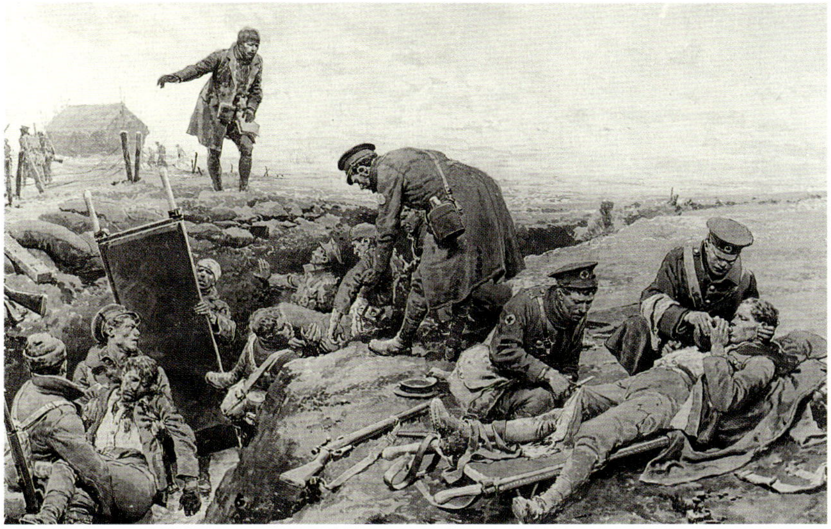

ABOVE Out of the horrors of World War I came advances in surgery. New methods of dealing with severe wounds and facial injuries were developed.

Most of the other broad principles of treating major injuries were established during World War I, for example, the importance of early splinting of fractures. Harvey Cushing *(1869–1939)* of Boston taught how gunshot wounds of the brain could be treated using gentle suction, and he also used powerful magnets to remove metallic foreign bodies from the brain. The importance of early surgery for abdominal injuries became apparent by 1915. Before then, missile injuries of the abdomen were almost invariably fatal. Dreadful injuries of the face, with extreme mutilation, were particularly difficult. The pioneering work of men like Harold Gillies *(1882–1960)* laid the foundations of modern plastic surgery by the development of pedicle flaps of skin from one part of the body to another.

World War II saw the last landmark in the treatment of wounds, again catalysed by war. Since the days of Lister, the dream had been to discover an agent that would kill bacteria that was spreading through the body without damaging the patient. In the early days of the war, Howard Florey *(1898–1968)* Ernst Chain *(1906–1979)* and a team of co-workers in the Department of Pathology at Oxford University began an investigation of the anti-bacterial properties of various types of fungi. *Penicillinium notatum* was chosen as the most promising, and by 1941 penicillin had been extracted in sufficient quantities to commence a clinical trial. Its value in combating wound infection was soon obvious, and by 1942 enough penicillin had been produced to enable supplies to be sent for use on wounded troops in North Africa. No substitute for the meticulous excision of the wound, its effects were nevertheless dramatic, both in the prevention and treatment of sepsis. This, complemented by the availability of blood transfusion, had significant effects on the morbidity and mortality of wounds of war.

BELOW Millions of lives have been saved by penicillin. Its discover was Sir Alexander Fleming, here painted by E Gabain.

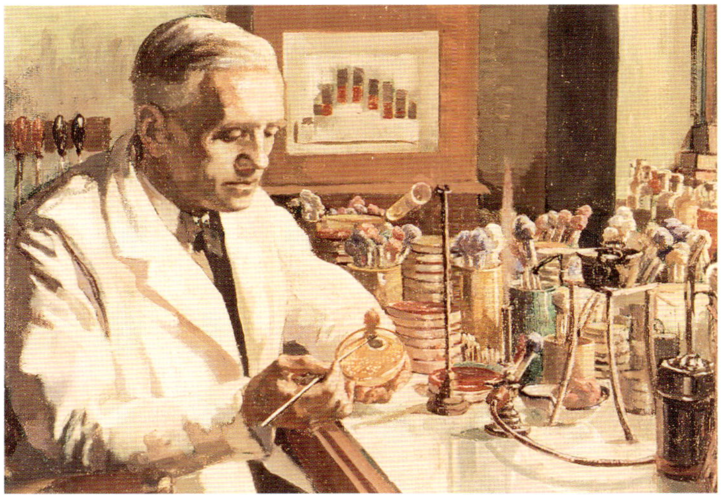

SURGICAL 'BREAKTHROUGHS' BEFORE ANAESTHESIA AND ANTISEPSIS

Before the anaesthetic era, which commenced in the 1840s, surgical operations were agonizing. Of course, if the patient had a broken leg or a major wound, there was nothing to do but submit to the surgeon's knife. Otherwise, non-emergency, 'elective' operations would only be undergone if the condition itself was so painful or life-threatening that the victim could even consider allowing surgery. Then, of course, the patient would choose the surgeon with a reputation for speed; a limb might be removed or a bladder stone evacuated in a couple of minutes. Moreover, before antiseptic surgery was gradually introduced in the 1860s and 1870s, there was the overwhelming danger of infection – suppuration, as it was termed – which again discouraged surgeons and their patients from hazarding anything other than the most pressing and dangerous of diseases to the process of surgical intervention.

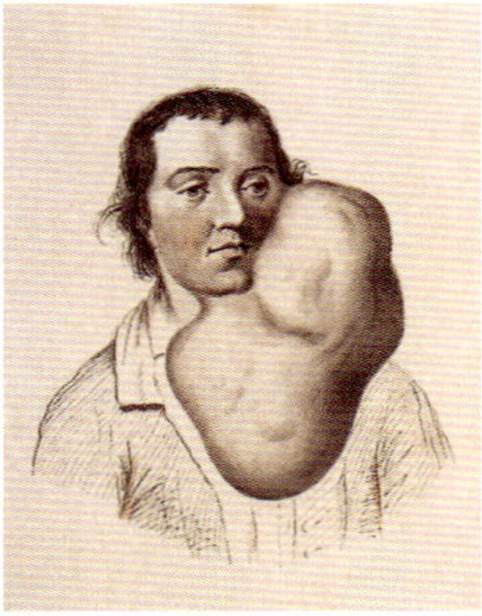

ABOVE This is the pre-operative drawing of John Burley and his parotid tumour 'the size of a common head'.

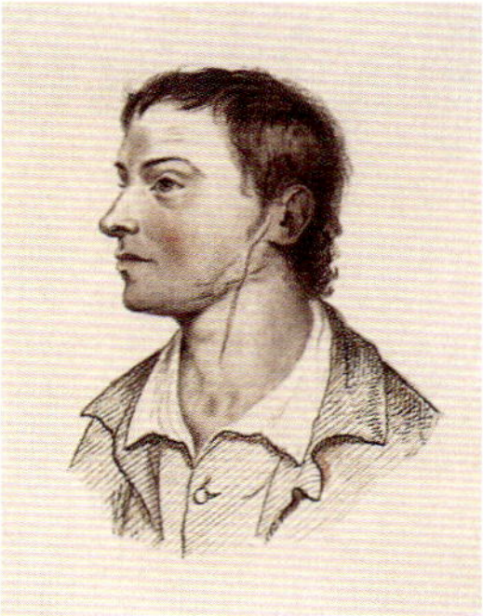

ABOVE John Burley after the eminent surgeon John Hunter had operated in 1785 to remove the tumour.

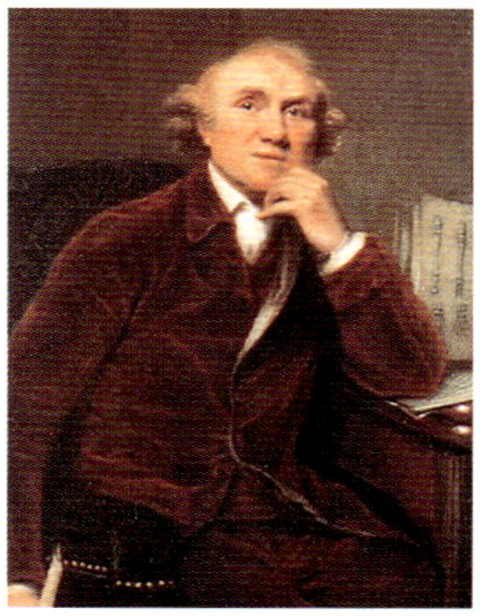

ABOVE This is the man who removed the tumour in John Burley's neck shown in the top picture – John Hunter.

Cancer of the breast was recognized from the earliest days, and the horrors of late disease encouraged surgeons in attempts at removal of the growth. Celsus, in the first century AD, recorded early attempts at surgery for this disease. He, like generations of his successors, was well acquainted with the poor prognosis of their endeavours: 'Some have used caustics, others the cautery, others cut them out with a knife. Notwithstanding, they have returned and occasioned death.' By the middle of the seventeenth century, total removal of the breast using either the amputation knife or the cautery was pictured graphically in the *Armamentarium chirurgicium* of Johannes Scultetus *(1595–1645)*, published in Ulm in 1653, eight years after the death of its author.

Over the next century or so, many surgeons advised complete removal of the breast together with the lymph glands in the armpit (axilla). In 1825, Sir Astley Cooper *(1768–1841)* in his *Lectures on the Principles and Practice of Surgery* wrote 'it will be sometimes necessary to remove the whole breast where much is apparently contaminated; for there is more generally diseased than perceived and it is best not to leave any small portion of it as tubercles reappear in them. If a gland in the axilla be enlarged, it should be removed and with it all the intervening cellular substance.' Cooper wisely noted that 'if several glands in the axilla be enlarged, their removal does not succeed in preventing the return of the disease'. By 1844, Joseph Pancoast *(1805-1882)* of the Jefferson Medical College in Philadelphia was advising still more radical surgery – that muscle should be removed, that affected portions of ribs should be cut out with the cutting forceps or a saw, and that the axillary glands should also be removed. These pioneering surgeons were masters of anatomy, their skill and speed at dissection honed by years of practice in the mortuary. Thus the principles of many of the major surgical procedures of today were gradually established.

John Hunter *(1728–1793)* is rightly regarded as the father of modern scientific surgery in Great Britain. His philosophy could be summed up by a famous remark he made in a letter to his friend and pupil, Edward Jenner (of vaccination fame): 'Why do you ask me a question, by the way of solving it. I think your solution is just; but why think, why not try the experiment?' In 1785 he operated on a man of 37 with an enormous tumour of the parotid gland. The operation 'lasted 25 minutes, and the man did not cry out during the whole of the operation. The tumour weighed 144 ounces'. The facial nerve, the principal supply to the muscles of the face, passes through the parotid gland and yet Hunter, master anatomist, obviously left the nerve undamaged, as can be seen in the pre- and post-operative drawings.

In 1824, Sir Astley Cooper of Guy's Hospital in London carried out the first successful amputation at the hip joint. The patient was a veteran from the Battle of Waterloo. His leg had been amputated at the thigh on the battlefield, and since then the stump of bone remained chronically infected (with osteomyelitis) and the patient's condition had steadily deteriorated. Cooper first tied the main artery at the groin and removed the limb in 20 minutes. Securing the blood vessels and the dressings occupied 15 more minutes. Apart from the inevitable infection of the wound, the patient slowly recovered and eight months later was convalescing in the country residence of Sir Astley.

Perhaps the most extraordinary example of these surgical endeavours was the first successful elective operation on the abdominal cavity. This was performed, not in some great hospital by a distinguished professor, but in the front parlour of the doctor's house in what was then frontier country, Kentucky. The surgeon was Ephraim McDowell *(1771–1839)*, who was born in Virginia but moved to Kentucky as a boy when his father was appointed a judge at Danville, the first capital of that state. His father had served as a colonel in the Revolutionary War. McDowell studied surgery in Edinburgh and returned to Danville in 1795 as its only surgeon. In December 1809, McDowell was called to see Mrs Jane Crawford, aged 44, who lived in a log cabin in the depths of the countryside. After a pelvic examination, McDowell diagnosed a massive ovarian cyst and offered to carry out an experiment if the patient were able to reach Danville. Mrs Crawford journeyed on horseback, and an operation was duly performed in McDowell's front parlour with the assistance of his nephew, who had graduated only a few months before. The patient was laid on the kitchen table, a nine-inch (23cm) incision was made through the abdominal wall, the contents of the cyst evacuated of 15lb (6.8kg) of gelatinous material and then the sac, which weighed 7½lb (3.4kg), was removed. The abdominal wound was closed, The operation, (performed without any form of anaesthetic), lasted 25 minutes and the patient made an excellent recovery.

McDowell performed two further successful removals of large ovarian cysts before publishing his cases, and in all he performed at least 12 operations for ovarian pathology. Since that time the stature of McDowell has grown and he is now acknowledged as not only the first to remove a pelvic mass, but also to be the father of gynaecological abdominal surgery.

BELOW **The world's first successful operation to remove an ovarian cyst was carried out in 1809 by Ephraim McDowell in the front parlour of his house in Danville, Kentucky. The patient made a good recovery and survived to live for many more years. This painting by George Kasson Knapp shows the scene with McDowell standing (left).**

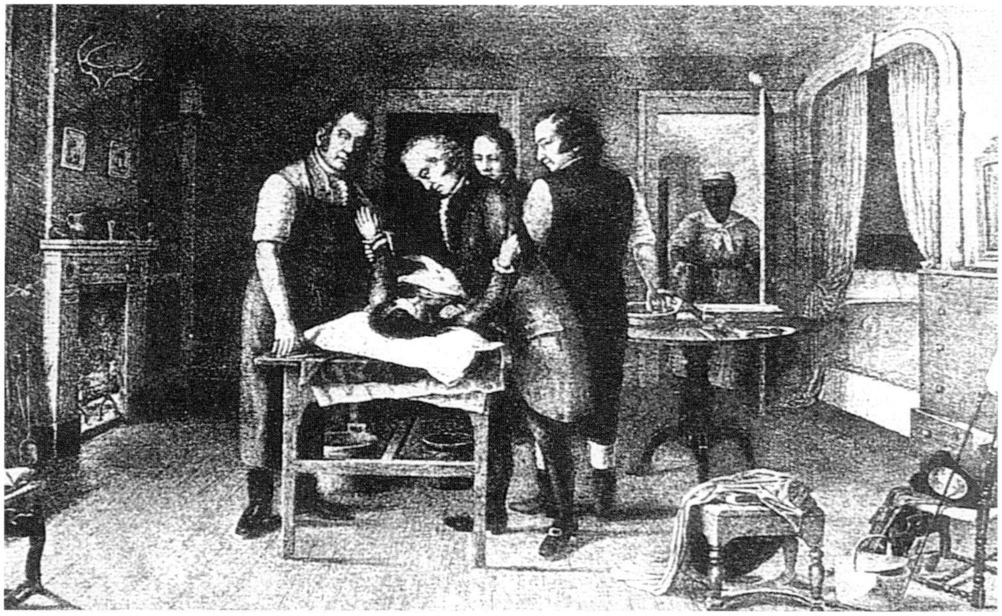

SURGERY ON DISEASED JOINTS

In Edinburgh, James Syme *(1799–1870)*, who was the head of clinical surgery at the University for 37 years, published a 'treatise on the excision of diseased joints' in 1831, in which he described some of the excision operations devised for the treatment of chronic infections of joints (usually tuberculous). In many cases this enabled the limb to be saved, with limitation of function it is true, but it was still preferable to the more drastic method of amputation. Of course, his operations were bedevilled by the risk of wound infection. It is interesting, therefore, that it was his son-in-law, Joseph Lister, who developed the antiseptic methods that enabled surgeons to perform these operations with safety.

POST-LISTERISM – THE MODERN ERA

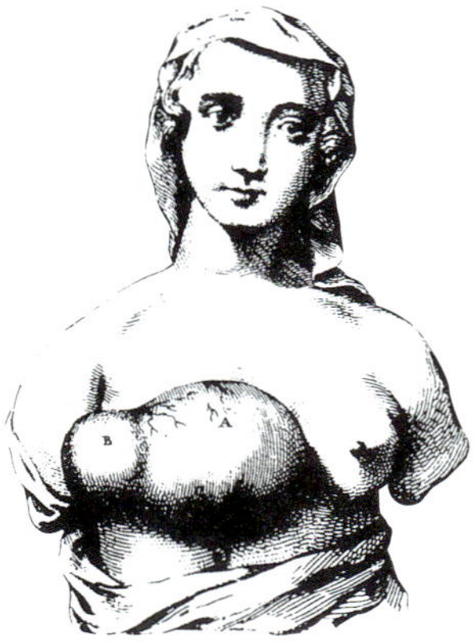

ABOVE In 1720 the German Lorenz Heister performed a mastectomy on this woman. Of course, pre-Lister, the wound became infected, but the patient did survive.

For some 2,000 years surgeons were quite aware of the immense possibilities of operative interventions; that major injuries could be repaired, tumours removed from breast, face and abdomen, arteries tied, amputations performed and so on. Yet they were held back by two things. First, the torture that these procedures involved. This was solved by the introduction of anaesthetic agents in the mid-nineteenth century. Second, the almost inevitable suppuration that would occur in the wounds produced either by injury or by the surgeon's knife itself. Infection was so common that the appearance of pus in the wound was actually welcomed by the surgeon. He called it 'laudable pus' – praiseworthy suppuration. Today we may laugh at this, but in thinking of the past we must always put ourselves in the position of the available knowledge at the time.

It was frequently noted that the risks of operations were much higher in the great hospitals than in the patient's own home. It was safer to have your baby in a cottage delivered by the local midwife than by the doctor in the maternity hospital in town. This, of course, we now know, was because of the great risk of cross-infection between one patient and the next from the filthy surroundings, septic wounds and indeed from the bacteria passed from one patient to the next on the surgeon's hands, instruments and dressings within the hospital environment.

The great breakthrough of Lister was to demonstrate that the cause of suppuration was not a mystery but was due to bacteria. The prevention of suppuration was possible by preventing bacteria from getting into the wound or by destroying them if already present. Lister did this by means of antiseptic agents such as carbolic acid. Later evolution of this antiseptic technique involved the aseptic ritual of modern surgery, which concentrated on the prevention of organisms reaching the wound.

As Lister's concept of the bacterial origin of wound infection slowly spread across Europe and the USA (and let us admit that it faced considerable opposition from many surgeons, particularly in Great Britain), the next stage of evolution was to progress beyond killing the bacteria that reached the wound by means of chemical antiseptics to the prevention of bacterial contamination by eliminating bacteria in the operating theatre – aseptic surgery. The use of steam sterilization of instruments, dressings and gowns, the wearing of masks, caps and gloves, air filtration and the other rituals of the operating theatre of today were introduced over the next couple of decades. Among the pioneers must be mentioned Gustav Von Neuber *(1850–1932)* of Kiel, and Curt Schimmelbusch *(1860–1895)* and Ernst Von Bergmann *(1836–1907)*, both of Berlin. In Great Britain, an important proponent of the new surgery was William Macewen *(1848–1924)*, who was a student under Lister in Glasgow and who became Regius Professor of Surgery in that city. Using aseptic surgery, Macewen was able to make considerable advances in the treatment of bone deformities, the surgery of mastoid infection and the first successful removal of the lung for tuberculosis, which he performed as far back as 1895. However, his greatest claim to fame must be as one of the founding fathers of neurosurgery. In 1879 he performed the first successful excision of a brain tumour (a meningioma) on a girl of 14.

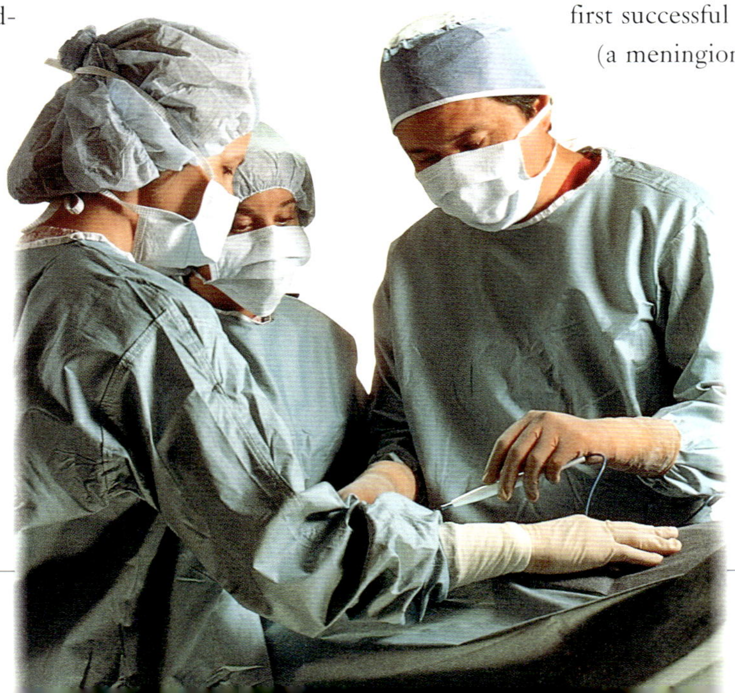

LEFT Aseptic surgery is based on the principle of preventing micro-organisms from being present in the operating theatre. The familiar picture of a modern surgeon using sterile instruments and wearing sterile gown, cap, mask and gloves has come about as a result of the work of the pioneers of asepsis in the latter part of the nineteenth century.

THE BURGEONING OF ABDOMINAL SURGERY

Lister himself never operated within the abdominal cavity. However, his antiseptic technique enabled others to perform abdominal surgery in relative safety. Earlier pioneers had established the broad principles of operations on the stomach, bowel and the other viscera; the pathologists had documented the disease processes that were there to be overcome, and the last 30 years of the nineteenth century saw spectacular advances in this field of surgery never experienced before or since.

Cancer provides some of the most difficult problems for the surgeon even to this day, and in the case of surgery of the abdomen, it was this condition which gave rise to some of the earliest operations. The first attempt at removal of a cancer of the stomach, the operation of gastrectomy, was performed in April 1879 by Jules Péan *(1830–1898)* of Paris. His patient was already seriously ill and died on the fifth post-operative day. In November 1880, Ludwig Rydigier *(1825–1920)* of Culm in Poland attempted the second gastrectomy in history, but his patient also died of exhaustion only 12 hours post-operatively. It fell to Theodor Billroth *(1829–1894)* to carry out the first successful gastrectomy. Billroth was Professor of Surgery at the great surgical university clinic of the Allgemeines Krankenhaus, Vienna. On 29 January 1881, the historic operation was performed on a woman called Thérèse Heller under chloroform anaesthesia. The abdomen was opened through an upper transverse incision, the tumour exposed, cut out and the gastric stump stitched to the duodenum. The operation lasted one-and-a-half hours and the patient's recovery was extremely smooth. The brave patient died of diffuse secondary deposits in the liver only four months later, yet the news that a patient could survive a major gastric cancer operation spread rapidly throughout the world. By 1890, Billroth and his team had performed 41 resections for gastric cancer with 19 successes.

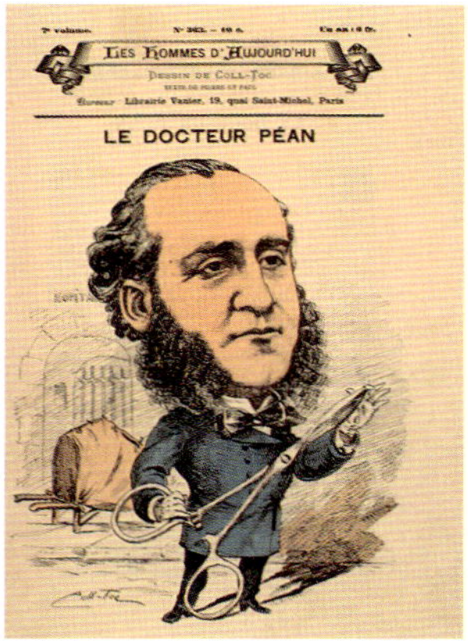

ABOVE Frenchman Jules Péan who performed the first successful elective removal of a spleen in 1867.

Meantime, Richard Von Volkmann *(1830–1889)* of Halle successfully removed a cancer of the rectum (1878). Paul Kraske *(1851–1930)*, Volkmann's assistant, perfected a method of resection of the rectum for cancer (1887). Gustav Simon *(1824–1876)*,

A SURGICAL GIANT

Theodor Billroth was undoubtedly one of the surgical giants of all time. He was the first to perform total removal of the larynx for cancer, pioneered excision of bladder cancers and tumours of the bowel, but more than that, he developed the concept of experimental surgery – taking problems first to the laboratory and from there to the operating theatre. He was the founder of the modern concept of reporting the total clinical experience of a department, to include operative mortality, complications and the five year follow-up, all so dear to the surgeon of today. Himself a great teacher, he produced a stream of surgeons who were responsible for the great German and Austrian school of surgery. Anton Wölfler *(1850–1917)*, for example, who assisted Billroth with the first successful gastrectomy, himself became head of surgery in Prague.

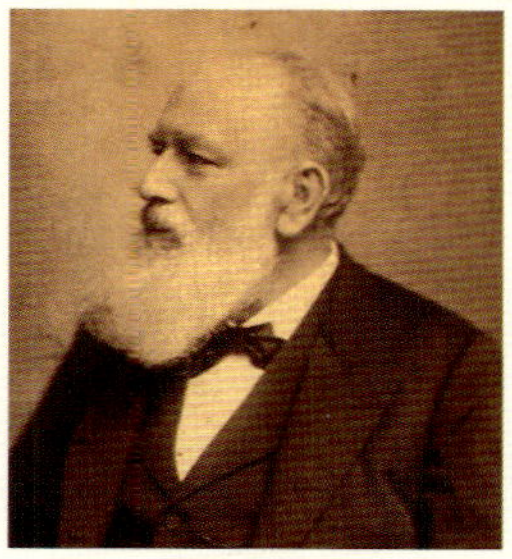

ABOVE Theodor Billroth extended surgery's horizons in the nineteenth century.

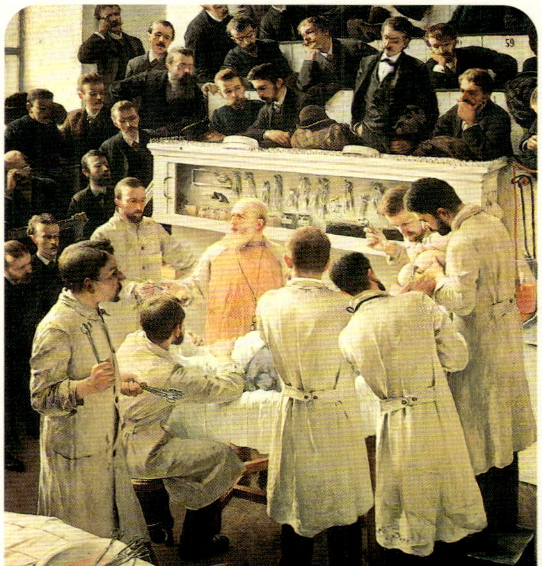

ABOVE Adelbert Seligmann's 1890 painting of Billroth operating at the Allgemeines Krankenhaus in Vienna. The patient is being anaesthetized.

in Heidelberg, reported the first successful planned removal of the kidney in 1870. In surgical operations of this type, the German and Austrian schools at first outran their colleagues in other countries. One reason for this was that they had at once adopted and vigorously practised the Listerian principles. In Britain, in contrast, Lister's teachings were regarded with disfavour by many surgeons and in London there was positive hostility to Lister's work. When once this antagonism had been overcome, British and American surgery entered these new regions, and in terms of dealing with acute abdominal emergencies, did some of the most important work.

THE FIRST APPENDECTOMY

The commonest cause of acute abdominal pain, inflammation of the appendix (appendicitis), was unknown as such in the middle of the nineteenth century. Although Thomas Addison *(1793–1860)* and Richard Bright *(1789–1858)*, physicians at Guy's Hospital, had clearly recognized that the appendix can be the site of acute inflammation, suppuration in the right lower abdomen continued to be described by the rather mystical name of 'perityphlitis'. Many patients died of perforation of the acutely inflammed appendix and general peritonitis. It was another physician, Reginald Fitz *(1843–1913)* of Philadelphia, who pointed out the vital necessity for early diagnosis and operation in this situation. He gave a lucid and logical description of the clinical features of the condition as well as actually coining the term 'appendicitis'. Fitz was unusual as a professor of medicine (at Harvard) in advocating early operation!

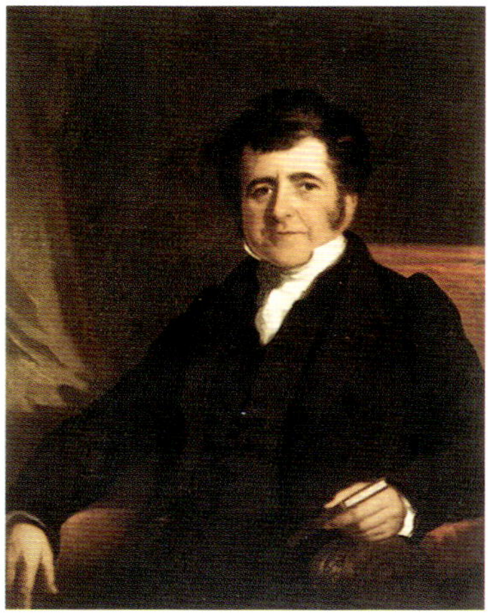

ABOVE The British physician Richard Bright. He gave his name to a type of kidney problem which is known as Bright's disease.

The first successful appendectomy was performed by British surgeon Robert Lawson Tait *(1845–1899)*. His patient was a young girl with a gangrenous appendix lying within an abscess cavity. The patient recovered, but he did not report the case until 1890. Thus, credit for the first published account of this operation (1886) must go to Rudolph Kronlein *(1847–1910)*, although his patient, a boy aged 17, died just two days later. In 1887, Thomas George Morton *(1835–1903)* of Philadelphia was first in publishing a successful appendectomy for a perforated appendix. Charles McBurney *(1845–1908)* of New York pioneered early diagnosis and early operative intervention, pointing out that in most cases of inflammation in the lower right abdomen, the appendix was the affected organ. He devised a useful incision located immediately over the appendix, which is used today and named after him, and he also described the point of maximum abdominal tenderness in this condition ('McBurney's point'). By publishing paper after paper on this topic, McBurney must be regarded, along with Reginald Fitz, as the pioneer for teaching surgeons how to diagnose and treat this important condition.

Another acute abdominal emergency, which, untreated, meant almost certain death, was perforation of an ulcer of the stomach. The first successful operation to close such a perforation was performed in a private house by Ludwig Heusner *(1846–1916)* of Barmen, Germany in 1892. The following year Hastings Gilford *(1861–1941)*, of Reading, England, did a similar operation with success, but did not publish his description of the case until after that of Thomas Herbert Morse *(1855–1921)* of Norwich, England, and within two or three

BELOW An abdominal operation being performed at London's Charing Cross Hospital in 1900. Surgical caps and masks were still not mandatory apparently.

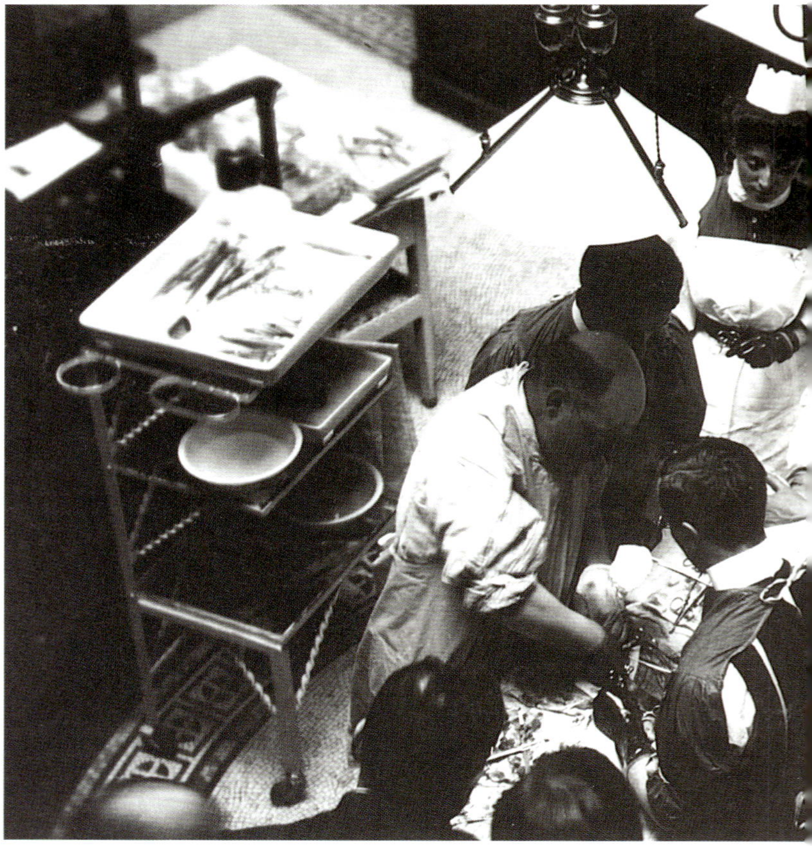

THE FATHER OF MODERN ABDOMINAL SURGERY

Robert Lawson Tait *(1845–1899)* was born in Edinburgh and was a pupil of the great Sir James Young Simpson *(1811–1870)*, who introduced chloroform into midwifery and surgery. He moved to Birmingham at the age of 25 and spent the rest of his active life there. Apart from his work on ectopic pregnancy and his early success with removal of the diseased appendix, he pioneered the surgery of ovarian cysts and tumours. In 1886 he was able to publish evidence of 137 consecutive cases of removal of such ovarian pathologies without a death. In 1879 he carried out the first removal of a diseased gall bladder in Europe, the second ever performed in the world, and within five years he was able to report 13 more cases with only one death. His contributions as a surgeon are summed up by William Mayo *(1861–1939)*, who wrote, 'The cavities of the body were a sealed book until the father of modern abdominal surgery, Lawson Tait, carried the sense of sight into the abdominal cavity'.

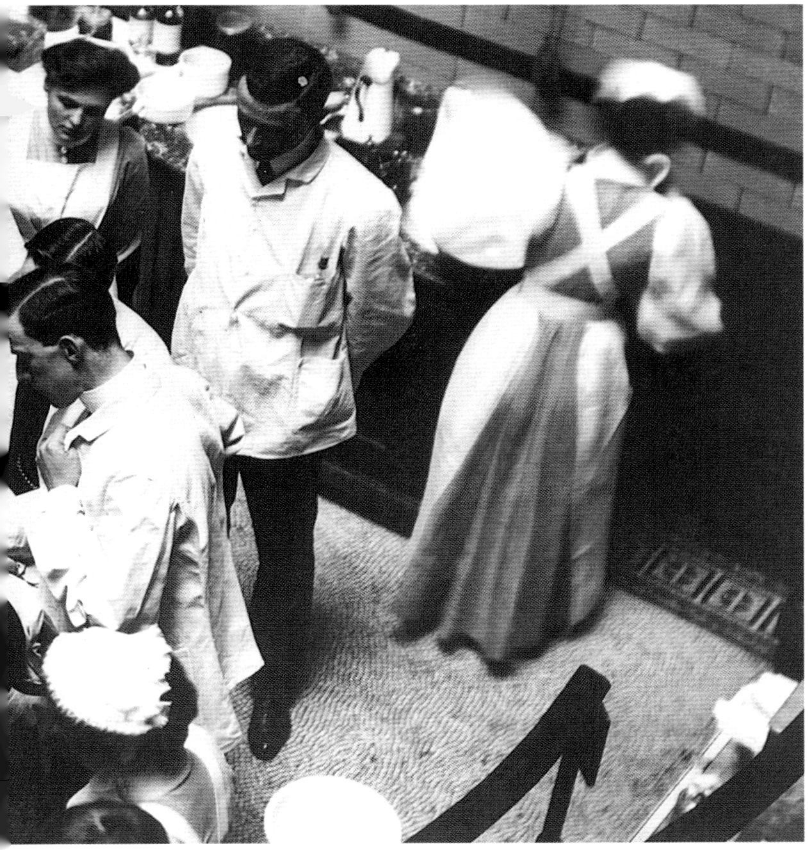

years of these publications the operation of suture of perforations of the stomach and duodenum became a routine part of the surgeon's armamentarium.

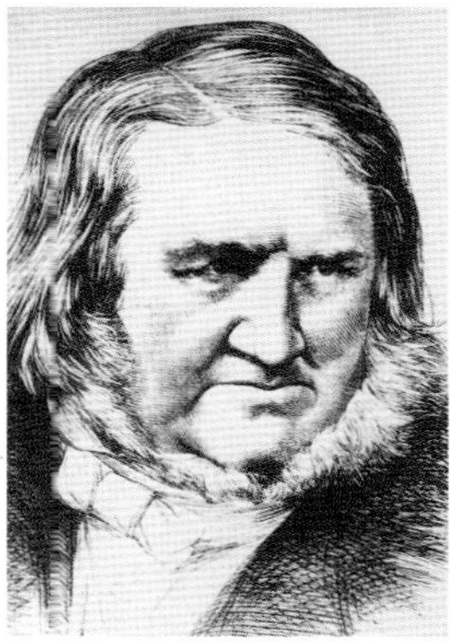

ABOVE Sir James Young Simpson, a leading nineteenth-century obstetrician and one of the founders of gynaecology.

From time to time the fertilized ovum, instead of implanting in the uterus, lodges in the Fallopian tube (causing an ectopic pregnancy). This cannot accommodate the enlarging embryo and ruptures after a month or two with catastrophic haemorrhage. Untreated, this is almost invariably fatal. In a book published in 1876 on this subject (by John Parry), we read, 'Here is an accident which may happen to any wife in the most useful period of her existence, which good authorities have said is never cured; and for which, even in this age when science and art boast of such high attainments, no remedy either medical or surgical has been tried with a single success'. When we read that eminent authorities were advising the use of electric shocks, the injection of narcotics into the sac of the embryo, and copious and frequent bleeding, we are hardly surprised at the rate of failure. Parry himself went on to suggest that the only remedy would be to open the abdomen and either tie the bleeding vessels or remove the tube entirely. The first surgeon to perform a successful operation of this kind was Robert Lawson Tait *(see box)*. It is interesting that the suggestion that he should operate on such cases came from a general practitioner dealing with such a patient in 1881. At the time Tait rejected the suggestion that he should open the abdomen and remove the ruptured tube, and a further haemorrhage killed the patient. In 1883, however, Tait had another chance; this time he operated, tied the tube and removed it. The operation was a success.

One by one the acute abdominal emergencies that had hitherto been almost invariavbly fatal were shown to be amenable to surgical intervention. In 1871, Jonathan Hutchinson *(1828–1911)* of the London Hospital operated on a female child aged two years who was desperately ill with intestinal obstruction due to an extraordinary condition in which a segment of the intestine pushes itself into the adjacent section rather like a sock turning itself inside out. Under chloroform, Hutchinson opened the child's abdomen, and easily reduced the six-inch (15cm) mass of obstructed bowel. The child made a good recovery from this three-minute operation.

The spleen is the most common organ to be damaged in closed abdominal injuries, particularly a severe crushing blow to the left lower chest or the upper abdomen; the most common cause of this today is a road traffic accident. Untreated, without surgical intervention, the majority of patients with this injury will die of haemorrhage. Rather surprisingly, there seemed to be diffidence by surgeons to open the abdomen in this condition in the pioneer days of abdominal surgery, and to remove the ruptured spleen. This fact is even more surprising since it had been shown centuries before that the spleen could be removed in animals and even man without any obvious loss of function.

For example, the Renaissance anatomist Andreas Vesalius had demonstrated that removal of the spleen in living animals was not fatal. In 1663 Timothy Clark removed the spleen from a stray dog who lived for a year, put on flesh, and was subsequently 'enthusiastic in its pursuit of sexual activity'. In 1676, he removed the spleen of a butcher who had tried to commit suicide by slashing his own abdomen. Through this horrifying wound the spleen protruded and, three days later, Clark removed the organ with complete recovery of the patient.

The first two unsuccessful attempts to remove the ruptured spleen after closed injury to the abdomen were reported by Sir William Arbuthnot Lane *(1856–1943)* of Guy's Hospital, London. Both were children injured in road traffic accidents but who survived only a few hours following the operation. It fell to Oscar Reigner, Chief Surgeon at the All Saints Hospital in Breslau, to have the distinction of performing the first successful splenectomy for closed trauma in 1893. The patient was a 14-year-old labourer who fell two storeys from scaffolding, striking his abdomen on a board. He was obviously dying from serious intra-abdominal haemorrhage when Reigner operated on him, removing the completely divided spleen. Of course, these were the days before blood transfusion, but the patient was given an infusion of normal saline. He had a stormy post-operative course, but eventually recovered after five months in hospital.

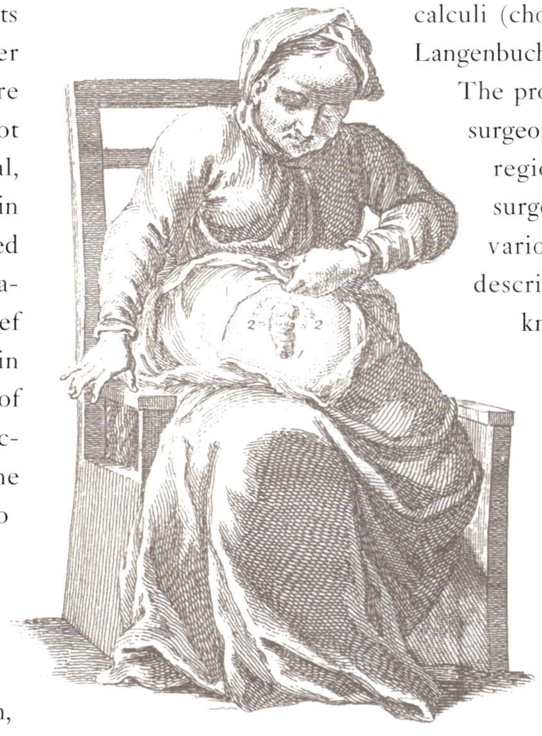

ABOVE **A picture of an intestinal fistula from William Cheselden's *Anatomy of the Human Body (1713)*. Huge advances in abdominal surgery were made in the late nineteenth century.**

GALL STONES AND HERNIAS

Solidified masses in the gall bladder, or gall stones, were mentioned by the Greek physician Alexander of Tralles in the fifth century AD. Arab physicians in the tenth century prescribed gall stones from the ox for epilepsy and various other complaints. By the sixteenth century, inflammation of the gall bladder due to stones was recorded at post-mortem by Vesalius, Fallopius and others. In 1743 Jean-Louis Petit *(1674–1750)* of Paris advocated that the gall bladder be opened after an abscess had formed and become adherent to the abdominal wall. He described several cases in which he and other French surgeons had successfully accomplished drainage of the gall bladder with the removal of stones in this manner, although few were brave enough to accept this advice. Opening the inflamed gall bladder and removing the offending stones, a technique called a cholecystotomy, was first performed successfully in 1867 by John Bobbs *(1809–1870)*, a surgeon from Indiana. The disadvantages of this operation are numerous, including recurrent infection, residual stones and recurrence of the stones themselves. The modern operation, removal of the gall bladder and its offending calculi (cholecystectomy) was first performed by Karl Langenbuch *(1846–1901)* in Berlin in 1882.

The problem of hernias in the groin had challenged surgeons for centuries. The complex anatomy of the region had been carefully studied by many surgeon-anatomists in the dissecting room. The various types and forms of hernias had been described and their complications were well known. However, apart from operating to relieve a strangulated hernia, which, left untreated, would be almost invariably fatal, treatment had made little progress. It usually comprised the fitting of an uncomfortable truss. With the adoption of antisepsis, radical repair of a hernia before strangulation occurred was now possible. However, early attempts at cure were not successful, with rapid recurrence often occurring.

The surgeon who pioneered the successful repair of groin hernias, based on meticulous anatomical reconstruction of the tissues, was Edoardo Bassini *(1844–1924)*, Professor of Surgery in the University of Padua. His technique is the basis of modern hernia surgery.

THE EVOLUTION OF THE SURGICAL SPECIALTIES

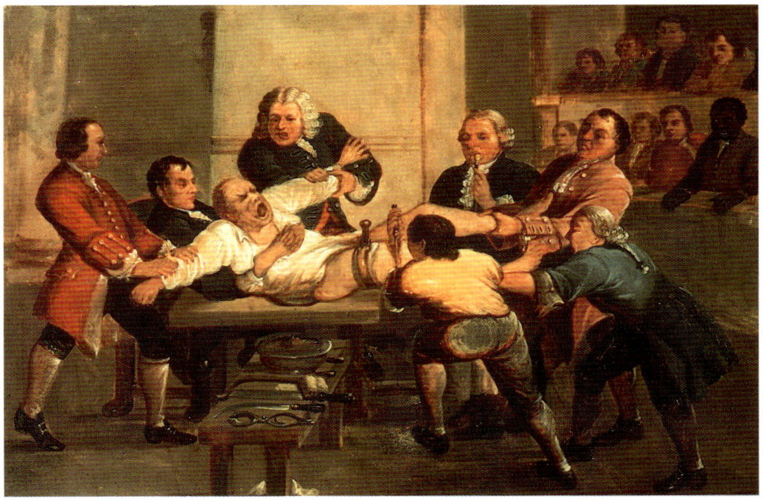

LEFT An eighteenth-century English painting that graphically illustrates the horrors of surgery before anaesthesia and antisepsis ushered in the modern era.

By the end of the nineteenth century, the enormous potential of modern surgery was already apparent. Few, however, could have foreseen the truly amazing and exciting progress that was about to be made. Massive areas of advance were undreamed of; the problems of the repair of heart defects, the transplantation of organs, the reconstruction or replacement of diseased blood vessels, the development of artificial joints, the cure for many forms of deafness and the alleviation of crippling diseases of the nervous system were all to be solved.

THE SURGERY OF MAJOR ARTERIES

Until recent times, vascular operations were confined to ligature of major blood vessels. We have noted the work of Ambroise Paré on the ligation of arteries in amputation and of this technique in dealing with aneurysmal dilatations (swollen weak points) of major arteries. For a torn or diseased blood vessel there was no other choice. Even if the patient survived the operation, this might often result in loss of the limb itself, since it was deprived of its major source of blood supply.

The first successful repair of a gunshot wound of a major artery was performed in Chicago by John Benjamin Murphy *(1857–1916)* in 1897. Murphy was undoubtedly one of the most colourful personalities in American surgery. Even his name reflects something of his character; he was born of humble Irish immigrants on a farm in Wisconsin and was christened plain John Murphy. However, when he went to school, he noticed that the majority of the other boys had at least two initials and so, determined not to be inferior to them, he added the 'B' to his name. After training in Chicago and spending two years in Vienna under Theodor Billroth, he became chief of surgery at the Mercy Hospital in Chicago, a position which he held until his death. His successful arterial operation *(see box)* was based on extensive and detailed animal experiments carried out on dogs, calves and sheep.

Although attempts had been made to reconstruct more peripheral aneurysms, surgeons long despaired of being able to deal with this disease when it affected the main artery of the

REPAIRING A GUNSHOT WOUND

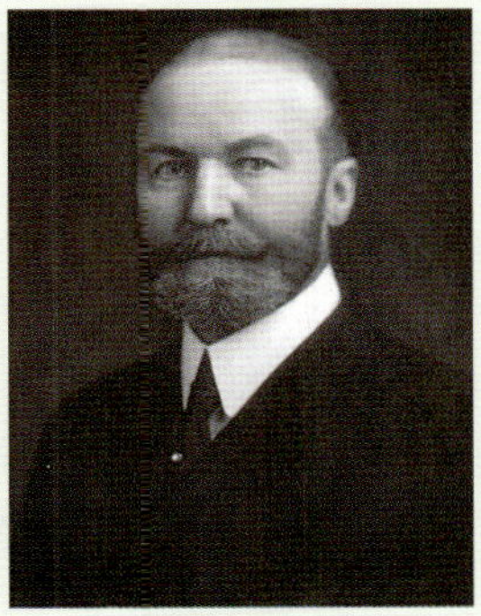

ABOVE John Benjamin Murphy, the American surgeon who successfully sutured a main artery.

JB Murphy's opportunity to put his experiments into clinical practice came when an Italian pedlar aged 29 was admitted, having been shot just below the groin. In the operation, both the main artery (the femoral) and vein to the lower limb were found to be torn and, indeed, much of the wall of the artery had been destroyed. The side-hole in the vein was sutured (stitched); one half-inch (13cm) of the damaged artery was cut away and the two ends of the vessel joined with interrupted sutures. When the clamps were removed, Murphy proudly reported 'not a drop of blood escaped at the line of suture'. The time for the operation was approximately two-and-a-half hours; the patient made an excellent recovery with full restoration of function of his lower limb.

body itself, the aorta. Indeed, even in my own young days as a surgeon, there was no alternative but to stand helplessly by and see these swellings slowly enlarge and rupture with the inevitable death of the patient. The first report of a successful resection of an aortic aneurysm greatly influenced general and vascular surgeons throughout the world and was carried out in 1951 by Charles Dubost *(1914–1991)*.

Dubost, a Parisian, used a graft from the aorta of a donor that had been preserved by freeze-drying. For decades before this, attempts were made to find a suitable replacement for an artery; materials such as glass or metal tubing proved to be disastrous failures. Freeze-dried arteries, harvested from the bodies of young accident victims, proved useful, but tended to degenerate with time. These have now been replaced either by using the patient's own superficial vein in the leg, (as in the commonly performed operation of coronary artery bypass), or by using woven or knitted tubes of synthetic fibre, such as teflon or dacron.

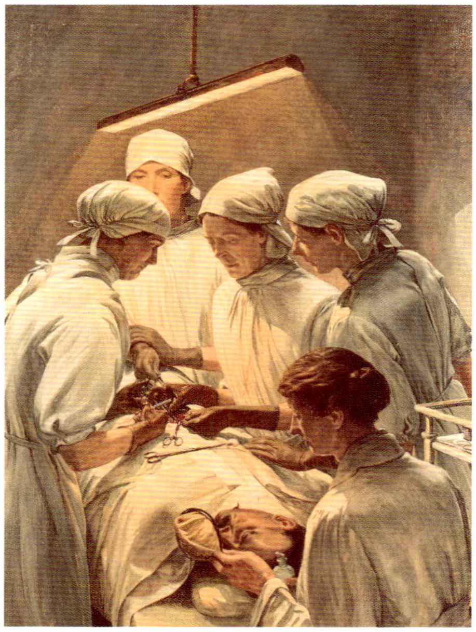

ABOVE **Dealing with war wounded inevitably advances the art of surgery. This is an operation at the Endell Street military hospital in London, painted by Francis Dodd.**

SURGERY OF THE HEART

The heart was long regarded as a surgical 'no go' area. Wounds of the heart were thought to be fatal and certainly beyond the help of the surgeon. Indeed, it was not until 1897 that Ludwig Rehn *(1849-1930)* of Frankfurt am Main performed the first successful repair of a cardiac injury. Even in World War I such operations were rarities, despite the fact that the operation is a perfectly straightforward procedure.

A commonly acquired disease of the heart is caused by stenosis, or narrowing of the mitral valve, so called because of its similarity to the shape of a bishop's mitre. It lies between two chambers, the atrium and ventricle of the right side of the heart, and is commonly involved as a complication of rheumatic fever. This was once a frequent disease of the Western world and is still common in developing countries. Adolescents are the usual victims. They present with breathlessness, greatly limited exercise tolerance and frequently with pulse irregularities; eventually, death supervenes from heart failure. Doctors long wished that a surgical treatment could be found for this mechanical problem and this was foreseen in 1902 by the Scottish pharmacologist Sir Thomas Lauder Brunton *(1844–1916)*. Experimentally, Duff Allen developed a most ingenious optical device which enabled him to view and divide the mitral valve of a cat using an approach through the atrium. Various knives were tested and eventually, in 1923, Elliott Cutler *(1888–1947)* in Boston succeeded in excising a portion of the stenosed (or constricted) valve by means of an ingenious valvulotome (a cutting tool), working through the thick muscle of the ventricle. The operation was, however, necessarily blind and somewhat dangerous. A considerable advance was made in 1925 by Sir Henry Sessions Souttar *(1875–1964)* of the London Hospital. The patient was a girl of 15, a labourer's daughter. The patient was severely ill and in the late stages of congestive heart failure. A large flap was raised to expose the heart and the stenosed valve dilated with the index finger passed through the auricular appendage of the right atrium of the heart; this was a much easier and safer approach than through the ventricle. The girl made an uneventful recovery and lived in fair health for five years.

Souttar's operation was ignored for more than 22 years, but was taken up again by Dwight Harken *(1910–1993)* of Boston. He had acquired a considerable experience of dealing with the removal of bullet and shell fragments from the hearts of wounded soldiers as a thoracic surgeon in World War II. In June 1948 he divided a stenosed mitral valve using his finger which had been fitted with a small knife. Later in the same year, the operation was performed again by Russell Brock *(1903–1980)* at Guy's Hospital in London, this time using only the surgeon's index finger. Reports of these successful operations rapidly spread; the remarkable return to normal function of these seriously ill patients gave great impetus to the development of cardiac surgery.

Congenital abnormalities of the heart and its great vessels are another common problem, which, untreated, usually result in severe disability and often in the death of the young patient. The first successful assays into surgical treatment were aimed at the great vessels, and could be carried out with the heart still beating. Robert Gross *(1905–1988)* of Boston reported the first successful ligation of a patent ductus arteriosus, a persistence of the shunt in the foetus between the aorta and the pulmonary artery, while Clarence Crafoord *(1899–1984)* of Stockholm in 1945 carried out successful resection and repair of cases of coarctation (constriction) of the aorta near its origin.

To permit open procedures on the heart itself under direct vision – to repair congenital defects, replace damaged valves and so on – means that the heart must be put out of circulation and stopped. This requires a pump system to keep oxygenated blood circulating, especially to the brain, without the pumping action of the heart itself. The American John Gibbon *(1903–1974)*, assisted in his work by his wife, constructed a prototype heart-lung pump that was used successfully in animal experiments in 1939. After a further 15 years of experiment he applied this successfully to a human, closing a heart defect under direct vision in 1953. Not only was it now possible to repair complicated congenital abnormalities of the heart, but also to replace diseased and defective valves within the heart.

ORGAN TRANSPLANTATION

Notwithstanding the story of the miraculous graft of a leg by Saints Cosmos and Damian in the third century AD, the transplantation of an organ from one person to another seemed beyond the realms of medical possibility. The first bona fide report of a successful replantation of a kidney into the neck of a dog was performed by Emerich Ullmann *(1861–1937)* in 1902. This autotransplant worked perfectly satisfactorily, but when a kidney was transplanted from one dog to another, it was rapidly destroyed, as was, even more speedily, a dog-to-goat transplant. Ullmann's work was taken up by Alexis Carrel *(1873–1944)*, a Frenchman working at the Rockefeller Institute, New York. Carrel worked out the technique for joining up fine blood vessels, which was necessary for such grafts (he was awarded the Nobel Prize in 1912), and confirmed Ullmann's findings in 1905. He was clearly aware that although he could overcome the technical surgical problems of transplantation of the kidney, he was defeated by the biology of the process. It was to be decades before these questions were, in fact, successfully answered.

The classical studies on skin grafting by Peter Medawar *(1915–1987)* and his group in Oxford during World War II clearly demonstrated that the rejection of a foreign tissue graft was an immunological mechanism. Peter Medawar, together with McFarlane Burnet *(1899–1985)* in Australia, shared the Nobel Prize in 1960 for their work in this field. The fact that skin grafts could be accepted between identical twins laid the basis for the exciting possibility that a sick identical twin might accept an organ graft from a healthy sibling. The first successful kidney graft between identical twins was performed in 1954 by Joseph Murray *(1919–)* and his colleagues in Boston. Murray subsequently received the Nobel Prize in 1990 along with Donnall Thomas for his work in this field.

There still remained, of course, the tremendous problems of the immunological barrier to transplantation. In 1959 Robert Schwartz and W Dameshek showed that the treatment of rabbits with a drug termed 6-mercaptopurine produced a long-lasting tolerance to human protein. After seeing this report, an English surgeon Roy Calne *(1930–)* showed that this drug could allow successful kidney grafts to be performed between unmatched dogs. Later, Calne, working with Joseph Murray in Boston, showed that azathioprine was more effective in suppressing rejection, and renal transplantation became accepted as treatment in patients in otherwise terminal kidney failure.

The first heart transplantation in man was performed in 1967 by Christiaan Barnard *(1922–)* in Cape Town. At first, results of heart transplantation were poor, but the use of new anti-rejection techniques, particularly the drug cyclosporin developed by Calne and his team in Cambridge, greatly improved the survival of this and other organ transplants. Thus today, heart, lung, heart and lung combined, and liver transplants are standard procedures, while grafts of small intestine and of pancreas (the last for refractory diabetes) are under active clinical investigation.

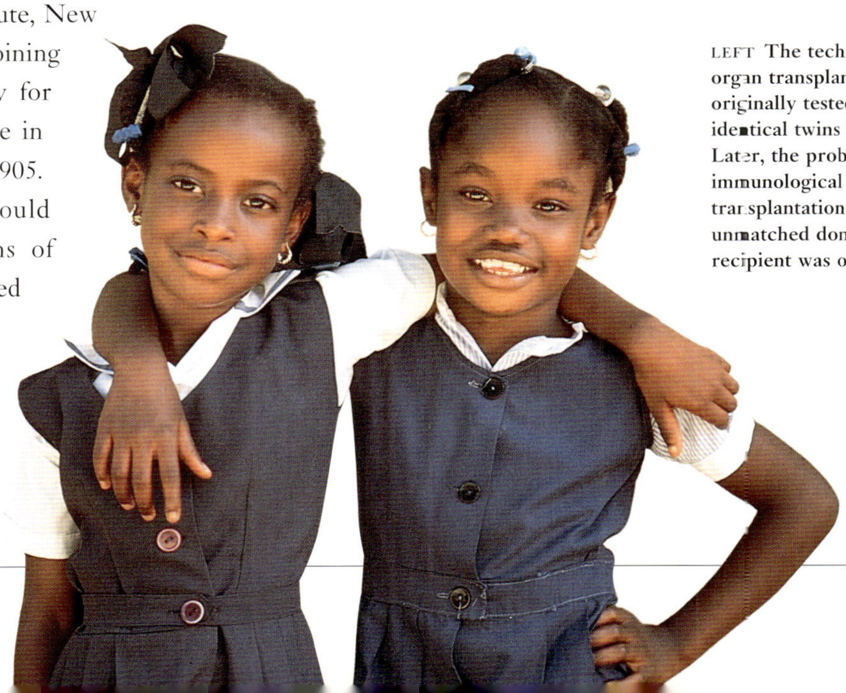

LEFT The technique of organ transplantation was originally tested on a pair of identical twins in 1954. Later, the problem of the immunological barrier to transplantation between unmatched donor and recipient was overcome.

ALTERNATIVES TO SURGERY

Over the centuries, alternative interventional treatments to what might be described as 'conventional' surgery have been and are being used. These can be defined as those techniques which are not based on our present day concepts of disease, which have developed as a result of studies of the physiology, pathology and bacteriology of man's illnesses. Acupuncture and the related technique of moxibustion were used by the ancient Chinese and are still in use today; fortunately, the red-hot cautery iron used by the Arabs is no longer employed. Even conventional medical practitioners of the past used techniques which were based on completely false concepts of disease and were harmful rather than beneficial to the patient.

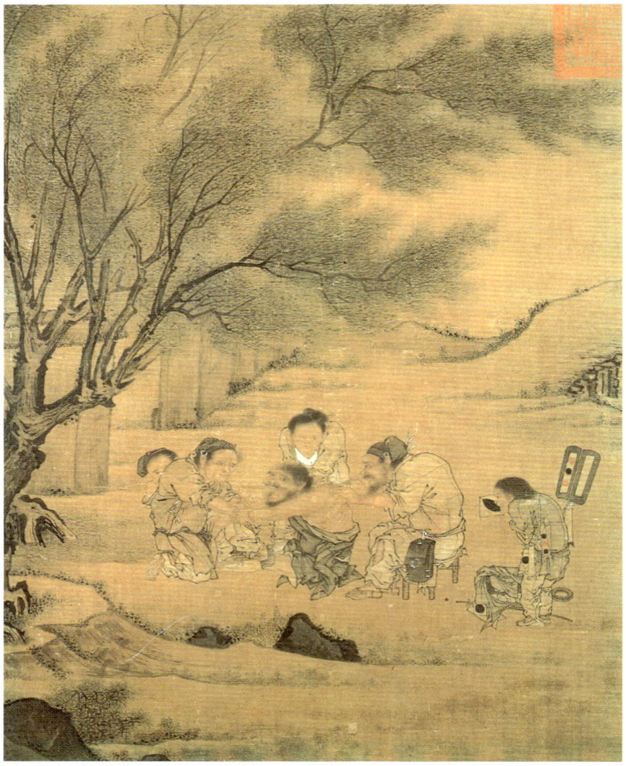

ABOVE A Chinese peasant being treated by a village doctor with moxibustion. The painting by Li Tang dates from the Sung Dynasty *(960–1279)*.

Since many people submit themselves to various alternative therapies, there must obviously be explanations for their popularity. These are not difficult, in fact, to find. First, something like 80–90 per cent of all ills which take patients to the doctor are self-curing or self-limiting. The common cold, most of the infectious diseases and many minor injuries are examples of problems that all resolve, whatever the treatment. Second, there is the well-known placebo effect of any treatment given with sufficient confidence by the practitioner. Third, recent studies have shown that a number of stimuli liberate the body's own morphine-like substances, termed endorphins, from the brain. Fourth, of course, is the possibility that the alternative explanation of disease is actually true. One problem in the assessment of the true value of many of these alternative therapies is the absence of double-blind controlled clinical trials. In these, patients are randomized between the treatment and a placebo, and neither the patient nor the doctor knows to which category he or she has been assigned. The patients are then followed up, the results assessed and statistically evaluated.

The nineteenth century saw numerous alternative systems of therapy flourish. Two treatments which involve manipulation are osteopathy and chiropractic.

The father of osteopathy was Andrew Taylor Still *(1828–1917)*. He had been a medical student in Kansas City, but left before qualifying to enlist as a soldier in the Civil War. Still elaborated a theory of disease that postulated that the living human body contains within itself the remedies necessary to protect it against disease and the correct functioning of the body requires a proper alignment of nerves, muscles and bones. He called the new science osteopathy, which literally means 'bone suffering'. By manipulation of the spine, disease could be cured. Considerable dispute developed between osteopaths and conventional practitioners, but over the decades the osteopaths modified their original principles so that the many schools of osteopathy in the United States now have virtually the same practices as regular schools of medicine.

Chiropractic is another healing system which ascribes diseases to derangement in the structure and the function of the vertebral column. It was founded in 1895 by Daniel D Palmer *(1845–1913)*. Proper adjustments of the spinal column by manual means are supposed to cure ailments of the internal organs.

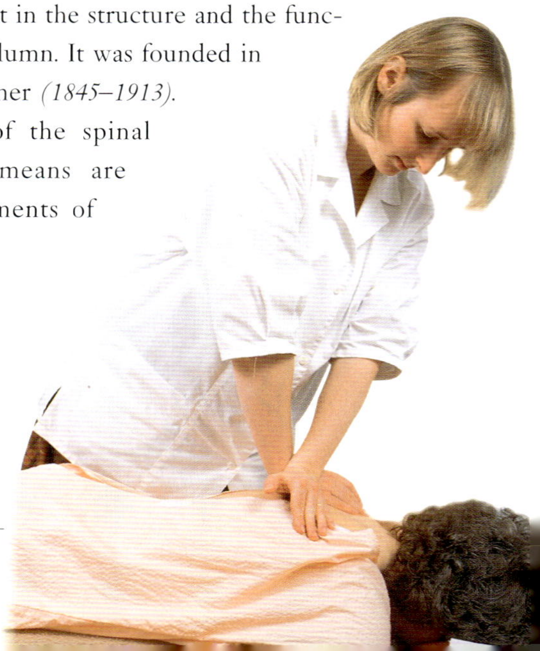

RIGHT A chiropractor manipulating the spine of a patient. The therapy aims manually to correct abnormalities in the alignment of the spinal vertebrae.

WHAT OF THE FUTURE?

One must be a brave person indeed, or a foolish one, to anticipate the future of surgery with any confidence in one's prediction coming true. Refinements in fibre-optic technology and engineering have produced the instruments which are already used for so-called 'keyhole' surgery. Fine tools can be passed into the abdominal and thoracic cavities so that many operations that previously required major incisions for exposure can now be performed through quite small puncture wounds.

Fibre-optic technology is allowing the development of instruments that pass along every tube in the body, for example to remove obstructions in the oesophagus, bile ducts, bowel, prostate and the major blood vessels. Plastic-tube replacement of the main arteries by passing these shunts through small puncture wounds is already in an advanced stage of development. Sophisticated engineering and imaging techniques are being developed to enable fine probes to be passed with great accuracy into the brain to deal with tumours, blood vessel abnormalities and even some psychiatric diseases.

Robots already find an important place in industry. The applications of robotic methods in surgery is also at an advanced stage of development, the aim being to have robotic equipment that can co-operate with the surgeon rather than replacing him totally. In orthopaedic surgery, for example, machines are being developed to drill the cavity in the patient's hip of the exact shape and size for placement of the prosthesis in total hip replacement surgery. The pre-operative planning in this system first builds a three-dimensional model of the patient's own hip by using data from computed tomography. The surgeon selects an appropriate implant to use based on several whose exact dimensions are stored in the system.

A voice-activated robot surgical assistant is being developed for laparoscopic (minimal access) surgery in the abdominal cavity. This device functions as a robotic cameraman for the surgeon. Like a human assistant, it obeys voice commands and will move the laparoscope to face the site of action as directed by the surgeon. In the future, operating rooms may be designed specifically to facilitate minimal access procedures and to incorporate all the necessary robotic and audio-visual technology.

Micro-robots may have applications in the world of surgery, which include sensory devices in the circulatory system, drug delivery systems, artificial sphincters to replace those damaged by injury or disease, valves for veins or the heart, and self-cleaning filters. One of the most interesting developments is the 'intelligent' micro-robotic endoscope. This is a 'mouse' that could propel itself within, for example, the bowel and videotape the journey for later study by the operator. At first the instrument would be purely diagnostic, but facilities might then be developed to take samples of tissue for microscopic examination or even to incorporate a laser for removing polyps and tumours. It may seem far-fetched, but only time will tell.

BELOW This surgeon has inserted an arthroscope into a patient's knee. A fibre-optic cable enables her to look inside the joint and to operate on damaged tissue.

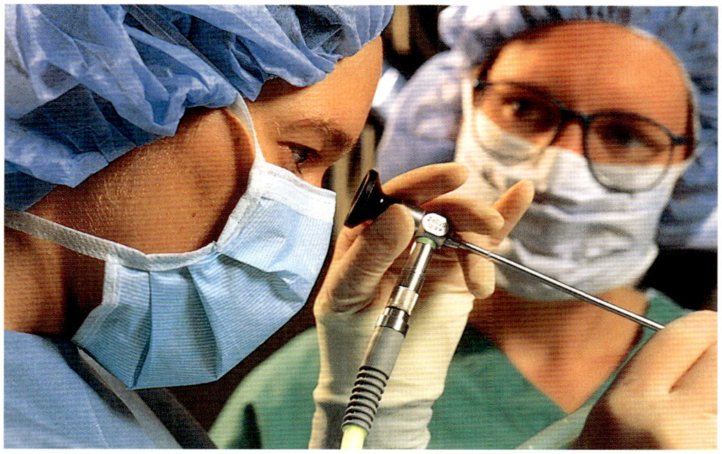

ROBOT SURGEONS

Eye surgery is another area which could benefit from robotic technology, since the movement required for some procedures depends on accuracy measured to the nearest micron. Computer-controlled tools have been designed to help in procedures which are beyond human ability to perform with hands and eyes, even if assisted by an operating microscope. Already a computer laser-scanning system has been developed for the treatment of refractive anomalies of the eye. In this system, a laser measures the shape of the cornea, while an ultrasound-pulsed laser performs the delicate cutting of the cornea to the correct dimensions.

CHAPTER SIX

HEALING AND THE MIND

MIND, BODY AND SPIRIT IN MENTAL MEDICINE

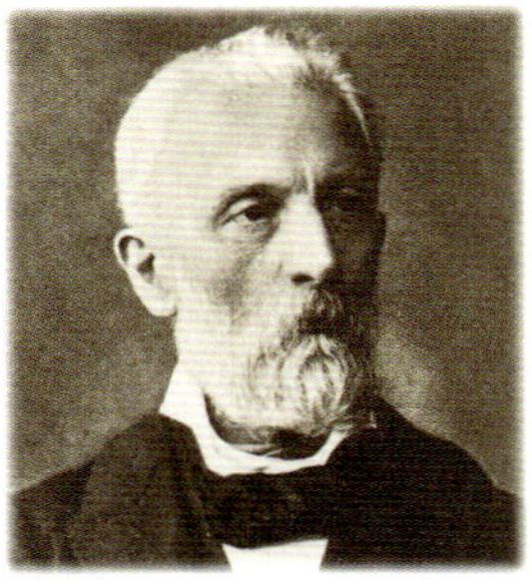

ABOVE Adolf Bastian *(1826–1905)* was born in Bremen. A prodigious traveller, he wrote more than 30 books.

DURING HIS FIELD WORK *in Guyana in the late nineteenth century, the German anthropologist Adolf Bastian fell ill one day. Suffering from a severe headache and fever, Bastian bid the local medicine man to treat him with his customary method. The medicine man, according to Bastian's account, requested he visit his lodge after dusk with his hammock and several leaves of tobacco. He was told to lie down on the hammock and not to move at all, lest he endanger his life. The medicine man, Bastian wrote, began by conjuring up the kenaimas (demons or spirits). Soon these manifested their presence by all kinds of noises, first low and soft, then louder and eventually deafening. Each of them spoke with its own voice, which varied according to the alleged personality of the kenaima. Some of them seemed to fly through the air; the patient could hear the rustling of their wings and feel a draft on his face. He even felt the touch of one of them and was agile enough to bite off a few fragments, which he later found to be leaves of boughs that the medicine man must have been swinging through the air.*[1]

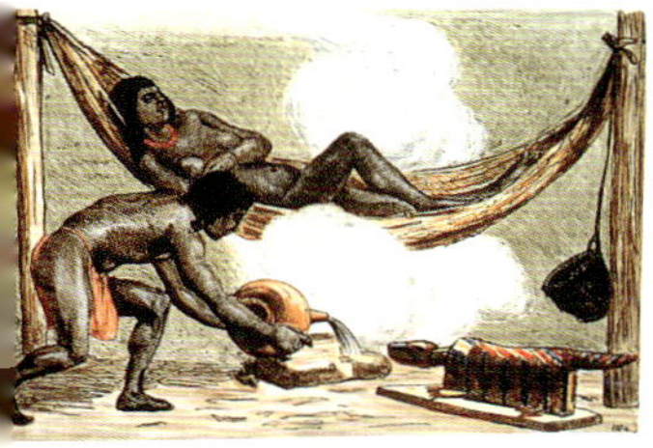

ABOVE A shaman smoking leaves under a sick patient as part of a magical healing ritual.

Bastian experienced the six-hour ordeal in a kind of hypnotic trance.. Although the medicine man's efforts did not cure Bastian of his condition, they left him with a lasting impression. Bastian, like many members of Europe's late nineteenth-century medical and scientific establishment, developed a keen interest in the medical practices of what were then considered primitive cultures, analyzing healing rituals in Africa and among the native peoples of North and South America. This interest, it must be emphasized, was far from purely academic, and even as Western medicine reached its professional and scientific zenith, magic, performance and ritual remained scientifically and therapeutically relevant.

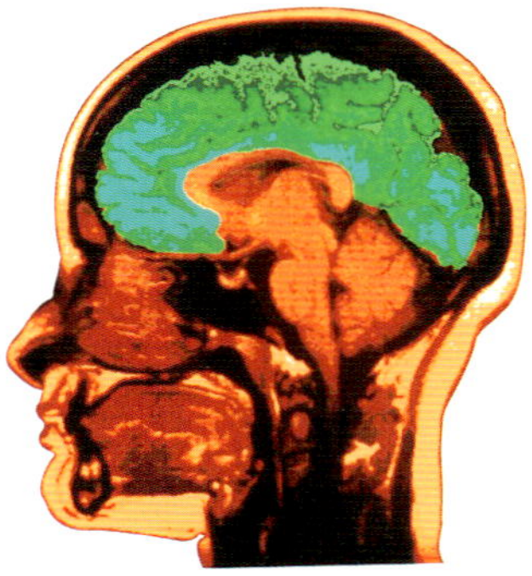

ABOVE A computer-enhanced magnetic resonance imaging (MRI) scan of a human head showing the brain. The green portion is the cerebrum, while the cerebellum is centre right, coloured orange. Below this is the brainstem.

Among medical specializations, psychiatry has been, arguably, most influenced by such ideas. Possibly this is because of the elusiveness of mental illness, and the glaring insufficiency of any single explanatory paradigm. Moreover, the difficulty of treating mentally ill patients and the perennially low rates of therapeutic success have motivated psychiatric practitioners to look elsewhere for inspiration and ideas; indeed, theories and treatments of the insane in the modern West often betray a deep debt to non-Western cultures. A third reason for this influence lies in the uniqueness of psychiatry as a modern profession. The belief that mental illness is a medical – as opposed to spiritual – condition is, in historical

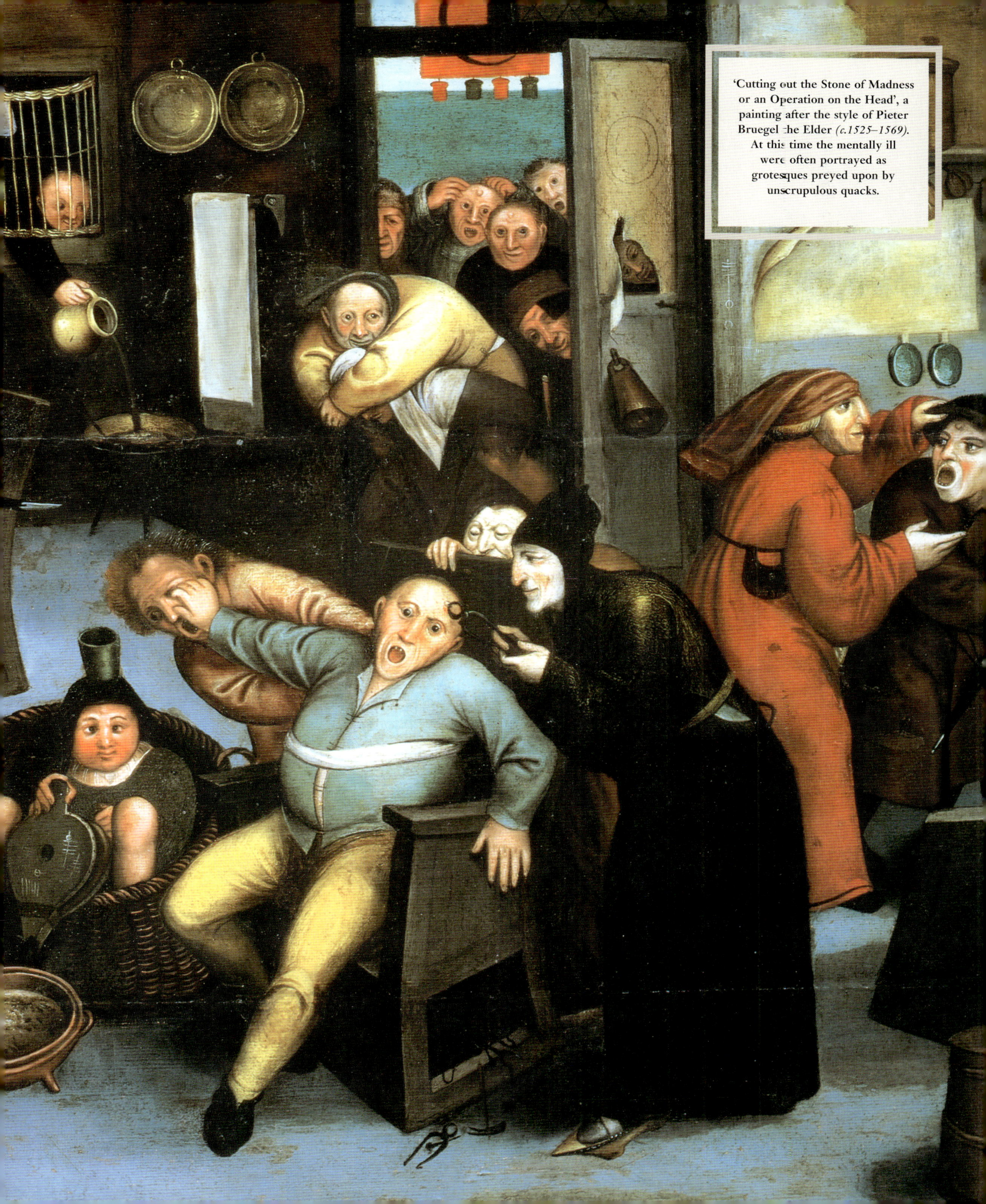

'Cutting out the Stone of Madness or an Operation on the Head', a painting after the style of Pieter Bruegel the Elder *(c.1525–1569)*. At this time the mentally ill were often portrayed as grotesques preyed upon by unscrupulous quacks.

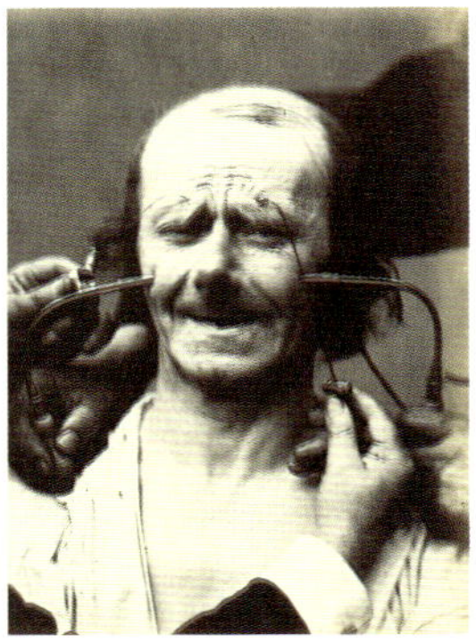

ABOVE Guillaume Duchenne *(1806–1875)* was a French neurologist. This photograph is from his work which sought to analyze 'electrophysiologically' the expression of emotions.

terms, a quite recent phenomenon, and psychiatry's religious roots, as well as mystical attitudes toward the mentally ill, linger even in contemporary times. Indeed, to this day psychiatric specialists continue to compete with religious doctrines on the one hand, and more mainstream medicine on the other.

Geographically, the existence of the psychiatric profession is a very isolated occurrence, unique to Western societies. In the East, in contrast, where the Cartesian dualism between the mind and the body which underpins much of Western medical thinking is not shared, the speciality did not develop indigenously. Mental illnesses – when recognized as diseases – fall within the province of general medical practitioners. Only with the arrival of European colonists did specialized psychiatric institutions arise in Eastern societies.

What we now think of as mental illness has been variously and alternately attributed by people of different cultures to the mind, the body, or external spirits, forces or toxins. Through examples selected from the history of psychiatry and mental illness, we will analyze shifting and historically contingent theories of mind, body and disease, showing how these ideas – and the corresponding treatments – fit into larger social and cultural formations. Loosely tracing the path of psychiatry to a modern scientific profession, we will focus on periods of change in how the mad are defined, where they are put and how they are treated. Today's psychiatric ideas, it will be argued, represent a phase in a long, cyclical process, a process that has been mediated by the relationships between doctors, patients, states, and societies and marked by the intriguing persistence of performative, ritualistic and magical approaches to therapy.

BELOW A detail from the painting shown on the previous page. The stone-cutter claimed to cure mental disorders by physically removing stones from the head of the tormented patient.

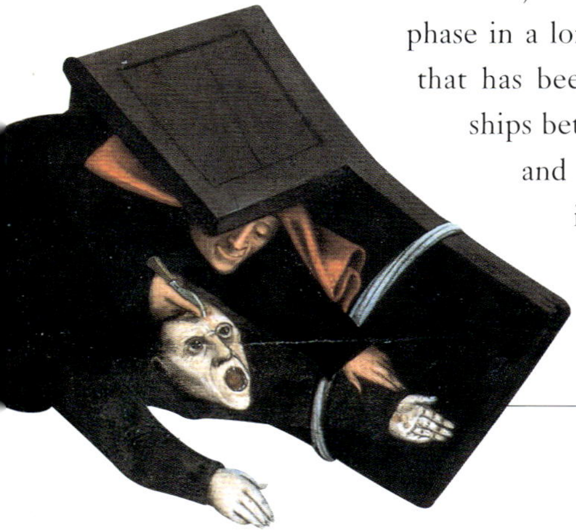

LITERARY MADNESS

Mental illness and mad people have occupied a central place in Western culture for centuries, stretching all the way back to the Bible and through to such contemporary classics as Ken Kesey's novel *One Flew Over the Cuckoo's Nest (1962).* Indeed, when Sigmund Freud sought to explain the notion of infantile sexuality, he turned to Sophocles' tragedy *Oedipus Rex* as the archetypal example. Over the centuries the mad have been portrayed in various ways that reflect prevailing cultural views of mental illness. For example, the Christian idea of the mad as holy innocents translates into depictions of child-like idiot-savants often possessing great wisdom. Renaissance theatre featured numerous fools and village idiots in its dramatis personae; at times, the mad are seen as essentially normal people driven to strange behaviour by the force of intolerable circumstances or overwhelming personal grief, as, for example, two of Shakespeare's most enduring and tragic characters, King Lear and, from *Hamlet*, Ophelia.

The image of London's Bethlem asylum, perhaps the oldest institution of its kind in the world, penetrated the culture of sixteenth- and seventeenth-century England. Bethlem, or Bedlam as it was dubbed in popular parlance, became synonymous with chaos, suffering and mismanagement; this struck a chord in a society that viewed itself as on the verge of madness. Alternatively, to take a nineteenth-century example, the mad character can be depicted as a loathsome brute, a hateful, mad-woman-in-the-closet type such as Mrs Rochester in Charlotte Brontë's *Jane Eyre.* Not long afterward French writers like Emile Zola and Charles Baudelaire, influenced by the theory of degeneration, voiced their dark diagnoses, expressing themes also visible in Feodor Dostoevsky's novels, notably *Notes from Underground.* The fascination with madness and mad doctors continues to thrive in today's culture, providing constant themes in works of literature, film and theatre.

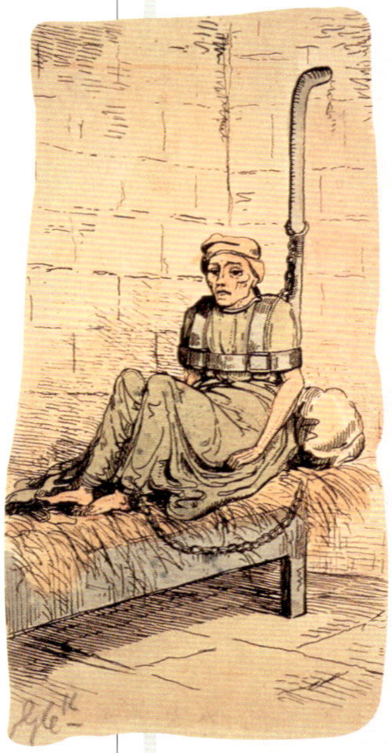

ABOVE An engraving by the British caricaturist George Cruikshank *(1792–1878)* of William Norris fettered in the notorious London asylum for the insane – Bethlem hospital.

FROM THE BODY TO THE MIND: THE MORAL TREATMENT

During the 'Reign of Terror' at the height of the French Revolution, a Parisian tailor publicly expressed reservations about the execution of Louis XVI, a confession which aroused the suspicion of his peers. Misconstruing a conversation he later overheard, the tailor became convinced that his death at the guillotine was imminent. Soon this delusion grew into an obsession which haunted his every act, necessitating his confinement in a lunatic asylum. The 'guilt-ridden tailor' ultimately found himself in the Bicêtre hospital in Paris, where he was treated by the celebrated alienist (the contemporary term for a mad-doctor) Philippe Pinel *(1745–1826)*.

Pinel prescribed a kind of occupational therapy, arranging for the tailor to mend the other patients' clothing for a small reward. Throwing himself into his work, the patient seemed quickly to recover from his delusional obsession, but the recovery proved temporary, and after several months he suffered a relapse. This time Pinel opted for a more creative approach that involved staging an elaborate spectacle; the alienist arranged for three doctors, costumed in magistrate's clothing, to appear before the inmate. Pretending to represent the revolutionary legislature, the three men 'officially' pronounced the tailor's patriotism beyond reproach, 'acquitting' him of any misdeeds. As a consequence of the faux trial, Pinel noted, the man's symptoms of guilt and distress disappeared at once, although, he had to admit, they did return again later.[2]

This case encapsulates a crucial shift in psychiatric ideas and treatments that occurred around the late eighteenth century. In the preceding period, doctors considered madness a thing of the body, originating variously in humours, physiological processes or nervous ailments. 'Every change of the Mind,' wrote the physician Nicholas Robinson, in a typical early eighteenth-century formulation, '...indicates a Change in the Bodily Organs.'[3] Yet, by the latter part of the century, a decisive shift of emphasis away from the body to the mind had occurred among French and British mad-doctors, marking a major turning point in the history of mental medicine. In 1789, for example, a British surgeon explicitly attributed insanity to the psyche, 'independent and exclusive of every corporal, sympathetic, direct, or indirect excitement, or irritation whatever.'[4] As such views gained increasing influence, they dictated a new focus on, in the words of the French alienist Jean-Etienne-Dominique Esquirol *(1779–1840)*, 'the ideas, thoughts, [and] projects of the lunatic.'[5]

BELOW The French alienist Philippe Pinel ordering the chains to be removed from patients at the Bicêtre, painted by Charles Muller *(c.1840)*.

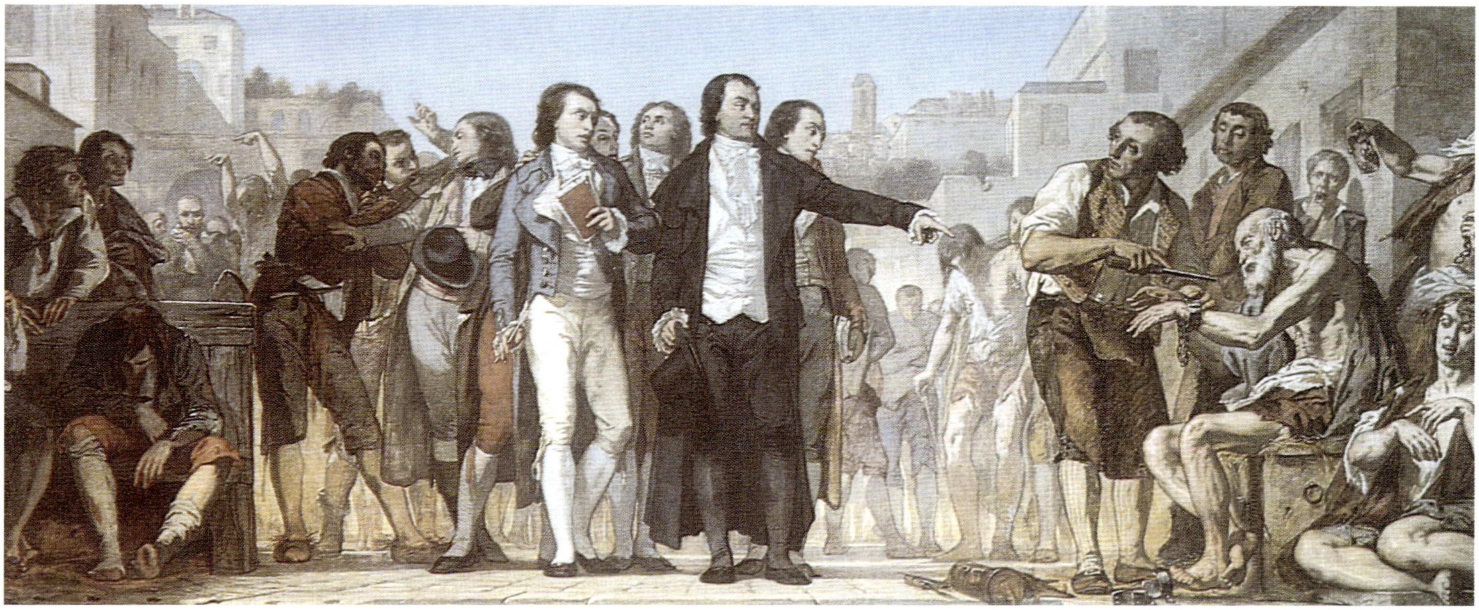

Accompanying this shift from the body to the mind was a change in therapeutic tactics and the rise of the 'moral treatment', a non-coercive and often highly theatrical doctor-patient encounter that in many ways foreshadowed the development of modern psychotherapy. The moral treatment is perhaps most noteworthy for its apparently humanitarian approach to the mentally ill; as such the new therapeutic regimen represented a revolution in psychiatric principles, hastening the end of the old regime of brutal confinements, tortures and various medicinal treatments. Instead, practitioners of moral treatment favoured psychological techniques over strictly medical methods, deriving therapeutic benefit from 'kindness, reason and tactful manipulation'.[6] As John Ferriar, a doctor at the Manchester Lunatic Asylum, observed in 1795, 'It was formerly supposed that lunatics could only be worked upon by terror. Shackles and whips, therefore, became part of the medical apparatus. A system of mildness and conciliation is now generally adopted, which, if it does not always facilitate the cure, at least tends to soften the destiny of the sufferer.'[7] In short, moral treatment literally unchained the mad, an act vividly, if rather misleadingly immortalized by subsequent European paintings of Pinel liberating the insane inmates of Bicêtre.

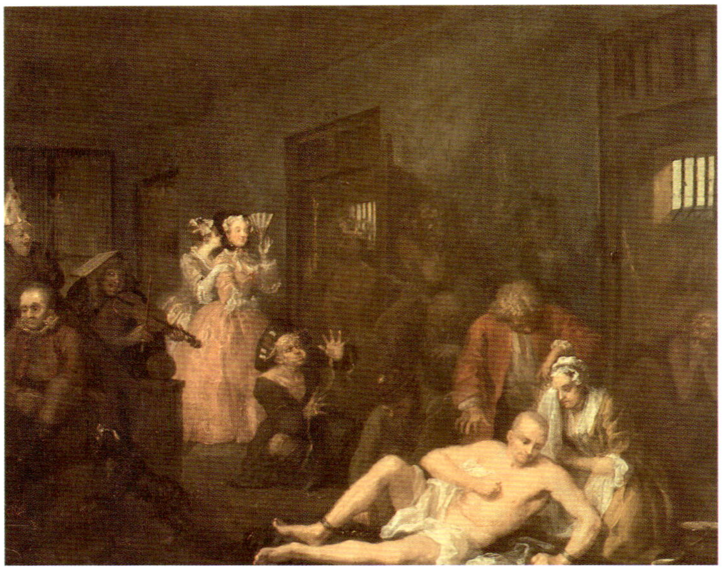

ABOVE William Hogarth captured the horror of Bedlam in his picture of the mad house in 'The Rake's Progress'.

MORE HUMANE TREATMENT?

This new approach to treatment – well illustrated by Pinel's 'guilt-ridden tailor' – derived from the assumption that mental disorders were caused by delusions or false ideas, and that if these ideas were corrected, the patient would return to normalcy. The lunatic, then, was often considered to suffer from an isolated 'monomania', a localized disorder which did not interfere with the rest of his functions. Such patients could be 'mad upon one subject', while retaining their ability to reason, their senses, and, in short, their humanity.[8]

Indeed, with the advent of these ideas, the mad were seen less as brutes or animals than as human beings who could and should be helped. This was in marked contrast to the preceding period in which the madman's alleged lack of reason – reason being the crucial faculty which accounted for human uniqueness – served to justify treatment of him as an inferior. As John Locke had observed at the end of the seventeenth century:

For [the mad] do not appear to me to have lost the faculty of reasoning, but having joined together some ideas very wrongly, they mistake them for truths, and they err as men do that argue right from wrong principles. For, by the violence of their imaginations, having taken their fancies for realities, they make the right deductions from them.[9]

JOHN LOCKE

Mental maladies were thus no longer seen as parallel to physical sickness; nor were they attributed to invasion or possession by an external entity; they were, in short, recast as a psychological – or even intellectual – problem. The lunatic, to an increasing number of doctors in late eighteenth-century Europe and North America, ceased to represent an unreachable species, and the border separating the mad and the normal suddenly became permeable, a change which opened up a host of treatment possibilities, ending the long period of therapeutic pessimism. As Dr William Battie, superintendant of London's St Luke's hospital, noted in the middle of the century:

Madness is… as manageable as many other distempers, which are equally dreadful and obstinate, and yet are not looked upon as incurable: and that such unhappy objects ought by no means to be abandoned, much less shut up in loathsome prisons as criminals or nuisances to society.[10]

DR WILLIAM BATTIE

Reflecting this new approach to the mentally ill, new asylums were constructed along the principles of domesticity, order and normality. These ideals were most famously embodied in the celebrated York Retreat, which William Tuke opened in England in 1796 for the purpose of providing humane care for insane members of the Quaker religious faith.

PATIENTS AND ASYLUMS

In the early nineteenth century, patients were increasingly integrated into the asylum 'community'; the idleness characteristic of life in earlier institutions was condemned and replaced by a range of new activities, summarized by the principle of occupational therapy. Undertakings such as nature walks, crafts, light agricultural work, reading or helping out in the kitchen all characterized life in the new asylums, as managers sought to distract patients from their morbidly solipsistic thoughts, to 'relieve the languor of idleness, and prevent the indulgence of gloomy sensations.'[11] In short, the approach to treatment in the new generation of asylums was reoriented around the principle of *management*.

But how was madness to be cured in such asylums? Moral management aimed to remove the delusion or moral (that is, mental) flaw at the core of the disorder, an act which often involved intense doctor-patient encounters and required, at times, a great deal of creativity and exertion on the doctor's part. In another case transcribed by Pinel, a devout Catholic, troubled by the Revolution's anti-clericalism, became obsessed with the idea of hell. Convinced that the only way to avoid eternal damnation was by following the asceticism of the ancient anchorite hermits, the man refused to take any food or drink. After the patient had fasted for four days, JB Pussin, the superintendant of the Bicêtre, came to him with several hospital attendants, all of whom were armed and noisily lugged heavy chains. Pussin demanded ferociously that the patient eat, threatening cruel punishments, and before long the man undertook to consume the soup he had been brought, after which he gradually resumed a normal diet and, according to Pinel, eventually fully recovered, regaining his former physical and mental health.

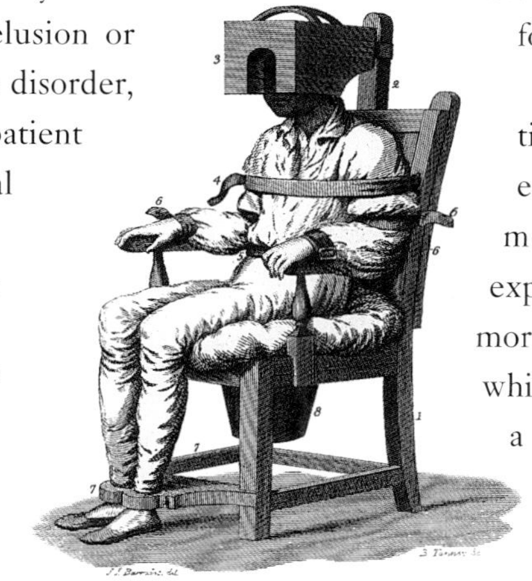

ABOVE **The restraining chair in which Benjamin Rush imprisoned his patients, sometimes for days on end.**

Although moral treatment removed the madman's physical bonds, it is important to note that it replaced the chains of the seventeenth-century asylum with a different type of bond by placing the patient in absolute moral and mental subordination to the doctor. Painful, coercive and threatening treatments remained very much in use – only in the era of moral treatment their effect was believed to be psychological rather than physical. The American physician Benjamin Rush *(1746–1813)*, to cite another case, was known to fetter patients for days with his infamous restraining chair, and the English alienist Francis Willis *(1717–1807)*, today chiefly known for treating King George III, intimidated his subjects with his fearsome stare.

These examples suggest that the diagnostic shift from the body to the mind was not necessarily a 'progressive' step; nor did it arise out of a purely enlightened or charitable impulse. Rather, it is a step that must be understood historically and viewed in terms of medical power and philosophical change. The moral treatment replaced the physical control of the older psychiatric model with a different and deeper kind of domination, by which psychiatric patients had to internalize a set of moral and social norms before they could be pronounced healthy and normal. 'Liberation from the racking of the body,' writes one historian, 'merely meant new tortures for the mind..., the imposition of more subtly terrifying "mind forg'd manacles" of guilt and self-control.'[12]

Psychologizing madness, finally, had a distinctively professional dimension; it served to differentiate mad-doctors from practitioners of general medicine by granting them a unique field of expertise and specialization. The asylum, furthermore, became the mad-doctors' domain, a space in which they had complete authority and control over a specialized patient pool. And this was truly the age of the asylum, a 'great confinement'; beginning in the late eighteenth century and accelerating through the nineteenth, new specialized institutions began sprouting up throughout Europe and North America. The psychological approach to madness can be seen in part as a consequence of these new asylums; as the contact between alienists and asylum inmates became more frequent, doctors paid increasing attention to their patients and began to take note of their moods and mental states.

THE SCIENCE OF THE PSYCHE: OUT OF THE CLINIC AND INTO THE LABORATORY

As the nineteenth century progressed, the 'great confinement' continued, and an ever greater portion of Europe's population was institutionalized in psychiatric asylums. In England, for example, the number of certified lunatics doubled in the years between 1844 and 1860, a period in which the populace as a whole increased by only 20 per cent; by the beginning of the twentieth century, the asylum population had reached more than 100,000. Likewise in Prussia, where a 'boom in insanity' was derisively declared, between 1880 and 1910 the number of asylum inmates more than quadrupled, from 27,000 to 143,000, while the general population increased from 27 to 40 million, or by only 48 per cent. In other words, out of every 100,000 Prussian inhabitants, 98 were admitted to asylums in 1880; by 1910 that figure had grown further, reaching the imposing sum of 356.

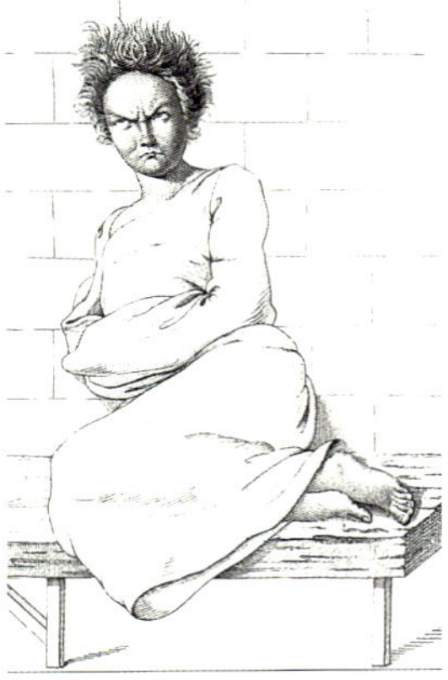

ABOVE Physical restraint of the insane was still practised in the nineteenth century despite the milder regimes that Pinel's 'moral treatment' had encouraged.

During this period of great asylum construction, individual asylums expanded as well, and the late eighteenth-century model of the cosy familial home gave way to a series of immense, faceless institutions that often accommodated as many as several thousand patients in appalling conditions. One early twentieth-century American asylum, for example, housed some 10,000 inmates; an even larger complex was to be constructed for London which would have facilities for accommodating nearly 12,000 pauper patients.

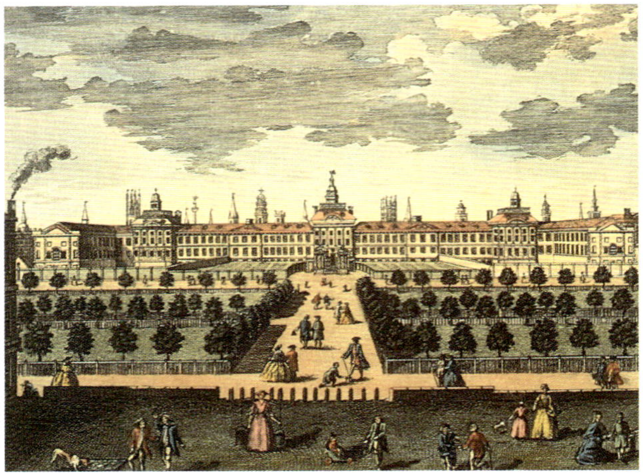

ABOVE The number of patients institutionalized in asylums soared in the nineteenth century. This engraving shows Bethlem Royal Hospital (colloquially known as Bedlam) at Moorfields in London.

By the middle of the nineteenth century, practitioners of the profession that soon came to be called psychiatry embarked on a new strategy for professional advancement, and correspondingly, adopted shifting approaches to mental illness as well. The turn from the body to the mind had come with a professional price. While successfully differentiating themselves from general practitioners, mad-doctors came into much closer contact with another group which posed a different kind of threat. With their regimen of psychological cures, alienists found themselves in the company of so-called charlatans and quacks, the non-licensed, often itinerant healers who made liberal use of magical cures and mystical methods often before enthralled audiences. It was not long before the profession changed direction and returned to the body and science as legitimizing strategies.

Over the course of the nineteenth century, the centre of psychiatric thought moved gradually eastward – first to Paris, and by the end of the century to German-speaking Central Europe. It was there that the psychiatric profession as we know it today came into being. Psychiatric medicine took quite a long time to constitute itself as a modern profession, as compared with other medical specializations. To take the case of Germany, psychiatry's main professional journal, the *Allgemeine Zeitschrift für Psychiatrie und Psychisch-gerichtliche Medizin (General Journal for Psychiatry and Psycho-forensic Medicine)* first appeared in 1844, but it would be another two decades before a professional organization, the Association of German Alienists, officially came into being. While only 32 doctors participated in the founding meeting in 1864, by the beginning of the twentieth century the organization could boast of 300 members, and on the eve of World War I, total membership had again doubled, reaching 627.

NEW WAYS OF CLASSIFYING MENTAL ILLNESS

The research of Griesinger and the other founding 'brain psychiatrists' (see below) coincided with a period of tremendous advancement in other areas of medicine. In the immediate aftermath of Louis Pasteur's and Robert Koch's celebrated microbiological breakthroughs, scientists had begun to isolate the microbes and bacilli that underlay numerous pathological conditions. Such groundbreaking achievements and the development of microscope technology exerted a profound influence on the way medical scientists approached all types of illness. Mental medicine was no exception to this trend, and toward the end of the nineteenth century, psychiatrists began to formulate new approaches to the diagnosis and classification of mental maladies, seeking to expose their common characteristics and underlying causes. As a consequence, out of the nineteenth century's Byzantine diagnostic arsenal emerged the neuroses and psychoses, and psychiatric classification began to take on a form recognizable to present-day practitioners.

At the middle of the century, Germany's universities had taken their place as the world's pre-eminent centres of scientific research, and German psychiatrists naturally pinned their greatest hopes for achieving professional recognition and scientific legitimacy on establishing a place within them. In 1865 psychiatry finally attained its first foothold when Wilhelm Griesinger *(1817–1868)* received a chair in psychiatry at the University of Berlin. Pioneering the establishment of mental medicine as a scientific, academic discipline in Central Europe, Griesinger famously declared, 'All mental illness is rooted in brain disease'. This conviction, along with his efforts to unify psychiatry with neurology, significantly reformed the study and care of the mentally ill. Griesinger's approach to mental illness became known as 'brain psychiatry'; he and his illustrious followers such as Carl Wernicke *(1848–1905)* and Theodor Meynert *(1833–1892)* sought to map human functioning onto brain anatomy and thus aimed to localize functional and behavioural disorders in cerebral lesions.

By explaining mental illness in terms of the *brain*, rather than the *mind*, Griesinger's views recast the mentally ill as 'regular', somatic patients (i.e., with physical disorders), not qualitatively different from the sufferers of any number of anatomical or physiological complaints. As such he granted psychiatric patients a degree of sympathy and dignity, removing much of the stigma that their maladies traditionally carried. Furthering a secularist, scientific approach to his patients, Griesinger demanded that they be treated with respect and humanity. Furthermore, he reversed traditional notions of asylum care, striving to subject it to the principles of reason and efficiency, and simultaneously relocating the psychiatrist from the asylum to the laboratory.

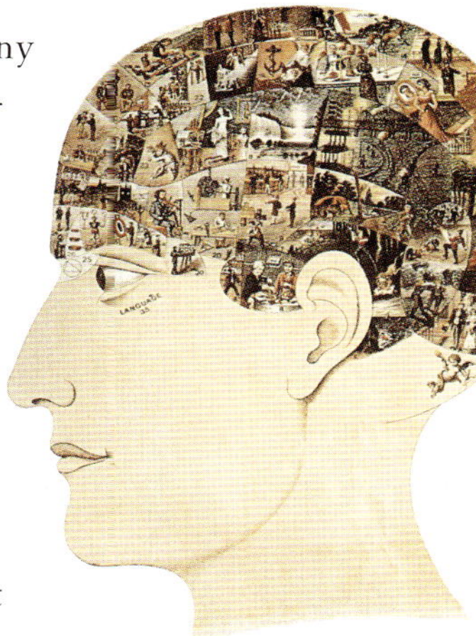

ABOVE Practitioners of phrenology believed that parts of the brain governed different human functions. In a curious way they anticipated the work of Griesinger and his school.

CHARCOT AND THE SALPÊTRIÈRE

The illustrious French neurologist Jean-Martin Charcot *(1825–1893)* played a unique role in the story of the new classification of mental illness *(see box)*. Charcot, known as the 'Napoleon of the neuroses', was chief physician at the Salpêtrière, a huge hospital in south-eastern Paris which served as a kind of clearing house for nervously and mentally ill patients from all over

BELOW The physician listening to a patient being percussed is thought to be Jean-Martin Charcot.

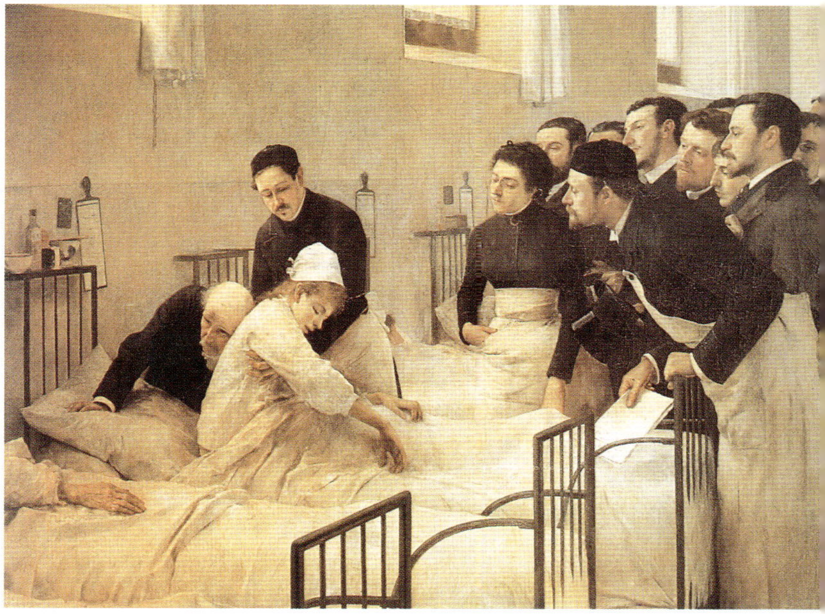

France. A worldly and charismatic man, Charcot was widely admired for his sumptuous Parisian receptions and his enthralling, dramatic lectures, held every Tuesday and Friday before packed crowds of physicians, students, writers and curious members of the public. Furthermore, his seemingly miraculous therapeutic abilities and his rapport with the Salpêtrière's female hysteria patients were renowned. As a Russian colleague recalled after visiting the master:

Many patients were brought to Charcot from all over the world, paralytics on stretchers or wearing complicated apparatuses. Charcot ordered the removal of those appliances and told the patients to walk. There was, for instance, a young lady who had been paralysed for years. Charcot bade her stand up and walk, which she did under the astounded eyes of her parents and the Mother Superior of the convent in which she had been staying.[13]

A LYUBYMOV

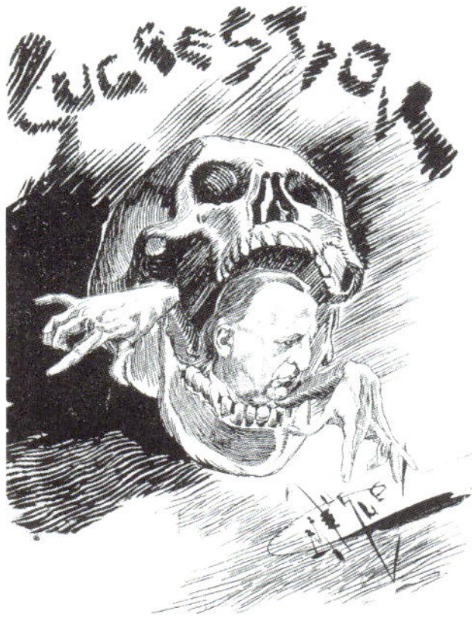

ABOVE A late nineteenth-century caricature of Charcot, renowned for his scientific analysis and classification of hysteria.

Charcot is perhaps best remembered for his positivistic project of conquering hysteria, a diagnostic entity which had been part of the Western medical tradition for centuries. First mentioned in classical times, hysteria derives from the Greek word *hystera*, meaning uterus, and it was originally seen as an exclusively female condition which resulted from the pathological wandering of the uterus and caused a host of mysterious symptoms, such as coughing, wild emotional fits, temporary or partial loss of feeling, sight or hearing. By the nineteenth century, these uterine explanations no longer held sway, but hysteria continued to be loosely linked to female anatomy and had become a general label for numerous unexplained symptoms and conditions. Whether the hysteria of ancient Egypt and Greece and the more modern conditions were the same disorder or simply shared a name is a matter historians and psychiatrists continue to debate.

Charcot took this impossibly broad disease category and subjected it to thorough scientific observation and classificatory rigour, seeking to unearth and elaborate its positive, universal laws. To study hysterical patients better, Charcot had his subjects sketched and, starting in the 1870s as camera technology improved, photographed, filling volume upon volume with his evidence.

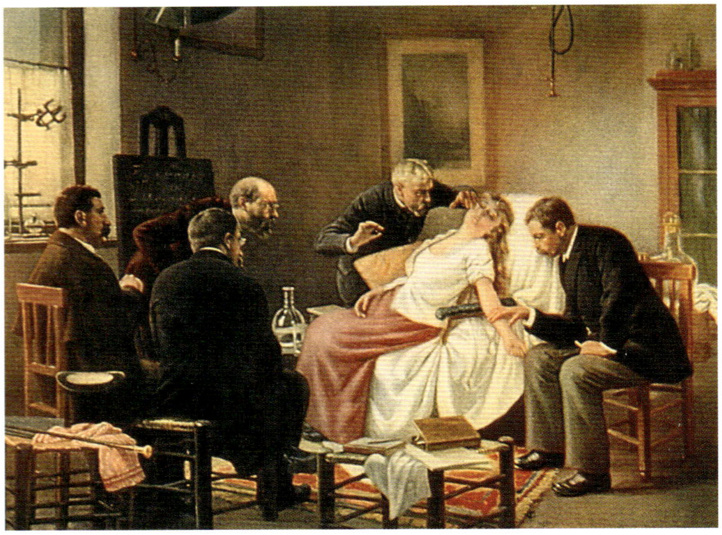

ABOVE In the nineteenth century, hysteria was still broadly held to be a female affliction.

Based on his observations of numerous hysterical patients in the Salpêtrière, Charcot concluded that all hysterical attacks followed the same pattern; each, he wrote, was characterized by four discrete phases: (1) tonic rigidity; (2) clonic spasms, the so-called 'Grands Mouvements' which produced clownish movements; (3) '*attitudes passionnelles*', that is, the physical acting-out of extreme emotional states; and (4) a final state of delirium. Charcot demonstrated these phases using his female subjects in his famous Tuesday lectures, presentations which could be described as circus-like and highly theatrical. However, a number of contemporaries, many of whom were Charcot's former students, began to criticize the master, denying that he had discovered hysteria's universal laws. In their view the charismatic Charcot had influenced his obedient patients to conform to his well-known ideas of the illness; under his suggestive spell they then mimicked the hysterical states that he had so influentially documented. Indeed, as contemporary observers often noted, a peculiar atmosphere permeated the wards of the Salpêtrière; it seemed that Charcot, his colleagues and his patients all seemed to influence one another suggestively. Moreover, according to critics and commentators, Charcot actually rehearsed the hysterical stages with his patients before the demonstrations, treating them like star performers and cultivating his suggestive 'hold' over them.

THE QUEEN OF THE HYSTERICS

Among the numerous female hysterics Charcot observed, none has occupied a more prominent place in the history of psychiatry than Blanche Wittmann. Wittmann, whose background and origins remain unknown, became one of Charcot's most famous patients, and an important model for his demonstrations, acquiring the nickname *'Reine des hystériques'*, or queen of the hysterics. She was known as a prima donna of sorts, who treated the Salpêtrière staff members with derision and disdain. However, Wittmann left the Salpêtrière for a while and was a patient at the Hôtel Dieu hospital, where the presence of a second personality, the so-called Blanche II became known. The second Blanche, a far more pleasant character, revealed that she had always been present, having hidden behind Blanche I during her demonstrations with Charcot. Jules Janet, Blanche's doctor at the Hôtel Dieu, kept her in this state – that is, as Blanche II – for several months, but ultimately she found herself back at the Salpêtrière as Blanche I. This time she was there as an employee working in the new photography laboratory, and in her prior, capricious personality, in which she denied her history as Blanche II and absolutely refused to discuss that phase of her life. She next found employment in the hospital's radiology laboratory where, tragically, she contracted cancer, and endured numerous amputations before finally succumbing to the fatal disease.

After formulating the laws of nervous disease, which Charcot asserted were 'valid for all countries, all times, all races', he turned his attention to the study of past phenomena. 'Hysteria has always existed,' he declared, 'in every time and place.' Indeed, in the zealously anti-clericalist atmosphere of the French Third Republic, the neurologist looked back to mystical and religious episodes of the past, such as witchcraft, possession and mystical ecstasy, and reinterpreted them through the hysteria diagnosis. Showing the physical correspondence between images of 'demonic' and 'ecstatic' episodes and the phases of hysterical attacks, Charcot endeavoured to expose Catholicism's canon of saints and demons as nothing more than undiagnosed cases of nervous illness, a view shared by Sigmund Freud as well as many of today's historians of psychiatry.

Late in the 1870s Charcot turned to another technique to aid his study of hysteria when he began a series of experiments with hypnosis. To many members of respectable scientific society, hypnosis seemed an unlikely, if not downright problematic preoccupation, but from today's standpoint it is clear that contact with hypnosis played a significant role in the evolution of mental medicine, highlighting psychiatric dilemmas that continue to this day.

HYPNOSIS AND MESMERISM

The association of hypnosis with charlatans and quacks hearkens back to Franz Anton Mesmer *(1734–1815)*, the late eighteenth-century Austrian physician who developed the notion of animal magnetism. Dissatisfied with the powerlessness of mainstream medicine in treating a whole host of maladies, Mesmer undertook a search for more effective therapeutic means and ultimately turned to astronomical theories. Believing that vital forces connected humans to their environment in the same way as magnets attracted metals, he began to see human beings as 'bipolar'. Mesmer came to attribute diseases to imbalances in these cosmic forces and thus sought to heal them by magnetically channelling these forces to his patients. Interestingly, he soon observed that his hand was just as effective a conductor as the magnet, and henceforth treated patients simply with a touch of the hand or his ever-present iron wand. Leaving Vienna for Paris, Mesmer began to treat patients in groups, staging elaborate healing rituals. But before long the increasingly popular medical performer incurred the wrath of French medical authorities. Having his practice condemned as fraudulent, he withdrew into obscurity in Switzerland at the end of the century.

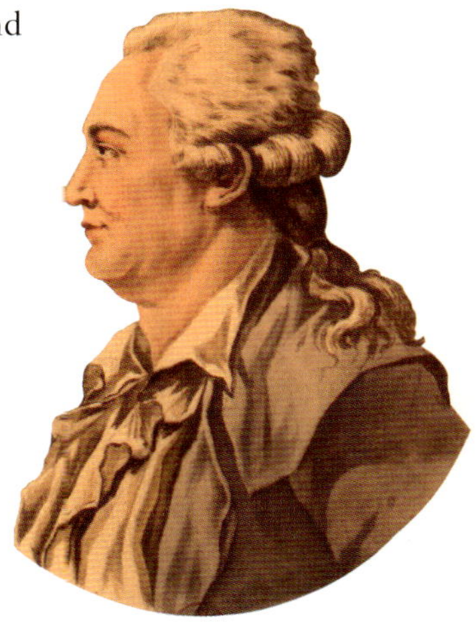

ABOVE Franz Anton Mesmer. Among his fashionable clients in Paris was Marie Antoinette.

The practice of what came to be called mesmerism and the related art of hypnosis continued to be regarded disdainfully by Europe's upright medical academies. However, after Mesmer's withdrawal, mesmerism attracted a considerable following. And its status changed dramatically, if only briefly, when a French physician named Victor Jean-Marie Burq *(1822–1884)* entered Charcot's Salpêtrière hospital three quarters of a century later. Burq had been practising a method he termed 'metallotherapy', with which he purported to cure hysterical women by applying

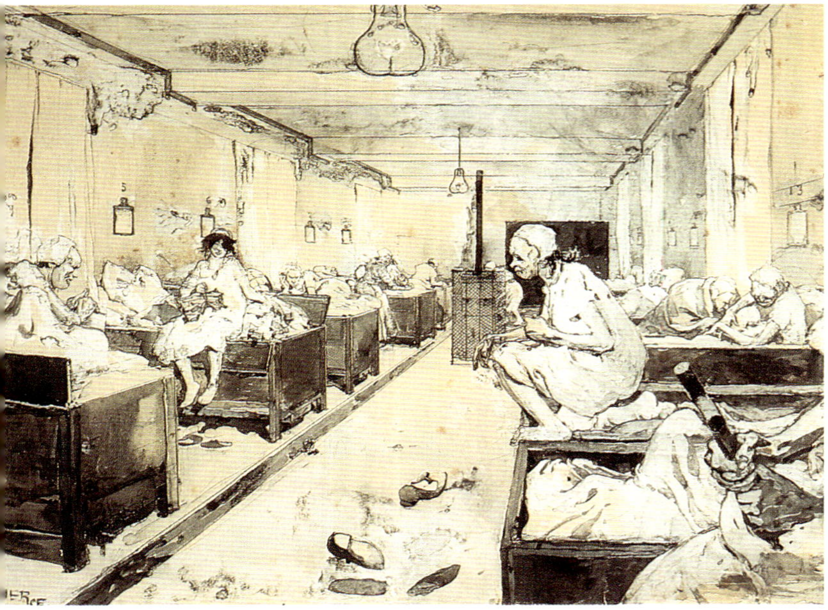

ABOVE A gouache painting by Daniel Vierge *(1851–1905)* of inmates at the Salpêtrière hospital in Paris, where Charcot used hypnosis to study hysterics.

metal plates to restore feeling to the affected parts of their bodies. Seeking official recognition in the eyes of France's medical authorities, Burq appealed to the French Biological Society, which invited him to the Salpêtrière, where his methods would be scientifically tested.

Over the years 1876 and 1877, Burq's techniques were carried out on a number of female patients who had been diagnosed with hysterical hemianaesthesia, i.e., numbness or loss of sensation in one half of the body. In fact, the method seemed to work, and a whole host of hysterical conditions were seen to be cured. Consequently, perhaps against its better judgement, the Society condoned Burq's techniques, deeming them therapeutically useful and worthy of further investigation.

It was through these experiments, in part, that mesmerism and hypnosis attracted the attentions of Charcot, who brought to it the same scientific and empirical rigour he had applied to hysteria. Though hypnosis remained suspect in the eyes of France's medical leaders, it was rife for colonization by neuroscientists. Just as Charcot had sought to demystify prophets and witches with the hysteria diagnosis, he turned his attentions to hypnosis, seeking scientific explanations and submitting it to the professional concerns and technical scientific vocabulary of the time.[16] Indeed, the tentative approval of the Biological Society and the interest of a doctor as respected and admired as Charcot legitimized the controversial art as a subject of research, if not as a therapeutic technique, and thus began an intense, though short-lived, dialogue between the realms of popular culture and scientific medicine over hypnosis, mesmerism and the occult.

Hypnosis and suggestion, in fact, became wildly popular topics in the 1880s, inspiring a great deal of not only medical and scientific, but also historical, anthropological and sociological investigations. Wars, miracles, religions and other puzzling events were attributed to the effects of mass suggestion by numerous late nineteenth-century psychologists and historians. In an age so dogmatically devoted to scientizing psychiatry, thinking about hypnosis, spiritism and the supernatural continued to play a conspicuous role in theories of the mind, and occupied such eminent psychological thinkers as Freud, Jung and William James, who turned to mediums and clairvoyants as a rich source for studying the human mind and personality.

Even Charcot, the zealous secularist, came to revise his earlier scepticism towards mystical practices and faith healing. Shortly before the end of his life the neurologist published an essay in which he upheld the value of so-called miracle cures for those physical diseases which were caused by the mind. 'Hysteric patients,' he wrote, 'possess an eminently favourable mental picture for the cultivation of faith healing... Among these individuals, both men and women, the influence of the mind over the body is sufficiently effective to precipitate a recovery from some diseases which, because of our past ignorance, were considered incurable.'[15]

But Charcot's interest in hypnosis was not pursued for therapeutic reasons. In his eyes, hypnosis was a valuable analytical method for understanding the hysterical constitution, for, in other words, seeing hysteria on the inside. According to one description, the work with hypnosis represented a kind of 'psychophysiological vivisection'.[16]

CRITICS OF THE HYSTERIA THEORY

Here Charcot again betrayed his intellectual debt to Burq and other mesmerists, who drew parallels between mesmeric sleep and hysterical states, observing that in both cases patients lost their ability to sense. Charcot conceived of the hypnotic state as essentially the same as hysteria, theorizing that an individual's susceptibility to hypnosis (suggestibility) meant the presence of latent hysteria. But Charcot's critics, most notably the French physician from Nancy, Hippolyte Bernheim *(1840–1919)*, rejected his hysteria theories, and found especially objectionable the connection he asserted between hypnosis and neurosis. As Bernheim derisively declared, of the thousands of patients Charcot had hypnotized, only one had actually conformed to the stages he outlined. In opposition to the great master, Bernheim and the other members of the Nancy circle disputed that suggestibility was a sign of mental pathology; in fact, their work showed that ordinary healthy persons, especially soldiers and others accustomed to obedience, were often quite easily hypnotized. The key lay not in their pathological condition, but rather in the power of suggestion, which Bernheim defined as 'the aptitude to transform an idea into an act.'[17]

Unlike Charcot, Bernheim, who coined the term psychotherapy, had become interested in hypnosis primarily for its therapeutic potential. He used the hypnotic state to render his patients receptive to external ideas which might resolve intrapsychic conflicts and relieve pain and suffering. Ultimately, Bernheim used hypnotic suggestion to treat not only nervous and psychic ailments, but also various chronic conditions of an exclusively physical nature such as rheumatism, ulcers, incontinence and menstrual cramps.

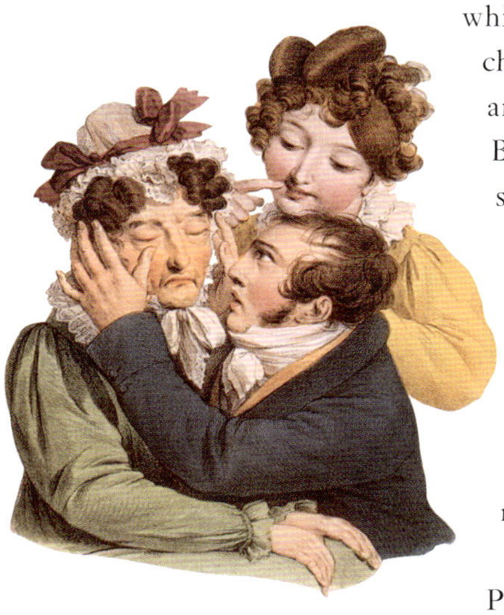

ABOVE Mesmer's ideas of animal magnetism exerted considerable influence. This lithograph from 1826 shows a doctor using 'magnetism' to heal a patient.

At the same time as the Paris and Nancy neurologists were debating the mysteries of the hysterical attack, books like *Trilby (see box)* fed the growing controversy about hypnosis in popular and political circles. These controversies ultimately led to an 1890 law that forbade the unlicensed public practice of the technique of hypnosis in France, and similar legislation was enacted around the same time in Austria, Italy and several German states. In the ensuing two decades, medical professionals across Europe began to turn away from hypnosis, a tendency most famously illustrated in the case of Sigmund Freud, who gave up the controversial practice around 1896. Certain clinicians, of course, continued to practise the method, but its magical and theatrical qualities were generally seen as incompatible with the modern science of psychiatry and inspired resistance among university medical scientists, who condemned it as crude, degrading and dangerous. Thus came to an end another phase in the long, cyclical history of hypnosis and its interactions with mainstream medicine.

HYPNOSIS AS POPULAR ENTERTAINMENT

Throughout the period of the late nineteenth century, hypnosis flourished in another form; not in the respectable halls of academic medicine, but rather as a popular street-level phenomenon. These years saw the proliferation of travelling hypnosis shows in numerous European cities and towns, in which the wonders of the technique were demonstrated on volunteers from the enthusiastic audiences. The shows attracted great popular interest, as hypnotists and mesmerists seemed uniquely able to make the deaf hear, the blind see and the paralysed walk. Yet rumours abounded that on occasion volunteers were permanently damaged, left in their hypnotic state, or even seduced or raped. Moreover, the idea spread – extrapolated from Bernheim's writings – that the mysterious powers of hypnotic suggestion could be used to exert one's will over other individuals and thus suggest them into carrying out unspeakable acts. As a result, numerous tales of murders and other crimes associated with the method appeared, further tainting hypnosis in the eyes of those involved in established medical science.

The scandals around hypnosis were reflected in the best-selling 1890s' novel *Trilby* by George du Maurier. In the novel, Trilby, the Parisian-raised daughter of an English lord, works as a seamstress and artist's model until she meets Svengali, a music teacher who hypnotizes her, trains her to sing beautifully, and marries her. But she can only sing this way in the hypnotic trance, and during her performance he sits in the theatre, fixing his eyes on her to perpetuate the hypnotism. Tragically, Svengali suddenly dies of a heart attack at the beginning of her premier performance, bringing her career to a catastrophic close.

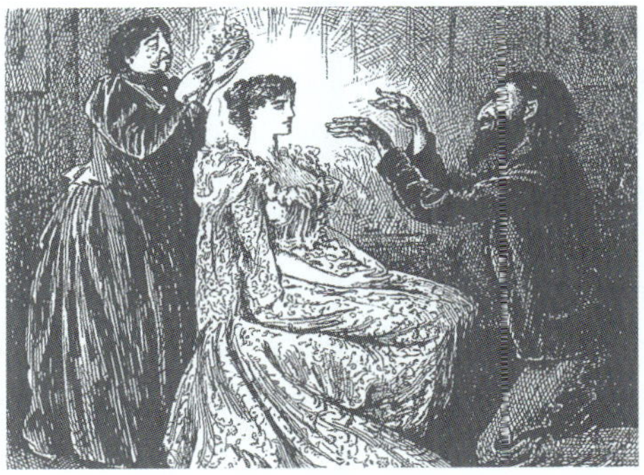

ABOVE 'Now sleep, my darling!' An extravagantly bearded Svengali hypnotizes Trilby, the heroine of du Maurier's novel.

EMIL KRAEPELIN'S INFLUENCE

The most significant German voice in the new psychiatric science belonged to Emil Kraepelin *(1856–1926)*, whose efforts in the late nineteenth and early twentieth century pushed psychiatric thought in a completely different direction. Like Charcot, Kraepelin strove for diagnostic clarity and rigour; but the similarities stop there. If Charcot was a psychiatric Bonaparte, conquering the most elusive of mental disorders, Kraepelin might be compared to Linnaeus, the great classifier. In contrast to the Frenchman's emphasis on visual observation and the external signs of nervous illness, Kraepelin devoted his greatest attention to internal constitution as he strove for a comprehensive system of classification for the maladies that afflicted the mind and nervous system.

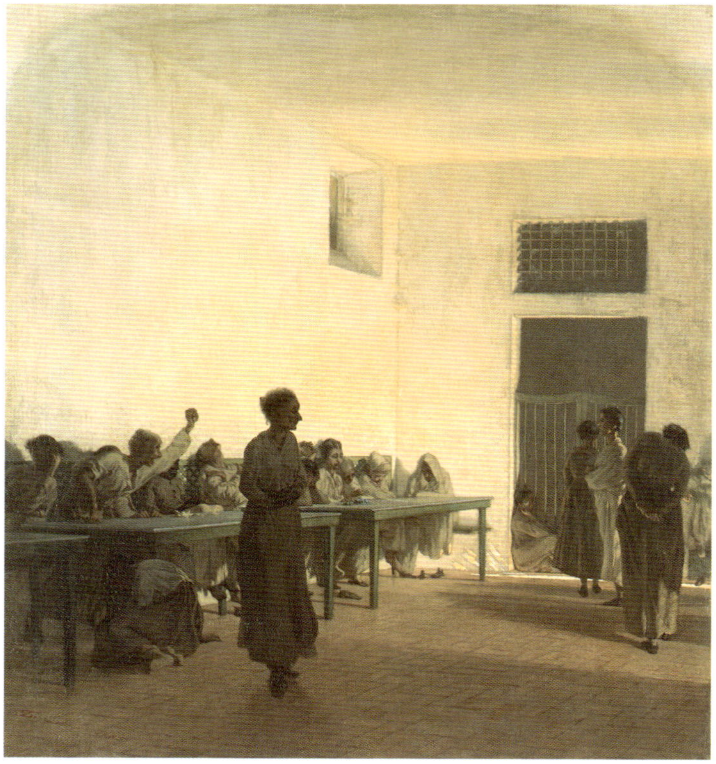

ABOVE **A bleak picture of a mid-nineteenth-century madhouse by the Italian Telemaco Signorini *(1835–1901)*. Despite the scientific successes of psychiatry, it did little to treat clinically the illnesses that it so rigorously classified.**

Kraepelin, whose influential Psychiatry Textbook can be seen as a forerunner of today's diagnostic and statistical manuals, emphasized the causes, or aetiology, of nervous and mental illnesses. He and his colleagues also brought statistics and the study of heredity into the psychiatric sphere. Furthermore, Kraepelin introduced the diagnosis of dementia praecox, the forerunner of schizophrenia, which in early editions of his book comprised the so-called degenerative psychological processes along with the diagnoses catatonia and paranoia. By early twentieth-century editions, however, dementia praecox constituted his major diagnostic building block and, along with manic depressive psychosis, comprised the bulk of his text. Dementia praecox emphasized a dulling of the senses, the withdrawal and listlessness that Kraepelin observed in his psychiatric patients, a condition which usually began in youth and gradually developed into full blown dementia. By 1911 the Swiss psychiatrist Eugen Bleuler *(1857–1939)* proposed the term schizophrenia as a substitute for dementia praecox; if hysteria and the neuroses were the most important psychiatric diagnoses of the nineteenth century, schizophrenia would assume this role in the twentieth.

Meanwhile, by the end of the nineteenth century, psychiatry's position at central European universities had grown increasingly secure. More and more universities began to open psychiatric teaching clinics and to create departments of psychiatry and neurology, and by the early 1900s psychiatry had become a requirement in the medical board exams of all German states. Yet, despite its rapid institutional growth, its scientific claims and increased resemblance to more mainstream branches of medicine, the young science of psychiatry had one significant failing; it remained powerless to treat the illnesses which fell in its professional domain.

The professional position of psychiatrists around the turn of the twentieth century was thus constantly plagued by a degree of insecurity and ambiguity. Despite accumulating observations and developing a refined and sophisticated diagnostic language, psychiatry had made few inroads into the clinical realm; the psychiatrist, according to one historian:

> *'...still suffered from the same ignorance of the causes of mental illness and he still had to be content with the same miserable methods of treatment... although anatomy and physiology had been so helpful to his medical colleagues, they had failed to teach him anything about the nature of these illnesses.' Not only were psychiatric patients prisoners of a sort, but '[the psychiatrist] himself was a prisoner caught up in the difficulties of the field in which he had chosen to work.'*[18]
>
> ERWIN H ACKERKNECHT

Despite their profession's rapid institutional expansion, as reflected in association membership, university departments hospital facilities and professional journals, psychiatry remained clinically stunted, and psychiatrists continued to be 'prisoners'of their chosen field. Indeed, issues of therapy and treatment were unpleasant subjects at best avoided; they comprised, for example, a tiny fraction of all lectures held at the annual convention of the German Psychiatric Association between 1891 and 1914. The great majority of presentations were devoted to more strictly 'scientific' concerns such as the classification and aetiology of mental illness. Kraepelin's *Lehrbuch*, for example, the most authoritative psychiatric text of the time, devoted little space to treatment in any of its eight editions. Nor was this therapeutic crisis limited to German-speaking lands; an ever-growing chorus of critics appeared in France, Britain and the United States, charging that the psychiatric profession had failed to deliver on its promise. Indeed, as the nineteenth century drew to a close, alienists could claim to cure a progressively smaller proportion of asylum inmates; death was a far more common escape route than return to society for the unfortunate residents of these immense institutions.

'When a future historian describes today's psychiatric era,' mused Georg Dobrick, an asylum doctor in what was then the Prussian city of Posen in 1910, 'he will come away with a curious impression. He will find an enormous blossoming of psychiatric literature alongside a low level of practical success. We know a lot and can do little.'[19] Psychiatrists seemed to respond to this crisis by moving even further away from the therapeutic realm; the asylum in turn became a repository, a kind of warehouse for those deemed unfit to participate in normal society. Indeed, if psychiatric interment did not cure patients, the vast and expensive asylum system had to be justified somehow, and it was in terms of this grimly pessimistic role that its function was redefined. Psychiatry henceforth became the 'defender of the social order', a profession charged with the formidable responsibility of policing the boundaries between the sane and insane, the normal and pathological.[20]

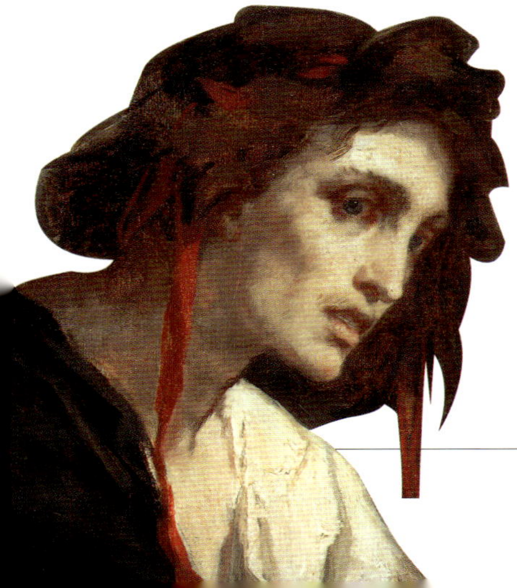

LEFT 'The Madman' by the French painter Thomas Couture *(1815–1879)*. At the end of the nineteenth century fewer and fewer of such asylum inmates were actually being cured.

JUDGING BY APPEARANCES

Correspondingly, psychiatrists devoted increased energies to determining precisely who fell into these categories, seeking to hone their diagnostic skills and observational technologies accordingly. Charcot's emphasis on observing his hysterical patients – an interest that coincided with improvements in photographic technology – helped inspire growing attention to the outward appearance of the mentally ill. Medical scientists had long sought to distinguish the insane from the normal based on their appearance, and their physiognomy in particular. And many late nineteenth-century psychiatrists, steeped in the somaticism of the day, came to believe that hysteria and other mental and nervous ailments were recognizable by particular external signs or 'stigmata', vaguely reminiscent of the *stigmata diaboli* thought to mark witches in the Middle Ages. Simply by examining a patient's facial expression, wrote Daniel Hack Tuke and John Charles Bucknill in an 1858 psychology

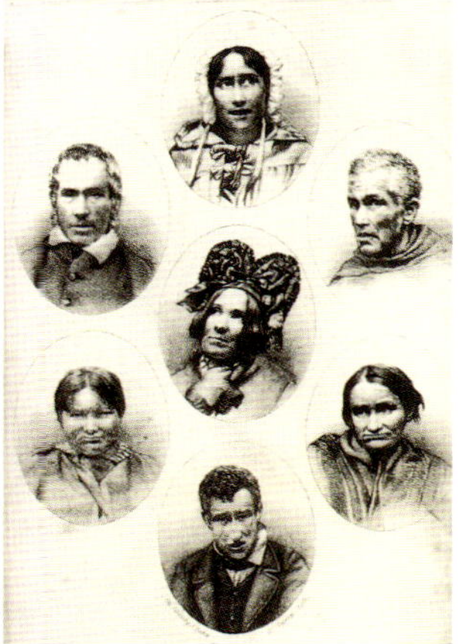

ABOVE **Photographs taken in a nineteenth-century asylum which purport to show 'Types of Insanity'.**

THE CAMERA AS A DIAGNOSTIC TOOL

'It may be stated,' declared the Viennese psychiatrist Richard Krafft-Ebing *(1840–1902)*, 'that every psychopathic state, like the physiologic states of the emotions, has its own peculiar facial expression and general manner of movement which, for the experienced, on superficial observation, make a probable diagnosis possible.'[21] The crucial difference was the invention and refinement of camera technology, which promised to turn the art of looking into an objective, scientific endeavour. And it was largely Charles Darwin who supplied the scientific grounding for this pursuit, basing his study of evolutionary emotions on dozens of photographic plates. The camera, henceforth, was considered an indispensable diagnostic tool, a visual parallel to the microscope, necessary for 'seeing' the insane and distinguishing them from the normal.

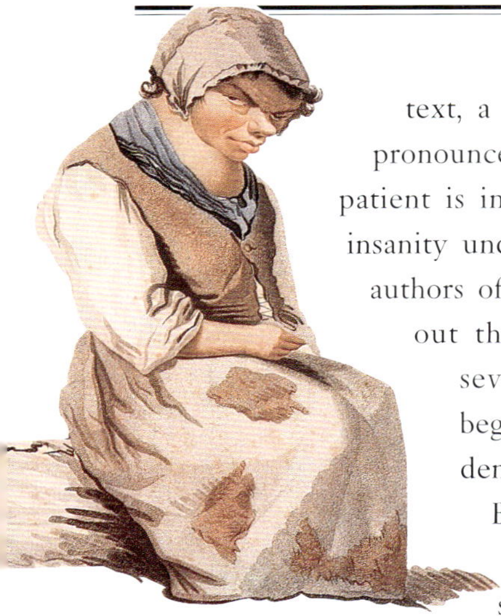

ABOVE A French textbook illustration of a sufferer from cretinism. At the end of the nineteenth century psychiatry was troubled by the apparent degeneration of humankind.

text, a perceptive doctor will 'be able to pronounce with accuracy, not only that the patient is insane, but the general form of the insanity under which he labours.'[22] While the authors of this treatise were careful to point out the limitations of visual diagnosis, several decades later such methods began to accommodate far more confident claims *(see box on previous page)*.

By the later nineteenth century, the optimistic, humane reformism of scientific brain psychiatry was giving way to escalating fears of decline and degeneration. A common assumption among psychiatrists and numerous other medical thinkers was that the vertiginous changes induced by modern life had taken their toll on the nervous and mental health of the people. Filthy and overcrowded factories and domiciles were seen as the causes of a perceived explosion in mental illness in Europe's rapidly expanding urban centres, as reflected by heightened rates of suicide and staggering increases in the numbers of admissions to mental asylums.

This alarmist atmosphere engaged the attentions of numerous doctors and social reformers by the early years of the twentieth century. At this time, eminent psychiatrists dedicated their research to problems such as mental disease and deviance among the urban poor and apparent increases in alcoholism, criminality, suicide and vagabondage. While one psychiatrist pointed to 'extraordinary fruitfulness of the big city in producing mental illnesses,' others noted the disproportionate numbers of paralytics, alcoholics, epileptics, psychopaths and suicidals who inhabited Europe's crowded metropolitan areas. Psychiatrists as well as anthropologists, criminologists, social reformers and numerous other groups bemoaned these conditions and turned increasing attention toward preventive and eugenic measures in the years before World War I.

Indeed, leading psychiatrists such as Kraepelin and Ernst Rüdin *(1874–1952)* count among the early, adamant advocates of this growing tendency that sought to promote national health and fitness by intervening directly in the human reproductive process. Kraepelin proposed (and eventually oversaw) an extensive research programme concerning the heredity of the nervous and mental illnesses, and in 1908 Rüdin became a co-editor of the *Archiv für Rassenhygiene (Archive of Racial Hygiene)*, the official organ of the eugenics movement in Germany. Influenced by the degenerationist theories of the French anthropologist Bénédict-Augustin Morel *(1809–1873)* – which diagnosed the inalterable biological decline of the human race – and alarmed by the declining birth rate and increases in infant mortality, German, French, British and American thinkers began to investigate radical solutions for preventing the heredity of mental illness and protecting humanity's genetic stock from what they saw as racial degeneration.

However, support for actually enacting eugenic measures was still tentative among psychiatrists. Most awaited the results of further research, hesitating to propose such radically interventionist programmes. While many searched for biological solutions to social and economic problems, at the same time other doctors concerned themselves with the mental and nervous health of members of the more affluent classes. Frequently condemning the turn of the century as a 'nervous epoch', German doctors in particular argued that material prosperity and peace had softened the populace, while fast-paced economic growth and new technologies progressively frazzled its nerves.

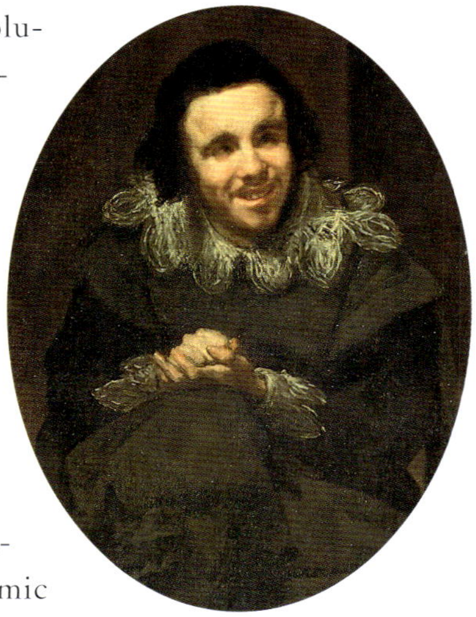

ABOVE 'The Idiot of Cori' by Velasquez *(1599–1660)*. In the twentieth century, supporters of eugenics were keen to find ways of eliminating 'degenerate' human beings such as this.

Neurasthenia, a nervous illness originally described by the New York doctor George M Beard, made its way to the European continent in the early 1880s. According to Beard's mechanistic conception of the nervous system, modern civilization exacted an enormous drain on the individual's finite reserve of 'nerve force'; as a result, neurasthenic symptoms such as fatigue, headaches, sleeplessness, dizziness, digestive problems, irregular heart beat and impotence had begun to appear with increasing frequency. Beard conceived of neurasthenia as a purely American phenomenon which he attributed to the country's peculiar social and economic relations, but his writings had great resonance in Britain, France, Germany and Russia as well, where thinkers endowed the illness with qualities peculiar to their own social, economic and geographical milieux.

PSYCHIATRY, COLONIALISM AND THE EASTERN WORLD

It was no accident that the developments described in the previous section coincided with a period of tremendous colonial expansion among the European powers. As France, Germany, England and Belgium raced to divide the spoils of the African continent, so grew the science of anthropology, which concerned itself with defining and distinguishing the characteristics of different 'races' and peoples of the world. The major target of these efforts was Europe's Jewish population, deemed to suffer disproportionately from numerous diseases, including hysteria, degenerative syphilis and psychopathology. In Africa and elsewhere, European racial science concentrated on observing, diagnosing and classifying native populations, deeming them to be mentally, morally and physically inferior to Europeans.

Western invaders were entering lands that often had highly distinct and well developed ideas of psychological sickness. As was explained in Chapter Four, Chinese civilization, to take one example, has a medical tradition of extreme antiquity, and it has shown an awareness of behaviours that we would call insane for more than 2,000 years. A description from a classical source (written in the period between 100 BC and AD 100) describes the mad patient in terms that would not be unfamiliar to Westerners:

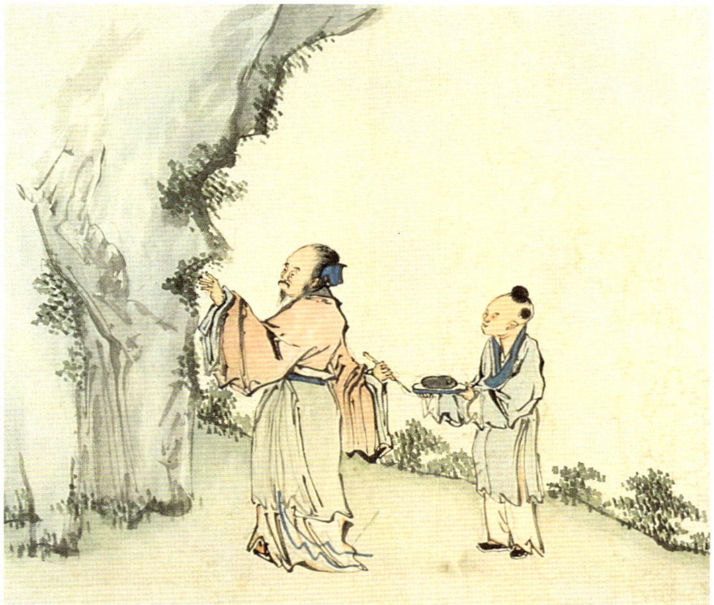

ABOVE Traditional Chinese medicine does not recognize the distinction between mental and physical disease that is characteristic of Western medical practice. It views mental disturbance as being a consequence of disruption of the harmony of the mind and body. Treatment might include acupuncture, moxibustion and the use of a variety of medicinal herbs.

...then he will discard his clothes and run about, mount heights and sing, or get to the point of not eating for several days. He will leap walls and ascend rooftops. In short, all the places he mounts are beyond his ordinary abilities...he will talk and curse wildly, not sparing relatives or strangers. Not wishing to eat he will run about wildly.[23]

QUOTED BY MARTHA LI CHIU

As a portrayal of what was called *k'uang*, this description of insanity remained representative, with little emendation for centuries.

Chinese medicine, of course, makes no distinction between psychological and physiological functioning, which is the very basis of modern Western psychiatry. In contrast to the Western therapeutic tradition, which since Graeco-Roman times has emphasized the curative effect of catharsis, Chinese tradition has regarded excessive emotionality as likely to cause disease. Treatment and prevention of emotional disorders thus involves efforts to preserve moderate, harmonious levels of feeling. It was necessary to preserve the mind-body harmony, Chinese healers believed, to maintain general health. Furthermore, according to Chinese medical theory, psychological and physiological functions are viewed as being combined in certain internal organs; the heart, kidney and lung are seen as particularly important for psychological processes. Thus patients suffering from psychological problems tend to focus on certain organs as the locus of their disorder. Anger, to take one example, is associated with the liver and thought to be due to heated blood, and it may be treated accordingly.

The first psychiatric hospital in China was opened in 1898 at the behest, unsurprisingly, of British missionaries. In the words of one observer, 'A party consisting of the doctor, a man carrying on his back an insane patient followed by the wife of the doctor, stood at the door of one of these buildings. A key was inserted in the door. It opened and for the first time in the history of China a mind-diseased patient was to receive special care.'[24] Despite institutional growth and the presence of Western teachers, psychiatry did not establish deep roots in China.

Psychiatry is, perhaps, more culturally bound than other branches of Western medicine; nor could its proponents boast of the tremendous therapeutic breakthroughs that made the adoption of other Western disciplines like surgery seem so attractive. Furthermore, the centrality of language to psychiatric treatment and teaching may have also hindered its spread in cultures where few Westerners speak local languages and dialects.

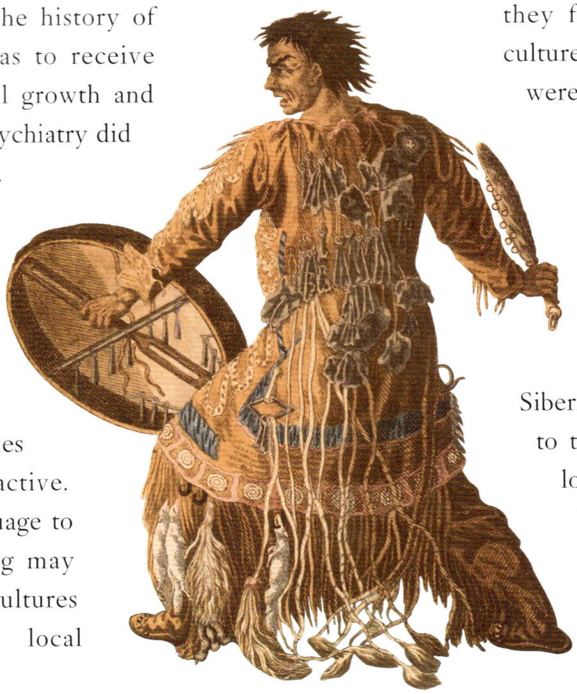

ABOVE A traditional dancing shaman from Kamchatka in Siberia. The shaman sings, drums and dances himself into an ecstatic trance to enable him to intercede with the spirit world.

OTHER CULTURES, OTHER PRACTICES

When European colonists arrived in other parts of Asia and Africa, they encountered very different disease conceptions. Maladies we now think of as mental illness were, in many lands, attributed to such causes as the intrusion of a foreign body, loss of the soul, demonic possession, breach of taboo, and sorcery. While Westerners may have dismissed these ideas as nonsense or quackery, they functioned very effectively in their own cultures and represented a system of beliefs that were shared by healers and patients.

In cases of soul loss, for example, the role of the healer is to locate the soul and return it to its rightful place. This theory, which accommodates an enormous amount of variation, can be found among the native peoples of Australia, the Philippines, and Indonesia, as well as Siberia and parts of Africa. Among the Siberians, to take one example, the belief exists that the lost soul ascends into the world of the spirits. The task of finding the soul belongs to a shaman, who acts as a kind of mediator between the physical and spiritual worlds. The shaman, like the medicine man who treated Adolf Bastian, must work himself up into an ecstatic state, expending enormous amounts of energy in hunting, bargaining with and often fighting with the spirit world for possession of the lost soul.

The theory of possession, according to which evil spirits have entered and taken hold of the subject's body, is enormously widespread. This is usually manifest by a sudden change of identity, personality and aptitude of which, like Blanche Wittmann *(see page 153)*, the individual is often aware. These symptoms, in fact, strikingly resembles what Western psychiatry calls multiple personality disorder.

Three modes of therapy present themselves: expelling the spirit physically; transferring it into another body by ritual means; and, the most common method, exorcizing it; that is, driving it out through non-physical means. Exorcism is a confrontation – an intense struggle between the exorcist and the invading spirit involving ritual prayers and incantations that may be repeated over a period of months or even years; it usually occurs in a sacred spot in the presence of witnesses. The exorcist acts as a representative of a higher power, and confident of his eventual victory, encourages the patient to give up the spirits possessing him or her.

BELOW An African counterpart of the Siberian shaman – the medicine man – performing healing rituals before his tribe.

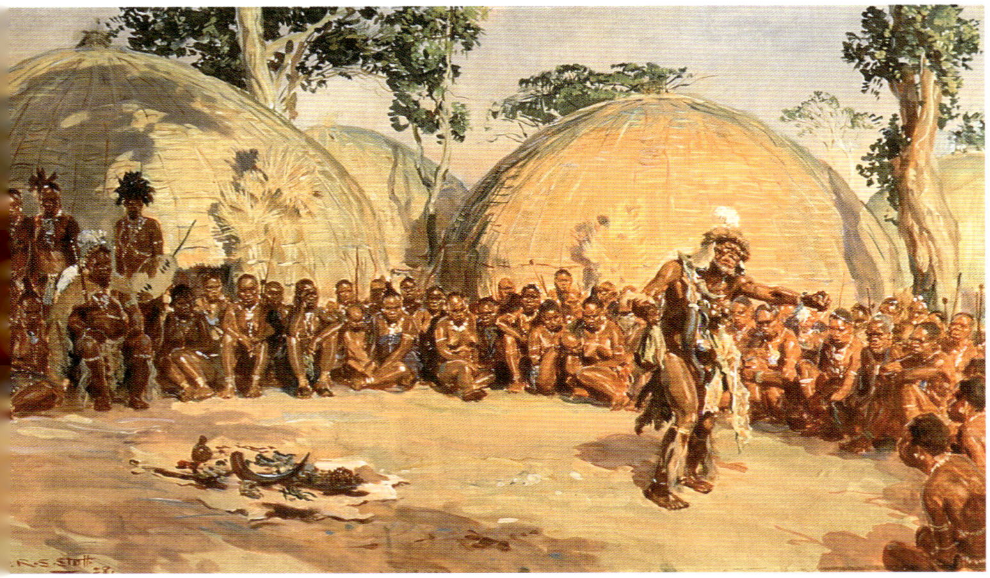

WAR, PSYCHIC TRAUMA AND THE RETURN OF SUGGESTION

Even as the new scientific psychiatry reached its zenith, and somatic systems held sway in the centres of Western medicine, a chorus of dissenting voices arose to challenge the new orthodoxy. The source of these new challenges can be traced in part to the study of psychic trauma and its mental health consequences. Once again, we turn to Charcot, who contributed to this tendency with his theories of traumatic hysteria.

At the Salpêtrière, Charcot observed numerous cases of hysterical symptoms arising in men, including headaches, heart palpitations, chest pain, irregular pulse rate, constipation, dizziness, fainting spells, trembling of the hands and neck, emotional and sleep disorders, and mental disorientation. These symptoms closely resembled those of his hysterical female patients; significantly, they seemed to arise after traumatic events, such as work-place accidents and train crashes. In women, on the other hand, Charcot believed that hysterical attacks were generally unleashed by emotions or passions; jilted lovers and weepy, romantic girls being a highly susceptible category.

Charcot developed a model to explain these symptoms in which an environmental *agent provocateur,* or traumatic stimulus, could act in the presence of an inherited, constitutional disposition, or *diathèse.* He attributed the onset of symptoms to a combination of factors, but gave primacy to the pathogenic effects of the emotions unleashed by traumatic experiences, in particular, fear. Both organic and emotional factors played a role, and Charcot posited that traumatic experiences could become superimposed on physical injuries or irregularities. Although he remained convinced that hysteria could only develop when the prerequisite physical and hereditary preconditions existed, Charcot thus cautiously introduced psychological elements into his disease model. These elements, as construed by several of his followers, set the stage for the collapse of the somatic model. While French neurologist Pierre Janet *(1859–1947)* formulated his theories of trauma and dissociation, or the splitting of the personality, the Austrian Sigmund Freud *(1856–1939)* elaborated on (but later denied) the long-term effects of childhood trauma on a person's subsequent mental health. If Freud helped propel and publicize this paradigm shift, it first found widespread acceptance during World War I.

THE ROOTS OF PSYCHOANALYSIS

Psychoanalysis began as a theory of hysteria, and the case which contributed the most to Freud's theory of hysteria was not even his own. It was, rather, his elder Viennese colleague Josef Breuer *(1842–1925)* who, along with the patient whom he called Anna O, made several of the fundamental psychological and therapeutic contributions to Freud's science of the psyche. Indeed, just as Blanche Wittmann became inextricably associated with the history of Charcotian hysteria and multiple personality disorder, Anna O was one of a mere handful of patients whose sufferings significantly contributed to the history of psychoanalysis *(see box overleaf).*

Freud drew heavily on the Anna O case as he formulated his first theory of hysterical neurosis in 1895. Still sharing the language of mechanical, somatic psychiatry, Freud wrote that when the mind was unable to discharge the effects of psychic trauma, particularly when the trauma had been suffered in a semi-hypnotic state, it repressed the memory in a manner that caused hysterical neurosis to develop. Soon thereafter, in a move that still evokes controversy, he shifted emphasis away from the memories of traumatic experiences and onto the repression of sexual fantasies, positing the existence of infantile

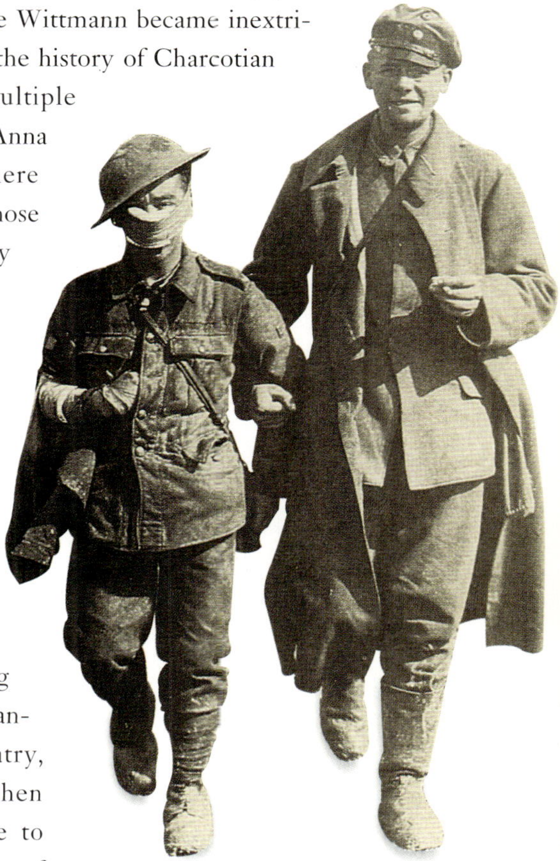

ABOVE During World War I, thousands of soldiers suffered psychological breakdown. Seen here on the left is the painter and poet Isaac Rosenberg. He paid the supreme price; he was killed in 1918.

THE CASE OF ANNA O

Anna O, or, rather, Bertha Pappenheim, was born to a comfortably bourgeois, traditionally Jewish Viennese family in 1859. By all accounts she was a girl of tremendous talent and ability, and, in fact, would grow up to become a brilliantly creative writer, a passionate and tireless social worker and the crusading leader of the German-Jewish feminist movement.

Her troubles began in 1880 when her father suffered a severe illness, and Bertha assumed much of the responsibility for taking care of him. One evening while waiting for his doctor to arrive, she experienced partial paralysis in her right leg. Soon the condition worsened, and she developed a whole variety of peculiar, debilitating symptoms, including contractures, partial temporary blindness, linguistic disorganization, and a splitting of her personality into a 'normal' melancholy personality and a crude, agitated person; in the second state she suffered from hallucinations of black snakes. Breuer, the family physician, visited Bertha in the evenings, and, after hypnotizing her, had her recount her hallucinations and daydreams. She found great relief in this activity, which she dubbed her 'talking cure', and she soon showed signs of marked improvement.

However, when Bertha's father died several months later, her condition took a sudden turn for the worse, and, strikingly, she lost the ability to speak her native German. Furthermore, the split between the two personalities grew more acute, and, as Breuer noted, one personality was reliving events that had occurred exactly one year earlier. Breuer continued his previous therapeutic technique with mild success, but began to see her for longer and more intense visits. At this point he made his key therapeutic breakthrough. He found that when Bertha narrated the conditions surrounding the onset of particular symptoms, the symptoms in question would mysteriously disappear. Thus was born the cathartic method. According to this radical idea, once the cause of particular symptoms were brought to consciousness, the symptoms would no longer persist.

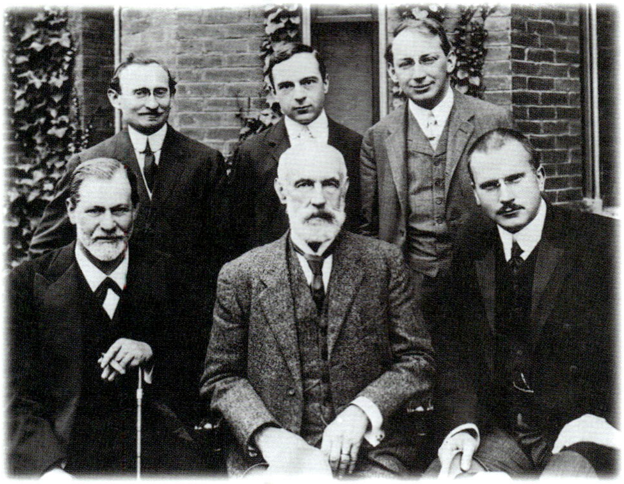

ABOVE **The founding father of the psychoanalytic movement, Sigmund Freud (front row, left), is seen here with Carl Jung (front right) at Clark University, USA, in 1909. Jung's collaboration with Freud ended in 1913 when their differences became irreconcilable.**

sexuality. Around the same time, Freud abandoned the practice of hypnosis, focusing instead on the patient's resistances and on the transference – and later counter-transference – that inhered between analyst and patient.

Over subsequent years, Freud expanded and developed his theory of hysteria, founding first a theory of the neuroses and gradually developing an entire therapeutic and aetiological system, which incorporated anthropological, historical and psychological investigations. Through the international psychoanalytic movement, Freudian ideas found fertile ground abroad, ultimately attracting growing numbers of followers in Europe and America and revolutionizing psychiatric thought and practice. Prominent among Freud's associates was the Swiss psychologist Carl Gustav Jung *(1875–1961)*, who drew heavily from religious and anthropological roots and incorporated the study of symbols, myths and archetypes into his system of analytic psychology. In contrast to Freud's nearly exclusive emphasis on the pathogenic role of the sexual, Jung examined the influence of broader cultural factors on the individual psyche, positing the existence of a 'collective unconscious'. He was named the director of the international pyschoanalytic movement, a post he held until he – like so many of Freud's early associates – split with the master in the years before the outbreak of World War I.

Freud was only the most significant of dozens of psychiatrists, psychologists and neurologists who developed psychogenic theories in the early twentieth century. For many of these pioneers, confirmation of their ideas occurred during World War I.

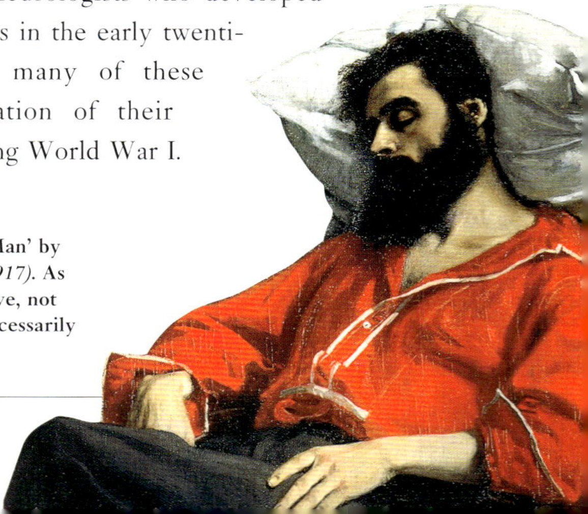

RIGHT **'The Wounded Man' by Charles Durant *(1837–1917)*. As World War I was to prove, not all wounds of war are necessarily physical in nature.**

THE TRAUMA OF WAR

Forced to experience the shattering effects of modern weaponry and to endure the inhumane conditions of trench warfare, hundreds of thousands of soldiers broke down psychologically, suffering from a condition known in the Anglo-American world as shell shock. By the war's first Christmas, doctors throughout Europe observed the startling onset of dramatic shaking, stuttering and disorders of sight, hearing and gait among mobilized soldiers, and began to question the connection between these puzzling symptoms and the manifold shocks and horrors of combat. Though Russian physicians had observed similar symptoms in the Siberian campaigns of the Russo-Japanese War of 1904, they remained largely unknown in Western European medicine. Significantly, no organic cause for these conditions could be found, and to explain their onset doctors looked increasingly to the psyche, becoming convinced that the mind converted the fears, terrors and traumatic memories of warfare into debilitating physical symptoms.

Because these men were so militarily and economically valuable to the belligerent nations, doctors were under enormous pressure to treat and rehabilitate them. Early attempts at curing involved treatments derived from the somatic paradigm; consequently, doctors aimed to calm soldiers' nerves through soothing baths, massages and gentle rest cures which were often aided by sedatives and nutrient-rich diets. But these methods met with little success, and a mood of therapeutic pessimism prevailed in psychiatric circles. As the ranks of shell-shocked soldiers grew and the need for manpower escalated concomitantly, the taboos against psychological cures were gradually lifted. Consequently, a number of psychotherapeutic and suggestive techniques came into practice. These methods, which military-medical authorities called active treatment, varied significantly in accordance with doctors' particular styles and preferences; they included techniques that range from the familiar, such as hypnosis and electrotherapy, to the obscure, for example, faux operations, deception cures, phoney wonder drugs, or the placement of a metal ball on the larynx to induce a shriek in functionally mute patients. But these diverse techniques were united by their common basis in the principles of suggestion; in all cases it was the suggestive effect that the doctor produced, rather than the material properties of the treatment, which was believed to act as the therapeutic agent. At times, active treatment involved elaborate stagings that are curiously reminiscent of the artifice and theatrical patient-doctor encounters that characterized Enlightenment-era moral treatment *(see box)*.

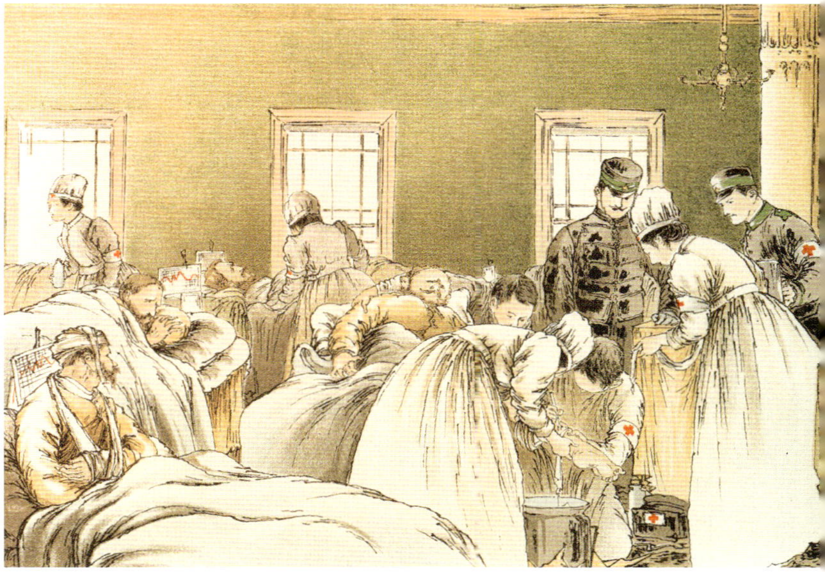

ABOVE Twentieth-century warfare added a new dimension to human suffering and a new concept – shell shock.

A German psychiatrist succinctly summarized the key to active treatment when he remarked, 'The doctor cures through his personality, not through his method.' Hence, little attempt was made by military or medical authorities to prescribe particular methods to the practitioners of active treatment; as with the moral treatment of the late eighteenth century, the charismatic powers and management skills of

THE POWER OF SUGGESTION

When treating patients with somatoform hysterical disorders – that is, the conversion of emotions and thoughts into physical symptoms – the neurologist Max Rothmann *(1868–1915)* pretended to administer a wonder drug which, he promised his patients, would cure their condition almost instantaneously. First Rothmann explained that, due to the painfulness of the medication, it would be administered with a short-term anaesthetic. He then put his patients to sleep and performed no operation whatsoever. After the patients awoke, he informed them that the operation had been a success and encouraged them to demonstrate that their disorders had disappeared, ordering them to move their temporarily paralysed body parts, for example. As Rothmann enthusiastically reported, the method worked almost effortlessly on the great majority of cases.

individual doctors were deemed therapeutically effective. The new war neurosis hospitals erected around Europe's battlefields in the middle of the conflict actually resembled early nineteenth-century asylums in a number of ways. The principle of moral management well characterizes the relationship between military psychiatrists and their soldier-patients, in which the moral and psychological value of fighting for the national cause was continually stressed. Moreover, the forms of occupational therapy introduced in the older asylums were utilized in the war setting as well, as doctors considered crafts, agricultural work and sport to carry tremendous therapeutic benefits.

These treatments, widely deployed by French, German, Austrian, British and Italian doctors starting around 1916–17, seemed to bring miraculous results, suddenly eliminating dramatically debilitating symptoms in thousands of men. Indeed, due to these sudden therapeutic successes, doctors often characterized the new methods as magical or 'miracle cures', falling back on language that seems out of step with the scientific ethos of the psychiatry of the time and reviving the debates on hypnosis and suggestion from the days of Bernheim and Charcot. Thus, in a manner akin to Charcot's sudden cures, in the following passage the Viennese psychiatrist Wilhelm Stekel describes the 'miracle cure' of a Hungarian soldier through a rudimentary form of hypnotic suggestion:

Among my patients there was a man who had lost his speech following a persistent artillery barrage. I promised to cure him in a few minutes. All the doctors of the hospital together with the chief surgeon and the head-nurse gathered together to witness this demonstration. I used a different method – fascination. The patient, a simple Hungarian peasant (I could not communicate with him as I do not speak Hungarian), was sitting opposite me in a chair. I looked persistently into his eyes for two minutes and then I intoned 'A-a-a.' Like an automaton he repeated the 'A.' Then I used other vowels, progressed to syllables, and finally he repeated a few Hungarian words I had learned at the hospital. At last the expected miracle occurred: he was cured. A stream of tears broke from his eyes.[25]

WILHELM STEKEL

It was not just 'simple peasants' who suffered. The traumatizing impact of war made itself felt in educated circles too, though these sufferers were treated with significantly more respect. In fact, several of Europe's leading literary figures succumbed to the illness, notably some British writers who suffered shell shock and left an enormous literary legacy which helped to shape subsequent perceptions of war, masculinity and mental illness.

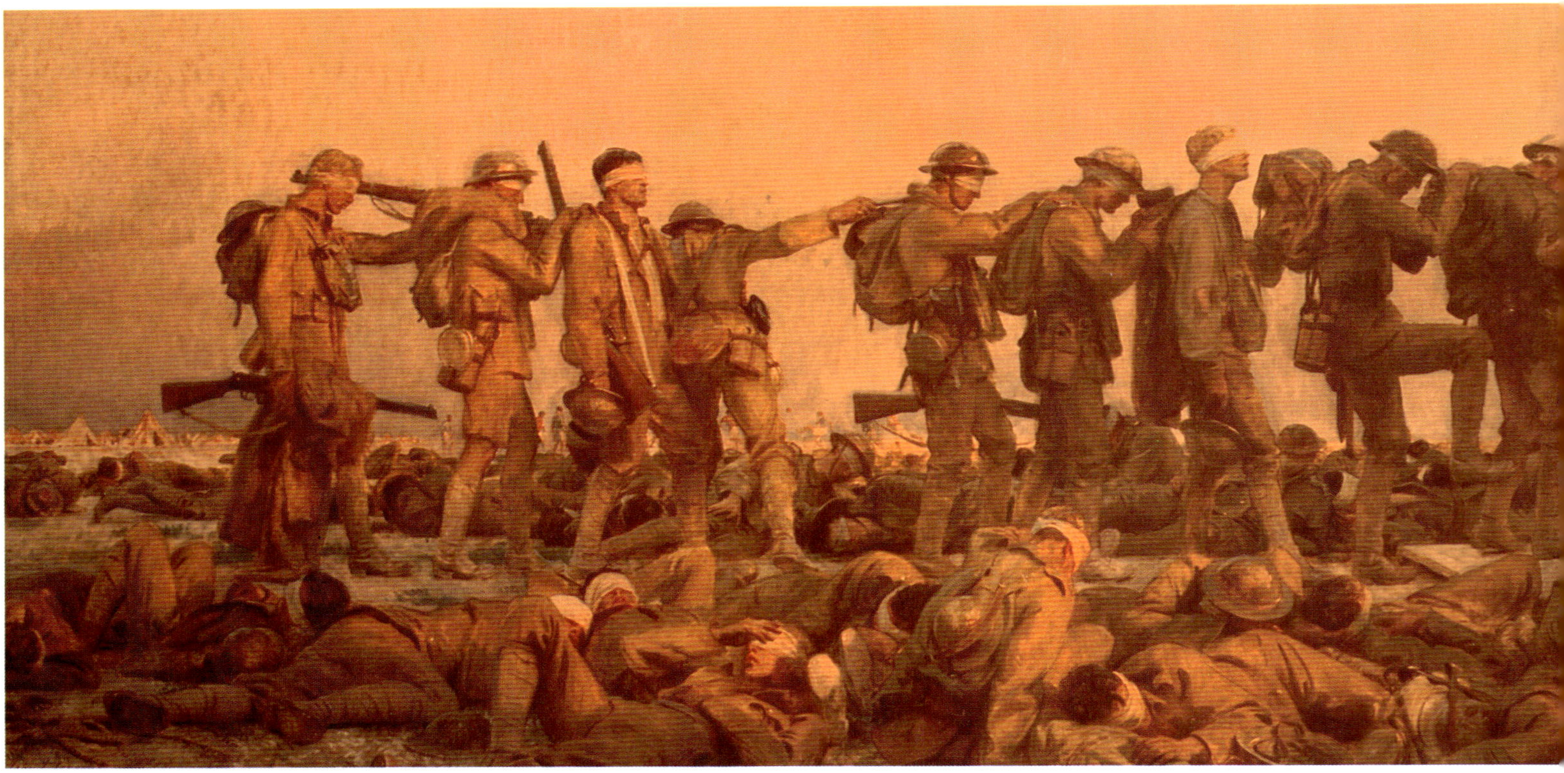

WAR AND THE MEMORY OF WAR

One legacy of World War I was a growing belief among both psychiatrists and lay people that ordinary, healthy persons, when exposed to particular conditions, could 'go mad'. When they returned from battle to their wives and families, men of all the belligerent nations, like Septimus Smith in Virginia Woolf's novel *Mrs Dalloway*, were observed to be somehow 'different', to have left behind their old, innocent selves on the fields of Flanders. Many continued to be tormented by traumatic war memories, which they could not prevent themselves from revisiting long after war's end. Yet it is one of the ironies of the war experience that to many, madness, because it provided an escape route out of the trenches and preserved an individual's life, represented the most sane, rational reaction to the horrors and dangers of combat. The line between madness and sanity, so increasing numbers of people began to believe, was blurry and fluid. While links between insanity and creativity had been long investigated, in this period madness was actively embraced as a form of expression by *avant-garde* artistic movements,

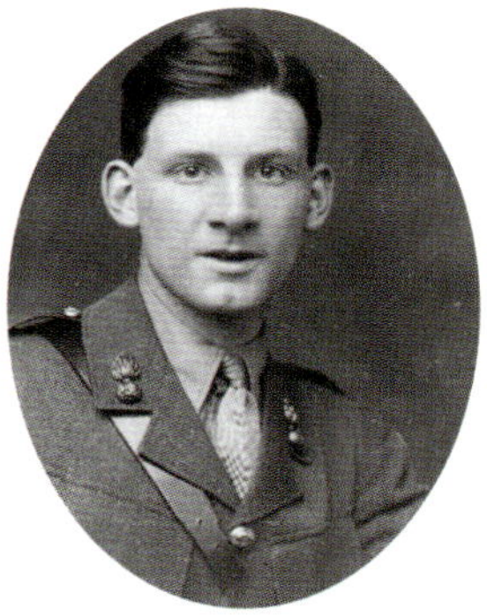

ABOVE Siegfried Sassoon was diagnosed as being mentally disturbed because he published an anti-war statement in 1917 entitled 'A Soldier's Declaration'.

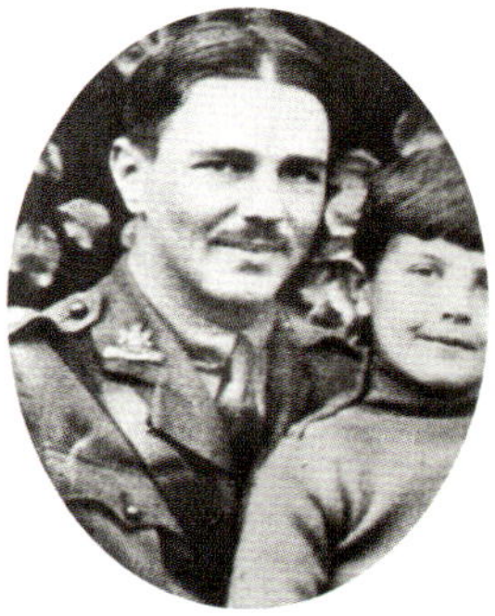

ABOVE Wilfred Owen met Siegfried Sassoon when they were both at Craiglockhart War Hospital. Owen had been sent there for treatment for shell shock. He recovered and eventually returned to the front where he was killed in November 1918. As he wrote in 'Anthem for Doomed Youth', 'What passing-bells for these who die as cattle? Only the monstrous anger of the guns.'

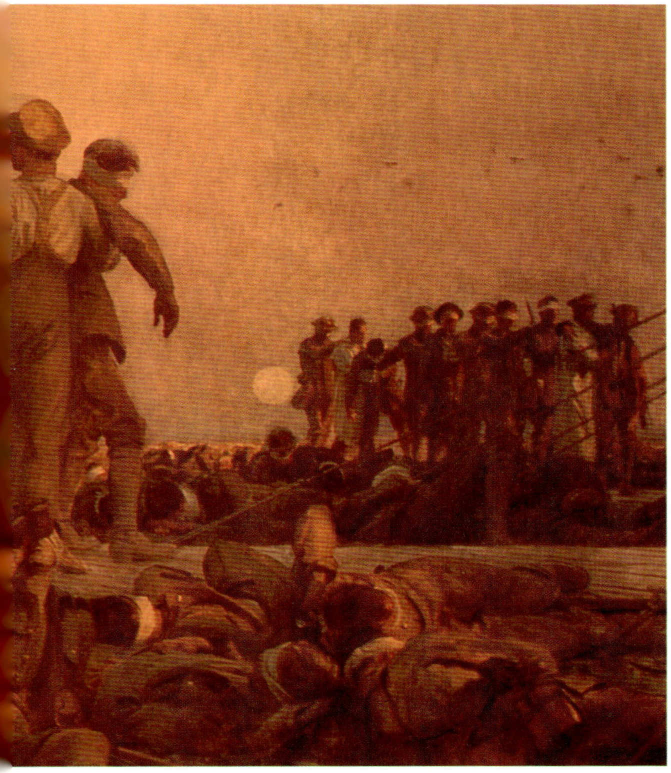

LEFT The painter John Singer Sargent *(1856–1925)* is best known as a portraitist of fashionable Victorian and Edwardian society. He was moved by the horrors of World War I to produce this powerful evocation of the battlefield. Entitled 'Gassed' it shows soldiers blinded by a gas attack being led from the front.

SHELL-SHOCKED

In a famously fraught clinical encounter, the poet Siegfried Sassoon was treated for three months by the English neurologist and anthropologist WHR Rivers at the Craiglockhart War Hospital near Edinburgh, where his fellow traumatized writers Robert Graves and Wilfred Owen were also housed. A second lieutenant, Sassoon had been a brave soldier who earned the Military Cross and the nickname 'Mad Jack' for his daredevil antics. He first got into trouble when, recovering from a war wound in 1917, he published 'A Soldier's Declaration', a pacifist treatise in which Sassoon characterized Britain's military conduct as a 'deliberately prolonged...war of aggression and conquest'. Instead of facing a military tribunal, however, Sassoon came into the hands of medical authorities. Diagnosed as a war neurotic, his anti-war sentiments were seen as evidence of mental illness, and he was sent to Craiglockhart in July of the same year.

To counter this condition, which Sassoon never believed he had, Dr Rivers applied a method loosely derived from psychoanalytic techniques, one that calls to mind the method first used in the case of Anna O. As in Breuer's case a quarter of a century before, Rivers' therapeutic strategy relied on catharsis; he sought to bring the symptoms' traumatic antecedents into the patient's consciousness, to discuss them and thus re-channel them in a healthier direction. After several months of treatment, Sassoon decided to return to service, not out of any political conviction, but out of concern for the men of his company. As he wrote in his haunting poem 'Sick Leave',

When I'm asleep,
dreaming and lulled and warm—
They come, the homeless ones,
the noiseless dead...
Out of the gloom they gather about my
bed.

such as the dadaists and surrealists. Indeed, many of their leading lights, such as German caricaturist and painter George Grosz and the montage artist John Heartfield, had fought in the war and experienced psychological breakdowns.

To many medical professionals, the war's legacy was to prove that madness could be brought on by purely psychological and emotional stimuli. These views represented the cyclical return of old ideas that have risen and fallen over psychiatry's long history. Their early twentieth-century revival stemmed, above all, from the war and its mental health consequences. Another medical consequence of the war and its psychiatric casualties was the growing belief that psychiatry had a role to play in daily life. No longer confined to the chronically mentally ill asylum population, psychiatrists began to treat patients straddling the precarious 'borderline' between mental illness and health. For the most part this patient pool consisted of the so-called neurotics, whose disorders and dysfunctions did not prevent them from carrying on with everyday activities.

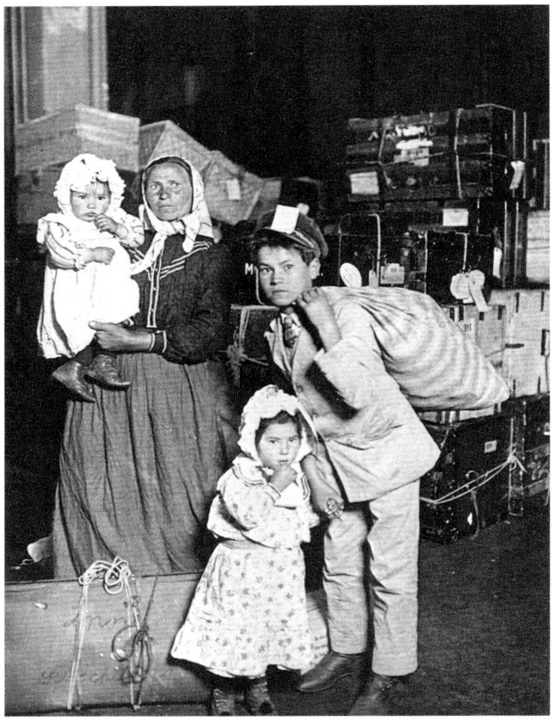

ABOVE **Italian immigrants arriving in New York in 1905. At around this time the mental hygiene movement was exerting influence in the United States. It sought to safeguard public health by preventing mental illness.**

One dimension of this new psychiatric activity was mental hygiene, an originally American initiative founded in 1908, which after the war became a widely influential international movement. Mental hygienists strove to intervene in the daily lives of 'normal' individuals, promoting measures to prevent the outbreak of mental diseases and to preserve society's productive capacity. Transmitting psychiatric teachings into schools, factories and offices, mental hygiene played a key role in shifting social and medical attention away from mental *illness* and onto mental *health*. The movement had perhaps its most profound effect in the Soviet Union, where both medics and political officials showed great concern with improving production and protecting national health as a way of preserving the young state.

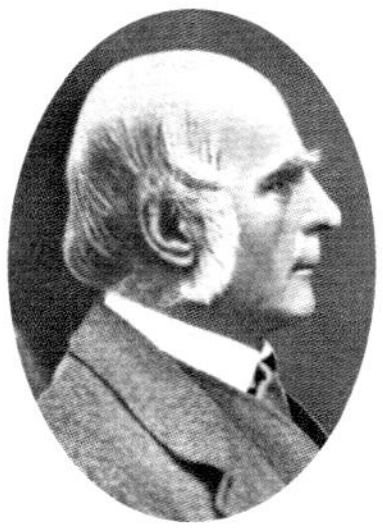

ABOVE **Sir Francis Galton** *(1822–1911)* **introduced the study of eugenics and heredity.**

EUGENIC PSYCHIATRY

Parallel with mental hygiene came the development of eugenic psychiatry, another pre-war idea which took on greater strength in the light of the physical and psychological consequences of World War I. Numerous medical thinkers declared that the war had performed a kind of evolutionary reversal, a non-natural selection, by allowing the majority of 'mentally deficient' men to escape combat through nervous illness, while their healthier counterparts bravely fought, often to their own detriment and even death. Amid the trying economic circumstances of the war's aftermath, these ideas brought issues of mental illness and heredity firmly to the fore. Growing belief in the biological, heritable basis of mental disease and concern with national economic health paved the way for one of the darkest episodes in the history of psychiatry.

The involuntary sterilization of mentally ill individuals began on American soil, where fears of being overrun by foreign immigration, disease and population degeneration took on particularly large dimensions early in the present century. In 1907 the American state of Indiana pioneered legislation allowing the sterilization of the mentally ill and criminally insane. Over the next two decades, 27 other states and one Canadian province followed, with the result that some 30,000 people were sterilized, often involuntarily, by 1939. The American programme was actually a model for German eugenicists, who sought to enact similar legislation in Germany in the 1920s.

Plans for eugenic psychiatry – on the verge of realization when the Weimar Republic fell – became reality in Germany when the Nazis assumed power in 1933. In their attempts to form a genetically pure, racially healthy nation state, the Nazis immediately passed legislation calling for the compulsory sterilization of large numbers of mentally and nervously ill, including schizophrenics, the severely alcoholic, the congenitally epileptic, and sufferers of 'congenital feeble-mindedness' *(angeborener Schwachsinn* in German terminology*)*. Most of these operations were carried out in the law's first four years; the Nazi regime, in fact, sterilized as many as 400,000 patients between 1933 and the start of World War II in September 1939.

Later in the 1930s, Nazi treatment of the mentally ill advanced to its next, unprecedently criminal phase in the so-called euthanasia programme, in which tens of thousands of psychiatric patients were brutally murdered. The idea that the mentally ill represented an enormous social burden which, because they cost the state more than they contributed, did not deserve to live, was first articulated during World War I. In 1919 a German psychiatrist, Alfred Hoche, and Rudolf Binding, a law professor, wrote a tract defending taking the life of the incurably insane, an idea which resonated in Britain and North America as well. Yet only in Germany were the political circumstances favourable to these radical measures, and beginning in 1938, German psychiatrists ordered and supervised the execution in gas chambers of mentally ill children and adults.

RECENT DEVELOPMENTS

The years since World War II have been marked by heated competition between the major schools of psychiatric thought. A vocal anti-psychiatry movement arose in Europe and America in the 1960s, charging that mental maladies were largely 'man-made' and criticizing psychiatric power and practices. Issues of trauma and memory have risen to the fore once again, most conspicuously since the 1970s, with the widely publicized psychological suffering of Vietnam War veterans. The topic continues to provoke great cultural, medical and legal controversy almost a century after Freud abandoned the seduction theory, as many psychotherapists claim to uncover repressed memories of childhood sexual trauma in their patients, who then often press for financial compensation or legal redress against their supposed abusers.

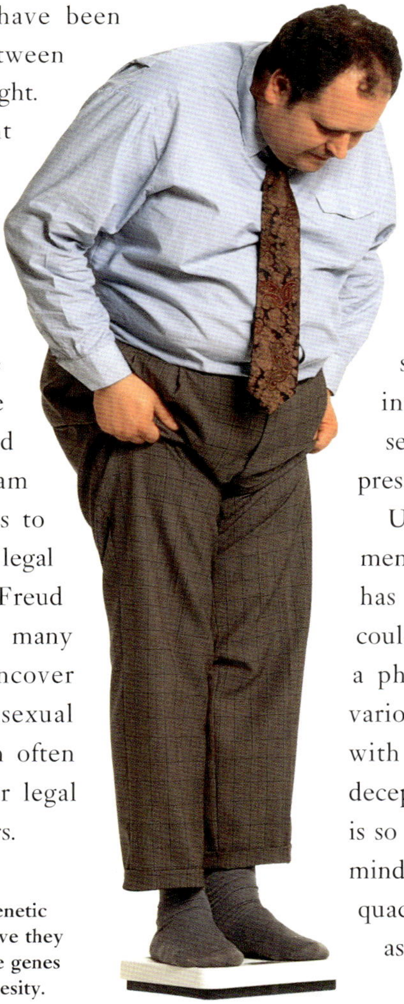

RIGHT Today's genetic psychiatrists believe they have identified the genes responsible for obesity.

Neo-kraepelinians race to document an ever-expanding array of disorders and syndromes, continually updating and reissuing their classificatory tome. Biological approaches to the mind are back, too, competing with and now seemingly overtaking psychological psychiatry and psychoanalysis for authority. Electric shock treatment, or electroconvulsive therapy (ECT), is experiencing a renaissance in North American hospitals as well. In contemporary Western science, the newly ascendent biological approach is primarily represented by two strands: genetic psychiatry and psychopharmacology.

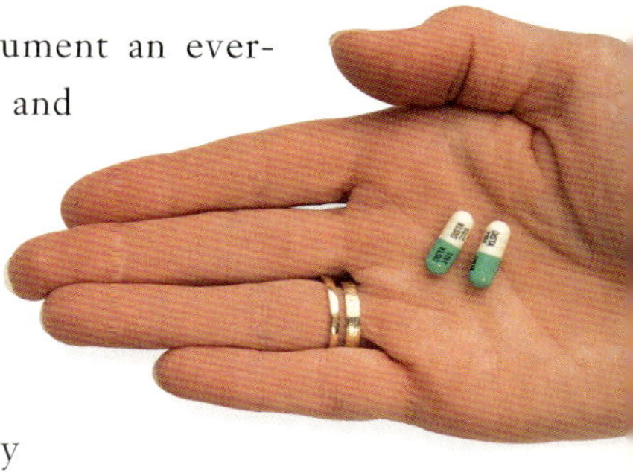

ABOVE Psychotropic drugs such as Prozac are currently prescribed in vast numbers in the Western world to help people to cope with depression.

Scarcely deterred by past precedent, today's scientists are searching for the genetic basis of mental maladies with renewed zeal. In their ambitious attempts to chart inherited human traits comprehensively (the humane genome project), scientists now claim to have found specific genes responsible for such behaviours and characteristics as obesity, schizophrenia and alcoholism. At the same time, pharmacology continues to expand rapidly; while medication has been used to deal with psychoses for several decades, more recently drugs have been developed for sufferers of less debilitating conditions like neuroses, anxiety and depression. Prozac and other psychotropic medications are sweeping the developed world, prescribed to ever-growing segments of the population who can no longer cope with the pressures and stresses of late twentieth-century life.

Undeniably, such psychiatric technologies have relieved the mental suffering of countless patients, and psychiatric science has made advances that Charcot, Kraepelin and Griesinger could never have dreamed of. But current ideas represent only a phase in a cyclical, historically contingent trajectory. In various times and places mental maladies have been treated with drugs, surgical interventions, talking cures, theatrical deceptions, mesmerism and shamanism. Understanding why this is so might throw into doubt conventional dichotomies between mind and body, science and magic, and legitimate medicine and quackery. More awareness of psychiatry's history can only help as late twentieth-century thinkers continue the challenge of comprehending and curing disorders that afflict the mind.

CHAPTER SEVEN

HEALERS IN HISTORY

A MULTI-CULTURAL PERSPECTIVE

HEALERS, *both in the East and the West, may categorically view the state of health as the absence of disease. Indeed, one modern medical dictionary defines health unequivocally in the following terms – 'The state of the organism when it functions optimally without evidence of disease or abnormality'. Disease, then, is an altered state from the 'normal' structure and/or function of the body. But are disease and illness synonymous? Generally, no. Disease more often implies a physical or medical process from the healer's viewpoint, whereas illness more precisely represents a patient's or a society's view of suffering caused by disease. However, despite the difference in perspective that the words imply, both of these terms certainly constitute part of what it means to be sick.*

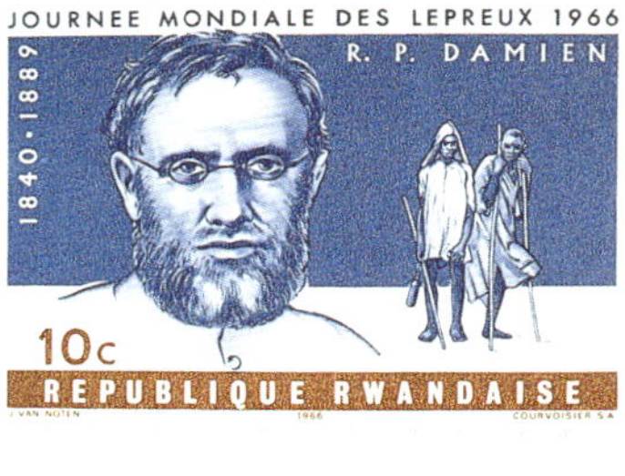

ABOVE Father Damien DeVeuster tended to leprosy victims at Kalaupapa until his death from the disease in 1889.

An example of the distinction between disease and illness is provided by Giuseppe Verdi's opera, *La Traviata (1853)*. In this impassioned work, the heroine Violetta suffered from a lung disease – a deviation from the normal condition of her lung – in which a germ was eating away or consuming the tissue and blood vessels, precipitating sporadic haemorrhages. Violetta and her companions recognized this *illness* from the occasional spots of blood she coughed up onto her handkerchief. For her physician, this *disease* was consumption, what we would call tuberculosis. From Violetta's viewpoint, she was gradually growing weaker, paler, and fainting more often. Her illness incapacitated her and prevented her from physically enjoying the life she had dreamed of leading with her suitor, Alfredo. Illnesses are generally viewed more subjectively, whereas disease is typically the healer's objectification of that same sickness. Both Violetta and her healer – together with many opera fans sobbing in the audience – knew that her sickness would be fatal, but they viewed the characterization of this sickness in different ways.

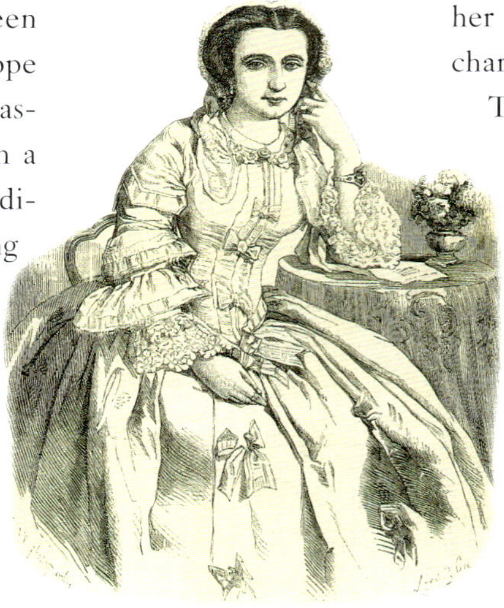

ABOVE In *La Traviata* Verdi's heroine Violetta knows that she is *ill*. Her doctor can diagnose the *disease* as consumption. Patient and physician naturally view sickness from different perspectives.

This chapter focuses upon key healers in different cultures throughout world history. After briefly reviewing different cultural views of sickness, formulating a working definition of 'healer', and reinforcing the proviso that the idea of a healer implies that of a patient as well, it surveys the ancient healing traditions of Egypt, Greece, India, China, Native America, and Africa. Important Biblical and women healers will also be discussed. The second portion of the chapter examines various cultural perspectives of the human body and the cultural exchange between particular healing traditions. Finally, the chapter reviews the evolution of modern healers. Topics discussed include alternative and complementary medicine, military and women healers, and the transmission of disease. A few 'parting thoughts' regarding the healer and death conclude the chapter.

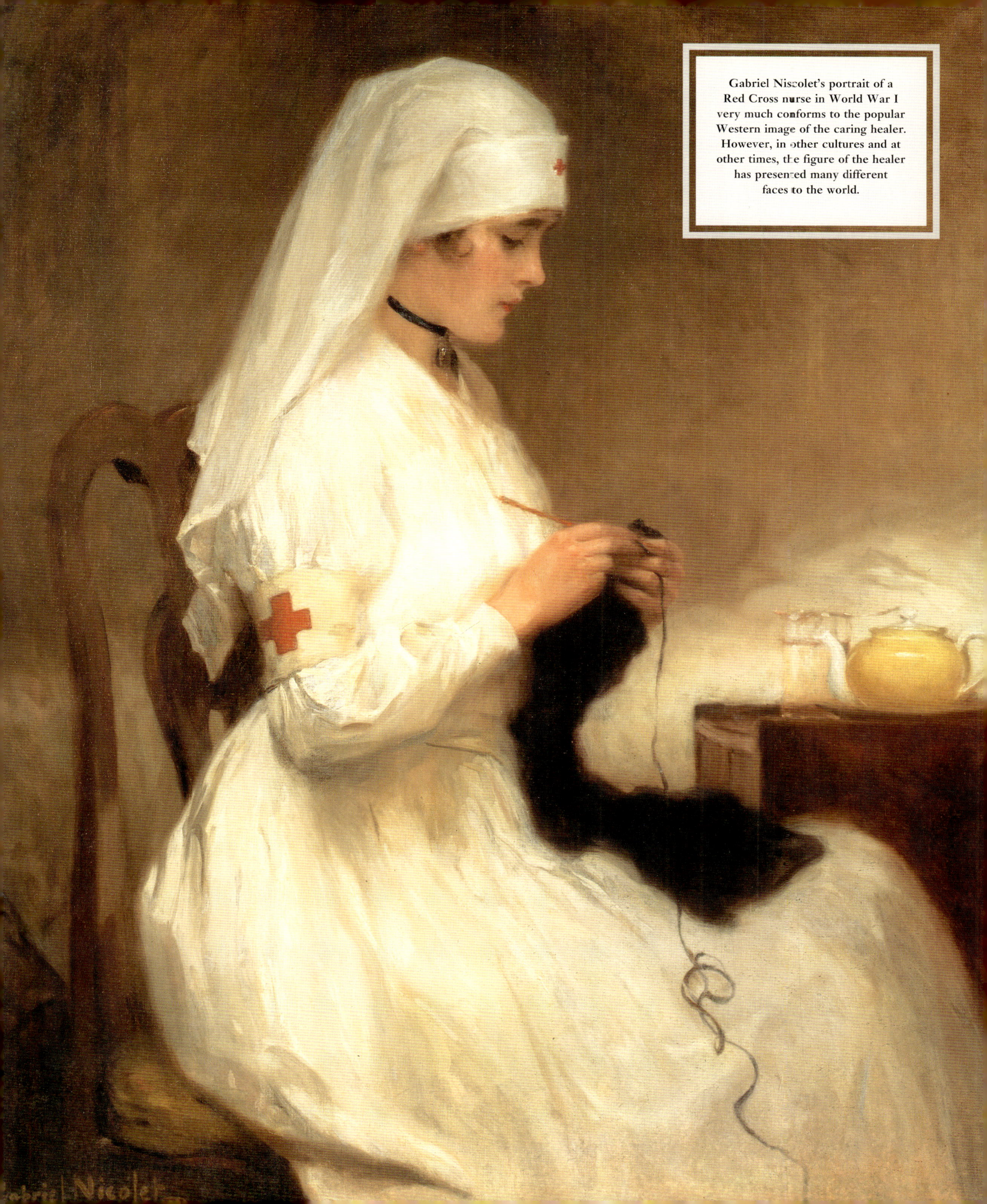

Gabriel Niscolet's portrait of a Red Cross nurse in World War I very much conforms to the popular Western image of the caring healer. However, in other cultures and at other times, the figure of the healer has presented many different faces to the world.

CULTURAL VIEWS OF SICKNESS

Illnesses may be viewed differently by different societies. Some cultures have viewed sickness as a disgrace, whereas others have seen the same disease/illness with grace. Socrates, the renowned philosopher of Ancient Greece, deemed bodily health and beauty to be the 'highest blessing possible'. Illness was disgraceful; the sick were not worthy of living. Understanding this unusual viewpoint may help to explain why the Greek philosopher Zeno hanged himself after having disfigured his otherwise beauteous body as a result of a broken finger.

Later cultures, particularly those in the Christian world, viewed disease as an opportunity for spiritual as well as physical cleansing or purification. The sick were, as medical historian Henry Sigerist noted, viewed as privileged. They were released from their obligations and they received special attention. Those who regularly laboured had, society believed, earned the assurance and insurance to have their disorders treated. Do you view the sick as having an elevated or privileged position in your society today? If so, do you think that people feign sickness, or perhaps even convince the medical community that they are suffering from vague symptoms that are difficult to measure clinically? Some critics have claimed that disorders such as Chronic Fatigue Syndrome, a.k.a. 'Yuppie flu', have actually been 'created' to fulfil societal needs.

Sigerist captured the essence of the societal views of sickness in a 1929 article, 'The Special Position of the Sick'. Sickness, Sigerist claimed, has often removed individuals from their otherwise daily routines and responsibilities. Some cultures, such as the Kubu of Sumatra, physically isolate the sick from society. Thereby, the sick were culturally 'dead' long before their physical decease. Lepers in various cultures have been similarly castigated throughout history. Such 'treatment' was rendered in Biblical times, as is recorded in the Book of Leviticus in the Bible, but it has also been practised in modern cultures as well. For an example from recent times, consider Hawaii.

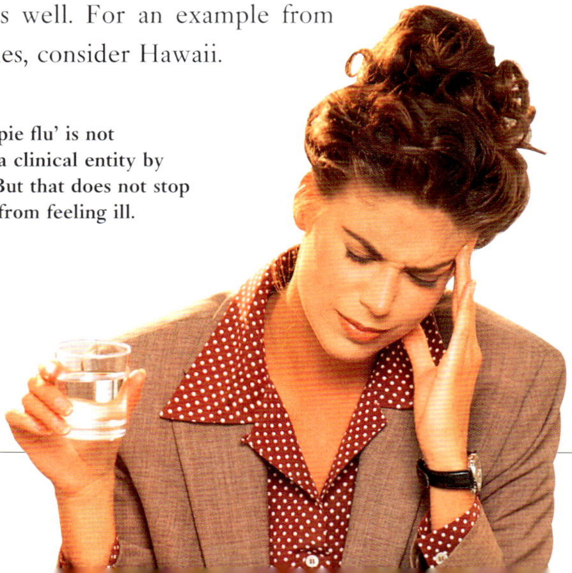

RIGHT 'Yuppie flu' is not accepted as a clinical entity by all doctors. But that does not stop its sufferers from feeling ill.

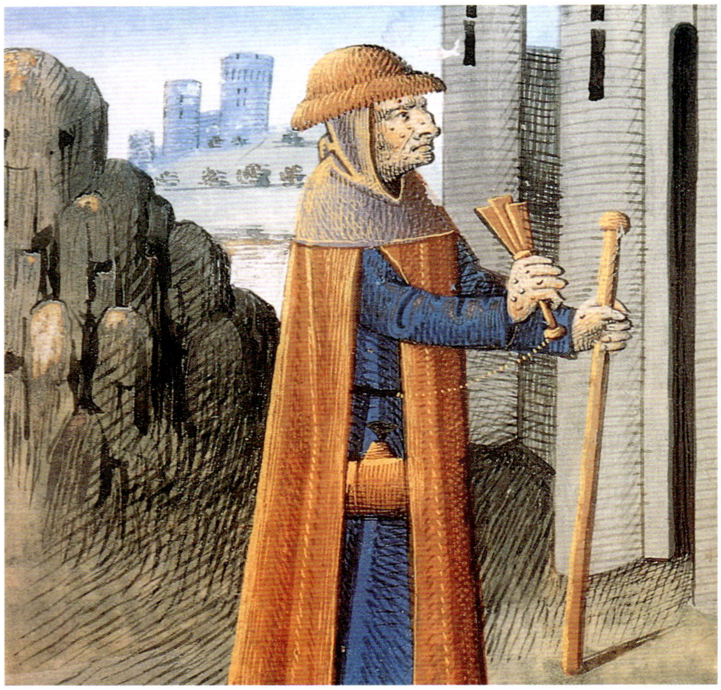

ABOVE Historically it was long the plight of the leper to be cast out from his culture and stigmatized as unclean. In this way some societies have evaded the burden of caring for the sick.

Hawaiians colloquially referred to leprosy as the 'separating sickness' because, as Stephanie J. Castillo has shown in her vivid 1992 television documentary, 'Simple Courage', the inflicted were forcibly removed from their families and transferred to a 'living tomb', the isolated leper colony of Kalaupapa on the island of Moloka'i. In the mind of some 'healers', this effort effectively quarantined the 'unclean' from contaminating the rest of society. It also enabled Hawaiian society leaders to more or less forget about the thousands of natives they had ostracized from their living culture.

As recently as 1986, the Cuban government enacted similar quarantine and removal policies for their citizens infected with HIV, the Human Immunodeficiency Virus associated with AIDS. As the Cuban Vice-Minister of Health, a physician, proclaimed, 'We have an opportunity to stop the disease in our country. It would be irresponsible if we didn't face the situation with courage, knowing we could stop it. We have an epidemiological opportunity that we are not going to lose.' Long-time resident of Kalaupapa in Hawaii, Olivia Robello Breitha, has adamantly opposed these isolationist measures in Cuba, pleading with responsible government and health policy leaders not to 'do to people with AIDS what you did to us'.

THE HEALER

Whether healers throughout history have typically acted in the best interests of their patients or have been governed by the greater interests of society remains difficult to ascertain. Who, indeed, were these healers?

'Healer' has implied many different meanings to cultures across the world throughout history. In many modern societies, licensed physicians, surgeons, and nurses are the individuals most directly responsible for the physical care of the ill or diseased. Their precise roles have varied in part due to their level of training. In other situations, their practices correlated with the types of diseases being treated. Surgeons, for instance, have long treated external, visible disorders whereas physicians have primarily treated diseases concealed under the skin. Both throughout history and today, 'healer' may imply one in solo practice or a member of a team, a generalist or a specialist, a man or a woman, a student of written or of oral tradition, and one who treats solely physical disorders or one who cares for the spiritual needs of patients, too.

Healing, itself, has frequently been regarded as a two-way process. That is, in order to have a healer, there must also be an individual in need of being healed. It may be easily imagined that people suffering from a large, outward tumorous growth, or experiencing persistent pain in the right abdominal region, or enduring an uncontrollable loss of fluids would readily seek assistance from one they viewed as a healer. Many conditions, however, are much more invisible to the sufferer. For instance, how does one distinguish a diminished ability to remember life experiences, something commonly known as a 'sign of aging', from early signs of Alzheimer's disease? I have often heard the humorous bantering that 'If I get Alzheimer's, would anyone really notice?' In other cases, healers typically expect sufferers to believe that they are inflicted with an infectious agent, perhaps a tubercle bacillus, or malarial parasite, or a polio virus which the sufferers have never seen for themselves. Regardless, many of the individuals carrying such infectious agents turn to a healer, swallow mysteriously named potions, and undergo extensive and expensive chemotherapy wholly upon trust.

Given this interaction, we must remember that throughout history a dialogue has existed between the healer and the one seeking this service. Unfortunately for historical accounts, the patients' participation in this dialogue has typically gone unrecorded. Thus, we are generally left with a one-sided history of healing, that describing the healer's point-of-view. In recent decades, historians like Roy Porter and Dorothy Porter in their *Patient's Progress: Doctors and Doctoring in Eighteenth-Century England (1989),* have begun to revise the previously lop-sided historical reporting by reintroducing accounts of patients' responses and responsibilities in the overall negotiation of health care delivery. Although limited space and lack of sources prohibit me from sharing many insights from the receiving end of healing, the reader should try to remember the sufferers' presence and importance in the healing scenario.

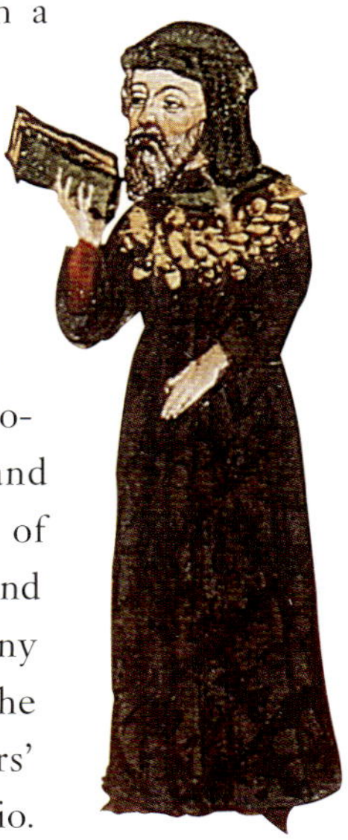

ABOVE The works of Rhazes (*c.864-925*) provided a cultural bridge between the healing traditions of Greece and the Arab world.

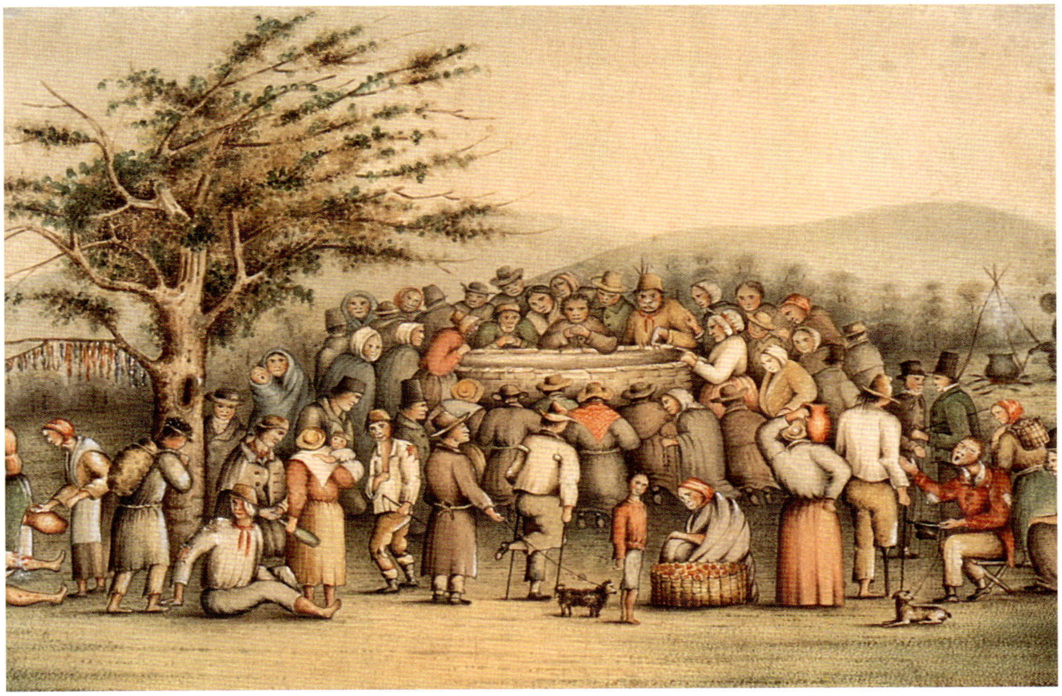

BELOW Healing implies the active participation of both healer and sufferer. Too often, history ignores the role of the sick in this equation.

ANCIENT HEALING TRADITIONS

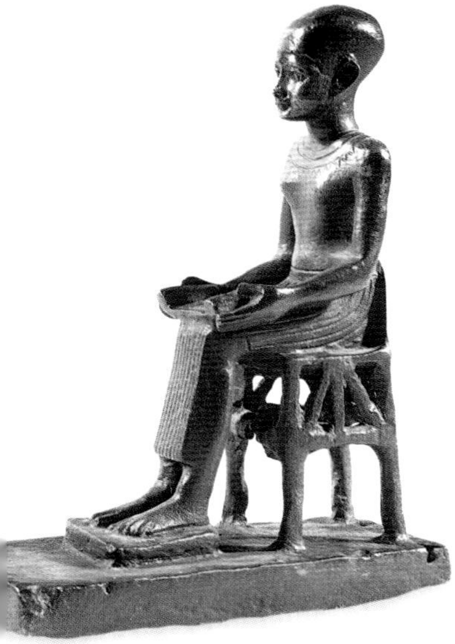

ABOVE A statue of the Egyptian Imhotep, the earliest known physician (*c.2980 BC*). He was later revered at Memphis as a god of healing.

This section reviews a selection of distinguished ancient healers and their practices from Egyptian, Greek, Indian, Chinese, Native American and African traditions. Although each culture will be examined individually, it is important to remember that distinct healing traditions have often coexisted at any given time.

EGYPT

Egyptian medicine may be viewed as two intertwined schools of thought: magical and empirical. The magical school incorporated religious ideas into medical practice; the empirical one was based on a sense-oriented approach to treatment.

Followers of magical medicine invoked the gods to protect the people. One such god was Imhotep, a mortal physician who worked under Pharaoh Zoser (*c.2900 BC*). After his death, Imhotep became recognized as a demigod after Egypt became a province of Persia around 525 BC. Ptah, the father of Imhotep, and Sekhmet, a female goddess, were also worshipped for the cures they delivered by a cult of healers who spread their wisdom across Egypt. Imhotep's influence in this culture is also found in the elaborate Egyptian 'Ritual of Embalming'. The Egyptian goddess Isis was also known for her healing powers. According to myth, Isis formed a serpent from the sun god Ra's saliva and mud. The next day, it stung Ra. Isis came to him demanding to know the secret name given to him so that no magician would have power over him. When he could endure the pain no longer, Ra took his secret name from his heart and placed it in Isis's, thereby giving her the power to heal.

At times, the two Egyptian schools of thought coexisted. Magical incantations were often recited in conjunction with the empirical use of drugs or surgery. The 'Ritual of Embalming' included empirical directions of chemical preservation together with prayer. This dual basis for healing was used throughout ancient Egypt until magic gradually became less prominent.

MAGICAL MEDICINE

Of the various temples erected to Imhotep, the temple at Memphis served as a place of worship, a hospital, and as a school of magical medicine. The following account depicts the use of magical medicine in this temple. Satmi Khamua, and his wife Mahituaskhit, had been unable to conceive a child. One night, the woman went to the temple and recited the following prayer,

Turn thy face towards me, my lord Imhotep,
son of Ptah;
it is thou who dost work miracles, and who art
beneficent in all thy deeds;
it is thou who givest a son to her who has none.
Listen to my lamentation and give me conception of
a man-child.

The woman then slept in the temple and was supposedly visited in her dreams. A voice told her to feed the herb colocasia to her husband. She followed these instructions and conceived a child.

ANCIENT GREECE

Greek healers provided the predominant influence on medical thinking and practice throughout Western history. The earliest information about ancient Greek medicine is derived from the writings of Homer in the ninth century BC. It is not certain whether Homer was one man, or a name given to work from a number of hands; Homeric accounts of medicine therefore vary. In the *Iliad*, medicine was deemed a 'noble art', and physicians were regarded as 'professionals and servants of the public'. This account also underlines the correlation between good hygiene and good health that existed in Greek medical thought. Wounds were dressed with compresses and bandages, and medicinal roots were applied. While tending the wounds, a song was sung, indicating a practice that combined elements of both empirical and magical medicine. However, in the *Odyssey*, Greek culture had begun to emphasize ways in which magic was considered the most useful way to treat the ill, reflecting society's changing view of healing.

Apollo became recognized as the 'god of healing'. The *Iliad* relates how he was considered as both 'the avenger' and 'the spreader' of plague. Homer described a situation in which one country took a priest's daughter as part of the spoils of war. The priest offered to trade his life for the life of his daughter but was turned away. He then offered prayers to Apollo, and Apollo visited plague on the victor's country until she was returned.

Other healing figures appear in Greek mythology. Paean was decreed the 'physician of the gods'. Chiron, a noted surgeon, had a pupil named Aesculapius. Legend leads us to believe that Aesculapius, a mortal, became part of Greek mythology. The legend of Aesculapius inspired a cult of followers who established a great medical school in Cyrene around 429 BC.

Aesculapius has long been linked with a serpent, the symbol of the healing art. As physician Robert Rakel described in 'One Snake or Two' *(Journal of the American Medical Association, 1985)*, 'In addition to representing wisdom, learning, and fertility,' the serpent symbolizes 'longevity and the restoration of health'. Egyptians visualized the serpent shedding its skin as representing the renewal of life. Earlier references are traceable to a serpent on the staff of the Babylonian healing god, Ningishzida. The twin-serpent staff of the messenger of the Greek gods Hermes (or Mercury in Roman mythology) – the caduceus – has, in many countries, gained popularity as a symbol of medicine from its aesthetic appeal. However, the single-serpent staff of Aesculapius remains the 'only true symbol of medicine'.

The next great school of Greek medicine stemmed from the age of Hippocrates, a Greek physician who practised and taught the art of medicine in the fifth and fourth centuries BC. The methods and philosophy of his teachings were recorded in a large collection of some 60 books collectively known as the *Hippocratic Corpus*, although the actual authorship of this work has been a matter of scholarly debate for many years. During the Golden Age of ancient Greece, medical knowledge was part of the training common to all well-educated men. Such men could turn to the *Corpus*, or at least to their memory of public lectures taken from the *Corpus*, to find guidance toward preserving their health and preventing disease.

Hippocrates viewed disease as a 'natural process'. The physician's goal, he argued, was to aid nature in healing the body. In order to determine the ideal state of health for each patient, Hippocratic physicians were taught to observe carefully the patient's natural surroundings. For example, *On Airs, Waters, Places*, one of the better-known works in the collected Hippocratic writings, states that a physician should be able to determine his patient's condition without ever questioning him. Specifically, factors such as the changing seasons, climate, and locale, together with the patient's life-style, offered valuable clues regarding the patient's health. In another well-known work, the *Hippocratic Oath*, the importance of morality, truth, and compassion in the practice of medicine is discussed. Today, many medical students around the world still make the pledges enshrined in the Hippocratic Oath (*see box*).

According to Hippocrates, no disease was thought to be 'sacred'. Rather, he argued that all disease owed its origin to natural causes. Specifically, disease occurred from an imbalance in the state of a patient's humours. In Greek thought, the universe was composed of four elements: air, earth, water, and fire. These four elements were linked to four humours in the body, respectively: blood, black bile, phlegm, and yellow bile. The body was considered to be in a state of disease (or dis-ease) when the equilibrium between these humours was imbalanced.

THE HIPPOCRATIC OATH

I swear by Apollo the physician, by Aesculapius, Hygeia, and Panacea, and I take to witness all the gods, all the goddesses, to keep according to my ability and my judgement the following Oath:

To consider dear to me as my parents him who taught me this art; to live in common with him and if necessary to share my goods with him; to look upon his children as my own brothers, to teach them this art if they so desire without fee or written promise; to impart to my sons and the sons of the master who taught me and the disciples who have enrolled themselves and have agreed to the rules of the profession, but to these alone, the precepts and the instruction. I will prescribe regimen for the good of my patients according to my ability and my judgement and never do harm to anyone. To please no one will I prescribe a deadly drug, nor give advice which may cause his death. Nor will I give a woman a pessary to procure abortion. But I will preserve the purity of my life and my art. I will not cut for stone, even for patients in whom the disease is manifest; I will leave this operation to be performed by practitioners (specialists in this art). In every house where I come I will enter only for the good of my patients, keeping myself far from all intentional ill-doing and all seduction, and especially from the pleasures of love with women or with men be they free or slaves. All that may come to my knowledge in the exercise of my profession or outside of my profession or in daily commerce with men, which ought not to be spread abroad, I will keep secret and will never reveal. If I keep this oath faithfully, may I enjoy my life and practise my art, respected by all men and in all times; but if I swerve from it or violate it, may the reverse be my lot.

INDIA

In contrast to the Greek emphasis on the physical basis of health, the people of early Indian civilization regarded the spirit as more important than the body. According to medical historian Henry Sigerist, the Indians believed that a person's 'present and future life, his happiness or misery, are determined by his own actions'. The sum of these actions, called Karma, not only determined a person's afterlife but could also inflict illness and pain in his or her present life.

One chief practitioner of Indian medicine was Siddhartha Gautama Shakyamuni, who lived in the sixth century BC. During one lengthy meditation he was tempted by Kama-Mara, the god of desire and death, to succumb to basic human desires, but he refrained. He awoke in what has been called the 'Great Awakening', and from that moment forward was known as the 'Buddha', which is Sanskrit for 'the enlightened'. Knowledgeable of the role of spirit in healing and Karma, Buddha professed 'love and compassion for all mankind' and also the 'peace of mind brought about by the abandonment of desire'. Following the teachings of Buddha, monasteries have been created for monks wishing to experience solitude to attune the body and mind. This philosophical basis of healing endures in Indian medicine today.

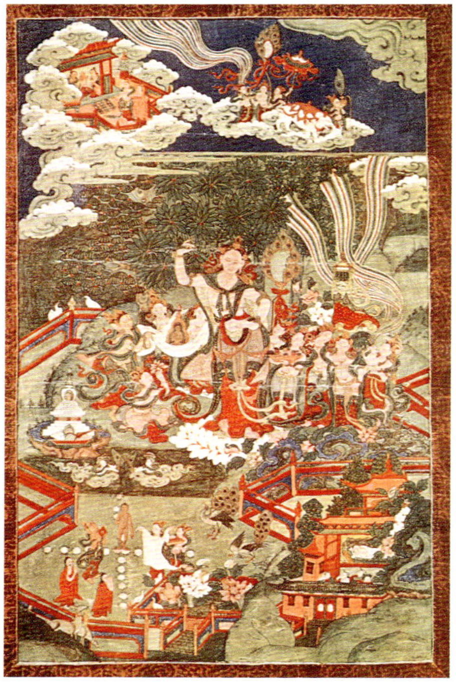

ABOVE A Tibetan painting representing the birth in Nepal of Siddhartha Gautama, the Buddha or 'enlightened one'.

Another Indian system of healing is based on the four Vedas of sacred lore. This system was thought to have been revealed by the godhead, Brahma. The four Vedas are a collection of hymns, prayers, incantations, and charms used to protect people. Together they form the basis of Vedic Medicine. One Veda, *Atharva*, includes a system of ancient Hindu medicine called Ayurveda, which is covered in detail in Chapter 4. Ayurvedic medicine was based on treatises written by Caraka and Suśruta. Caraka lived at the beginning of the Christian era; the great surgeon Suśruta lived during the first millenium AD. The *Caraka Samhitā* describes medical practice whereas the *Suśruta Samhitā* is devoted to surgery. A typical surgeon, or vaidya, seated in a hut surrounded by a garden of medicinal herbs, would pass on his learning by reciting verses of the Ayurveda to several young apprentices who stood by steadfastly. As no copy of the *Suśruta Samhitā* was printed at that time, surgeons had to learn their art from another surgeon who already had this work memorized.

The vaidya developed a comprehensive understanding of external anatomy, but had limited exposure to internal structures since dissections were not permissible. Some Vedic rites included human sacrifice, but this provided only minimal knowledge of internal anatomy. Apprentices, in order to gain surgical expertise, practised their techniques on fruits, meats, and dead animals. Indian surgeons harnessed nature to assist in all parts of healing. Natural substances, such as a honey-butter paste, provided a favourite healing ointment. As a different and more direct example of nature at work, surgeons would tie a rope attached to a bent tree branch to an arrow penetrating a patient and allow the branch to spring back its original position, thereby extracting the arrow.

In contrast to the four Hippocratic humours, Indian medicine was based on the belief that 700 vessels carried three basic 'doṣas' in addition to blood. The doṣas were *pitta* (bile), *kapha* (phlegm), and *vāta* (wind). The flow of *rakta*, the blood, was disrupted when the three doṣas were imbalanced. The Indian practitioner knew of 107 vital points, or *marmas*, which corresponded to various body regions or functions. For instance, *kukundara marmas* on either side of the spinal cord were known to cause paralysis if they were penetrated.

CHINESE MEDICINE

Traditional Chinese Medicine (TCM), one of the oldest known forms of practice, is also the most unique. The earliest Chinese medical work is *Huangdi Neijing (The Yellow Emperor's Inner Canon)*, dating from the Han Dynasty in the third century BC. The dialogue in this work between the 'Yellow Emperor', Huangdi, and his chief minister, Ch'i Po, reveals the basis of medical thought and practice. This work described three essential beliefs that have established themselves as the basis of TCM: tao, yin and yang, and the five elements of life. The philosophy of tao, founded by Lao-tzu, is conceived as the pathway guiding a person's conduct on earth to match the demands of the afterlife.

Yin and yang are considered to be the basis of life. Said to have been divided from chaos by the god Pan Kua, yin and yang are the two opposing and complementary forces of life present throughout nature. Disease is considered to be a disturbance in the balance of yin and yang. According to *Neijing*, 'All happenings in nature as well as in human life were conditioned by the constantly changing relationship of these two cosmic regulators.' In Chinese thought, the microcosmic body is interconnected with the greater macrocosmic universe. The anonymous authors hoped to create an eternal masterpiece. They achieved their goal in that much of the medicine described in their book forms the basis of TCM teaching and practice today.

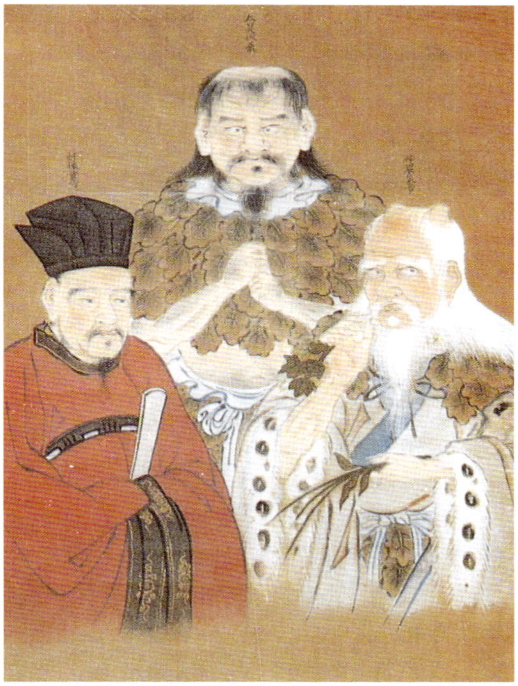

ABOVE **An eighteenth-century painting on silk, 'The Emperors of Chinese Medicine'. The figures illustrated are (left to right) Huangdi, Fu Hsi and Shen Nong.**

Shen Nong, one of the three ancient Chinese healers, was known as the 'Divine Agriculturist'. He searched for herbal remedies for various ailments, and tested the effects on himself. His records formed the basis of China's long-standing emphasis on herbal treatments.

CONFUCIUS AND TCM

K'ung Fu-tzu *(551-479 BC)*, or Confucius, is one of the greatest intellectual contributors to Chinese history. Confucius' work contains important references to the five elements. These elements, the basis of all life, include water, fire, wood, metal, and earth. As in other traditions, the proper balance of elements is considered necessary for health in the Chinese system.

Other than herbal medicine, the most widely-known form of TCM still in use today is acupuncture. This practice is based on the view that meridians or channels carry qi, a form of vital energy, throughout the body. Unlike arteries, veins, and nerves, the channels form an invisible network uniting all parts of the body. Inserting acupuncture needles at various points on the skin affects corresponding bodily function. Healers can choose from 365 acupoints on the skin to correct excesses of yin or yang in order to renew the balance between the two within the body. Bian Que, a physician in the fourth century BC, claimed to have brought a prince out of a coma using acupuncture.

Moxibustion is another method for balancing yin and yang in the body. In moxibustion, the herb 'moxa' is twisted into a cone, placed upon needles inserted into specific channels, and burned in order that the heat produced should stimulate qi in afflicted bodily parts. This procedure resembled in practice the cupping employed in conventional Western medicine throughout much of history. Heated glass cups were placed upon the skin to produce a blister with the intent of drawing off bodily humours.

One significant difference between TCM and medicine practised elsewhere in the world was that, in China, taking the pulse has long been a common and critical diagnostic tool. Wang Shu-ho composed the 12-volume *Mei Ching (Book of the Pulse)* in AD 280. In this work, 'the human body is likened to a chord instrument, of which the different pulses are the chords. The harmony or discord of the organism can be recognized by examining the pulse, which is thus fundamental for all medicine'. Unlike the experience many Westerners receive in a modern clinic, the traditional Chinese examination of the pulse was a complex process. The healer would measure the pulse of the patient and compare it with his own. Great care would also be taken to determine the character of the pulse. For example, a pulse may be described as being 'sharp as a hook, fine as a hair, ... dead as a rock, smooth as a flowing stream, ... the front crooked and the back delayed, ... and sharp as a bird's beak'. Specifically, three different tests are incorporated using light pressure, medium pressure, and heavy pressure. The Chinese have identified about 200 kinds of pulses to be used in diagnosis. Seventeenth-century British physician John Floyer learned this intricate pulse method, reported the knowledge back to Europe, and devised the earliest known pulse watch.

TCM was founded at a time when dissection was prohibited. Critics claim that modern 'barefoot doctors' practising TCM in China, having gained their know-how from one of over 2,000 TCM hospitals, remain biased towards ancient philosophy rather than attempting to gain an empirical understanding of the body which Western scientific medicine can provide.

FAITH HEALING

New Testament Biblical accounts attest to many acts of healing performed by Jesus. He healed physical ills, exorcised demons, and cleansed individuals from sin. In the Christian Era, many sick individuals viewed treatment of their illness as an opportunity to become purified. As medical historian Owsei Temkin noted, disease was 'a portal through which man acquired eternal salvation'. ('Health and Disease', *1973).* For the Christian healers, it was a duty to care for both the physical and spiritual well-being of the sick.

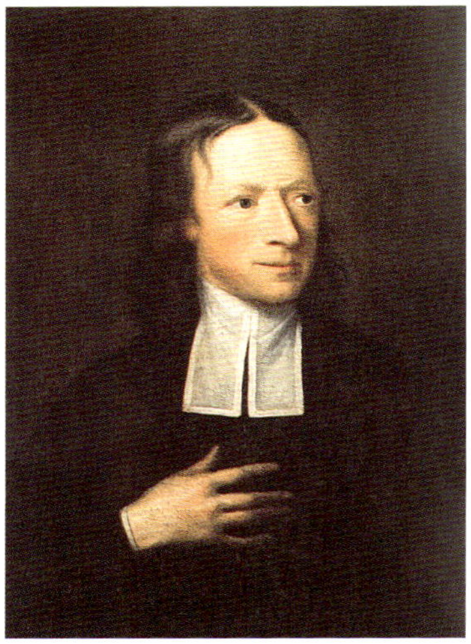

ABOVE The spiritual and physical healer, and founder of Methodism, John Wesley. The portrait by Robert Hunter dates from 1765.

Christian monasteries often provided hospice services, and 'cleric-physicians' have, for centuries, been the primary care givers in many communities. One such practitioner, the eighteenth-century founder of Methodism, John Wesley *(1703–1791)*, healed both the spiritual and physical ailments of his followers. He provided the lay public with a manual, *Primitive Physic (1747),* designed to be neither 'too dear for poor men to buy', nor 'too hard for plain men to understand'. His prescriptions contained 'only Safe and Cheap and Easy' ingredients so that any literate individual could compound medicines for his or her own use.

Nearly 2,000 years AD, spirituality as part of physical healing remains controversial. Numerous frauds have been exposed relating to faith healing and psychic healing. Still, many healers prescribe the power of prayer as part of their armoury. Recent support of spiritual healing in orthodox Western medicine is evident in a 1996 *Mayo Clinic Health Letter* report that 'a growing number of physicians are considering the idea that spiritual practices and beliefs might strengthen traditional medicine when accompanied by realistic expectations'.

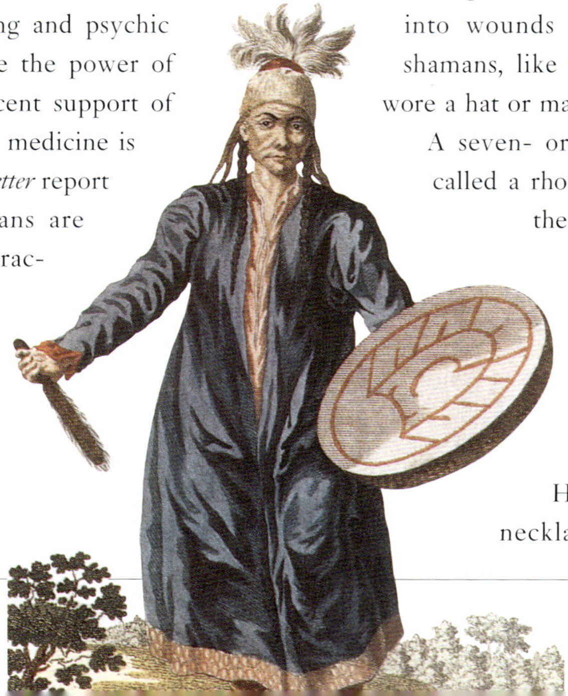

RIGHT Shamans feature in many healing traditions. This female figure is Russian; women shamans are also active in Native American cultures.

NATIVE AMERICAN HEALERS

Medicine men, or shamans, have been the primary healers in Native American culture. Throughout history, shamans were considered to be healers, sorcerers, seers, educators, and priests, thereby serving both medical and spiritual needs. Their god-given supernatural powers allowed them to cure the sick, perform ritualistic magic, impose their will upon others, and enlist the gods to ensure successful crops, hunts or village raids.

Either men or women could be shamans. One Apache woman became a shaman after surviving two mishaps, first being attacked by a mountain lion, and then being struck by lightning. Anyone who could survive such circumstances, the Apaches claimed, was thought to have the supernatural powers necessary for healing. Most shamans, however, achieved their positions through some type of apprenticeship.

The Ojibwa tribe, like many others, had several classes of medical personnel. The herbalists, many of whom were women, knew the medicinal properties of a wide range of plants, herbs, roots, and berries which he or she would apply to the sick for a fee. According to ethnographer Walter Hoffman, Ojibwa medicines were thought to be 'distasteful and injurious to the demons who are present in the system and to whom the disease is attributed' ('The Midé'wiwin or Grand Medicine Society', *1891*).

Shamans typically used the following tools in their trade: a special costume made of animal skins, a drum or rattle, a medicine bundle containing charms and healing amulets, 'medicine sticks' to serve as an offering, warning, or invitation, and a bag of herbs. He or she might also use a bleeding or scarifying instrument made of flint, obsidian, or snake fangs. Hollow bones were used for sucking out poisons, a mortar and pestle for mixing medicines, and a syringe for injecting medicine into wounds or giving an enema to patients. Some shamans, like the Apache Nan-ta-do-task, traditionally wore a hat or mask when performing healing rituals.

A seven- or eight-inch (18 or 20cm) piece of wood called a rhombus, bull-roarer, or whizzer was used by the Walapi, Pueblo, Zuni, Navajo, and Utes tribes. This wood was fastened to a horse-hair or leather thong and whirled rapidly above the head to invoke wind or rain, which was believed to enhance crops and cure the sick.

Medical necklaces were also used. High Wolf, a Cheyenne shaman, wore a necklace strung with eight left-hand middle

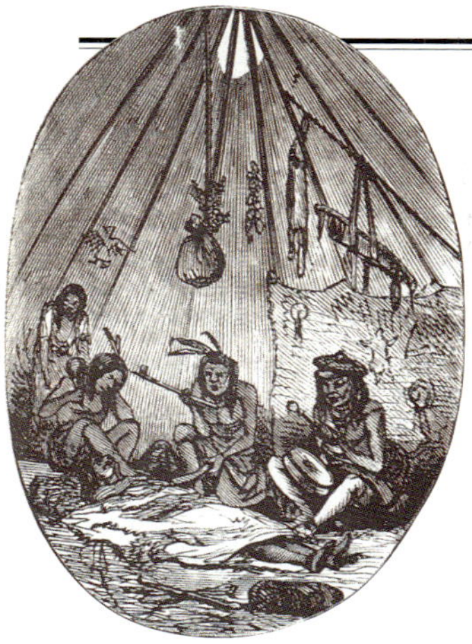

ABOVE Medicine Lodge from *Harper's Illustrated Weekly*, 1868. A patient is attended by a medicine man.

fingers from enemy warriors and five arrowheads which he had removed from his own body. This necklace, thought to possess supernatural powers, also contained four pouches made from human scrota.

From the spiritual healing viewpoint, the medicine bundle was the shaman's most important tool. It was made of animal skin and contained amulets like deer tails, dried fingers, and the maw (stomach, mouth or gullet) stone of a buffalo. The charms were used both to ward off evil and as healing agents. Healers offered a special chant over a bundle and over each of the articles contained inside. These precious bundles were handed down from father to son or to newly initiated shamans from their teachers.

Shamans have often successfully treated both native Americans and Caucasians. Anthropologists, physicians, and others have attributed much of this success to psychological factors including faith and the power of suggestion. Medical historian and ethnographer Erwin H Ackerknecht claimed that 'the participation of the community in the healing rites, and the strong connection between these rites and the whole religion and tradition of the tribe, produce certain psychotherapeutic advantages for the medicine man which the modern physician lacks' ('Primitive Medicine: A Contrast with Modern Practice', *1946).*

AFRICAN MEDICINE

Like healers in native American cultures, the African shamans serve as intermediaries between the material and spiritual worlds by seeking out the spiritual cause of physical and emotional problems. According to geographer Robert Voeks, African patients are thought to increase their susceptibility to health problems by straying from the 'cosmic equilibrium imposed by the spirit realm' ('African Medicine and Magic in the Americas', *1993).* They may also become inadvertent victims of direct intervention by dead ancestors or, more likely, of purposeful manipulation of the spirit realm by magicians or sorcerers. For example, if a doctor explains to a patient that she has malaria because she has been stung by a mosquito carrying malaria parasites, she would want to know why the mosquito stung her and not someone else. A typical reply would indicate that someone sent the mosquito to sting only her. Therefore, shamans need to discover the cause of the sickness, identify the 'criminal', diagnose the nature of the disease, apply the correct treatment, and ensure that the misfortune will not recur.

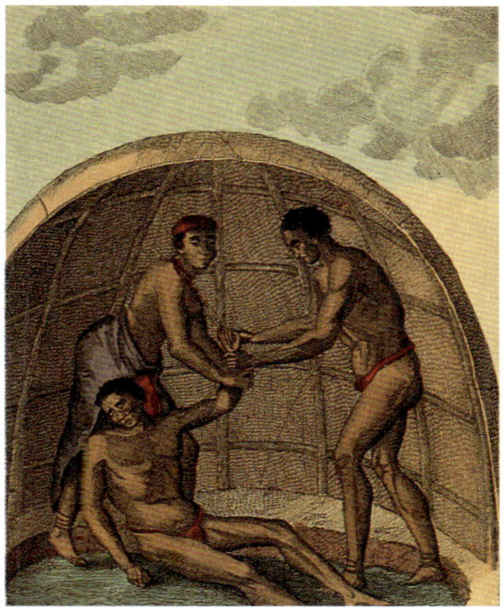

ABOVE African medicine combines physical with spiritual therapies. Here a medicine man is operating on a man's hand.

Cures, whether to restore spiritual equilibrium or neutralize black magic, are obtained mostly through offerings to the ancestors and spirits, the observance of taboos and through fasting and seclusion. As part of their therapeutic regimen, shamans give massages, use needles or thorns, and bleed patients. They may jump over the patient, go into trances, recite incantations and use ventriloquism. They might also ask a patient to sacrifice animals. This is in addition to using medicine prepared from herbs, bones, and minerals.

INVOKING THE HOLY PEOPLE

Navaho Indians who exhibited 'asocial behavior' or violated 'sacred observances' upset the gods, whereupon they were inflicted with disease (Jim Faris, 'Visual Rhetoric: Navajo Art and Curing', *1986).* Accordingly, since humans brought disease upon themselves, they appealed to the Holy People to cure their disorder. The healing process of calling upon the Holy People included prayers, songs, dances, and paintings made from sand. Holy People had the power to forgive transgressions, whereby health was restored. Healing ceremonies such as the nine-day Nightway were used to cure physical disorders including blindness, deafness, paralysis, headache, as well as various mental problems. In the Nightway the shamans instructed other members of the tribe to produce a dry sand painting. Later, sand from the painting was applied to the patient. The healing ceremony also included the use of sacred cigarettes, prayer sticks, topically applied and ingested medicine, massages, and sweat baths.

According to Swiss minister and professor John Mbiti's *African Religion and Philosophy (1990)*, African shamans are considered the 'greatest gift' to their societies. Every African village has a shaman nearby who is accessible to everyone at almost all times. There is no standard age for a 'calling' to become a shaman; the calling may come when one is young or old. Sometimes shamans pass their position on to a son, daughter, or other relative. In a way that recalls the ethical strictures of the Hippocratic Oath, they are expected to be trustworthy, morally upright, friendly, willing and ready to serve, able to discern people's needs, and not to charge excessive fees. These claims are based upon the practices of shamans in the Gold Coast, Nigeria, the Congo, Angola, Madagascar and South Africa. Shamans have also practised for a considerable time in other African countries south of the Sahara.

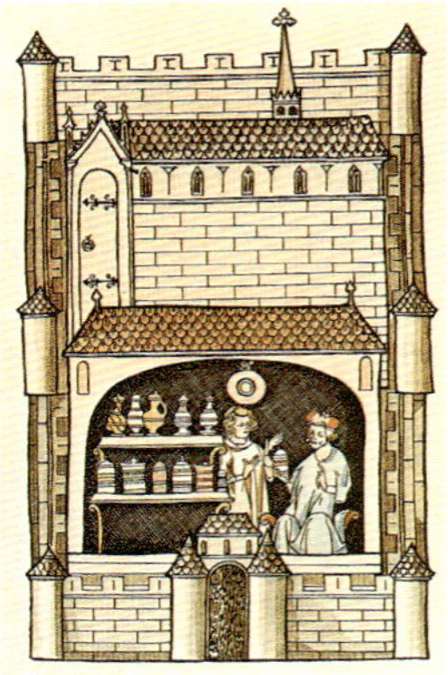

ABOVE Biographical details of Trotula are scant, but she is known to have written extensively on women's health, obstetrics and midwifery. The historian Kate Campbell Hurd-Mead believes that she is one of the figures depicted in this illustration of the medical school at Salerno in Italy.

WOMEN HEALERS

Many women are celebrated among ancient healers, but two particular women of the medieval period deserve special consideration. One of these was the eleventh-century Italian physician Trotula. Although little is known about her private life and only fragments of her original manuscripts exist, Trotula is known for composing the first complete work on women's health. This work, *De passionibus mulierium (On the sufferings of women)*, remained the authoritative writing on the subject for over 700 years. Trotula, also known as Trotta, Trocta, Trotolla di Rugerio, and Eros was a practically-oriented physician. Her diagnoses were based on careful observations of urine, pulse and facial expression, and she taught her students to use the same methods. She believed in making her patients comfortable and prescribed only the medicines that they could afford.

OBEAH MEN

There are a variety of shamans in African cultures called, variously, myal, conjure doctors, voodoo practitioners, and obeah men. *Obeah* is derived from the word *obayi* which means 'witchcraft' in the Akan language of Ghana, West Africa. An obeah man casts spells and sells deadly charms. One expert commentator, Donald Hogg, writing in 1961 in his book on magic and science in Jamaica, provided the following observations:

> *The obeah man employs ghosts as active agents, using the materials and spells to summon them, aid them and supplement their efforts. He secures the services of these spiritual assistants by performing various rituals over the bones of dead men, and in return for their help he feeds them, houses them in altars, and pays them for each job with rum, silver, and often sacrificial feasts. Each obeah man has several such ghostly partners, with whom he maintains intimate and permanent relations.*
>
> DONALD W HOGG, *MAGIC AND SCIENCE IN JAMAICA*

> *When you reach the patient, ask where the pain is, then feel his pulse, touch his skin to see if he has fever, ask if he has a chill, and when the pain began, and if it was worse at night, watch his facial expression, test the softness of his abdomen, ask if he passes urine freely, look carefully at the urine, examine his body for sensitive spots, and if you find nothing ask what other doctors he has consulted and what was their diagnosis, ask if he ever had a similar attack and when. Then, having found the cause of his trouble, it will be easy to determine the treatment.*
>
> TROTULA

Trotula also composed one of the first paediatric treatises, as well as completing a work on skin disease which contains one of the first descriptions of the outward manifestations of syphilis.

Another women healer of note was Hildegard von Bingen. In 1098, Hildegard was born in Germany near Bingen on the Rhine. At the age of eight, she was sent to study under her Aunt Jutta, an abbess at Disibodenburg on the Nahe River, where she learned German and Latin. According to medical historian Kate Campbell Hurd-Mead's *History of Women in Medicine (1938)*, Hildegard's abbey companions claimed that she 'miraculously cured all diseases'. Although she had described having strange daydreams or visions since childhood, her spiritual gifts were not fully recognized until she gained a position within the church. When she was 30 years old, she was chosen to succeed her aunt as abbess, and she began writing medical and psychological treaties as well as hymns, prophesies and religious instructions. After 1163, Hildegard began writing medical books, including *Causae et curae (Causes and cures)*, a work on holistic healing, and *Physica*, a natural history of man, animals and plants. Although Hildegard did not attend medical school, her writings are considered to be among the most complete and greatest medical works of the Middle Ages. Despite what may be considered as a distorted sense of anatomy, many of her ideas became more fully appreciated long after her death.

HILDEGARD'S REMEDIES

Hildegard attributed all of her medical knowledge to God. Knowledge about the medicinal properties of plants was regarded as a manifestation of God's way of revealing special healing gifts to mankind. Among her own medical remedies, Hildegard prescribed a concoction of peony, carline thistle, galgant and pepper to cure stomach pains, and the cooked womb of a cow or sheep to correct a woman's infertility. She also described cures for paralysis, fevers and mental diseases such as epilepsy, always relying heavily on herbs, plants, and most especially, God for these cures. Revered by popes and kings in her own day, scholars have only recently begun to recognize her importance.

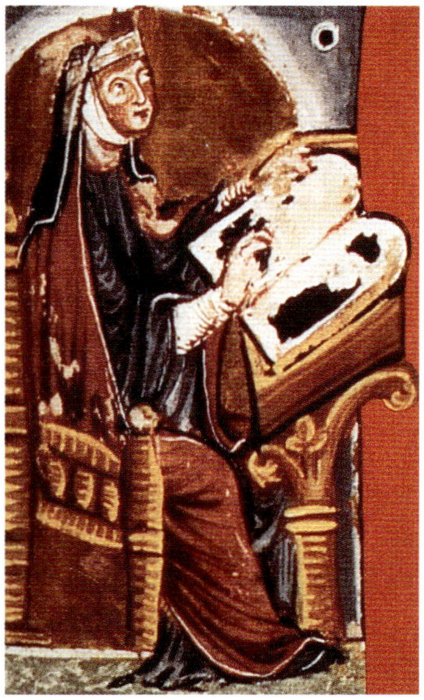

ABOVE Hildegard von Bingen was a mystic and visionary who also wrote an influential book of natural and holistic healing entitled *Causae et curae*.

Women like Hildegard were quite rare among the healers. More typically, women who were called to the healing arts practised midwifery. Midwives such as Shiphrah and Puah are mentioned in the Bible for their role in delivering and protecting Moses. Later we find people such as Louyse Bourgeois, who wrote *Observations*, a book on midwifery, in 1609, and also delivered French kings. The majority of midwives, however, attended the births of poor and middle-class women. In 1671, physician William Sermon claimed that a midwife should possess the following qualities:

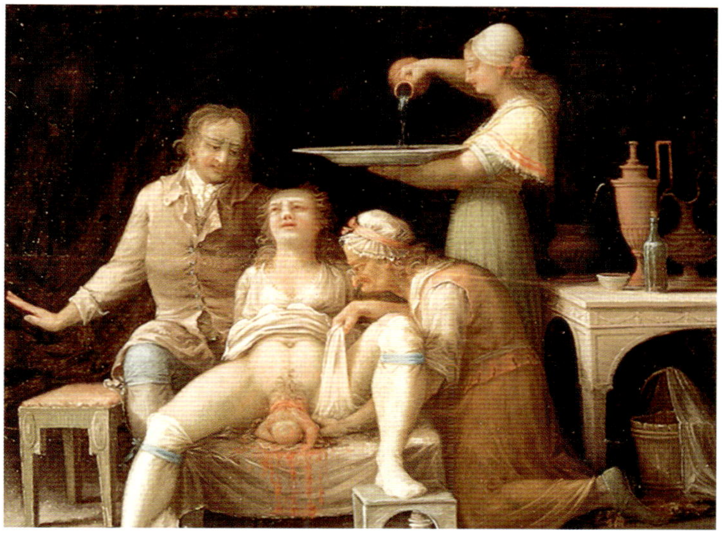

ABOVE Before the establishment of formal schools of midwifery, most women in labour were attended by midwives who had often learned their skill from their forebears.

> *As concerning their Persons, they must be neither too young, nor too old, ...well composed, not being subject to diseases, nor deformed in any part of their body... their hands small, and fingers long ...Touching their deportment: they must be mild, gentle, courteous, sober, chaste, and patient... As concerning their minds; they must be wise, and discreet....*
>
> WILLIAM SERMON, *LADIES COMPANION*

Midwives generally gained their know-how through informal apprenticeships. Most midwives were illiterate and learned their skill through oral tradition while assisting a more experienced midwife. The only standard requirement was that a midwife should already have children. Most midwives were married, middle-aged women who followed their mother's practice. In addition to attending routine deliveries, midwives were required to extract and baptize any child whose mother died in childbirth. Laws prohibited them from inducing abortions and from concealing any births of children by unmarried mothers.

THE HUMAN BODY AND CULTURAL EXCHANGES BETWEEN HEALING TRADITIONS

THE HUMAN BODY

One difference in the cultural responses to 'illness' and 'disease' stems from various views of the human body. From the earliest recorded history, humans have expressed keen interest in the structure and function of the body.

One Roman physician, Galen of Pergamum, *(AD ?131–201)* dissected and vivisected a variety of animals during the second century AD to further his knowledge of anatomy and physiology. Among his experiments, he opened the arteries of living animals in order to examine blood flow and tied the ureters (i.e., the tubes connecting the kidneys with the bladder) of live animals to prove that urine came from the kidneys. Again using live animals, he separated the spinal cord at different locations in order to determine what types of paralysis occurred in them.

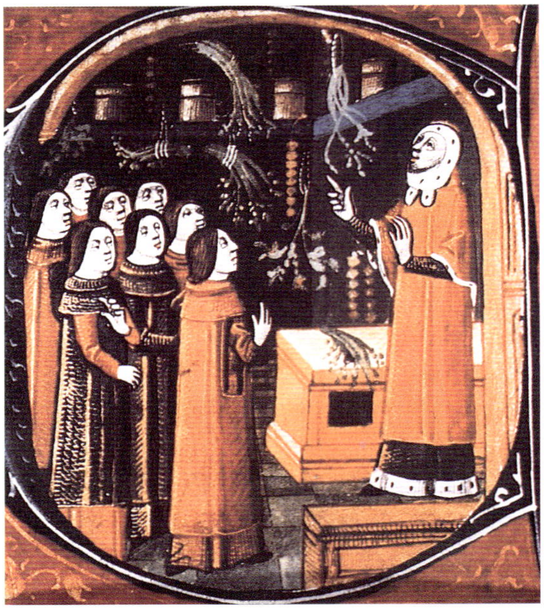

ABOVE **Galen, the foremost Roman physician. His medical philosophy and his medicinal compounds were deeply influential.**

Early in life, Galen was assigned to treat injured gladiators. The gladiators butchered one another in public arenas, and then the citizens fought for a piece of the dead gladiator's body. A segment of a gladiator's liver, for example, was thought to possess curative powers for epilepsy. Utilizing his position, Galen tested many different forms of surgical treatments. He found a tourniquet less likely to stop extreme bleeding than directly applying pressure to the vessel. If this still was not effective, he urged surgeons to 'grasp the part from which the outflowing blood is coming' with a hook and 'twist it around'.

Later in life, Galen devoted more time to writing philosophy. He gradually came to accept that the Creator of life was infinitely wise. He viewed every tissue, disease, and body function theologically as well as physiologically. The dualism implicit in this way of studying the body is evident in his book, *On the Usefulness of the Parts of the Body*. Uncovering the physical mystery of the human form was 'in no way inferior' to the pursuit of those initiated into some 'sacred rite'. Nor is the body 'less able' than priests to 'show forth the wisdom, foresight, and power of the Creator'. He urged readers to follow his discourse 'closely…as it explains the wonderful mysteries of Nature'.

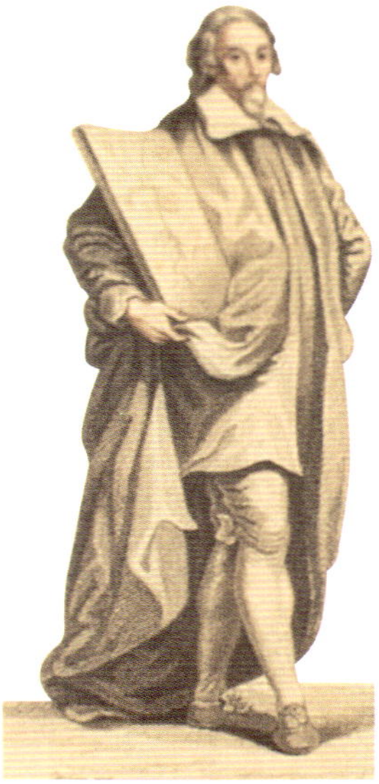

ABOVE **William Harvey drew a parallel between the human microcosm and the macrocosm of the universe.**

Medieval and Renaissance healers extended the Greek and Roman anatomical notion of the human body as 'an image in miniature of the Cosmos itself'. In diagnosing and treating disease, medieval physicians relied upon 'Zodiac Men' images, in which each zodiacal sign in the heavenly bodies was thought to hold special curative power over a corresponding part of the human body. In the Renaissance, selecting the site for blood-letting, for instance, might be based upon the understanding of a particular heavenly constellation's influence. British physician William Harvey *(1578–1657)* popularized the macrocosm/microcosm analogy in his conceptualization of the heart as the centre of a circulating system of life-sustaining blood, much like the life-giving Sun at the centre of the Copernican universe.

During the Renaissance, dissection became increasingly important in the training of physicians and surgeons. The obsession with obtaining an internal view of the human form reflected contemporary thought. Renaissance philosophy directed individuals to turn their gaze away from scholastic writings towards the inner make-up of the natural world. Nature's secrets, they claimed, would be revealed by peeling away its structure layer by layer. Renaissance physicians used anatomical dissection to identify signs or reference points of the inner physiological working of humans that were not always visible on the surface. This display also allowed them to view nature's 'parts' directly, interpreting correlations between anatomical structure and physiological function for themselves without being constrained by tradition to follow only ancient doctrine.

Dissection gradually led some healers to adopt a 'soul-less' view of the human body. The human body, according to Enlightenment French physician Julien Offroy de La Mettrie *(1709–1751)*, is 'a machine that winds its own springs: the living image of perpetual movement'. The growing man-machine image stemmed primarily from the work of French philosopher René Descartes *(1596–1650)*. In *L'homme machine*, Descartes depicted man as a dynamic, physiologically functioning machine. Blood circulated, food was digested and humans reproduced via purely mechanical means. The body was composed of material parts which worked together according to physical, mechanical laws. According to some accounts, God acted as the engineer behind this great terrestrial machine. The question remained, however, as to whether God could intervene at any stage of malfunction or whether humans functioned entirely by a predetermined course or by free will. Healers who intervened with God's work in order to fix the broken machine were sometimes charged as atheists.

Particular views of the human body have also shaped ideas about who was eligible to practise medicine. For women to become physicians in modern Western culture, they had to gain admission into recognized educational programmes. At the close of the nineteenth century, the prevailing medical view, as Harvard physician Edward Clarke vividly described in *Sex in Education; or, A Fair Chance for the Girls* (1873), was that a woman's 'reproductive machinery' could not become fully 'manufactured' if she pursued academic studies. Clarke argued that the 'force' needed for reproductive development would be diverted to the brain. The male-dominated medical profession used this argument to restrain women from pursuing higher education in order to preserve the state of the family and society; only a privileged few sat the qualifying exams in Switzerland (1865) and Germany and France (1869).

In contrast, women were included in the very first class of osteopathic medical training, which was held in 1892 at the American School of Osteopathy (ASO) in Kirksville, Missouri. Andrew Taylor Still *(1828–1917)*, the founder of osteopathy and the ASO, was a firm believer in the equality of the sexes. To Still, women had proved that 'if man is the head of the family, his claim of superiority must be in his muscles and not his brain'. He noted that women performed 'well in the [Osteopathic] classes, clinics, and practice', and proved 'as well worthy of diplomas as any gentleman'.

By 1900, the machine-image of bodily workings became more popularly known as the 'human motor'. Andrew Taylor Still shared this view of the body working as a motor-driven machine. He incorporated motorized machine imagery within the actual practice of osteopathy. His use of mechanical leverage, manipulating bones as levers to relieve pressure on nerves and blood vessels within the human frame, formed the foundation of osteopathic medicine. All 'remedies necessary to health', Still exclaimed, 'exist in the human body'. They can be efficaciously 'administered by adjusting the body in such condition that the remedies may naturally associate themselves together ...and relieve the afflicted'.

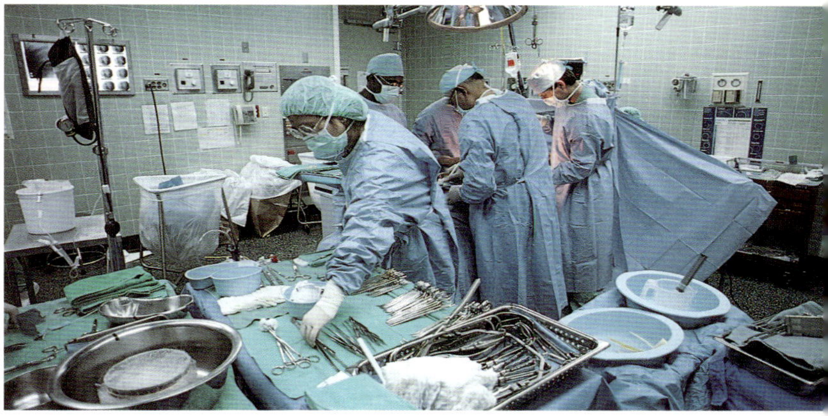

ABOVE Transplant surgery presupposes a Cartesian view of the body as a machine made up of replaceable parts.

Although confronted by opponents on many fronts, the mechanical, man-machine image of the body overcame the opposition and continues to be upheld by many healers today. Perhaps the most visible manifestation of this presupposition lies in the robot-like devices used in contemporary clinical practice. Supportive 'vital' functions have been taken over by iron lungs, artificial limbs, mechanical hearts and kidneys, as well as skin grafts and 'living organ' transplants. The body, once viewed as ideally individual, has become an assemblage of replaceable units. As medical science has discovered further uses for human organs, tissues, and cells, the human body has become, in a sense, public property. As Russell Scott argued in *The Body As Property (1981)*, citizens are viewing it more as a 'duty' to make their dead bodies available for the aid of the living. Claims upon the dead have already become something of a public entitlement, and the human body is, in some countries, a marketable commodity.

More so than in any preceding century, twentieth-century ingenuity has resulted in a more complex understanding of human form. Technology has enhanced our power to visualize bodily components infinitely smaller than the naked eye could perceive. At such a microscopic level of visualization, the twisted chain ladder of our genetic code engineers our entire bodily make-up. With the discovery of the molecular structure of DNA in 1953, the mystery of our genetic selves began to unravel. Not only did this newly deciphered body give healers insight into the process of heredity, but within decades it offered the potential for creating 'more perfect' variations of living forms. Visualizing a perfectible level of humanness may empower some to re-engineer human form and function. Designer bodies, often imbued with Frankenstein-like forms, are one possible ramification of the Human Genome Project. This project, the largest funded international medical collaboration in history, is designed to map out all of the genes on each of the human chromosomes. While results of this project may unlock the secrets of previously incurable genetic afflictions, the ethics underlying human manipulation of human form has provoked many to question whether Aldous Huxley's 1932 *Brave New World* vision of humans created in high-tech hatcheries will be our twenty-first century reality. Such technological leaps have transformed the image of a healer.

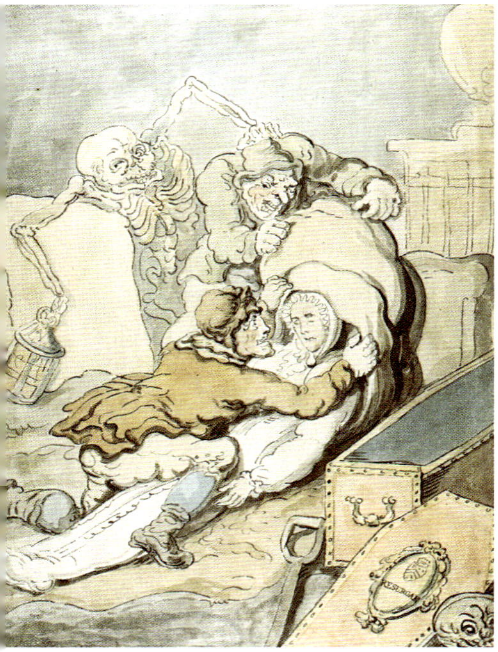

LEFT Such was the demand for bodies for anatomical dissection in England in the late eighteenth and nineteenth centuries that gangs of criminal 'bodysnatchers' grew up to supply the trade. They would dig up recently buried corpses and sell the bodies for dissection. The most notorious of these felons were Burke and Hare, who murdered people to provide specimens for Robert Knox's anatomy classes. This watercolour of bodysnatchers *(1775)* is ascribed to the artist Thomas Rowlandson.

THE FIRST HEART TRANSPLANT

Perhaps the best known episode of human engineering was the first human heart transplant. Christiaan Barnard *(1922–)*, an Afrikaner, spent several years in the 1950s developing techniques for open-heart surgery, correcting congenital heart malformations in children, and perfecting artificial heart valves. He secured a heart-lung machine which artificially oxygenated blood outside of the body and transported it back to the body, working in the place of the heart and lungs. This process increased the amount of time that surgeons could use in an open-chest operation.

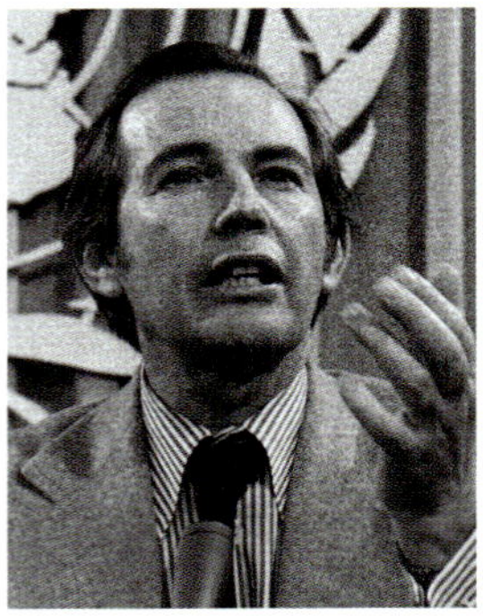

ABOVE A graduate of Cape Town medical school, Christiaan Barnard spent some time researching in the United States before returning to South Africa to practise surgery.

After perfecting the technique on dogs, Barnard performed a human heart transplant at Groote Schuur hospital in South Africa on 3 December 1967. His patient, the 55-year-old Lithuanian emigrant Louis Washkansky, had suffered a series of heart attacks in the previous seven years. When he was admitted to Groote Shuur in November 1967, doctors gave him only a few weeks to live. Washkansky survived until a suitable donor was found. The donor, 25-year-old Denise Darvall, had been hit by a car, was pronounced 'brain dead' and was placed on a respirator.

Washkansky survived the operation, but died 18 days later from pneumonia. Still, the operation was deemed a success, and it opened the doors for the hundreds of lives annually saved by this technique today. The uniting of South Africans, Americans and Lithuanians allowed this frontier of medicine to reach fruition, and it demonstrates one way in which interactions between different cultures have contributed significantly to modern medicine.

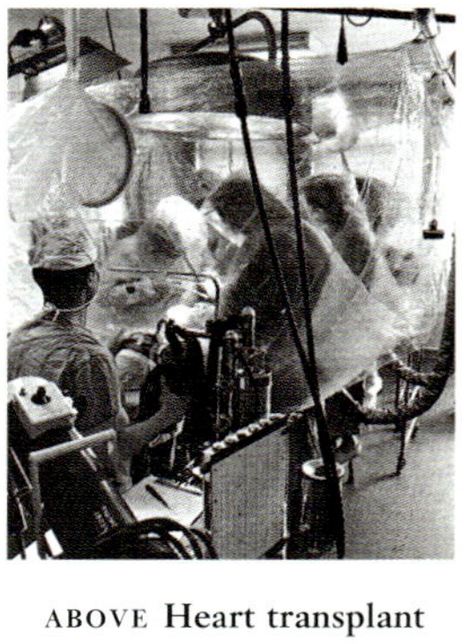

ABOVE Heart transplant surgery was headline news in the 1960s. Today the technique is routinely used to save lives.

CULTURAL EXCHANGES BETWEEN HEALING TRADITIONS

Cultural exchanges between different theories and practices of healing have existed for centuries.

One example, the Persian physician Avicenna (ibn Sina) *(980–1037)*, often called Islam's 'Prince of Physicians', practised humoral medicine in the eleventh century. He was the first scholar to create a complete philosophical system in the Arabic language, and he claimed that logic was a better guide to medical success than first-hand investigation. His *Canon of Medicine*, written for general practitioners, was an encyclopedia of medicine that served as an authoritative text in multiple language translations throughout Europe until the 1500s. It included diagnostic methods based on urine samples and the pulse, techniques for blood-letting, and prescriptions for preventative medicines.

Moses Maimonides *(?1135–1204)*, a pupil of the Arab medieval physician-philosopher Averroës (ibn Rushd) *(1126–1198)*, developed a medical practice using components of both Greek and Galenic traditions. An itinerant practitioner, travelling from Cordoba to Egypt, Maimonides ultimately worked as court physician to Saladin, Sultan of Egypt and Syria, providing him with advice on personal hygiene and dietetics. Most importantly, Maimonides integrated natural philosophy and medicine into Jewish culture. Jewish medical institutions around the world today still recognize the importance of the name Maimonides.

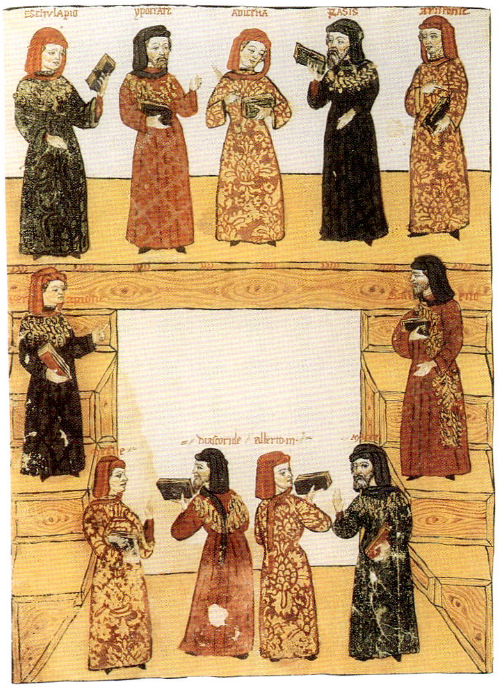

ABOVE The frontispiece of a fifteenth-century Italian manuscript showing the fathers of Western medicine. Avicenna (ibn Sina) is top centre.

One unlikely practitioner, explorer Álvar Núñez Cabeza de Vaca *(?1490–?1556)*, was instrumental in transporting Old World medicine to the New World. In 1527, Cabeza de Vaca left Spain with explorer Pánfilo de Narváez for the planned conquest of Florida. After having fought disease and natives in Florida's interior, the expedition departed in an attempt to reach the Spaniards already in Mexico.

The destitute party, now with Cabeza de Vaca in command, followed the Gulf coast and landed at present-day Galveston, Texas. Cabeza de Vaca recorded that they were 'so emaciated we could easily count every bone and looked the very picture of death' *(Cabeza de Vaca's Adventures in the Unknown Interior of America, 1988)*. Natives began to care for these woeful men. Soon, half of these Indians were dead from a disease thought to have been acquired from the Spaniards They planned to kill the disease-bearers until one Indian reasoned: if the Spaniards indeed had the power to kill the Indians with this disease, why would they have let so many of their own die en route? The Indians suddenly viewed the Spaniards as healers.

Cabeza de Vaca claimed that 'their method of cure is to blow on the sick, [whereby] the breath and the laying-on of hands supposedly casting out the infirmity. They insisted we should do this too and be of some use to them. We scoffed at their cures and at the idea that we knew how to heal.' To encourage their compliance, the Indians denied the Spaniards food until they acquiesced. This presented a religious dilemma to the Spaniards. According to their Catholic faith, they would lose their souls for practising pagan rituals. However, not complying with the Indians would cost them their mortal lives. The solution? They combined Catholicism with the Indian healing ceremony. 'Our method', according to Cabeza de Vaca, 'was to bless the sick, breathe upon them, recite a paternoster and Ave Maria and pray earnestly to God our Lord for their recovery.' Their method worked.

As time passed, the Spaniards once again became ill, and the tribes lost faith in their healing powers. They were enslaved but later escaped and were peacefully taken in by a tribe near present-day Austin, Texas. There the Spaniards were housed with the medicine men, because the Indians had 'heard of us and the wonders our Lord worked by us'. By the first evening, people were already asking to be healed by the Spaniards.

Despite having left Europe to conquer foreign lands, Cabeza de Vaca gained high regard for native Americans. Several years later, when Coronado's expedition passed through what is now New Mexico, native people sang the praises of Cabeza de Vaca, a 'great doctor … who gave blessings [and] healed the sick'.

AFRICAN MEDICINE

African medical beliefs travelled to the Americas when Europeans shipped slaves to their colonies, notably during the seventeenth and eighteenth centuries. The Africans brought their knowledge of traditional healing practices with them from their homeland and later borrowed successful herbs and techniques from the European and Amerindian cultures that they encountered in the New World. Slave medicine, therefore, was created by a blending of cultures.

A variety of healing practices developed among Afro-Caribbean cultures. The variations were partly due to differences in natural geography. 'Coastal medicine', for instance, employed the use of sea water and evoked the spirits of the sea to assist in healing. This was distinct from 'highland medicine', which was strictly based on the herbs and folklore of mountainous regions.

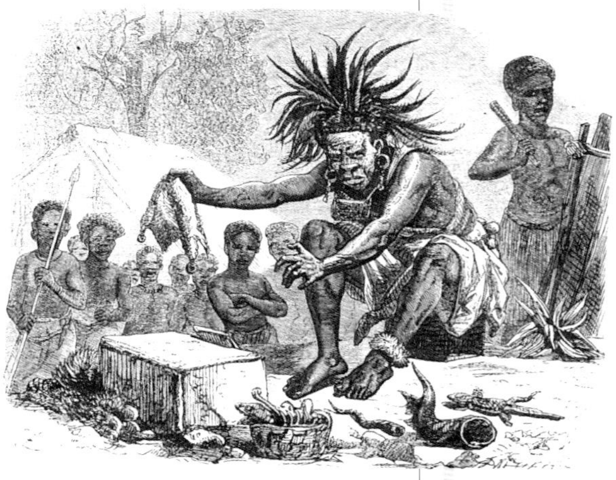

ABOVE An African shaman casts out a demon. The slave trade carried African medicine to the Americas.

In Barbados, slaves kept their medical knowledge 'a secret from the white people, but preserve[d it] among themselves by tradition with which they sometimes perform notable cures', according to William Hillary's *Observation on the Changes of the Air and the Concomitant Epidemical Diseases in the Island of Barbadoes (1766).* In *Afro-Caribbean Folk Medicine (1987),* author Michel Laguerre posited other reasons why slave practitioners kept their medical practice private. They did so, he argued, 'to avoid being the victim of the master's hostility and also because of the role of the healer as someone who could both cure and hex'.

Still, some Caucasians sought care from slave practitioners. In Brazil, some of the aphrodisiacs, philtres and fertility agents of the Africans were desired by white slave masters. Roman Catholics in Venezuela asked African shamans to exorcize the devil from their parishioners.

African medicine retains its presence in the Western hemisphere today. Pocomania healers in Jamaica treat patients with African-derived herbal baths and infusions combined with Christian prayers. Umbanda medicine now has followers in much of Brazil; Obeah magic has spread from Jamaica to Panama, Belize, Florida, and the Bahamas.

MEDICINE AND VOODOO

Typically, the slave medical practitioners served their societies in a threefold role. First, they were the ones to whom slaves turned for treating illnesses which white doctors could not treat. They also were capable of inflicting illnesses upon other individuals by casting spells. Finally, they could effectively remove spells or hexes that had been cast upon an individual. These practitioners came to be known under a variety of names including hoodoo doctors in the United States, voodoo priests in Haiti, myal and obeah men in the Anglophone Caribbean Islands and quimboiseurs, magicians or conjurers in the French Antilles.

In the 1790 Haitian revolution, the high priest Boukman performed voodoo chants and rituals to immunize his followers against the 'white man's magic'. His work was successful; the French army was eventually defeated, reinforcing local belief in voodoo medicine. In South Carolina, the African-born shaman Gullah jack was an important conspirator in the Vesey slave revolt of 1822. However, the failure of his magic may have weakened the faith of his followers.

JAPANESE MEDICINE

Another cultural exchange between healing traditions is found in the development of Japanese medicine. Traditional Chinese medicine had long been practised in Japan, where it was known as *Kanpo.* The 52-volume Chinese herbal, *Pên- ts'ao-kang-mu,* was a particularly useful medical guide. Western medicine reached Japan beginning in 1600 with the Dutch who congregated on Deshima, the small 'going-out' island in Nagasaki Bay. The Jesuit missionary physician, Christavaõ Ferreira – known to the Japanese as Sawano Chuan – compiled information about Western surgery in several seventeenth-century Japanese treatises. However, the earliest work of lasting influence was Narabayashi Chinzan's *Kōi geka sōden (Surgery Handed Down),* published in 1706. Narabayashi borrowed extensively from the well-known Renaissance surgical writings of the Frenchman Ambroise Paré *(c.1510–1590)* and incorporated insights from his own study under Willem Hoffman, the Dutch physician at Deshima from 1671 to 1675.

Hollander Wilhelm Ten Rhyne *(1647–1700)* was the first physician at Deshima to describe his professional experiences with *Kanpo* in the seventeenth century to Eastern readers; most importantly, he provided detailed descriptions of acupuncture and moxibustion. After perusing key Western anatomical writings and acquiring a working knowledge of Dutch, two Japanese physicians, Maeno Ryōtaku and Sugita Gempaku, translated Johann Adam Kulmus' *Ontleedkundige Tafelen (Anatomical Tables)* into the Japanese *Kaitai Shinsho (A New Book of Anatomy)* in 1774. According to Akihito, the current Emperor of Japan, himself a scientist by training, the elaborately illustrated *Kaitai Shinsho* was crucial, as it 'revealed errors in Chinese medical books that had previously been the sole source of information for Japanese physicians and illustrated the importance of learning by direct observation and of having an open mind' ('Early Cultivators of Science in Japan', *Science, 1992).* Dutch physician Carl Pieter Thunberg, a disciple of Linnaeus, introduced a systematic study of materia medica to Japan, a country whose physicians he claimed were 'very little acquainted with the remedies which they prescribe' *(Travels in Europe, Africa, and Asia, 1795-96).*

Of all Western healers, Philipp Franz von Siebold's *(1796–1866)* influence in Japan has been the most enduring. Soon after his arrival in Japan in 1823, Siebold claimed not to find an illness that Japanese healers' 'lack of skill' had 'not aggravated or worsened'. Thereupon, he set out to 'systematically teach and demonstrate' the benefits of Western medicine to them, explicitly deploring the diagnoses and treatments of *Kanpo* medicine. Siebold, known in Japan as Shiboruto, through both his direct influence and that of his pupils, established Western medical education in Japan. His legacy forged, as his epitaph states, 'such a strong bridge' between healers of the East and West.

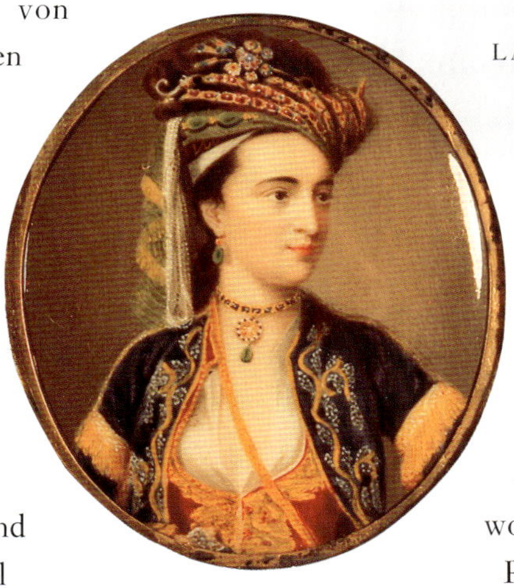

ABOVE **Lady Mary Wortley Montagu, an early proponent of the benefits of inoculation against smallpox.**

LESSONS FROM THE MIDDLE EAST

Elsewhere in the world, the West gained great benefit from an understanding of healing practices in the Middle East. Smallpox was the plague of the eighteenth century with a mortality rate over 50 per cent. No one was immune. Mary, Queen of England contracted it in 1694, and France's Louis XV died from it in 1774. Those that survived were often hideously scarred.

Lady Mary Wortley Montagu *(1689–1762)*, wife of the British Ambassador to Constantinople, reported that severe attacks of smallpox in Turkey had been prevented by inoculations. She described this treatment in a letter to a friend dated 1717.

Apropos of distempers, I am going to tell you a thing that will make you wish yourself here. The smallpox, so fatal and so general among us, is here entirely harmless by the invention of engrafting, which is the term they give it.

There is a set of old women who make it their business to perform the operation every autumn in the month of September when the great heat is abated.... They make parties for the purpose... the old woman comes with a nut-shell full of the matter of the best sort of smallpox, and asks what veins you please to have open'd.

She immediately rips open ...and puts into the vein as much [smallpox] matter as can lie upon the head of her needle.

LADY MARY WORTLEY MONTAGU, LETTERS

After her return to Britain in 1722, Montagu had her children inoculated. Britain's King George I, acting under advice from physicians Hans Sloane *(1660–1753)* and Richard Mead *(1673–1754)*, offered freedom to incarcerated criminals who would test the effects of inoculation. Caroline, Princess of Wales, also grew interested in having her children inoculated, but first wanted the method tested on 50 charity children. Those inoculated exhibited a mild infection, but it was not fatal and did not scar. They appeared to be immune from smallpox. Although Montagu had no medical training, her elevated social position and careful observation introduced an early form of smallpox prevention. English physician Edward Jenner *(1749–1823)* modified this method with a process called vaccination, whereby he introduced a milder form of the related disease, cowpox, into uninfected patients beginning in 1796. This method of preventing smallpox became widespread throughout the world.

EVOLUTION OF 'MODERN' HEALING TRADITIONS

ALTERNATIVE OR COMPLEMENTARY MEDICINE

In the eighteenth and nineteenth centuries, much like today, many people searched for healers who promised cures that conventional medicine did not provide. Physicians at this time commonly used harsh practices and strong medicines to treat common complaints. Unsatisfied with the results, many people embraced new ideas ranging from electrical therapy to the power of suggestion. Some of these new practices focused simply on good hygiene or preventative medicine, whereas others promised cures for disease. Often, healers advocated a combination of therapeutic approaches to produce a healthier mind and body.

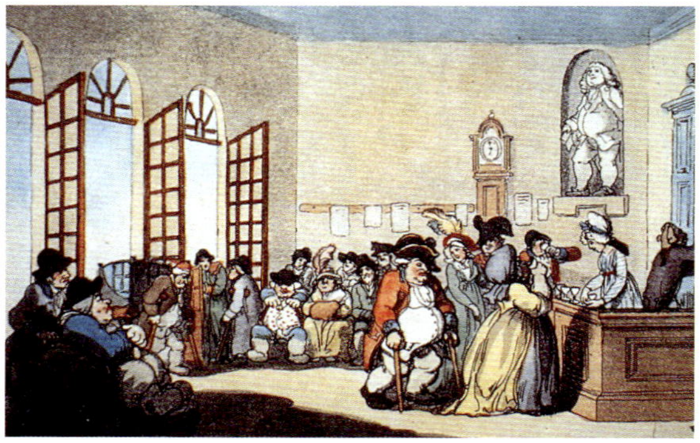

ABOVE Water cures, which had been practised in Roman Britain, gained popularity again in the eighteenth century. Taking the waters at Bath was both fashionable and therapeutic.

Some healers, like Franz Anton Mesmer *(1734–1815)*, resorted to nature to effect cures. In the eighteenth century, Mesmer considered that the movements associated with gravity and the tides resulted from a 'fluid permeating the entire universe and infusing both matter and spirit with its vital force' (Maria M. Tatar, *Spellbound: Studies on Mesmerism and Literature, 1978)*. He envisioned similar fluids flowing through the body and employed magnets in an effort to remove any bodily barriers which, by disrupting the flow, caused pain or nervous disorders. Later, he held fashionable group sessions in ornately furnished treatment rooms in Paris where patients were gathered around a central tub filled with 'magnetized water'. Patients grabbed iron rods protruding from the sides of the tub, placing them near their diseased bodily part. During the treatment, many patients were supposedly 'cured' through a convulsive fit while others were 'mesmerized' into a hypnotic trance.

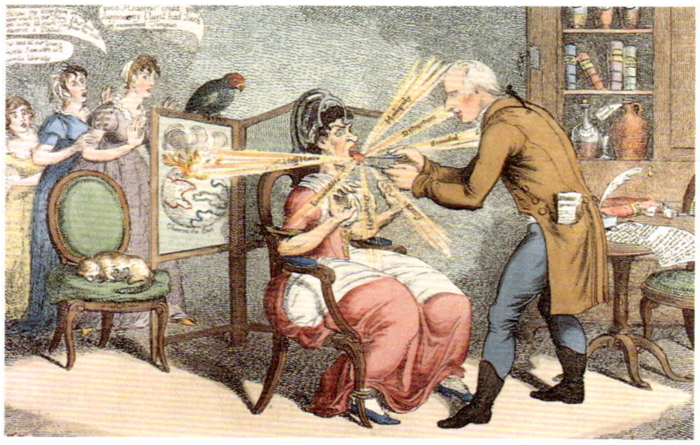

ABOVE An eighteenth-century cartoon by Thomas Rowlandson satirizing the enthusiasm of numerous self-authorized healers for electrical cures.

Water was a common component of other cures. Hydrotherapy used water, not to combat specific illnesses, but to enhance natural vitality in patients. In Europe, water therapy began as a cold-water cure; in the US, sitz baths, drinking mega-doses of mineral water and applying ice packs were all available options. People accepted hydrotherapy because it was natural and, when combined with other therapies, formed a complete 'hygienic system'. Hydrotherapy held particular appeal to women after Marie Louise Shew's publication of *Water-Cure for Ladies* in 1844. This magazine focused on women's health issues and popularized water cure in pre-natal care.

Viennese medical student, Franz Joseph Gall *(1758–1828)*, created the study of phrenology in the nineteenth century. He envisioned the brain as composed of 37 separate 'organs', each of which was responsible for a particular trait. These organs were organized into four categories or basic temperaments: vital, active, muscular, and nervous. Importantly, Gall believed that the size and shape of these organs could be modified and, therefore, the presence of a particular characteristic could be altered.

People embraced phrenology because of the possibility of controlling or reforming their personalities after a phrenological analysis. Travelling 'professors of phrenology' or 'bump doctors' gave lectures and analyzed heads across the country. The Fowlers (Orson, Lorenzo, Charlotte, her husband Samuel Wells and their children), a nineteenth-century family of famous lecturers, entertained their audiences while demonstrating their trade. They also composed the *American Phrenological Journal* and the widely read *Water-Cure Journal,* which linked water cures to

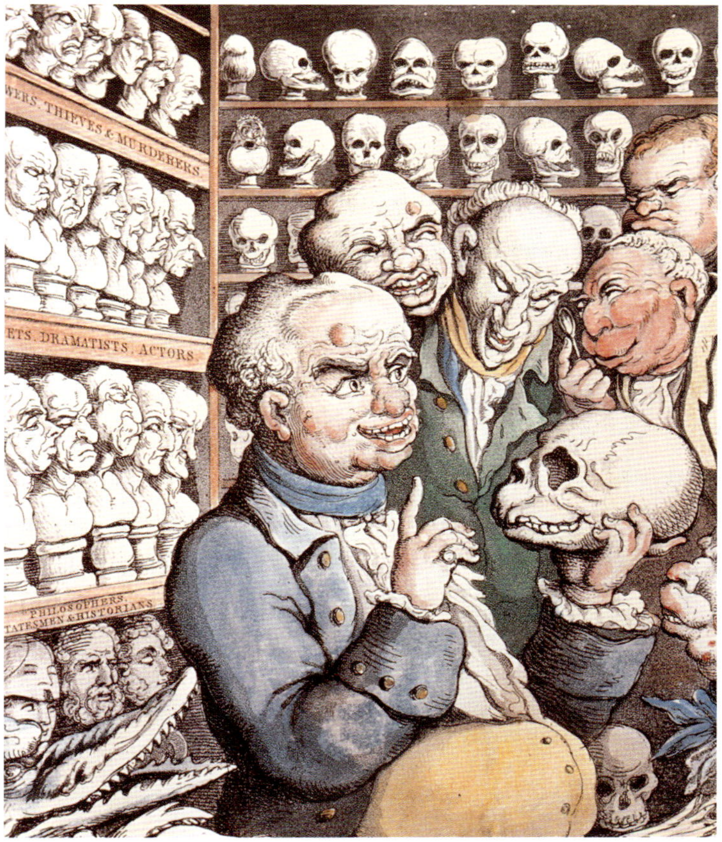

ABOVE **A caricature of Franz Joseph Gall, the inventor of the would-be science phrenology, which enjoyed quite a vogue in the nineteenth century.**

PATENT MEDICINES

Contrary to the expectation aroused by their name, patent medicines were not regulated for safety or effectiveness by government authorities. These medicines, which were particularly popular in the United States and Britain in the period between 1750 and 1930, were distinct for their striking advertising. Printed advertisements in magazines, newspapers, and even trading cards often used key words such as 'natural' or 'vegetable'.

One well-known remedy, Lydia E Pinkham's Vegetable Compound, pictured Lydia's own grandmotherly face on the label. This effective marketing ploy apparently made the compound seem natural and safe, even though it contained as much alcohol as most other popular cures. In the 1900s, the American Medical Association and federal food and drug acts contributed to the decline of patent medicines by demanding that proprietors support their claims and list the ingredients on the labels.

phrenology and other health reforms of the time. By the 1920s, phrenology had died out in the US due to criticism by the established medical community, the death of the first generation of Fowlers, and the emergence of Freudian theory.

In the 1800s, homeopathic medicine challenged the prevailing drug therapies. German physician Samuel Hahnemann *(1755–1843)* conducted experiments on himself and his family to determine the minimal concentrations of medicines needed to cure disease. He believed disease to be 'a disruption in the body's ability to cure itself', and he sought to administer the least concentration of a drug necessary to promote healing.

After the introduction of homeopathy into America in the 1820s, many physicians converted to homeopathy, and 22 schools taught Hahnemann's theory as written in the *Organon of Homeopathic Medicine (1810)*. A century later, those homeopathic colleges had been closed after coming under criticism from the American Medical Association and other policing organizations. Today, homeopathy has regained popularity in the United States and commands even larger followings in Great Britain, the Netherlands and India.

Mary Baker Eddy *(1821–1910)*, sickly since childhood, turned to alternative methods of healing, including mesmerism and homeopathy, seeking possible cures. While recuperating from a fall, she claimed to have actually healed herself through divine revelation after reading the Bible. Later, in 1875, she promoted her method of healing, Christian Science, through her book *Science and Health With Key to the Scriptures (1875)* and at her school, the Massachusetts Metaphysical College. Most of her 4,000 students who attended classes throughout the school's eight years of operation were women, possibly because women were typically precluded from conventional medical training.

Mrs Eddy taught that the 'divine mind' of the Deity worked through the healer and then to the patient. She also stated that the 'mental state prepares one to have any disease whenever there appear the circumstances which he believes produce it'. In other words, a patient is not sick, she only believes that she is sick. Mrs Eddy declared that 'malicious animal magnetism', or evil thoughts, could be directed toward the followers of Christian Science. Her followers, who compared Mrs Eddy to an earthly Jesus, grew from a small sect to an established church in the 1880s and 1890s. It remains an influential movement in many countries to the present day.

THE SEVENTH-DAY ADVENTISTS

The Seventh-Day Adventists were founded in 1836 in Michigan by a woman so opposed to orthodox medicine that she declared, 'If there was in this land one physician in place of thousands, a vast amount of premature mortality would be prevented.' Ellen Gould White *(1827–1915)* had faith in many therapies – the healing power of prayer, hydrotherapy, and phrenology – but she initially held no trust in physicians and their medications. Prone to visions, Ellen White claimed to have received a God-given message to found a religious following with strict dietary and health habits. She placed prohibitions among her followers on the consumption of tobacco, coffee, tea, alcohol, prescription drugs and hot spices. Sexual relations within the bounds of marriage were restricted to a minimum. Her accepted diet included fruit, vegetables, nuts and grains combined with a regime of outdoor exercise, fresh air and clean water. Distraught with contemporary female dress, she claimed women 'must dispense with heavy skirts and tight waists if they value health.' To meet this need, she devised her own lightweight bloomers.

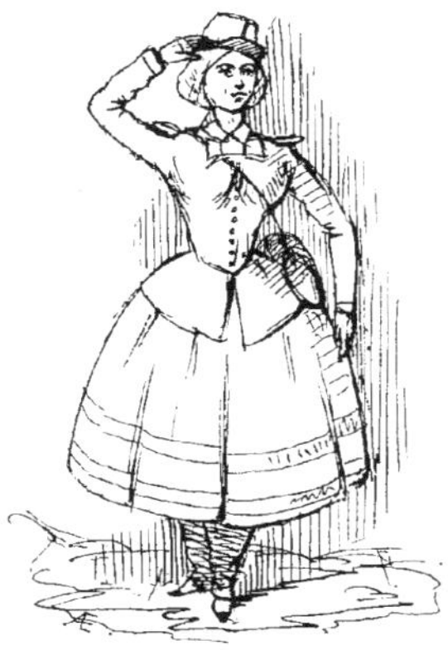

ABOVE **Women like Ellen Goukd White, founder of the Seventh-Day Adventists, campaigned to emancipate nineteenth-century women from restrictive clothing.**

In 1866, White established the Western Health Reform Institute outside Battle Creek, Michigan, and in 1878, the Rural Health Retreat in California's Napa Valley. Given the success of these institutions, she opened another Adventist sanitarium in Loma Linda, California, in 1905. Soon thereafter, having gained faith in the new standards of medical practice, she opened the College of Medical Evangelism to train Adventist physicians in Loma Linda in 1910. Today, the Adventists operate one of the largest Protestant health-care systems in the United States.

In the early years of the Adventists, White hired the young John Harvey Kellogg to help set type for her writings including *Health: Or, How to Live.* Kellogg, after medical training, became chief physician for the Western Health Reform Institute in 1876, changing its name to his own Battle Creek Sanitarium a year later.

DIETARY REGIMES AND HEALTHY EATING

Around the turn of the twentieth century, both JH Kellogg and CW Post promoted the cold, packaged cereals Cornflakes and Postum, respectively, as an alternative to the heavy, fatty foods Americans typically ate for breakfast. Physician John Harvey Kellogg also developed a health reform and treatment sanitarium in Battle Creek, Michigan *(see box)*. Known as the 'San', this institution, which was a combination of hospital, spa, and lecture hall, became popular with the wealthy.

Kellogg emphasized the importance of restricting diet, dress, alcohol, and sexual activity. He also expressed concern over preventing 'autointoxication', which caused constipation. He relieved this disorder through regimented diet and regular colonic irrigation, as well as surgery. He used ethical arguments, such as animal rights, and Biblical quotations to convince his patients to choose meatless meals. He also lauded the peformance of vegetarian athletes to demonstrate the benefits of their dietary choice.

BELOW **A fit-looking John Harvey Kellogg pictured in 1938 when he was 86. A living advertisment for the benefits of his dietary regimes, he lived to the advanced age of 91.**

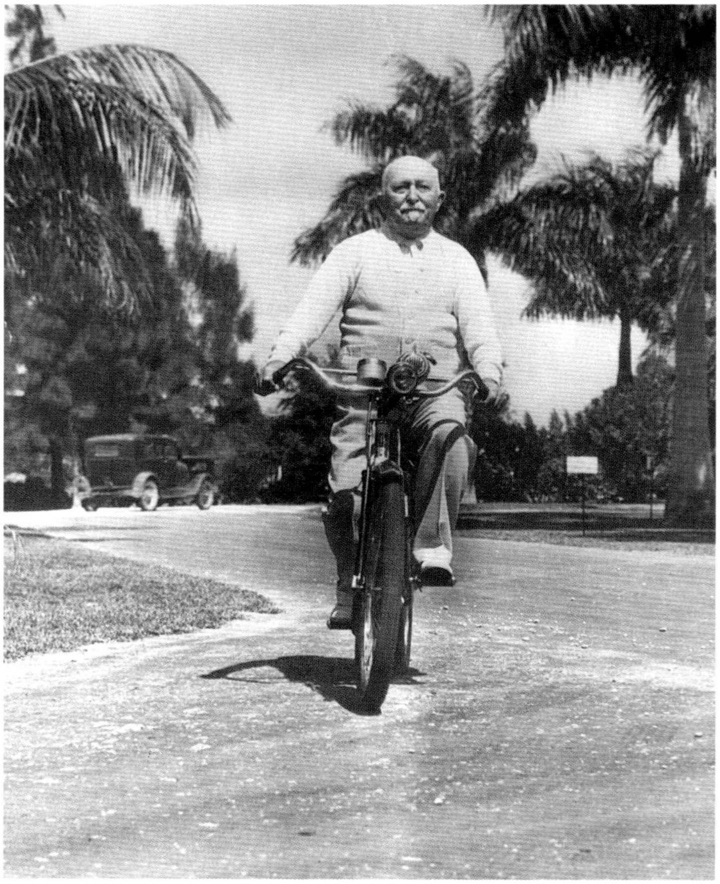

CHIROPRACTIC AND OTHER THERAPIES

In the final years of the nineteenth century, American Daniel David Palmer *(1845–1913)* claimed that the pain caused by a mis-aligned spine impinging upon the nerves could be relieved by manipulation. This theory became the educational basis of the Palmer School of Chiropractic, which he founded in Davenport, Iowa in 1899. (The name derives from the Greek words 'cheiro' and 'praktikos' meaning 'performed by hand'.) His son, BJ, helped spread chiropractic methods through advertisements, books, and the school's annual lyceum of entertainment and chiropractic knowledge. Although conventional or allopathic physicians have long criticized chiropractic practitioners or 'bonecrackers' on account of their lack of scientifically-based techniques, these healers have become so widely respected that today many health insurance companies are prepared to cover chiropractic care.

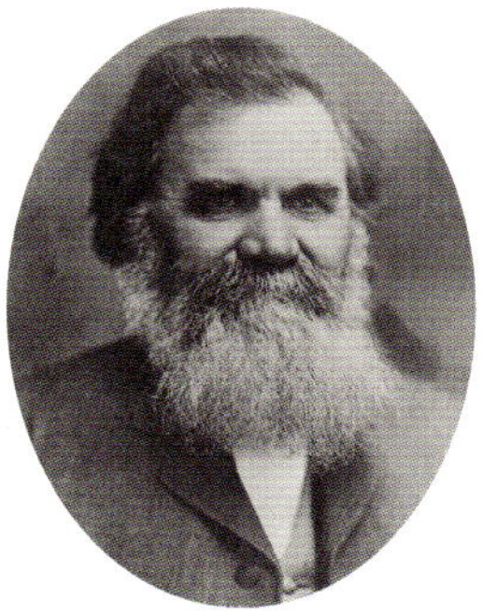

ABOVE Daniel David Palmer, the founder of a new form of therapy that he called chiropractic.

BELOW The nineteenth century was a time of firm belief in the therapeutic effects of mountain air. It was one of the reasons why sanitoria for tuberculosis sufferers were often sited up in the mountains. Its causative agent, the tubercle bacillus, was identified by Robert Koch in 1882.

In recent years, vitamins and antibiotics have become 'panaceas' or 'cure-alls' in the minds of many patients. Earlier in this century, oxygen was considered a similar 'cure-all'. Kansas City physician Orval J. Cunningham was concerned by reports that people in the US mountains generally succumbed to the influenza epidemic of 1918 that cost millions of lives across the world. This seemed paradoxical, for mountain air was considered to have exceptionally healthy qualities and was readily used in tuberculosis treatment.

To test the effect of oxygen, Cunningham began treating his patients with a variety of artificially-induced high pressures of this gas. His patients recovered, and he soon began using this therapy to treat a whole variety of conditions including arthritis, glaucoma, pernicious anaemia, syphilis, diabetes and cancer. Despite his own assiduous self-publicity, the national medical policing agencies found no scientific evidence to support his treatments.

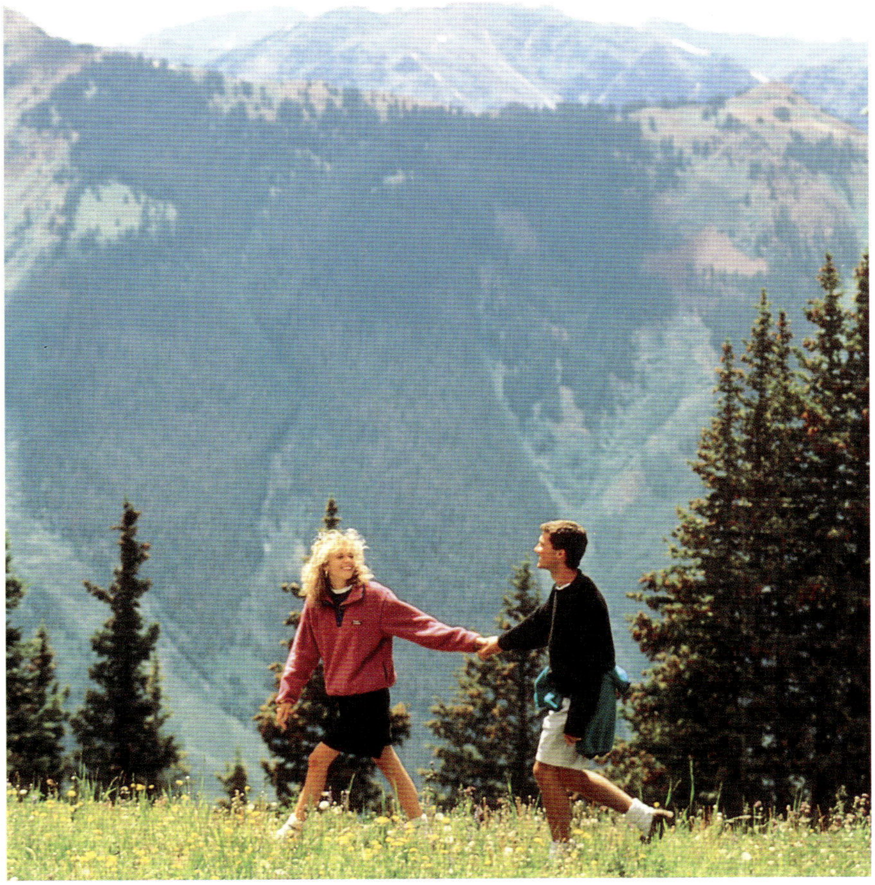

GOAT-GLANDS FOR HEALTH

In the search for youth and fertility, many men visited the office of physician John R. Brinkley in Milford, Kansas. Brinkley obtained 'glands' from goats and, in a brief surgical procedure, replaced or added this gland to the male testicles of his patients. Brinkley called this operation 'the goat-gland proposition'. Goats were chosen because of their ancient symbolism as lively, active animals. The operation was not promoted as a cure–all, but one that would treat high blood pressure, insanity, and skin diseases, as well as 'rejuvenating' the gland recipients.

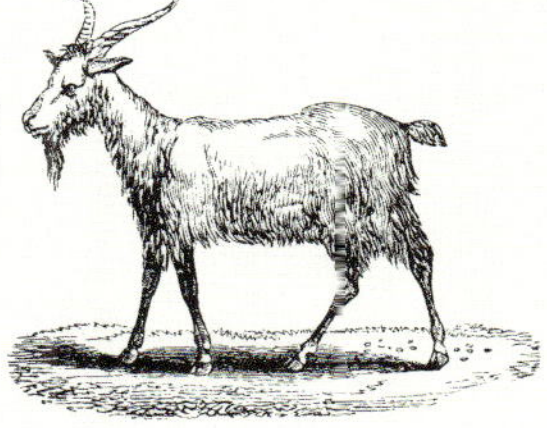

CURRENT CONTROVERSIES

During this last decade of the current millennium, controversy has arisen in the US reminiscent of the patent medicine venture a century ago. 1990s' investigative reports claim that 'medical mistreatment' is rife in nearly all of the Amish, Old Order Mennonite and Hutterite communities. Kansas City Star newspaper medical writer Alan Bavley argued in a 1996 account that the Amish, a group of 'plain people' who 'do a lot of physical labor, eat unprocessed food, rarely drink or smoke.... ought to be the picture of health'. Despite their predilection towards health, it is precisely these people, raised to follow their cultural values to 'trust, obey and submit', that are particularly susceptible to exploitation by modern day 'quacks'.

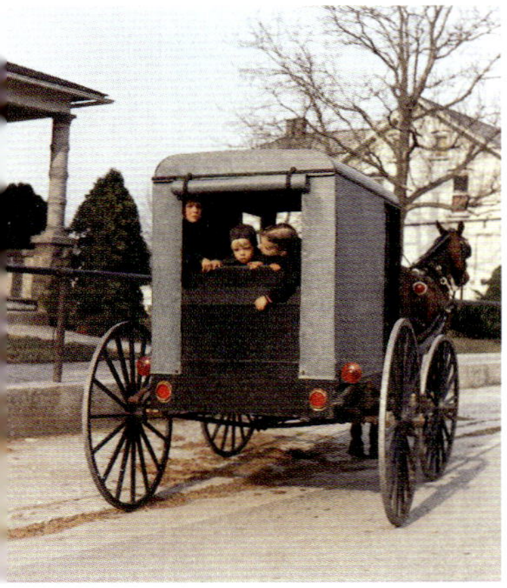

ABOVE Amish communities have, somewhat uncritically, embraced alternative therapies with enthusiasm.

The 'plain people' have readily accepted a wide variety of alternative medical therapies, including reflexology, iridology and naturopathy. They are often persuaded that colonic irrigation, mega-doses of vitamins and shark cartilage food supplements are the best way to sure health. One Amish grocery store proprietor, acting as the community healer, proffers 'health elixirs' made of blue-green algae, claiming that they will 'keep your brain working at its best'. Others have been lured south of the border, to the mecca of alternative medical treatment, Tijuana, Mexico. Here, patients may receive treatments from a variety of self-proclaimed healers. One such vendor, Geronimo Rubio of the American Metabolic Institute, touts a special cancer cure. Rubio draws a patient's blood, injects it into a goat, draws it from the goat and reinjects it as an 'anti-cancer serum' back into the patient.

Few have done more than American news journalist Bill Moyer – whether to his credit or his credulity – to advance the cause of alternative medicine. Moyer's television series, *Healing and the Mind*, which was screened in the United States in 1993, reinitiated a boom in alternative healing. Perhaps the best advice regarding the reputation of healers today is, 'When in doubt, check it out'. One source that investigates reputed fraudulent healers around the globe is the Health Claims Subcommittee of the Committee for the Scientific Investigation of Claims of the Paranormal in Amherst, New York.

MILITARY PRACTITIONERS

Throughout history, military personnel have made significant contributions to the healing arts. One example from the eighteenth century serves as a typical example. Scurvy killed many sailors aboard both commercial and military vessels at this time. English naval physician James Lind *(1716–1794)* composed a detailed account of the symptoms and prevention of this disease in his *Treatise of the Scurvy (1753)*. Lind concluded that an unbalanced diet was chiefly responsible for this sickness and that fresh fruit rations would balance sailors' diets, thereby preventing scurvy. In the 1770s, Captain James Cook expanded Lind's findings and noted other foods that also prevented scurvy on his three Pacific voyages. Although Lind's and Cook's experiments were quickly published, lemon juice did not become an obligatory preventative agent in the British Navy until 1795.

Another military healer, American Army Surgeon William Beaumont *(1785–1853)*, became interested in food, particularly the process of human digestion. Beaumont was fortunate to be presented with an extraordinary view of digestion entirely unavailable to others. Alexis St Martin, one of his private patients, received a gaping shotgun wound to his stomach that never fully healed, enabling Beaumont to observe the workings of the stomach first-hand. Given this literal insight into digestion, Beaumont performed numerous experiments beginning in 1833. In one experiment, he inserted various foods tied to a string through the opening into the stomach, periodically checking their degree of digestion. He also studied the stomach's movements during digestion, the composition of gastric juice, and the impact of mental states upon secretion and digestion.

The United States experienced an unprecedented need for healers during the American Civil War *(1861-1865)*. Many of the 'surgeons' in these conflicts gained their entire medical training on the battlefield. Wounded soldiers were left lying on the field, unless they could transport themselves to an area hospital or medical tent. Antiseptic technique was not yet standard procedure, and surgeons operated on successive patients with the same blood-covered knife and pus-stained hands. Infection also spread throughout overcrowded hospitals, especially where ventilation was lacking.

William A Hammond *(1828–1900)*, Surgeon General of the North, dedicated himself to improving the conditions in army hospitals. In hospitals, he observed that disease, not wounds, was the primary cause of death. His initial concern was to improve ventilation. A constant movement of fresh air through the hospital, he reasoned, would prohibit stagnant, disease-filled air from

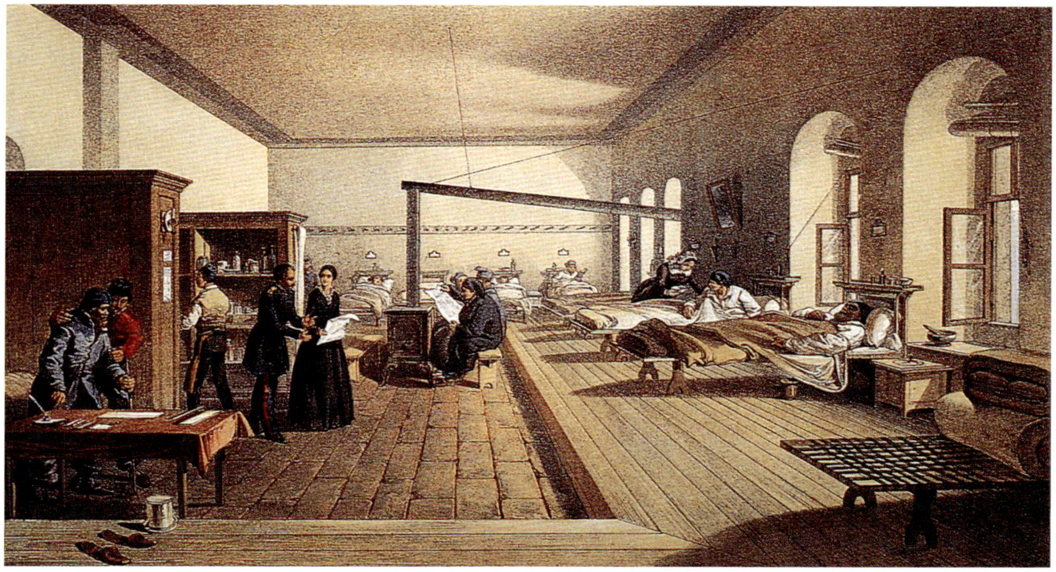

LEFT **Florence Nightingale, the pioneer of women's nursing, in the hospital wards at Scutari during the Crimean War, in a linograph from an 1856 engraving by William Simpson.**

infecting patients. He also arranged a pavilion setting whereby distinct wings of a centralized building each housed patients with specific medical needs.

Jonathan Letterman, Medical Director of the Army of the Potomac, created an ambulance service. His was not the first in history, however, as Dominique-Jean Larrey *(1766–1842)* and Pierre-François Percy *(1754–1825)* had developed similar systems in Napoleon's army. Letterman's plan required that every regiment had three ambulances equipped with designated drivers. Eventually the entire Union army put this efficient transport system into effect during the American Civil War.

WOMEN HEALERS

War also revolutionized the practice of nursing. Prior to the 1850s, nurses had the unenviable reputation of being low-class drunken thieves. Although some religious sisters had been long engaged in nursing the sick, their emphasis on spiritual care played little part in the emerging nineteenth-century hospital system. Typically, hospitals relied on lower-class women to serve as nurses. In most cases nurses received little, if any, medical training and, in some, the only requirement to be a nurse was to have been a hospital patient.

The British pioneer of nursing, Florence Nightingale *(1820–1910)*, was born in Florence. Although her desire to pursue nursing initially met with objection, Nightingale persevered and received sporadic nurse's training beginning in 1851 in Kaiserswerth, Germany, and later with the Sisters of Charity in Paris. However, it was the Crimean War that transformed Nightingale from a local nurse into a national hero.

By October 1854, word of the deplorable hospital conditions in the Crimea became public knowledge. Sidney Herbert, Britain's Secretary of War, wanted to send a group of nurses to Scutari, Turkey. Herbert wrote, 'There is but one person in England that I know of who would be capable of organizing and superintending such a scheme.' This person was Nightingale, and by 4 November 1854, she, 38 nurses, and Charles Holte Bracebridge and his wife, Selina, arrived in Turkey shortly after the Battle of Inkerman. With newly wounded men continuously being admitted, the nurses soon encountered drastic shortages of water, soap and linens for bedding and bandages. Upon their arrival, the nurses busied themselves making bandages, pallets, shirts, pillows and slings. In her 14 November 1854 letter to surgeon William Bowman, Nightingale recorded the following statistics:

> *...on Thursday last [Nov 8] we had 1715 sick & wounded in this hospital (among whom 120 Cholera patients) and 650 severely wounded in...the Gen[eral] Hospital...when a message came to me to prepare for 510 wounded...who were arriving from the dreadful affair of the 5th of Nov[ember] from Balaclava...I always expected to end my days as Hospital Matron, but I never expected to be a Barrack Mistress.*
>
> FLORENCE NIGHTINGALE, LETTER OF 1854

The war ended in February 1856, and the hospitals were closed the following August. Nightingale then returned to England, where illness and fatigue turned her into a veritable hermit who abandoned most of her social ties and devoted herself entirely to work. In 1861 she opened the Nightingale School of Nursing at London's St Thomas' Hospital.

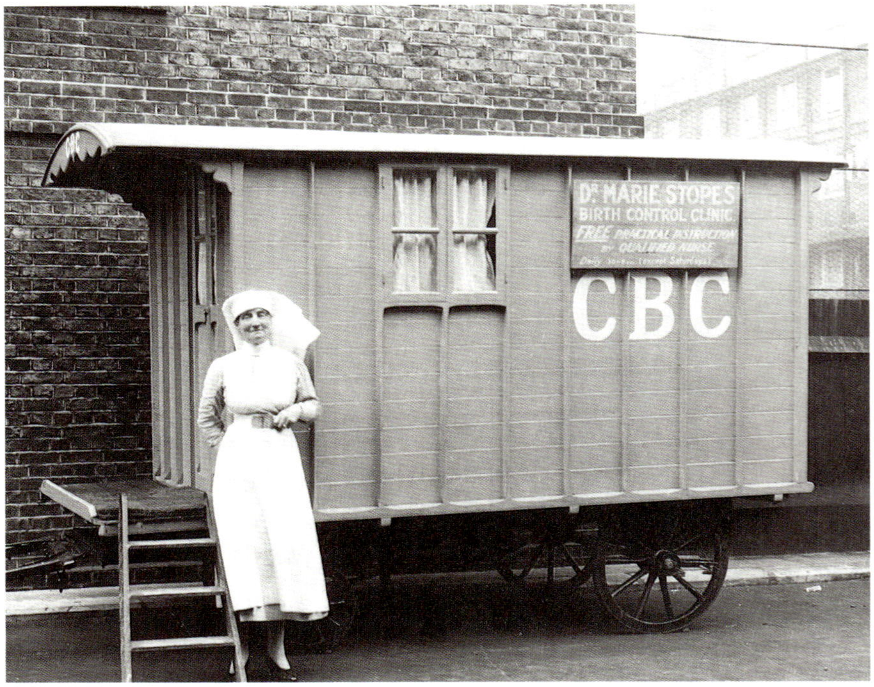

ABOVE **Marie Stopes founded Britain's first birth-control clinic in 1921. This mobile unit is pictured in the late 1920s.**

Up until relatively recent times, midwifery was principally a female-centred practice. Parturient women were, in most Western cultures, attended by 'neighbourhood women' and female relatives who delivered children as part of their family, medical and community responsibilities. The early 'art' of midwifery was typically passed down through oral tradition. In the eighteenth and nineteenth centuries, the growth of 'man-midwifery' challenged the more traditional practices. Previous traditions became classified as bad, dirty, superstitious and life-threatening, whereas male midwifes, and the eventual male-dominated obstetrics profession, represented their practice as good, clean, scientific and life-saving. A 'midwife debate' erupted, one which continued into the twentieth century when midwifes were essentially legislated out of existence in the United States and brought under regulation by the medical profession in Great Britain.

Over the last quarter of a century, obstetricians' authority over childbearing has been increasingly challenged. The impetus for this challenge arose largely from consumers. When 'natural childbirth' techniques within the physician-controlled hospital setting failed to meet some women's expectations for a humane and satisfying birth experience, they started looking for alternatives to the medicalized obstetrical approach. They rediscovered an insight of previous generations: midwifery provided a safe and satisfying birth experience. Writings, including Suzanne Arms' *Immaculate Deception: A New Look at Women and Childbirth in America (1975)* and Ina May Gaskin's *Spiritual Midwifery (1977)*, presented statistical accounts supporting their perceptions and experiences that midwifery was at least as safe as obstetrics.

To target the contraceptive needs of working-class women, Marie Stopes *(1880–1958)* opened the first birth-control clinic in England in the early 1920s. She offered free consultations and contraceptives. Examinations were performed by a midwife and, if necessary, patients were referred to the clinic's female physician. As a model, Stopes looked to Dr Aletta Jacobs' clinic, established in Amsterdam in 1882. After speaking with Margaret Sanger *(1883–1966)*, a birth-control movement leader

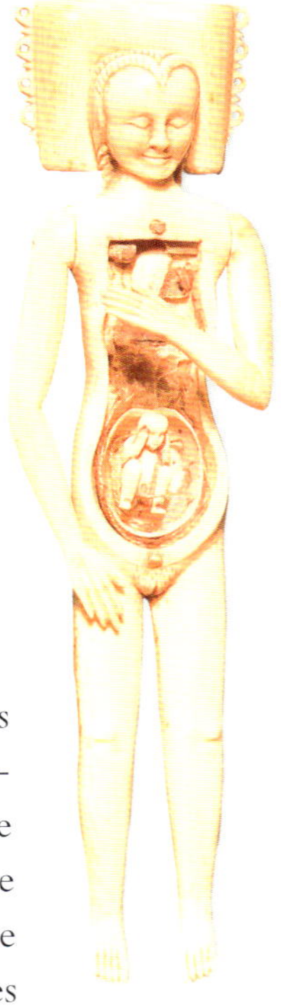

ABOVE **An antique model of a pregnant woman created for students of obstetrics.**

SISTER KENNY'S THERAPY

Elizabeth Kenny *(1886–1952)*, widely known as Sister Kenny, served as a bush nurse in early twentieth-century Australia. While caring for patients suffering from polio, she became convinced that physicians were treating the disease incorrectly. Physicians regularly applied splints and casts to immobilize the affected limbs and limit the interaction between weakened and strong muscles. On the other hand, Sister Kenny promoted a vigorous regimen of physical therapy and hot packs from the first signs of muscle spasm. Although she successfully treated polio patients in numerous hospitals, Australian physicians criticized claims that her patients experienced fewer permanent crippling effects than theirs. Frustrated by these unrelenting criticisms, she travelled to the US and established the Sister Kenny Institute in Minneapolis, Minnesota. Sister Kenny's therapy was taught across the country and was employed as one measure to battle the polio epidemic.

from the US, Stopes turned her attention to contraception in her books *Married Love (1918)* and *Wise Parenthood (1918)*. In this writing she criticized the use of a 'safe period' and promoted the cervical cap as means of reliable contraception.

Across the ocean, Margaret Sanger worked as a nurse in low-income sections of New York. In her everyday work she cared for women's physical and psychological complications from self-induced abortions and unwanted pregnancies. Her patients, however, had no information on dependable birth-control methods. She disseminated information about effective birth-control procedures through her birth-control clinic, her popular writing, including *The Birth Control Review* and *Woman Rebel*, and the American Birth Control League.

TRANSMITTING DISEASE

Throughout the ages, myriad opinions have been offered regarding the origin of diseases. As early as Girolamo Fracastoro's 1546 publication, *De contagione*, healers have speculated as to whether direct contact was responsible for transmitting disease. Others proposed that diseases spread as a result of environmental disturbance, such as changes in the quality of the air. Some air was healthy, they argued, whereas other air was deemed of poor, bad or 'mal' quality.

Some healers began to investigate the possibility that diseases were caused by tiny living germs. Before microscopes were invented, distinct micro-organisms and bacteria were not known to exist. In the late seventeenth century, the Dutch optician Antoni van Leeuwenhoek *(1632–1723)* observed 'little animals' under a microscopic lens in scrapings taken from between his teeth. The appearance of these tiny organisms on human surfaces suggested their role in disease. This observation was extrapolated to the idea that diseases actually resulted from the growth of germs in the body. For the next 200 years, this idea was often refuted until Louis Pasteur *(1822–1895)*, Joseph Lister *(1827–1912)* and Robert Koch *(1843–1910)* helped to solidify the 'germ theory of disease' in modern medical science.

Pasteur, a chemist by trade, performed research that eventually convinced the scientific world of the germ theory's validity. In the 1860s and 1870s, Pasteur demonstrated that microbes actually caused fermentation. Previously, fermentation was considered to be a spontaneously occurring event. Pasteur's eventual discovery of specific microbial activity demonstrated that not all bacteria induced disease. Pasteur's work not only provided crucial support for the germ theory, but it also inspired other healers whose work enhanced the ability to cure

PASTEUR'S BREAKTHROUGH

As part of his contribution to the eventual germ theory, Pasteur performed research on two diseases: pébrine, a silkworm disease, and rabies, a disease typically fatal to humans. In his work on pébrine, he discovered that a specific protozoan was only present in diseased silkworms, thus supporting the idea that one organism causes a particular disease. In his 1885 essay 'Prevention of Rabies', he announced his discovery that he could 'incubate' the germ responsible for the disease by transmitting it from rabbit to rabbit via injection. Once he had accomplished this, he explored various methods of preventing rabies. For example, he inoculated dogs with different sterilized portions of the diseased rabbit's spinal cord. Sterilizing the tissue had, in effect, deactivated the germ, and the injection did not induce rabies in these dogs. When he followed this injection with inoculations of increasing virulence over a period of days, the dogs did not contract the disease. To Pasteur, this indicated that the dog had become immune to rabies. He received the opportunity to test his preventative technique on a human after seven-year-old Joseph Meister had been severely attacked by a rabid dog. His treatment was a success, and he later noted that '...three months and three weeks have elapsed since the accident, ... [and Meister's] state of health leaves nothing to be desired'.

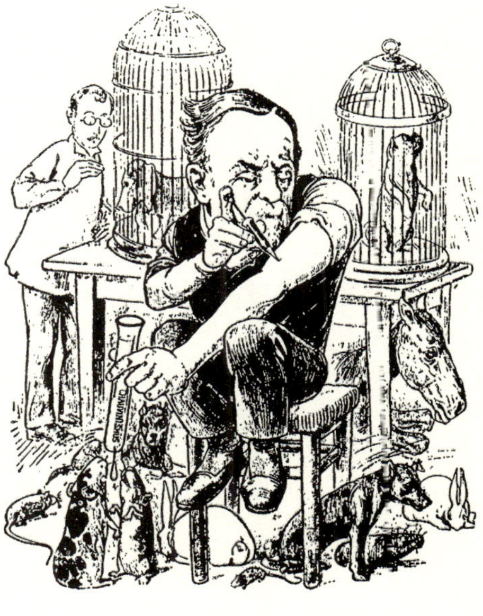

ABOVE A caricature of Louis Pasteur, who produced an effective rabies vaccine in 1885.

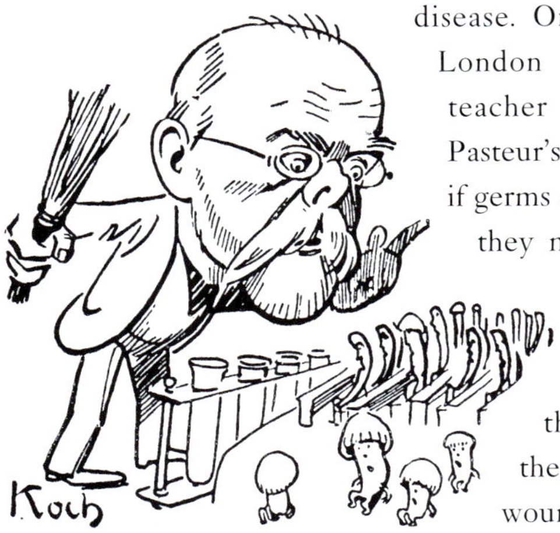

ABOVE **Robert Koch 'culturing' bacteria. He received the Nobel Prize for Medicine in 1905.**

disease. One such individual, the London surgeon and medical teacher Joseph Lister, studied Pasteur's work and reasoned that if germs could cause fermentation, they might also be responsible for the putrefaction commonly seen in wounds. He considered that the germs present in the air could fall into open wounds. As a result, he set out to determine methods to protect against such an infection. Lister read of the success experienced when carbolic acid was used to treat putrefying sewage. Unaware of French surgeon François-Jules Lemaire's previous similar findings, Lister applied carbolic acid dressings in the treatment of compound fractures in which bones penetrated through the skin, thereby creating an environment ripe for infection. His technique of inserting carbolic acid-soaked cloth into the wound saved the limbs of nine of his first 11 patients. He further tested carbolic acid as a spray in the operating room, but he abandoned its use having concluded that germs on clothing and skin were far more responsible for wound infection than germs in the air.

Robert Koch's work was also paramount in advancing the germ theory of disease. Koch's most influential research came from the study of *Bacillus anthracis*, the causal agent of anthrax. Prior to Koch's investigation, microscopic rod-shaped bacteria had been found in the blood of animals infected with anthrax. Some healthy animals that were experimentally injected with infected blood died before rods were found in their blood stream. He concluded that although the rods actually caused the disease, it was spores formed from the germs that actually communicated the disease to other individuals. Therefore, if the infected blood did not contain the infective spores, then the inoculated animal's blood would not show the presence of the disease. His discovery of the varied infectivity of different stages of a pathogenic organism's life-cycle was of vast importance.

Identifying the germ causing the disease was one step; understanding its natural transmission was another. During the 1890s, Ronald Ross *(1857–1932)* of the Indian Medical Service studied malaria and, in 1897, discovered that the parasite responsible for this disease was found in the *Anopheles* mosquito. He then proposed that the mosquito served as the vector for the disease, transmitting it whenever a mosquito drew the blood of an infected animal and subsequently attacked an uninfected human. Only after understanding the transmission process of parasite and germ-born diseases could preventative measures against these diseases be significantly improved.

Distinguishing whether genetic components or environmental factors are the predominant precursors of disease presents a great dilemma to modern healers. Having provided a glimpse into studies of genetics, attention now turns to environmental concerns. Biologist Rachel Carson *(1907–1964)* informed the public about the harm of pesticide use through her best selling book *Silent Spring (1962)*. Concentrating on the widespread use of DDT, Carson demonstrated that many chemicals were haphazardly used without regard to the health of the surrounding animals, plants and humans. She also attempted to link particular cancers to specific chemicals used in the workplace and found in the foods we regularly eat.

ARCHIBALD GARROD AND 'METABOLIC ERRORS'

Although in 1900 germs were thought to be the cause of most diseases, one London physician, Archibald Garrod *(1857–1936)*, considered that some sicknesses might arise from heritable 'metabolic errors' in the body. Like the medieval physician 'piss prophets' interested in urinoscopy, Garrod, too, was interested in chemical changes which altered the colour of urine. To test his idea of hereditary disease, Garrod turned his attention to a pregnant patient suffering from alkaptonuria, a disorder thought to be caused by an intestinal germ which, among other complications, discoloured the sufferer's urine. True to his thinking, this patient delivered a child who soon began to produce blackened urine – the diagnostic sign of alkaptonuria.

Garrod's work received little attention until the 1940s, when George Beadle, Boris Ephrussi and Edward Tatum developed a working model, the fruit fly, in which inborn errors (actually genetic mutations) could be experimentally tested. This later work sparked many healers to contrive methods to alter genetic mutations and correct 'inborn errors' in the hope of preventing disease. Similar hopes are desired from the ongoing Human Genome Project.

Following the release of *Silent Spring*, citizens demanded information about ways in which spraying infected the natural world around them. A federal committee was established to investigate pesticide use and its consequences. Rachel Carson's testimony before this committee helped change the views of influential government officials and create the US Environmental Protection Agency (EPA) in 1970.

The EPA maintains an inventory of data on toxic substances and their effects on the human body. Today, if a toxic area is identified, the EPA commissions studies to investigate both the location and chemical effects on the surrounding community, then co-ordinates state and local agencies to act on the research results. Federal funds are available through the EPA's 'Superfund' legislation to evalute and clean up these dangerous toxic waste sites. Through the efforts of Rachel Carson and her environmental disciples, indiscriminate pesticide, toxin and chemical use has become a concern to the lay public and is now regulated by government policy.

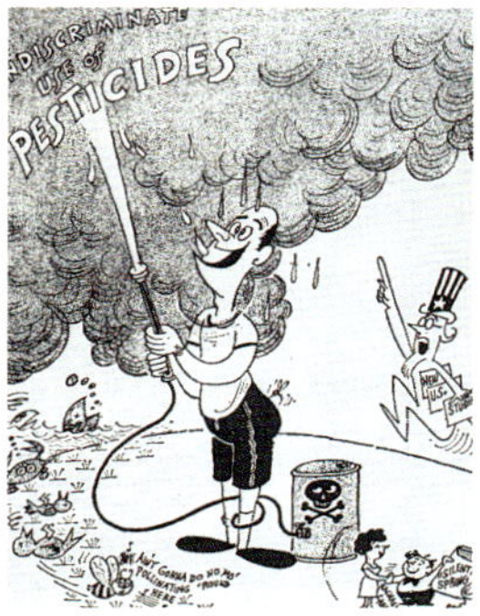

ABOVE Rachel Carson's efforts to ban pesticides led to the formation of the EPA in the USA.

PARTING THOUGHTS

In many modern health-care delivery systems, particularly in the West, death is viewed as a healer's failure to combat a disease successfully. Such a view, however, is the result of a paradigm shift in attitudes regarding the art of dying. Prior to the past 50 years, death with dignity was much more common. Social historian Philippe Aries noted in his 1974 *Western Attitudes Toward Death* that earlier Western society allowed the dying to play an organizational role in death. Death was family-centred, occurring in one's home accompanied by much public ceremony and spiritual sanctity. Russian author Aleksandr Solzhenitsyn picturesquely captured this ideology in his Nobel-Prize winning novel *Cancer Ward (1968).*

[The old folk] didn't puff themselves up or fight against it and brag that they weren't going to die – they took death calmly. They didn't stall squaring things away, they prepared themselves quietly and in good time, deciding who should have the mare, who the foal … And they departed easily, as if they were just moving into a new house.

ALEKSANDR SOLZHENITSYN, *CANCER WARD*

In more recent decades, healers – at least in Western society – have recreated death as a technologically-based, solitary, sanitized and secularized phenomenon centred within a hospital and hidden from public view. Critics argue that such a scene unnaturally abandons the very individuals which healers *should* recognize to be the most in need of humane care. Surgeon Sherwin Nuland, in his widely acclaimed *How We Die (1994)*, attempts to 'demythologize' the medicalization of death, both for healers and the general reading audience. 'Doctors rarely *want* to give up', Nuland claims. 'As long as there is any possibility of solving The Riddle, they will keep at it, and sometimes it takes the intervention of a family or the patient himself to put an end to medical exercises in futility.' 'Do Not Resuscitate' orders exemplify that families must explicitly *refuse* the otherwise mandatory healer's intervention.

Some healers, however, have recognized the patient's desire to depart with dignity. Not all, however, have proposed such controversial actions as Jack Kevorkian's physician-assisted suicide. In 1967, physician Dame Cicely Saunders reintroduced the age-old concept of 'hospice' with her founding of St Christopher's Hospice in London. She explicitly sought to create a setting for dying without the god-like interventions which many healers enacted with their aggressive life-preserving procedures in hospitals. According to one patient's account:

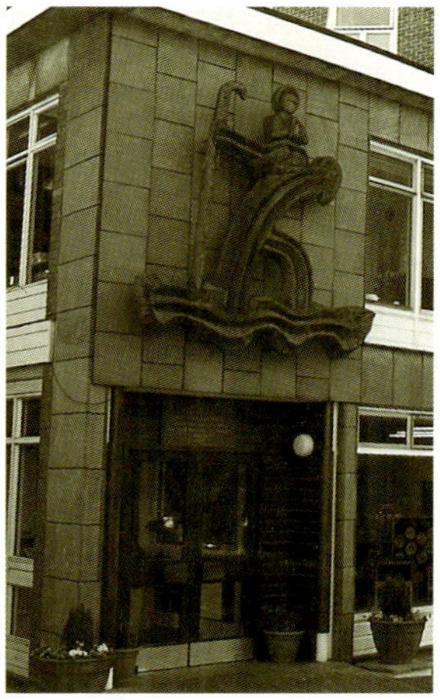

ABOVE The work of Dame Cicely Saunders reintroduced the concept of a hospice for care of the terminally ill.

Hospice has turned an eternal secret into a living principle; that what's truly important is life lived richly, deeply, meaningfully for as long as it lasts. Dignity, family, comfort and caring are hospice, an idea whose time has come.

HOSPICE PATIENT, *ALL ABOUT HOSPICE* (PAMPHLET OF THE FOUNDATION FOR HOSPICE & HOME CARE, *1991*)

Having come full circle, healers are beginning to once again accept that dying – like healing – is a two-way process. A dialogue exists between healer and patient. We have recognized the patient's voice as part of death. Perhaps the patient's voice will also become more a part of the future historical record of healing.

CHAPTER EIGHT

EAST MEETS WEST

THE EMERGENCE OF AN HOLISTIC TRADITION

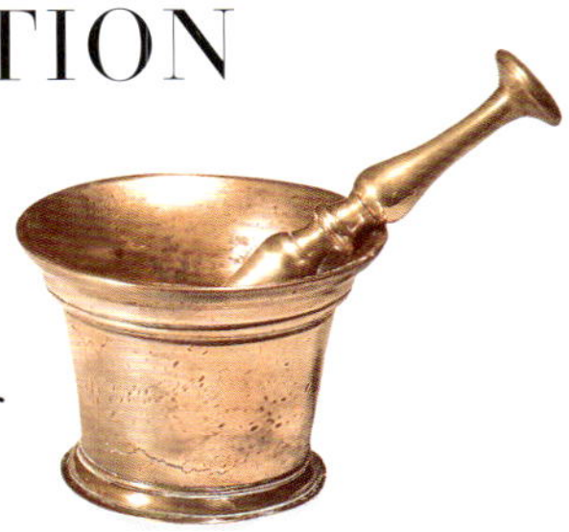

ABOVE Western and Eastern pharmacists alike use a pestle and mortar.

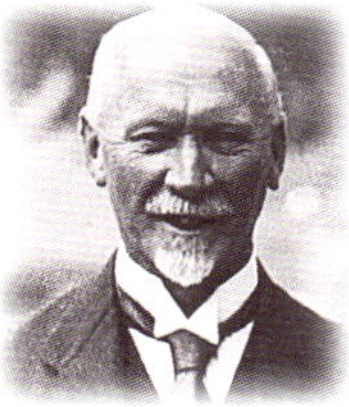

ABOVE Jan Smuts first coined the term 'holism' in the 1920s.

THE PAST 30 OR 40 YEARS *have seen a progressive re-emergence of the holistic tradition in the Western world – paralleling that which has been more consistently established in the East over many centuries. The concept of holism itself has not been defined in a single way to everyone's satisfaction, but it can be taken to be based on the involvement of the whole person in the promotion of health and the prevention of illness – in which the interplay of mind, spirit and body is perceived within the wider social context. The notion of holism itself in modern times derives from Jan Christian Smuts (1870–1950), a South African philosopher and statesman – he served twice as South Africa's Prime Minister and helped found the League of Nations. He developed the term as a counter to the reductionism of Western natural scientific thought. Holism in his definition makes the important recognition that the whole is greater than the sum of its parts.*[G4]

Holistic traditions in this sense have long been pivotal to health care and indeed to life itself in the East, based on philosophies linking mental and physical processes. This is best highlighted by such time-honoured practices as traditional Chinese medicine and Indian Ayurvedic medicine, which see mental and physical processes as existing in harmony in a healthy person.[K2] These medical traditions can be broadly viewed as holistic approaches, as they recognize that the patient is a whole being and they are centred on person-focused care. They are also based on the connection between the individual and his or her broader environmental setting. This is an important background for discussing the question of East meeting West, although in an historical sense Eastern and Western health philosophies, as will be seen, can only really be depicted as being in serious tension in this respect with the rise of scientific biomedicine in developed societies in the modern Western world.

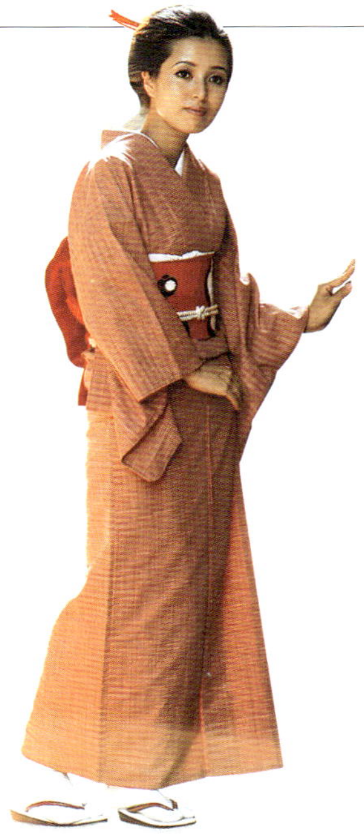

ABOVE An image that suggests a body in balance and a calm mind. Holism recognizes the interplay of mind, body and spirit.

Holism is in fact by no means a new concept in relation to health care in the West; it derives in part from the Greek physician Hippocrates who, as early as the fifth century BC, acknowledged the relationship between illness and the environment and the emotions.[A2] Building on the philosophy of ancient Greek medicine, which also has resonances in the East, health care in the Western world has a long subsequent history that in many respects echoes the ancient Greek Hippocratic tradition. This is no more apparent than in the Greek doctrine of the need to balance the four humours in the body to achieve health, in which the elements of fire, water, earth and air of Greek cosmology were adapted to explain the state of health in the microcosm of the human being.[K2] An holistic frame of reference that can be traced back

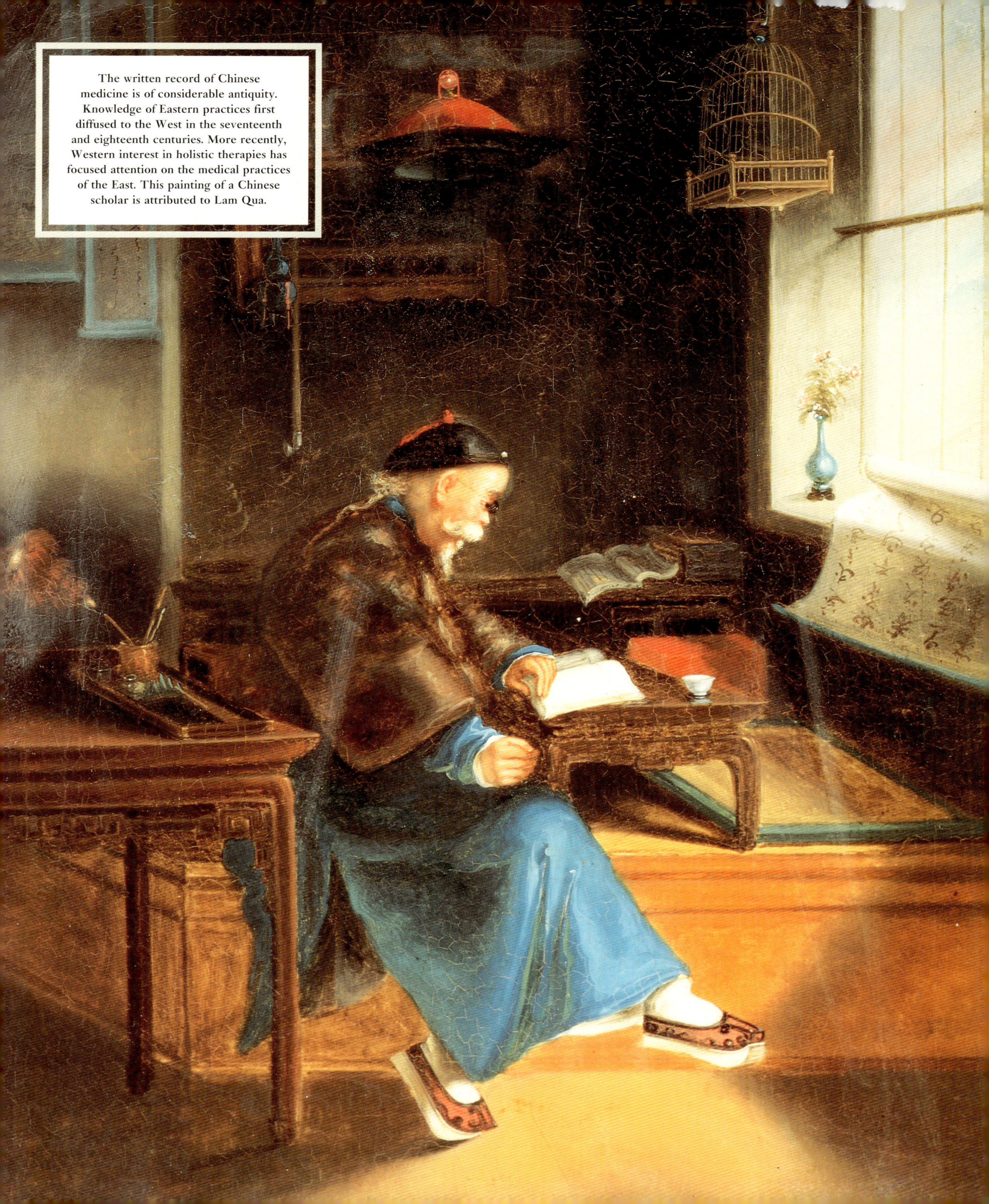

The written record of Chinese medicine is of considerable antiquity. Knowledge of Eastern practices first diffused to the West in the seventeenth and eighteenth centuries. More recently, Western interest in holistic therapies has focused attention on the medical practices of the East. This painting of a Chinese scholar is attributed to Lam Qua.

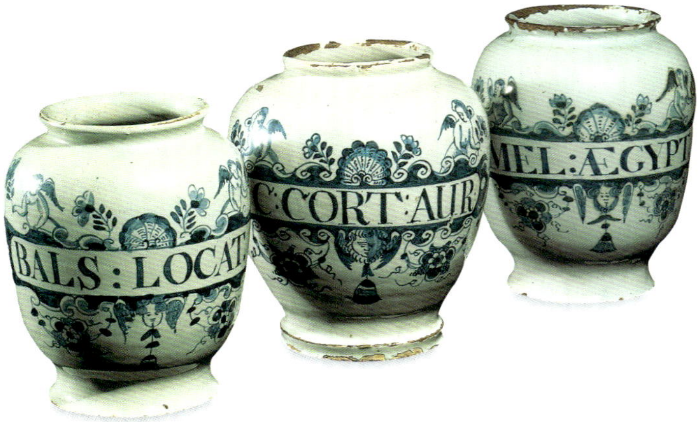

ABOVE Eighteenth-century apothecaries' drug jars. The health-care 'market' at this time embraced a wide variety of treatments – many holistic in nature.

to the Greeks in this sense certainly exerted an influence over the Western medical tradition.

In sixteenth- and seventeenth-century Britain, for example, a diverse range of holistically-oriented treatments were on offer, including charms and incantations, herbal preparations, astrology and magic – which were often provided on a self-help basis.[L1] A wide array of practitioners from bonesetters to healers were actively selling their wares on the developing health-care marketplace by the eighteenth century.[P5] In this period even regular practitioners and their patients viewed illness as a result of the malfunctioning of the individual constitution in which vital forces were in disequilibrium. The theory of humours in particular emphasized that this could occur if the system became too hot or cold, dry or wet, or if too little or too much blood was produced. Any imbalances needed to be remedied by such actions as blood-letting and/or an improvement in life-style, which might involve recommended changes to diet and taking exercise.[P4]

In the United States, early forms of medicine were also centred on the idea of helping nature to deal with the underlying causes of illness, with the family/community context and prevention being regarded as pivotal to a person's health.[L2] The United States, too, had its range of holistic practices, the most prominent of which involved the use of botanical medicines that became strongly associated with the populist Thomsonian movement in the early nineteenth century (*see page 88*). These were used not only by the colonialists, but also selectively by many native North American tribes, who employed them mainly on a symptomatic basis in order, among other things, to reduce bleeding and to serve as purgatives. It is clear from this example and the growing number of pills and tonics that were taken on a similar basis at this stage on both sides of the Atlantic that even in earlier times not all traditional health-care practices could be regarded as genuinely holistic.[R3]

EASTERN INFLUENCES AND WESTERN PRACTICES

The gradual diffusion to the West of Eastern healing methods linking mind, spirit and body had some impact on the prevailing patterns of health care, as international communication networks slowly began to develop. This is illustrated by acupuncture which – having initially diffused from China to other Eastern countries like Korea and Japan – began to spread from the Orient to parts of Europe by the seventeenth century. This mainly took place through the influence of Jesuit missionaries and Western doctors working abroad for the East India Companies. The merchant and explorer Marco Polo *(1254–1324)* also played a part in the transmission of knowledge from East to West at a much earlier date. Knowledge of acupuncture finally reached North America through

BELOW Marco Polo and his entourage are shown on this Catalan map. His account of his travels in China *(1275–1292)* stimulated European interest in the East.

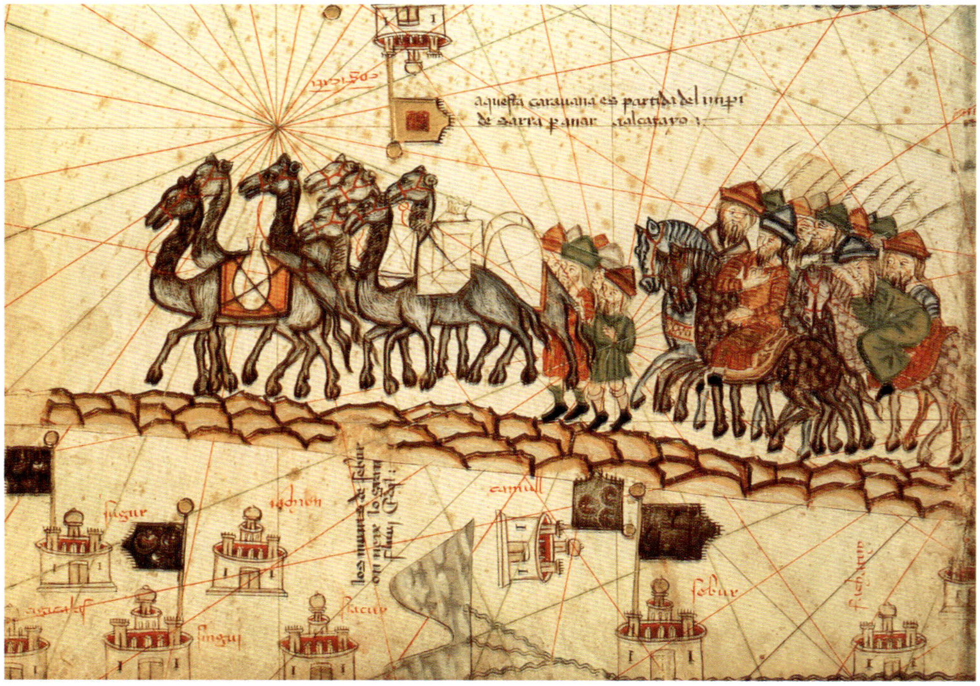

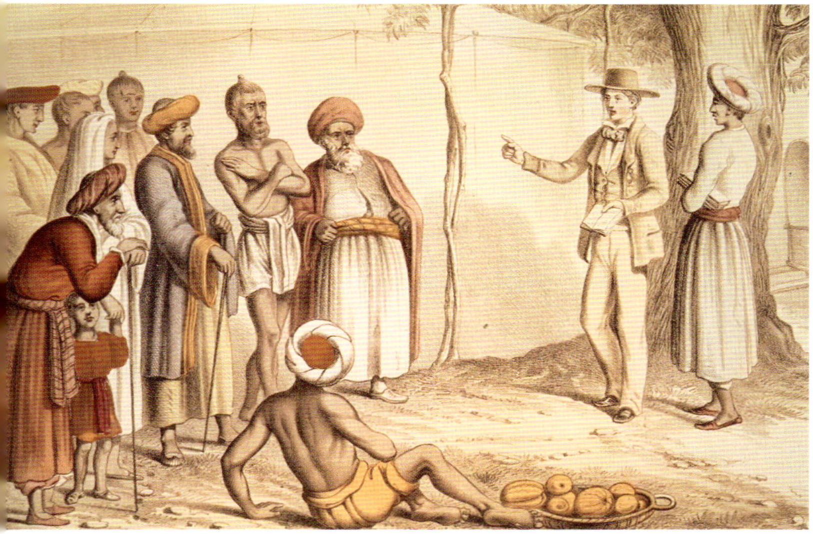

ABOVE The influence of European missionaries and teachers working abroad ensured that knowledge of Eastern practices found its way back to the West.

Europe by the early nineteenth century. The influence of such developments in medical circles, however, was limited; as witnessed by the fact that the traditional philosophical tenets underlying the practice, and its broad scope of application, were only vaguely understood at this stage *(see also Chapter Four)*. It was primarily used in the West in a very specific manner to deal with cases of pain, in contrast to its broader Oriental employment within a philosophical framework centred on holistic balance.[S4]

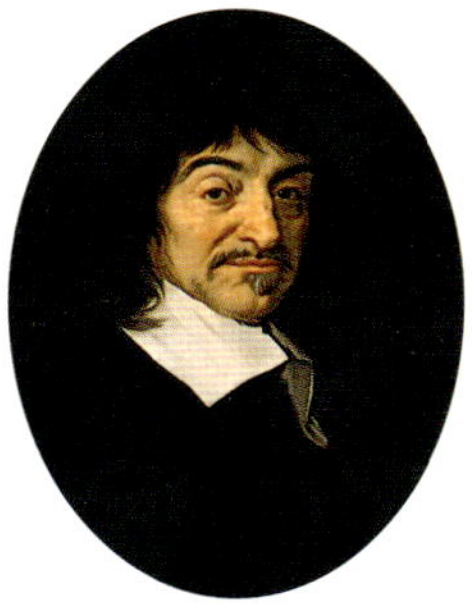

ABOVE Descartes' argued that mind and body are distinct; his dualism undermined holistic philosophy.

However, following the Enlightenment in Europe in the eighteenth century, the rise of biomedicine progressively squeezed out the more holistic tradition in the West, especially in the nineteenth and first half of the twentieth centuries. Biomedicine in this sense is seen as deriving from the classic philosophical distinction between mind and body propounded by René Descartes *(1596–1650)*, which contrasts with conceptions of health and illness based on the whole person. The body in the Western biomedical frame of reference is seen as the predominant focus. It is treated as though it is divisible into parts that can be repaired if they break down, through such means as drug therapy and surgical intervention. Crucially, the biomedical approach tends to be geared more towards the physical aspects of health and illness than the mental processes and the broader environmental factors that affect an individual – with little recognition of the uniqueness of the patient who is being treated.[M1]

The transition to biomedicine in the West was associated with the emergence of an officially designated medical profession which has gained a virtually monopolistic status in health care – not least in Great Britain and the United States.[B2] The biomedical approach, with its emphasis on 'scientific rationality', has played a key part in advancing the rise of doctors to power with state support in the Anglo-American context. Their role in the West has been further reinforced by the emergence of nurses and other professional groups subordinated to medicine in the wider health-care division of labour. The consequence of this has been the marginalization of both more holistic forms of therapy and of groups of alternative practitioners who are associated with an holistic approach. The latter were placed in a disadvantaged position in the health-care division of labour,

THE DECLINE OF A WESTERN HOLISTIC APPROACH TO HEALTH CARE

The shift away from holism can be seen to have taken place in three historical phases in the West. The initial phase was based on the practice of 'bedside medicine', where rich, fee-paying clients in the seventeenth and eighteenth centuries could shape their own diagnosis and treatment by medical practitioners in an holistic manner. It is important to emphasize that at this stage aspects of the patient's emotional and spiritual life, as well as the physical disposition of the individual, were seen as central by the practitioner in making a diagnosis within the established system of health care.

This frame of reference was progressively replaced, however, as the nineteenth century wore on with the move in Western medicine towards 'hospital medicine'. This new phase was characterized by concentration by doctors on the generic classification of diseases that were manifested in the patient, which meant that doctors moved away from the earlier focus on the individual as a whole person. The third phase that emerged as the twentieth century unfolded was the development of 'laboratory medicine', which removed diagnosis and therapy even further away from the whole patient – who came to be medically conceived as little more than a depersonalized object, comprised of a complex of cells.[J1] sometimes being completely prevented from practising within the restrictive legal framework that eventually emerged in the West – including many countries in continental Europe and several states in the United States of America.[S2]

The influence of biomedicine in the early to mid-twentieth century is also evident in the way in which it has affected the East, not least through the consequences of Western imperialism. The initial impact of Western expansionism in this regard arguably affected health adversely by, among other things, importing disease, destroying and syphoning off harvests and introducing colonial production systems that had deleterious effects on the indigenous population. On the other side of the coin, some of the positive features of biomedicine increasingly became available through the work of a relatively small number of Western health personnel in countries such as India and East Africa. Their focus, however, seems to have been primarily directed towards the care of the Western colonialists and only secondarily to the native population – and, when the latter group were treated, it was mainly in relation to mass conditions like malaria and sleeping sickness that might, if allowed to run unchecked, spread from the latter community to the former.[D1]

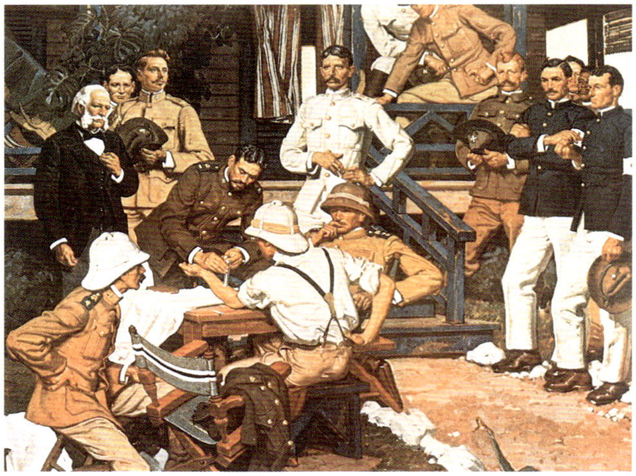

ABOVE Western biomedicine has had a beneficial impact on other cultures, not least in the virtual eradication of mosquito-borne diseases.

The effect that biomedicine and the related work of missionaries actually had on indigenous Oriental healing traditions, many of which were based on a more holistic approach, was limited. Much depended on the stance adopted by the governments formally in power in Eastern countries, especially with regard to their policies on the overall balance of health care provided by local health workers. In some Eastern settings, such as in China under the Kuomintang Nationalist Government in the period from the 1920s to the 1940s, the increasing use of Western biomedicine was seen as synonymous with the effective modernization of the nation. Accordingly, as in Meiji Japan in the nineteenth century, the employment of traditional medicine like acupuncture and herbalism was formally banned, even if in practice traditional therapies continued to hold considerable sway with some practitioners and the general public at a grass-roots level.[S4]

Just as more holistic forms of health care retained their importance in the East, despite the impact of biomedicine in the period leading up to the mid-twentieth century, so the newly defined alternative forms of holistic medicine did not completely disappear in the West in this period, notwithstanding the powerful influence of orthodox medicine. The medical profession certainly consolidated its position of power and become increasingly well organized in the West during the first half of the twentieth century, backed by further state support – which resulted in the numbers of rival alternative practitioners generally declining in face of the ideological assault by the medical establishment on homeopaths and other groups of fringe practitioners both inside and outside the profession.[N1,K3] However, this attack did not totally eliminate the range of alternative approaches; for instance, therapies from water cure to Christian Science were still available. The latter, indeed, was particularly prevalent in this period in the United States, where alternative therapies tended to be especially buoyant, in part because of the stronger populist pioneer tradition that prevailed in this country.[W1]

Some of the therapies on offer in Western societies even at this stage were influenced by the East. Hypnotism, for example, was given significant momentum by the work of James Esdaile *(1808–1859)*, a Scottish surgeon who had employed a mesmerist in Calcutta in the mid-nineteenth century to assist in performing operations on the employees of the East India Company. In addition, there were also the more immediate influences of migrant populations living in Chinatowns and other ethnically based communities in the West in which traditional health-care practices persisted.[I3] These and other more holistic approaches formed part of a minority subculture in the first half of the twentieth century in many Western societies. However, from the 1950s onwards – the period on which this chapter focuses – the nature and scale of this subculture, as well as the extent of the Eastern influence on it, grew dramatically in the West, bringing it closer to becoming part of a new integrated medical orthodoxy.

THE RECENT DEVELOPMENT OF THE WESTERN MEDICAL COUNTERCULTURE

There has been increasing public interest in alternative medicine throughout the West in the latter part of the twentieth century. This has been reflected in fast-rising demand for consultations with alternative practitioners in Western Europe and the United States.[S7,E2] The form of the therapies which are most popular vary from country to country – ranging, for example, from homeopathy in the Netherlands and France and spiritual healing in the Netherlands to chiropractic in Canada.[F1,C6] Similarly, there is a national variation in the extent of participation in such therapies, with between a fifth and one half of the population of Western countries typically going to consult an alternative therapist at some point in their lives. The overall trend nonetheless is in the same direction: the popularity of alternative therapies is rising rapidly and many people appear to want them included within the formal health-care system. The number of their practitioners is also rising correspondingly. This trend is also mirrored in the quantity of health foods and other preparations associated with alternative health care that are bought over the counter of health-food stores by today's consumers.[S2]

This development is part of a wider movement related to self-help and the growing empowerment of the consumer, and it particularly needs to be seen in the context of the increasingly overt counterculture that emerged in the West in the 1960s.[R2] At this time, the notion of scientific progress in medicine and other areas came under attack, as alternative life-styles developed – in an era when established traditions of all kinds were being critically scrutinized. This trend was linked with rising interest in Eastern mysticism, including transcendental meditation and the use of hallucinogenic drugs. It was reinforced by the stronger cultural links that were forged not only with India, but also countries like China as traditional boundaries were breached in the early 1970s with President Richard Nixon's visit to China in 1972, and the development of what was termed 'ping-pong' diplomacy with the West. Although many influences shaped the growth of a counterculture in health and other fields, the impact of the philosophies and practices of the East cannot be understated, as global communication networks expanded and traditional barriers based on political divisions receded.

While the development of a counterculture – prompted in part by the influence of the East – helps to explain the impetus for the expanding interest in a number of alternative therapies in some Western societies from

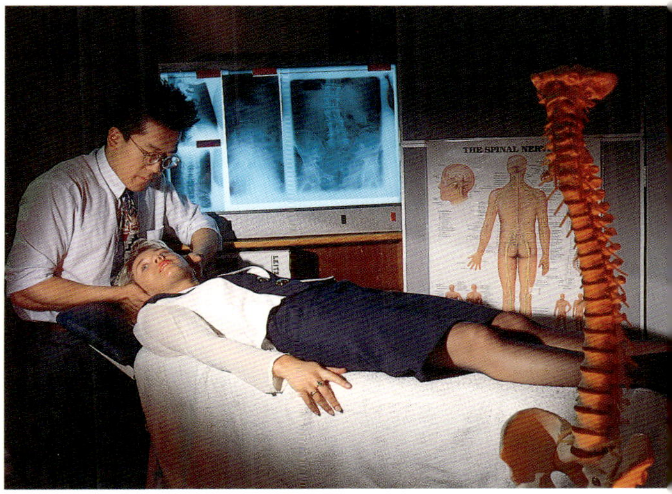

RIGHT In recent years, more and more Westerners have turned to practitioners of alternative medicine for the relief of pain and illness. This woman is being treated by a chiropractor, who seeks to promote well-being by manipulation of the spinal column. Note the X-rays of the patient's spine in the background.

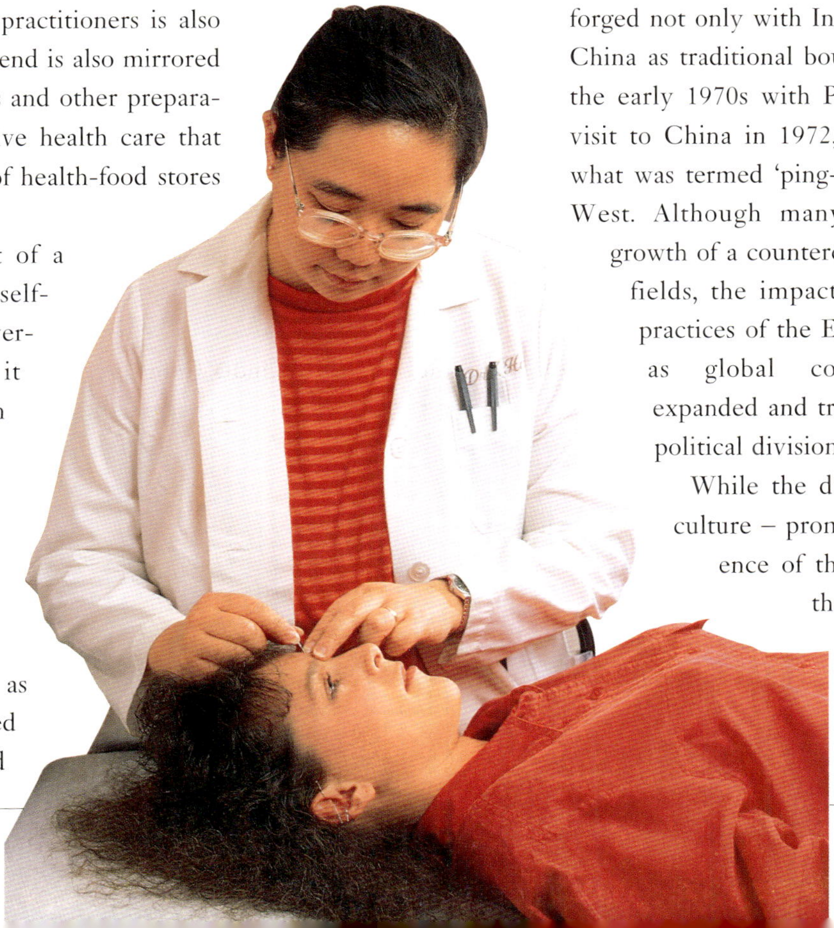

BELOW A Western woman is treated by a Chinese acupunctrist for headache and sinusitis – a picture that symbolizes the convergence of Eastern and Western medical practice that has characterized the latter part of the twentieth-century. Closer cultural links, diplomatic rapprochement and the growth of the counterculture in the West have all helped this process.

the mid-twentieth century onwards, their rising popularity also has roots in the shortcomings of orthodox medicine. At one level, the critique of Western biomedicine is based on its dehumanization of patients and the limitations that it imposes on their active involvement in their own health care. At another, it centres on the technical failure of biomedicine to live up to its own promise in terms of curing illness and enhancing the quality of life, especially as far as chronic illness is concerned. The fragility of its achievements became ever more apparent from the 1960s onwards, following awareness that even high-technology drugs and surgery could be both ineffective and unsafe – as highlighted by the thalidomide tragedy, in which thousands of babies were born with physical malformations after their mothers had taken this drug in pregnancy, and also in the number of hospital admissions following routine medical treatment. This has been underlined by contemporary research showing that over the last century the establishment of adequate diets and improvements in hygiene and sanitation have played a far more important role than biomedical interventions in improving health in the West.[P3]

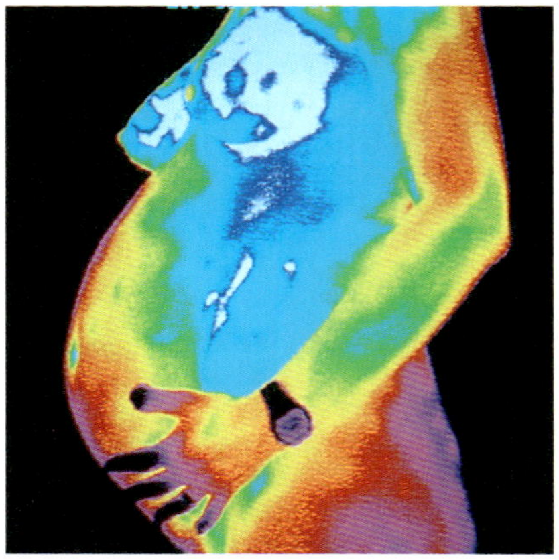

ABOVE A false-colour thermogram of a pregnant woman which reveals visually variations in body temperature. Western medicine now tends to rely heavily on such technology.

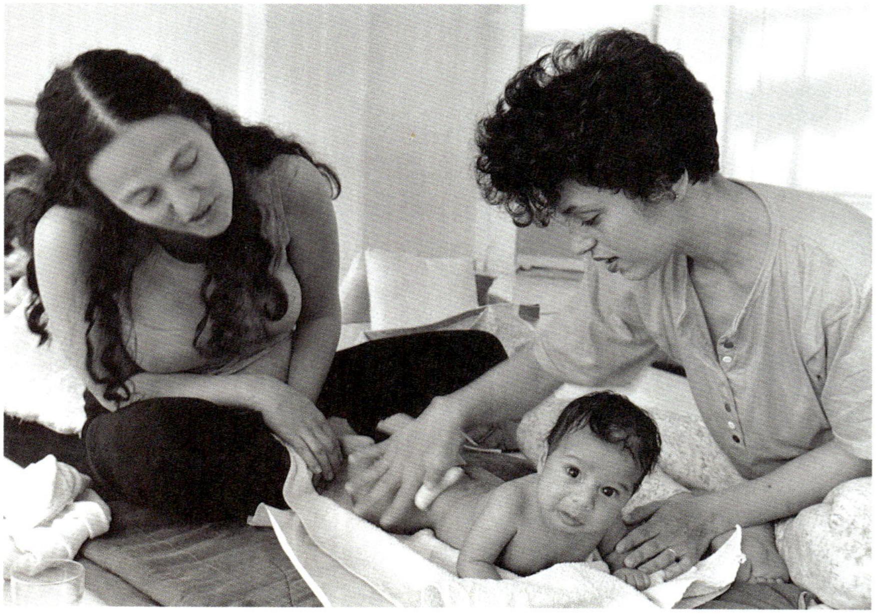

ABOVE A Dutch instructor teaches a mother how to massage her young baby. Touch therapies such as this enable parents to feel involved with the health and welfare of their children.

PUBLIC APPROVAL

The explanation of the upsurge of Western interest in alternative therapies, including those that have been heavily influenced by the East, however, is not straightforward. Some consumers are evidently committed to specific forms of alternative medicine as a first resort, but in practice such approaches seem to be largely used not so much instead of modern medicine, but as a complement to it – with the patient more typically seeking such help only when orthodox treatment has failed to deal appropriately with his or her condition.[T2,E2] Caution is, therefore, needed in assessing the commonly voiced view that the popularity of alternative therapies has resulted from a wide ranging and radical New Age shift in public consciousness. The increasing public interest in such therapies may be based more on disaffection with the shortcomings of contemporary biomedicine than a significant shift in social values,[C7] despite the current attractions of a culture based on individual self-determination in health care and the more interactive relationship that has developed between practitioner and client.[B1]

For whatever reason, though, interest in the West in alternative therapies has rapidly risen. This has been given further impetus by the still limited, but growing, political support received by such therapies. In Britain this is highlighted by the establishment of the all-party Parliamentary Group for Alternative and Complementary Medicine and the creation of special ministerial responsibilities in this area.[S2]

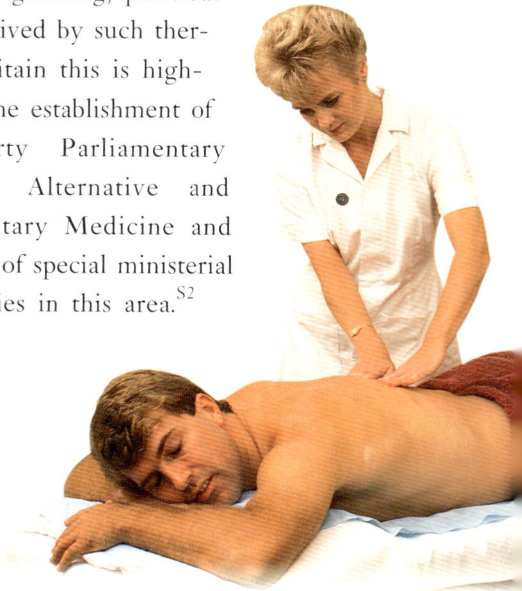

RIGHT Alternative therapies do not necessarily replace orthodox medical practices – they can exist alongside and complement them.

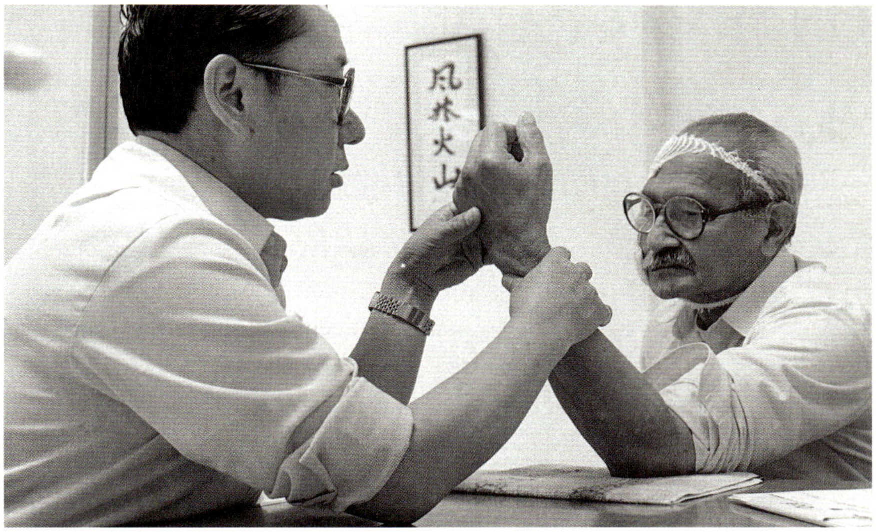

ABOVE European countries such as the Netherlands and Germany are actively researching the efficacy of alternative medicine within their systems of health care. Here a Dutch practitioner of Tibetan medicine takes the pulse of his patient.

In Europe more generally, a number of governments, including those of Denmark, Finland, Hungary, Italy, Norway, Slovenia, Spain, Switzerland and Great Britain, have recently joined forces to support a five-year European Commission Council of Science and Technology project examining the possibilities, limitations and significance of unconventional medicine. This has extended the thrust of politicians in countries like Germany and the Netherlands in sponsoring such research into the medical alternatives within their own national boundaries.[F1] In the United States, evidence of political backing in this area is apparent from the recent federal initiative to create what is now the Office of Alternative Medicine for funding purposes and the licensing of a number of alternative therapies at the state level.[E2]

CHOICE AND VARIETY

It is crucial to note, though, that the concept of alternative medicine in the West is broadly based, including a wide spectrum of therapies ranging from aromatherapy and acupuncture to herbalism and healing. These therapies, moreover, do not form the cohesive whole that is often suggested – not least because they have been established for varying lengths of time and can involve very different principles of operation. Indeed, there are national variations in the manner in which even the same therapy can be practised in different countries. However, what collectively distinguishes the medical alternatives is that they have hitherto tended to lie outside the mainstream educational and research framework that underpins orthodox Western biomedicine and its associated support structures.[S1] We should now look in more detail at the nature of what are defined here as alternative therapies, with special reference to the Eastern influences on them.

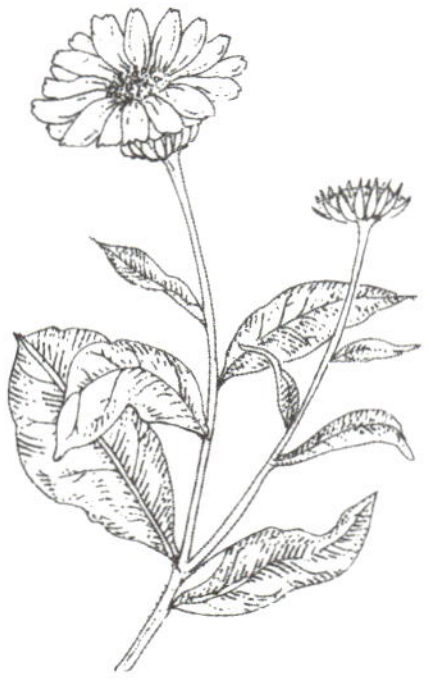

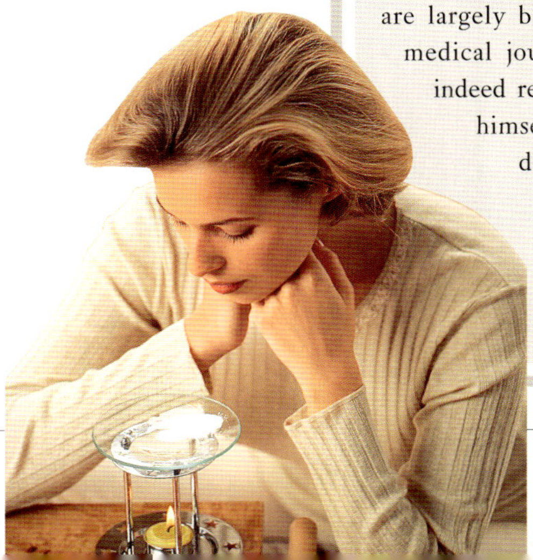

BELOW Aromatherapy involves the use of essential oils derived from plants. It is one of a wide range of alternative therapies that are popular in the West.

THE CRITIQUE OF MODERN MEDICINE

The critique of modern medicine has perhaps been most controversially set out by Ivan Illich *(1926–)*, a leading thinker at the height of the emergence of the counterculture. In 1976, he argued that Western medicine had reached a watershed in which the medical profession itself had become a major threat to health.[I1] He believed that there were three main types of iatrogenesis – or doctor-induced disease – that have made modern medicine counterproductive. The first he termed clinical iatrogenesis, based on the claim that the medical system is now producing clinical damage which far outweighs its benefits. The second is that of social iatrogenesis, which relates to the negative social effects of the increased dependency fostered by the growing over-medicalization of the life span. The third type of iatrogenesis, is that of structural iatrogenesis, which refers to the medical destruction of the ability of people to deal with pain, disease and death in a personal, autonomous way. Although Illich's arguments have been criticized for being overstated, they are largely based on evidence drawn from medical journals themselves. They have indeed recently been reiterated by Illich himself, following his reflection on developments in medicine over the past twenty years.[I2]

THE CONTEMPORARY WESTERN ALTERNATIVES TO MEDICINE

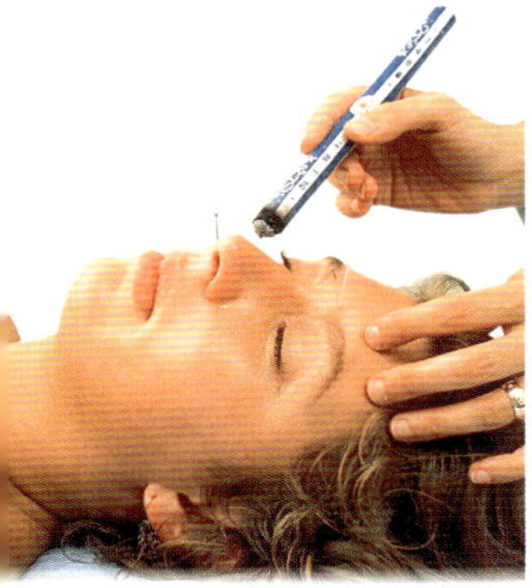

Two of the major Eastern influences on contemporary Western alternative therapies are traditional Chinese medicine and the Indian system of Ayurvedic medicine. These are rooted in ancient texts, based on the idea of individualized treatment and the concept of unity of existence. Both, too, are broad-ranging approaches in which the individual is expected to play an active part in ensuring his or her own well-being. Aside from the general holistic thrust implicit in the Taoist philosophy of harmony that underpins it, on a practical level traditional Chinese medicine is associated with such specific therapies as herbalism, moxibustion and acupuncture – from which other loosely related treatments like the Japanese method of shiatsu derived. The Hindu system of Ayurvedic medicine is equally associated with practices ranging from therapeutic fasting and dieting to herbal medicine and yoga. It may also be seen as a base from which other alternative therapies like homeopathy have more distantly developed.[S8]

The Eastern origin of a number of the more popular Western alternative therapies is well exemplified by acupuncture. In its classical Oriental form it is based on the premise that the life-force (qi) circulates through meridians, invisible channels that link the twelve key organs of the body, along which needles are inserted at specific acupuncture points to balance yin and

LEFT Moxibustion is a technique used by acupuncturists; a needle inserted in one of the body's acupoints is warmed by the application of a burning stick of the moxa herb to stimulate the flow of qi.

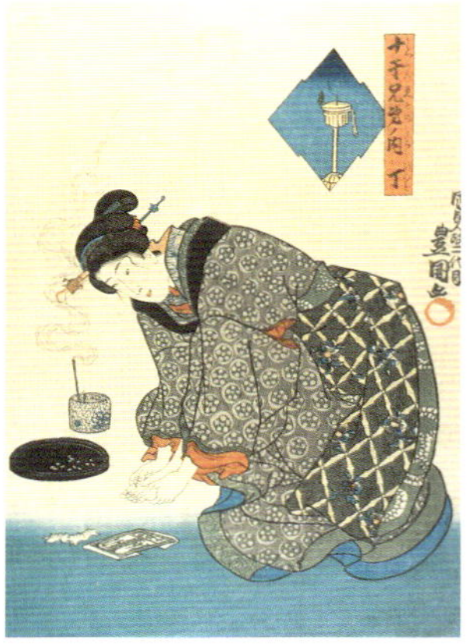

RIGHT A Japanese woodblock print showing another method of moxibustion. In this case, small cones of moxa are applied to the skin, then lit and allowed to burn down, so causing a small blister.

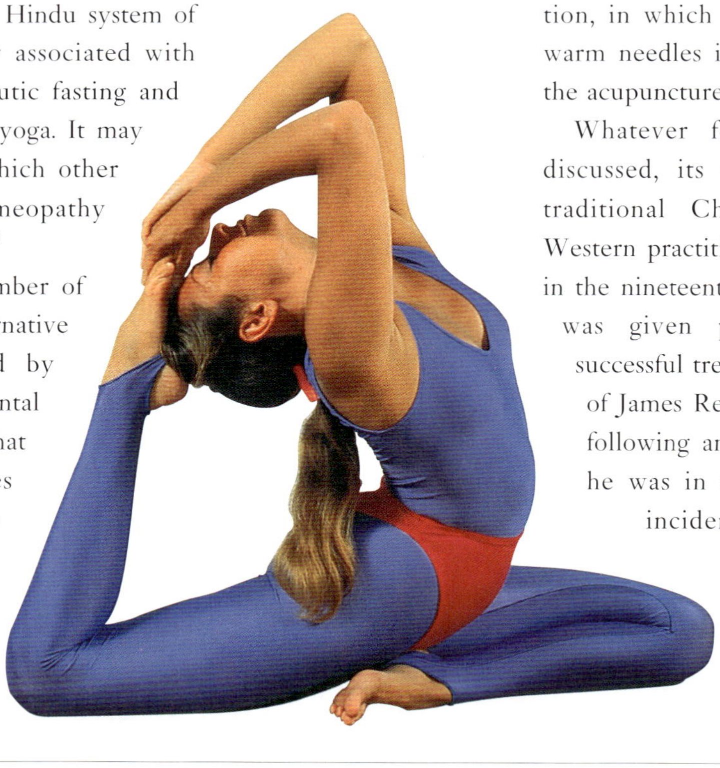

BELOW Yoga exercises are part of the traditional Indian system of Ayurvedic medicine. They are recommended not only to calm and energize the body and mind, but also as a means of achieving spiritual enlightenment.

yang. There are many different types of acupuncture practised in the West, ranging from its traditional Chinese form to a narrower, Western, medicalized type of formula acupuncture. There are major debates between its practitioners about such issues as where the acupuncture needles should be inserted for specific conditions and which illnesses can be treated with acupuncture. There are also a number of variants of acupuncture used in the West, including those based on the Japanese technique of shiatsu, which involves applying finger pressure to the acupuncture points, and, less commonly, moxibustion, in which the dried herb moxa is used to warm needles inserted in, or burned just above, the acupuncture loci.[S4]

Whatever form of acupuncture is being discussed, its roots undoubtedly go back to traditional Chinese medicine. While some Western practitioners of acupuncture were active in the nineteenth century, interest in the therapy was given particular momentum by the successful treatment for severe stomach cramps of James Reston, a *New York Times* journalist, following an operation for appendicitis while he was in China in the early 1970s. This incident stimulated teams of invited doctors from the United States and other Western countries to travel to China with a brief to investigate this phenomenon further.[13]

POPULAR FORMS OF ALTERNATIVE MEDICINE IN THE WEST

Some of the many currently popular forms of alternative medicine practised in Western societies are listed and described briefly below.

ACUPUNCTURE The insertion of one or more needles into the body for therapeutic purposes.

AROMATHERAPY The use of essential oils from plants for massage or inhalation.

BIOFEEDBACK Self-monitoring using an electronic apparatus designed to give the individual information to gain greater control over his/her mind and body.

CHIROPRACTIC A form of manipulation of the spinal and other joints based on stimulating the nervous system.

HEALING An approach, using the laying-on of hands, based on the transmission of energy to the client or the marshalling of the subject's energies for therapeutic purposes.

HERBALISM The use of plants to prevent and treat illness.

HOMEOPATHY An approach centred on the principles that 'like cures like' and that the more dilute a homeopathic substance is, the greater is its medicinal effect.

HYDROTHERAPY The use of water as a therapy as in taking health-giving baths and drinking spa water.

HYPNOSIS The employment of the artificially-induced state of semi-consciousness as a therapeutic technique.

MASSAGE The manipulation of the body to improve health.

NATUROPATHY An approach to prevention and treatment centred on enhancing life-style, involving dietary regimes and exercise.

OSTEOPATHY A form of manipulation of the spinal and other joints based on realignment.

RADIESTHESIA The use of dowsing with a pendulum to diagnose and treat illness.

REFLEXOLOGY The therapeutic massage of the feet, the sensitivity of parts of which is also employed in diagnosis.

SHIATSU A body therapy bringing together finger pressure and massage.

YOGA An approach based on exercise and posture aimed at enhancing spiritual development and health.

The definitions have been derived from various sources. These and other therapies can be explored more fully through such texts as Campbell and Stanway (*see Notes*).

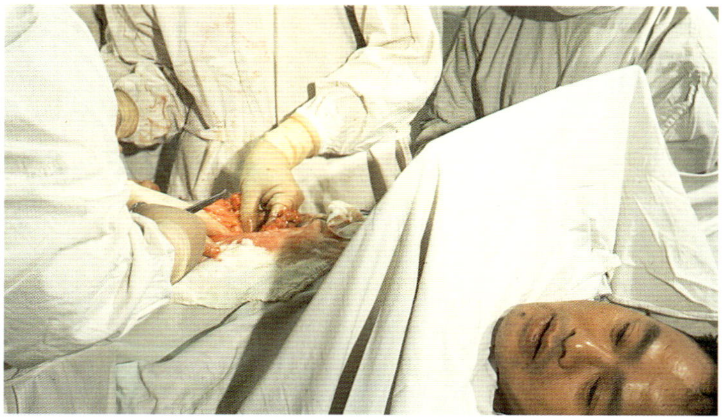

ABOVE **A patient undergoing a surgical operation in China while under acupuncture anaesthesia. He remains conscious, eyes open, throughout the operation.**

Particular attention was paid at this time to the Chinese technique developed in the 1950s of 'acupuncture anaesthesia', in which visiting medical teams witnessed dramatic operations for the removal of brain tumours and open heart surgery without the use of conventional anaesthetics. Pictures of these operations were beamed back by satellite to television viewers watching in the Western world.[S4]

INFLUENCES ON HERBALISM

Herbalism certainly draws on Eastern influences, as illustrated by the currently fashionable use of ginseng (and other herbs with clear Oriental origins) in the West. Central to this form of alternative medicine is the notion that the whole plant, rather than a refined and purified extract, is critical to its operation. The nature of herbalism today is complex, encompassing many different approaches drawn from indigeneous Western herbal folk lore systematized by influential early herbalists such as Culpeper and others, as well as elements of traditional Chinese medicine and Ayurvedic medicine from the East. Often these traditions are combined, with the primary focus concentrating on the relative empirical worth of a given remedy in practice. There are also other historical influences on its application, such as those deriving from Africa and South America. As evidence of the latter, Peruvian bark (cinchona) is particularly well known as the substance from which quinine is derived which is now used within orthodox medicine to treat malaria.[13]

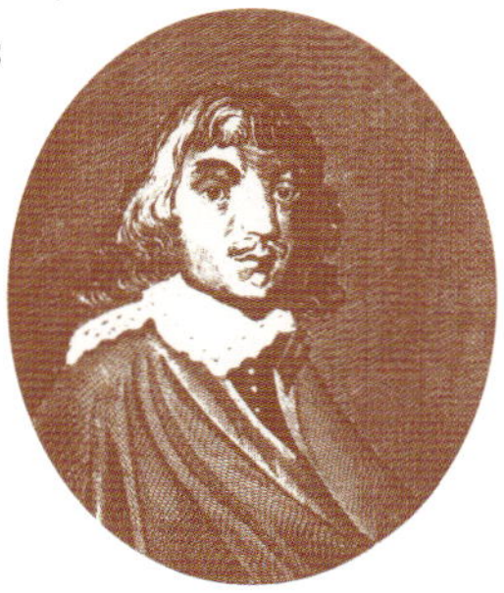

ABOVE **Nicholas Culpeper, the author of an immensely influential herbal.**

Alongside the herbal tradition, mention should also be made of homeopathy, which has proved popular in both North America and Europe. This is less specifically Oriental, however, since its direct origins can be traced back to Samuel Hahnemann *(1755–1843)*, the founder of homeopathy in early nineteenth-century Germany. Homeopathy itself is centred on the principle of treating clients with very small doses of substances (many of which are derived from plants), with the substance in question typically having been diluted to an infinitesimal degree through the processes of either trituration or succussion, in the case of solids and liquids, respectively. The homeopathic philosophy further emphasizes that the patient needs to be given the dose in diluted form to produce similar symptoms to the disease itself, with the aim of holistically stimulating the body's defence mechanisms.[C1] Its philosophy is summed up in Hahnemann's celebrated dictum *'Similia similibus curentur'* ('Like cures like'). The holistic approach is seen as pivotal by classical homeopaths who, like traditional acupuncturists and herbalists, base their practice on the diagnosis and treatment of the whole individual, including such personality characteristics as whether people are tidy, anxious and fearful, unlike most practitioners of orthodox biomedicine who typically have a disease-oriented approach.

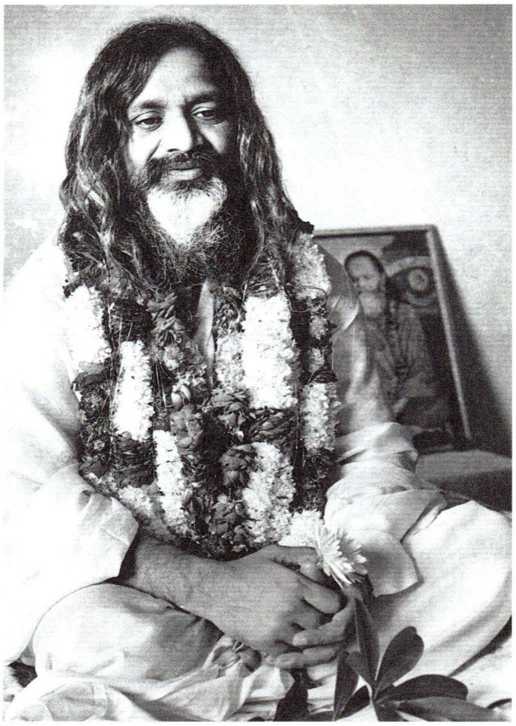

ABOVE **The Maharishi Mahesh Yogi became a familiar figure in the West in the late 1960s. His association with the Beatles made Transcendental Meditation headline news.**

It is also possible to link part of the current vogue for exercise in the West to Oriental influences. This is particularly true of those who engage in qigong, traditional Chinese exercises designed to strengthen and transform qi energy in a manner beneficial to health.[H1] A parallel Eastern influence on alternative medicine is also more directly apparent in the use of meditation to purify the body as a unified entity, which is clearly linked to Asian health traditions. Meditation has sat fairly comfortably with Western technology in relation to the recently established practice of biofeedback. Biofeedback originated in the late 1960s when an experiment was conducted at Harvard Medical School on the effects of Transcendental Meditation, a form of yoga that was introduced to the West by the Maharishi Mahesh Yogi who came to popular attention through his association with the Beatles. The Harvard experiment suggested that TM could lower blood pressure, which in turn led to the development of electronically operated monitoring devices displaying alterations in a patinet's mental condition on a screen. With the information generated, people are variously able to control their own responses to stresses and tensions to enhance their health through the benefits of relaxation.[I3]

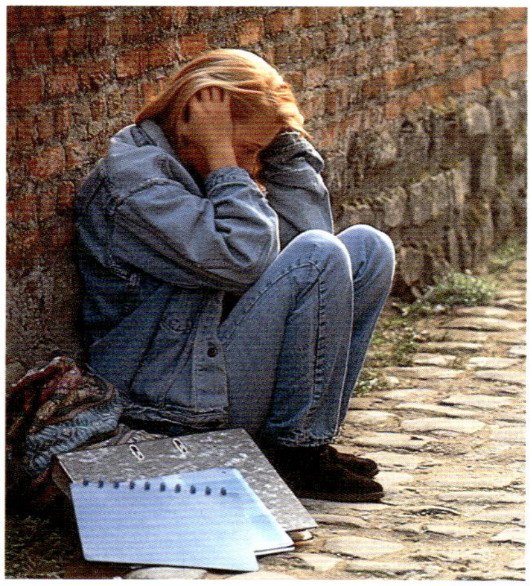

LEFT **An homeopath's diagnosis of an anxious person, like this, would take her personality type into account. Homeopathy does not merely respond to symptoms.**

Another illustration of the strong association between Western alternative medicine and Oriental thought is provided by the work of Deepak Chopra *(1946–)*, who has come to assume the status of a contemporary guru in the West. He has blended his version of Ayurvedic medicine with Western science and sold millions of copies of his books translated into many languages on such topical themes as increasing health and energy levels. His work is centred on the principle that individuals have different Ayurvedic body types with varying proportions of vata, pitta and kapha, which control movement, metabolism and digestion, and physical structure and fluid balance, respectively.[C3] More indirectly, many of the more popular Western alternative therapies, like aromatherapy, hydrotherapy, naturopathy, radiesthesia and reflexology – and even less mainstream approaches like colour therapy, which is primarily based on the use of coloured light to produce a healing effect – have also been influenced to varying degrees by Ayurveda and other Eastern medical traditions.

It should be stressed, though, that not all currently fashionable alternative therapies display such a clear East/West lineage. Good examples of this are osteopathy and chiropractic, which are at present very popular in the West, particularly in dealing with chronic back complaints. The founders of these systems were nineteenth-century pioneers from the United States and Canada – Andrew Taylor Still *(1828–1917)* in the case of osteopathy and Daniel David Palmer *(1845–1913)* for chiropractic. Although they both emphasized the holistic foundation of these therapies and the wide range of conditions that they could address, in recent years their exponents have tended to stress the importance of placing them within a Western scientific frame of reference, in terms of the way the education syllabus, training methods and practice is formally organized.[G2]

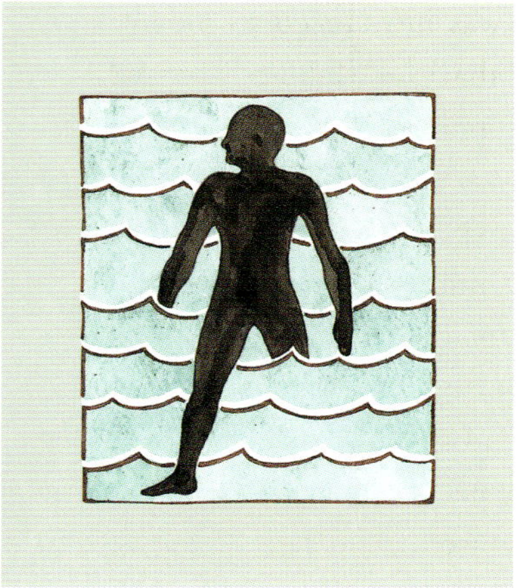

ABOVE Religious shrines, such as that at Lourdes, have a reputation for miraculous water cures that attracts the faithful to them.

Similarly, spiritual healing and faith healing, which are based on a belief in supernatural powers by the healer and patient respectively, do not have straightforward links with Eastern practices. Indeed, they can be technically separated from Oriental influence in so far as they are focused primarily on mainstream Western religious systems of belief, especially Christianity. This is manifested not only in the one-to-one relationship between healer and client, but also in the pilgrimages that millions of believers make annually to Lourdes in southern France and other holy shrines in the West on a self-help basis.[S8] Even here, though, there may still be a loose connection with mainstream strands of Eastern thought in so far as there is a common holistic concern with uniting mind, spirit and body, irrespective of the specific religious nature of the form of healing under discussion.

On the other side of the coin, it should also be noted that some Eastern types of therapy are not necessarily completely at odds with the Western medical tradition. Thus, in the case of acupuncture, for example, there are parallels between classical Oriental beliefs about energy flow and the long-standing Western theory of humours emphasizing the need for the body to be maintained in equilibrium and its four elements and humours mirror the five elements of the Chinese system. Measuring the flow of energy within the body is not unknown in modern Western biomedicine – and the acknowledgement of the presence of such energy led to the development of the current technique for electromyography, which records electrical activity in muscles. Eastern medicine and Western science are also coming together in relation to acupuncture itself, as traditional manual acupuncture is increasingly giving way to electroacupuncture, which involves the stimulation of acupoints with an electrically charged needle.[S4]

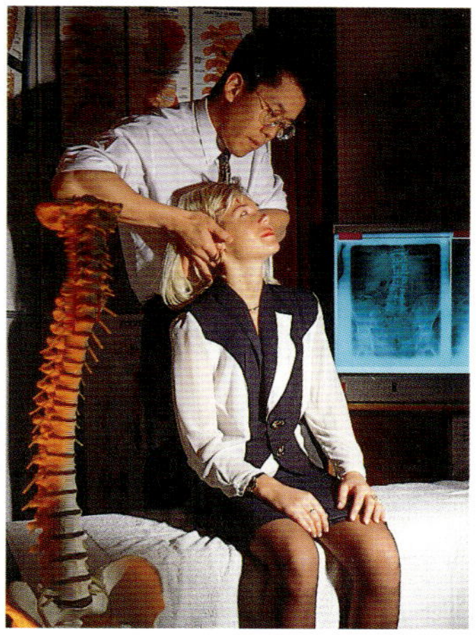

ABOVE Chiropractic is an example of an alternative therapy that developed in the West with little cross-cultural influence from the practices of the East.

Conversely, it should not be assumed that simply because Western alternative therapists usually label themselves as holistic that their practice necessarily always fits this mould, whether it is influenced or not by Eastern philosophies. Holism is an ideology which has helped unite the field, but the idea is not always translated into reality. The concept of alternative medicine covers many diverse therapies in the West. These vary in the degree to which they can be regarded as holistic, as illustrated by comparing the narrow mechanistic practice of some osteopaths with the broader approach of the traditional homeopath.[S1] Divergences in this respect can also arise according to the extent to which Western alternative therapists cooperate with other medical practitioners and show awareness of the wider socio-political setting in which they operate.[M1] In much the same way, while self-help in health care can be holistic, as the activities of the Boston Women's Health Collective have clearly shown,[P2] this is not invariably the case, as some self-help groups choose to work within a framework that is more disease-centred and biomedically orthodox.[V1]

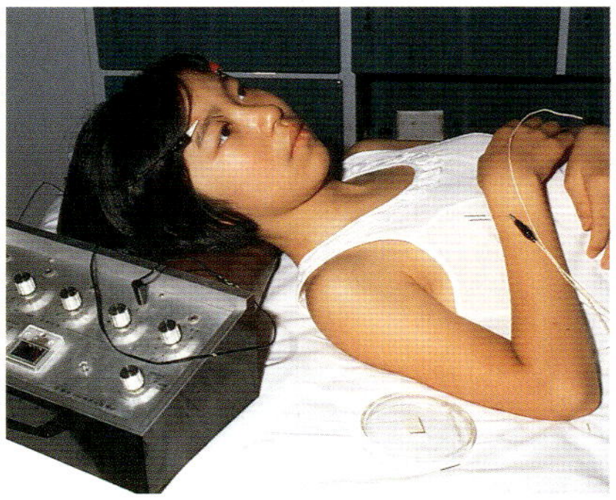

LEFT Electroacupuncture is increasingly popular with Chinese physicians because it is less time-consuming than manual needling.

ALTERNATIVE MEDICINE AND NON-MEDICALLY QUALIFIED PRACTITIONERS

The link between the more holistic elements of alternative medicine and biomedicine in the West in the latter part of the twentieth century has tended to come about through the actions of the consumer, rather than the medical or allied health practitioner. Having said this, in France doctors have long practised acupuncture in its traditional Oriental form to treat a wide range of maladies.[S4] In Germany, too, since the 1930s state licensing of the *Heilpraktikers* (or health practitioners), who are engaged in elements of alternative practice, has played an important part in health care.[A1] In Britain there is also a long tradition of involvement of a small group of doctors in homeopathy, sponsored by well-publicized royal patronage and highlighted by the current existence of five homeopathic hospitals in the UK's state-funded National Health Service.[N1] These cases, however, must be viewed as the exceptions that prove the rule, for the overarching medical response in the West to alternative therapies since the mid-twentieth century has tended to be oppositional. This is well illustrated by the long-running campaigns that have been waged by the American Medical Association and the British Medical Association against accepting such therapies into the medical mainstream.[B5,B3]

Some of this consumer-led demand for alternative therapies relies on self-help routines, particularly through the use of simply acquired techniques like aromatherapy and massage, and the purchase of over-the-counter preparations. However, the most significant thrust towards the integration of alternative and orthodox practices has come about through people consulting the many tens of thousands of alternative practitioners who are not medically qualified now operating in Western societies, in parallel with their normal visits to doctors and other health personnel. In understanding the coming together of Eastern and Western traditions, therefore, it is worth exploring the organizational relationship of practitioners to the therapies concerned. Firstly, however, it should be stressed that most alternative practitioners tend to be working in a disadvantaged position. Although the legislation is not always fully enforced, in Western European countries like Spain and Greece only officially designated health professionals can legally practise – and in France and Belgium the employment of alternative therapies such as homeopathy is not formally open to those without medically recognized qualifications.[F1] This applies to acupuncture, too; in many states in the United States this particular therapy has been defined as a medical technique, from the practice of which unlicensed practitioners are firmly excluded.[S4]

Even in situations where non-medical practice is officially permitted, however, there are variations in the level of funding for treatment from such practitioners that can be obtained by consumers from the state and private sector. This inevitably tends to generate financial, geographical and other inequalities in access to these therapies. Thus, in a country like Britain, where non-medical alternative therapists

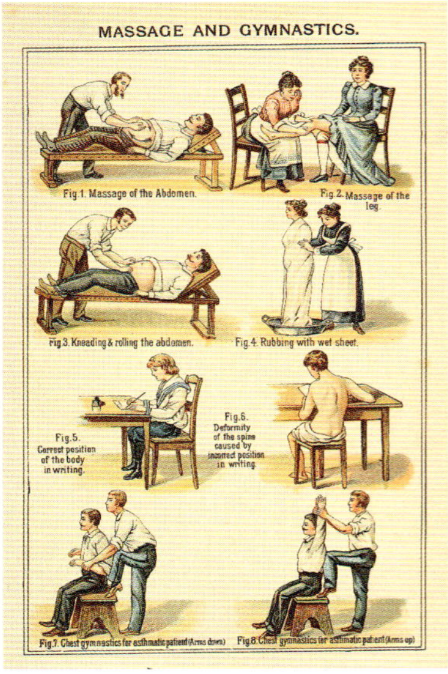

ABOVE This magazine illustration from 1898 celebrating the virtues of 'Massage and Gymnastics' shows that enthusiasm for alternative medicine is not just a modern phenomenon.

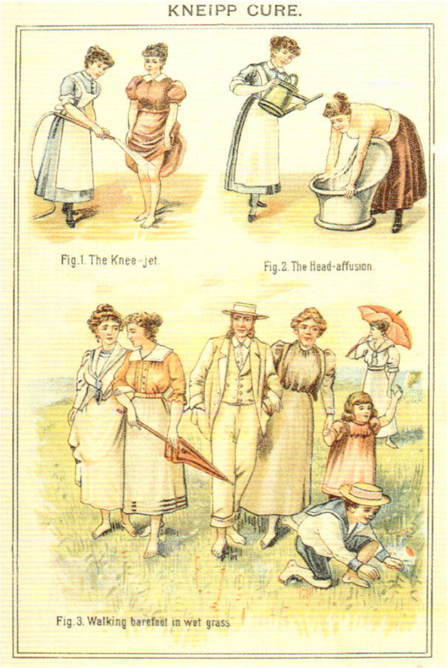

LEFT The Kneipp cure was a type of hydrotherapy conceived at the end of the nineteeth century by a German priest, Father Kneipp.

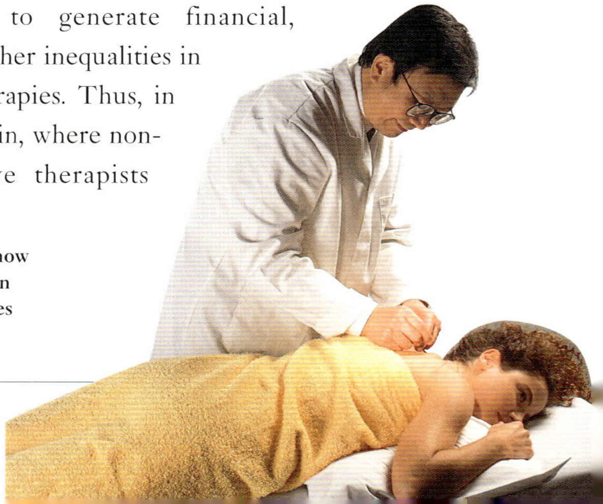

RIGHT Acupuncture is now quite strictly regulated in many European countries and certain US states.

THE POPULARITY OF ALTERNATIVE THERAPISTS IN THE WEST

The use of alternative therapists in Western societies is very widespread. It has been estimated that in the United States, for example, consumers make some 425 million visits each year to practitioners of unorthodox therapies, which is greater than the number of annual visits to all primary-care physicians put together. Recent statistics suggest that those using such therapists represent some ten per cent of the population over a twelve-month period, and some 19 visits are typically undertaken by each consumer.[E2] In Western Europe, meanwhile, the proportion of the population estimated to use practitioners of alternative medicine over any twelve-month period ranges from six to seven per cent in the Netherlands, eight to ten per cent in Britain, up to 15–20 per cent in Finland and 24 per cent in Belgium, which is probably the highest rate in Europe.[S7] It should be noted, though, that there are difficulties in interpreting such data because of international variations in the legal standing of alternative therapies. Nonetheless, the figures clearly indicate the trend towards extensive use of alternative therapists in the West.

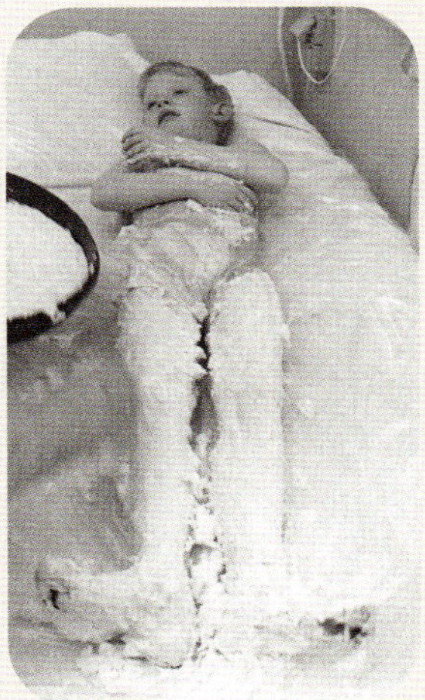

LEFT This Dutch child is being treated for asthma with parapack, a therapy that involves profuse sweating. Up to seven per cent of the population of the Netherlands are thought to use alternative medicine.

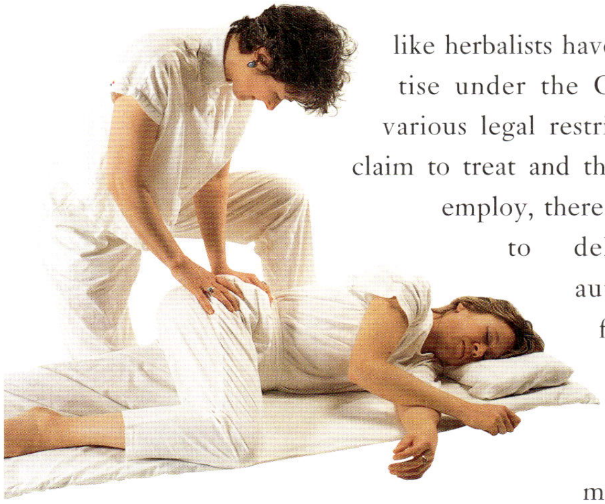

ABOVE Of Japanese origin, the technique of shiatsu uses finger pressure and manipulation to stimulate the body's acupoints to promote healing. Like many other alternative therapies, the training and qualifications of its approved practitioners may be regulated.

like herbalists have the opportunity to practise under the Common Law subject to various legal restrictions on what they can claim to treat and the remedies that they can employ, there are limits on their ability to deliver such therapies autonomously within the framework of the National Health Service.[H2] In the United States, state regulation of unorthodox medical practices such as acupuncture means that even well-qualified practitioners must operate under physician supervision. However, there are some states where both physicians and non-physicians can practise independently, albeit subject to providing reasonable evidence of their educational qualification in the alternative therapy concerned.[C4]

This position of disadvantage can be at least partly explained in terms of the power and interests of the medical profession in protecting its own territory against competitors in the health-care marketplace. However, it should also be acknowledged that legitimate considerations regarding the public interest in relation to the level and type of training of practitioners of both Western and Eastern styles of medicine do exist, which may have restricted the position of non-medically qualified alternative therapists. In addition, there are potentially wider forces at work, including the influence of powerful multinational pharmaceutical companies that can view the rise of alternative therapies as a threat to their commercial interests. Also, non-medically qualified alternative practitioners are not a cohesive group, and they have not always presented their case in as well-coordinated a manner as they might in order to gain wider acceptance.[S5]

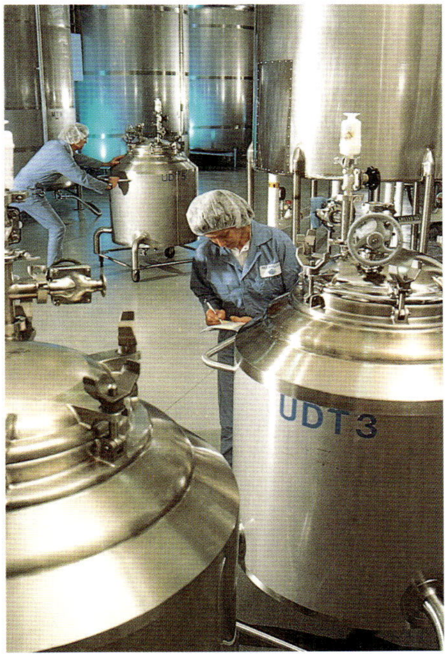

ABOVE Multinational pharmaceutical companies exert influence over the health-care market. They may not view the popularity of alternative medicine with unqualified approval.

THE MOVE TO COLLECTIVE ORGANIZATION

This relative lack of coordination is largely because the tradition of alternative practice has been individualistic. Although there are exceptions as, for example, in the case of chiropractors in the United States, who have been strongly organized historically at a collective level,[W2] typically there has been little coherence among unorthodox Western practitioners in organizational terms, even in specific therapeutic fields. However, this situation has changed considerably, particularly over the past two or three decades when a range of bodies representing particular alternative therapies have grown up in the West. Nationally, these have taken the form of organizations ranging from the Canadian Naturopathic Association[C5] to the Society of Homeopaths in Britain,[C2] while on a wider front they have included such bodies as the International Association of Colour Therapists and the International Association of Aromatherapists.[F2] Although there is evidently a desire to improve public standards of treatment, this development also seems to be aimed at ensuring that alternative therapists gain the most favourable legal standing in the marketplace.

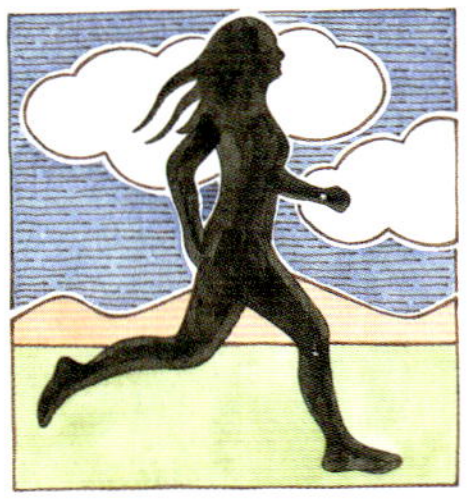

ABOVE Naturopathy is a therapy that concentrates on life-style, diet and exercise regimes. Qualified naturopaths typically have to undergo several years of training at a recognized college of naturopathy to receive accreditation.

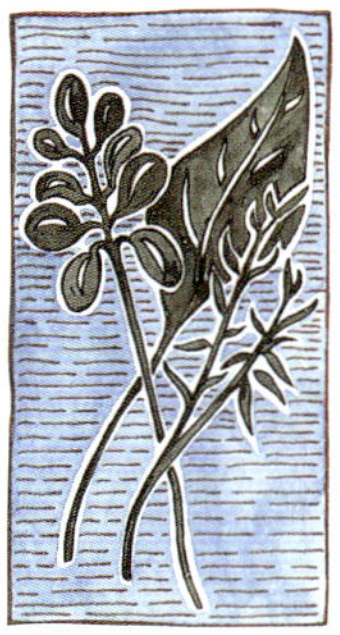

ABOVE Herbalism can be practised in a self-help way in a family context, but potential hazards suggest that it is sensible to consult qualified practitioners.

This has been a particular concern in Europe, where some therapists fear that tighter controls may be introduced as a result of harmonization, following the creation of the European Union.[F1] The enhancement of the organizational structure of alternative medicine has been especially evident in Britain, where the regulation of this area has hitherto been amongst the most liberal in the Western world. Here, on an even greater scale than in many other Western societies, a number of practitioner groups are actively engaged in the professionalizing process. Their enthusiasm has been raised by recent legislation that has given both osteopaths and chiropractors the right to maintain a register and protection of title.[S2] The process is, however, best illustrated in this context by developments in Britain associated with acupuncture, one of the therapies with the

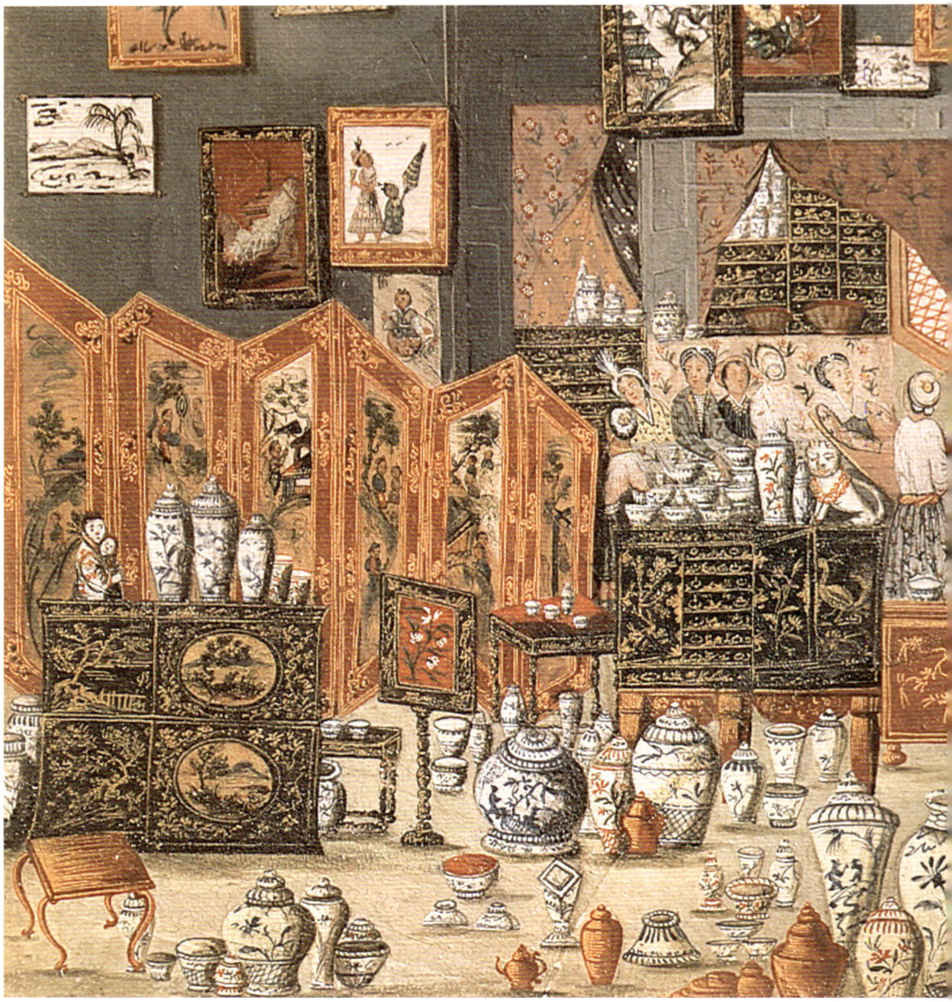

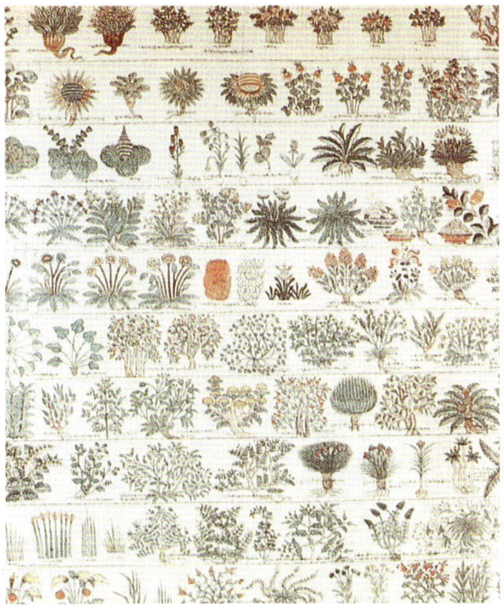

ABOVE Herbs illustrated and classified in an Indian pharmacopoeia. On occasion, herbs may be prescribed by unlicensed practitioners who have no formal qualifications.

strongest Eastern roots. Here the various mainstream non-medical acupuncture organizations have come together under the single administrative umbrella of the British Acupuncture Council and it has established a common standard for educational requirements and codes of ethics in a search for legal recognition for this discipline.[S3]

In spite of these general trends, a number of unorthodox practitioners still operate individually without formal qualifications, legally or illegally, in Western societies. This has certainly been the case, for instance, in relation to some hakims, practitioners of the Unani system of medicine. This derives from the Muslim parts of India and Pakistan, has some roots in ancient Greek medical thought and common links with Ayurvedic health philosophies. Hakims engage in diagnosis and treatment on the basis of classifying both the patient and potential remedies in terms of their heat, dryness, coldness or wetness. Such practitioners, like their Hindu counterparts who practise Ayurvedic medicine, have often learned their skills with herbs and other substances through an apprenticeship model centred on the principle of family transmission, rather than through the medical colleges in Asia that run formal courses in this kind of alternative medicine. Nonetheless, Unani practitioners have a captive market among the migrant Asian population in many Western countries – as well as an increasing number of other consumers, as the popularity of Eastern therapies rises in the Western world.[E1]

However, concerns have been voiced in the West about the safety of some Oriental forms of alternative medicine in untrained hands – as, for example, in relation to the toxic heavy metals contained in certain tonics used by hakims and the potentially fatal threat posed by outbreaks of hepatitis B and collapsed lungs from the insertion of acupuncture needles.[E1,S4] Nonetheless, in part

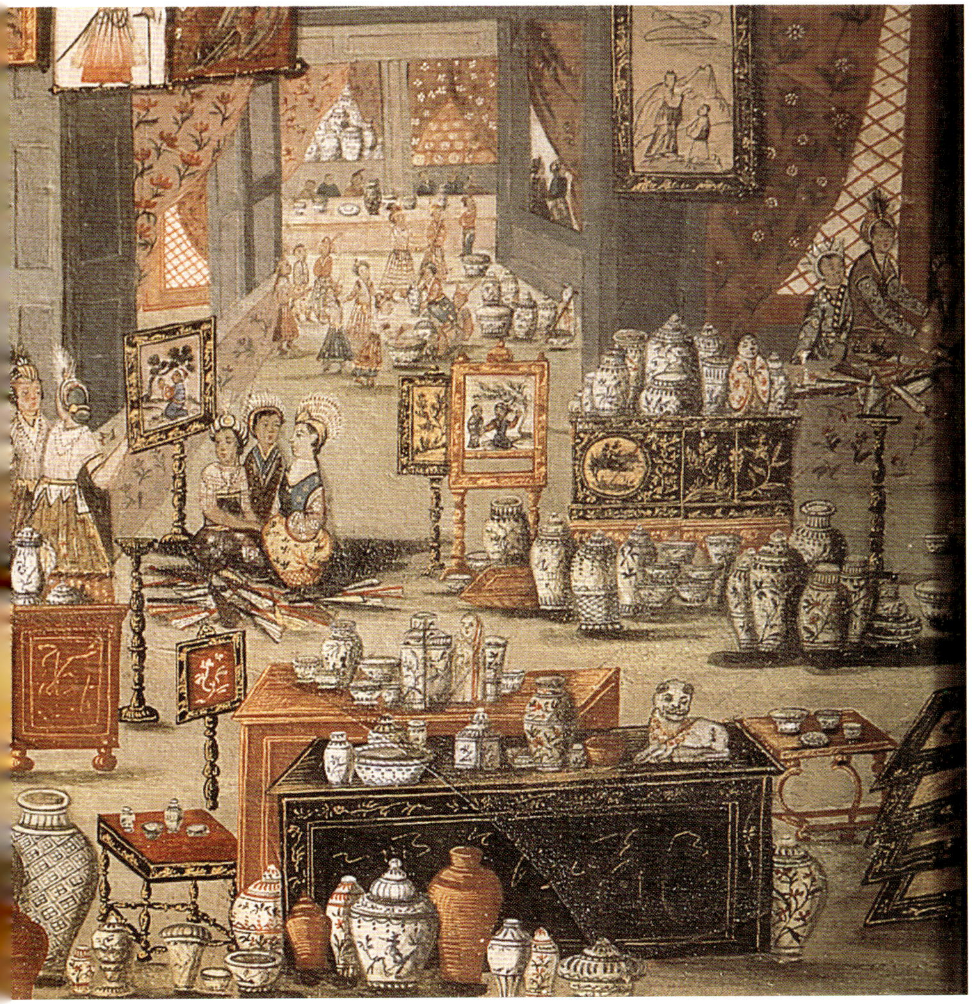

LEFT Eastern influences spread to Europe as early as the nineteenth century. This picture of a Chinese dealer's shop was probably painted in Holland.

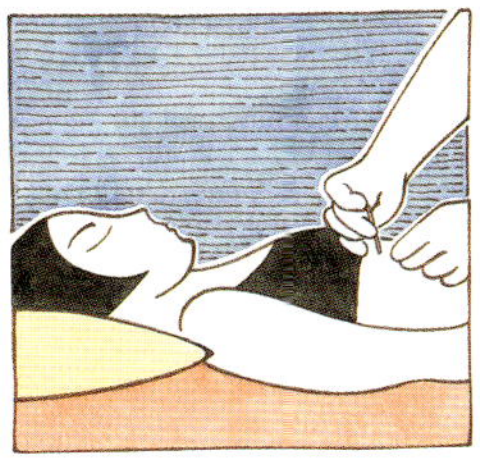

ABOVE The insertion of needles into a body is not without risk. It is important that practitioners of acupuncture are professionally competent.

because of the general moves of non-medical unorthodox therapists to put their own house in order, the medical profession has become more favourably disposed to cooperation with practitioners of alternative medicine. This is clearly indicated in Britain by the shift of the position of the British Medical Association from the earlier blanket condemnation of such therapies as primitive non-scientific superstition in 1986[B3] towards its expression of support in 1993 for collaborating with alternative therapists.[B4] This trend has been paralleled in the United States, as can be seen by the way in which chiropractors have now followed in the footsteps of osteopaths in gaining both state licensure and the right to reimbursement within the Medicare and Medicaid schemes. The American Medical Association has also been legally compelled to moderate its longstanding campaign against them.[W3]

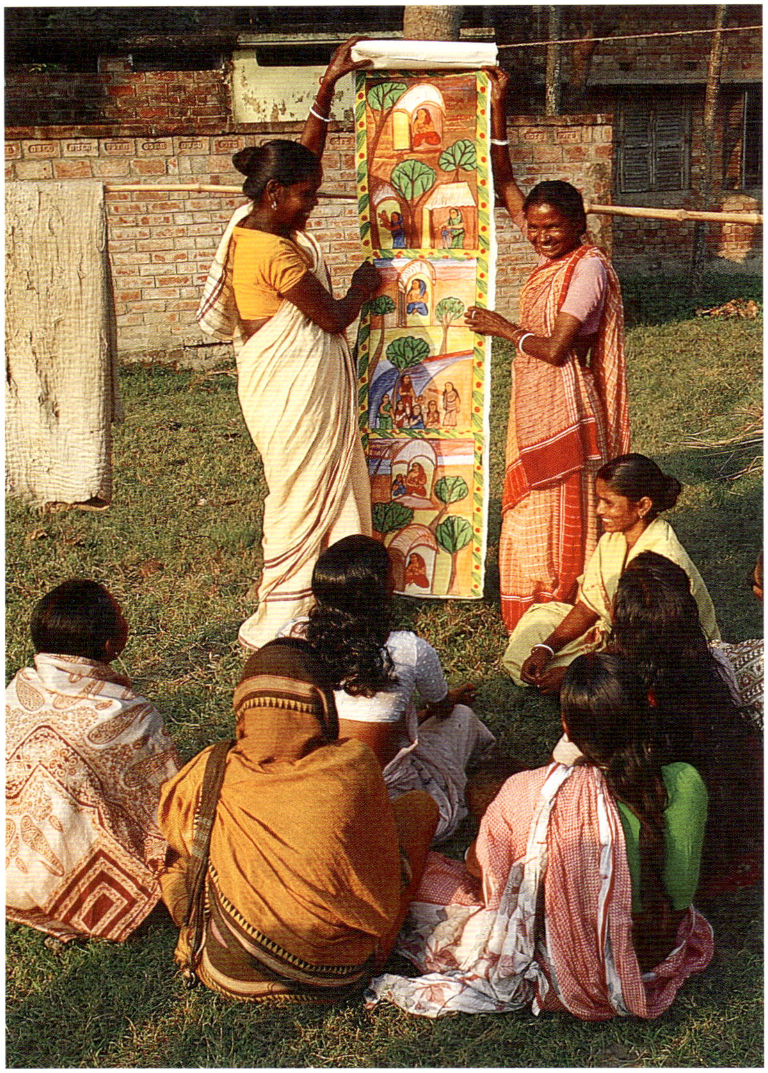

ABOVE Cutural exchanges between East and West have brought about changes in the way health care is practised in both cultures. Here women are taught about the benefits of breastfeeding their babies by local community health advisers.

Such changes clearly also reflect the pressures which have been brought to bear by the public and politicians alike on the side of more holistic unorthodox approaches to health care, as the holistic health movement has gained support on both sides of the Atlantic.[A2] In consequence, improved cooperation between doctors, allied health personnel and non-medically qualified alternative practitioners – coupled with stronger referral networks – has come about in both Europe and North America in recent years. There is, of course, still a considerable way to go at a time. For example, in the United States, a study carried out in 1990 revealed that some nine out of ten consumers consulting an alternative practitioner did so without being recommended to by their doctor, and three-quarters of these did not tell their doctor about their use of such therapy.[E2] However, the growing recognition of the benefits of greater interprofessional cooperation between practitioners and doctors, as part of the pursuit of holistic health, is testimony to the way in which Western and Eastern approaches to health care are now beginning to converge in the West.

In such circumstances, it can be argued that the vested interests of leading figures in the medical establishment in many Western countries – in terms of the protection of their power, income and status – have played a key part in this process. Establishment opinion has increasingly shifted from outright opposition to alternative therapists to an acceptance of incorporating them on a subordinated or otherwise limited basis within the orthodox division of labour, in much the same way that other occupational groups like nurses and midwives were drawn under the wing of medicine in earlier decades.[S2] Of course, organizational shifts in the balance of Western health care have not just occurred in the relationship between orthodox and unorthodox practitioners, but also within medicine itself. More specifically, there has been a growing tendency not only for Western biomedical and Eastern-inspired alternative practitioners to co-exist, but also for Western and Eastern approaches increasingly to be combined in the curriculum of the medical doctor, who may work in association with allied health personnel in the orthodox health-care system in a complementary fashion.

THE HOLISTIC REFORM OF WESTERN ORTHODOX MEDICINE

Doctors at grass-roots level in the West have often been more ready to recognize the benefits of the holistic alternatives to medicine than those in elite positions in their profession.[S2] There has been a growing willingness among such practitioners to incorporate holistic practices within Western medicine, including Eastern therapeutic approaches. This has particularly, but not exclusively, applied to those working in general practice in community settings where doctors themselves have increasingly either taken up the practice of alternative therapies in their own right, or integrated them into their own practice through delegation to other members of the health-care team. While there are some Western doctors who claim that holism has always been central to good medical practice, therefore, the recent limits on this development in an age dominated by biomedicine should be recognized.[S6] Equally, however, there are encouraging signs that a more holistic approach to patients' needs is gradually emerging out of this development as Eastern and Western approaches to health care come ever closer together in the West.

At a wider level, it is important to note the rapid expansion of holistic health care centres since the 1960s, often with active medical involvement. This trend has been much in evidence across the United States, where there are many models of such centres. Their key characteristics are as follows: they aim to address the physical, psychological and spiritual needs of the individual; to mobilize the capacity of the individual for self-healing and self-care; to acknowledge the role of consumers in the wider social system; to stress health promotion and wellness; to emphasize the importance of diet and exercise; to use the therapeutic potential of the care setting involved; to build a partnership between consumers and care givers; to involve a wide range of health personnel in the day-to-day management of the centre; to ensure the personal growth of staff and clients; to engage in the ongoing training of staff; to include indigenous healing systems and healers in the operation of the centre; to provide an environment where change is facilitated; and to self-evaluate their own performance.[G3]

ALTERNATIVE MEDICINE AND WESTERN DOCTORS

The employment of alternative medicine, including therapies with Eastern roots, by doctors themselves, is becoming increasingly widespread in the West. This is highlighted by recent research studies which have provided the following information on a number of countries.

BRITAIN Approximately one third of general practitioners have been trained in alternative therapies, with many desiring further training and up to 37 per cent using homeopathy, one of the most frequently practised therapies.

FRANCE More than one third of general practitioners use alternative therapies, and five per cent of such practitioners employ these exclusively, while 21 per cent use them often and 73 per cent occasionally.

THE NETHERLANDS Almost one half of general practitioners employ alternative therapies, with a range spanning from 40 per cent using homeopathy at the highest point to four per cent employing acupuncture.

THE UNITED STATES Doctors in the United States also variously make use of alternative therapies, although comparable data on the extent of this practice on a national basis are not readily available.

For further discussion of the international use of alternative therapies by Western medical doctors see, amongst others, Fisher and Ward (1994), from which the above is derived.

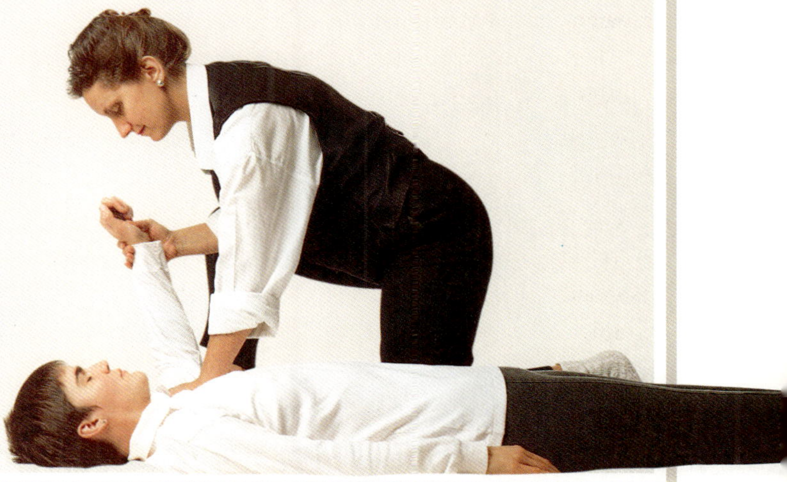

RIGHT One of the traditonal therapies from the East enjoying popularity in the West is *shiatsu*, a massage technique originated in China and developed in Japan.

Centres such as the Bresler Center in Los Angeles and the Kripalau Center in western Massachusetts broadly follow mainstream Oriental philosophies, a point underlined by the fact that they frequently include such Eastern practices as acupuncture, massage and qigong exercises – as well as a range of other locally based alternative therapies and a myriad more orthodox biomedical treatments, all offered in synthesis. However, such centres are by no means unique to the United States in the Western world. This is illustrated by the well-known Marylebone Health Centre in Britain, one of several in Western Europe. This Centre very much fits into the holistic health-care mould by bringing together alternative therapists, such as herbalists and homeopaths, with orthodox doctors, nurses and midwives in a multi-disciplinary fashion under one roof. It also encourages clients to participate in the running of the Centre and in the administration of self-help activities that it promotes, such as yoga and meditation.[P3]

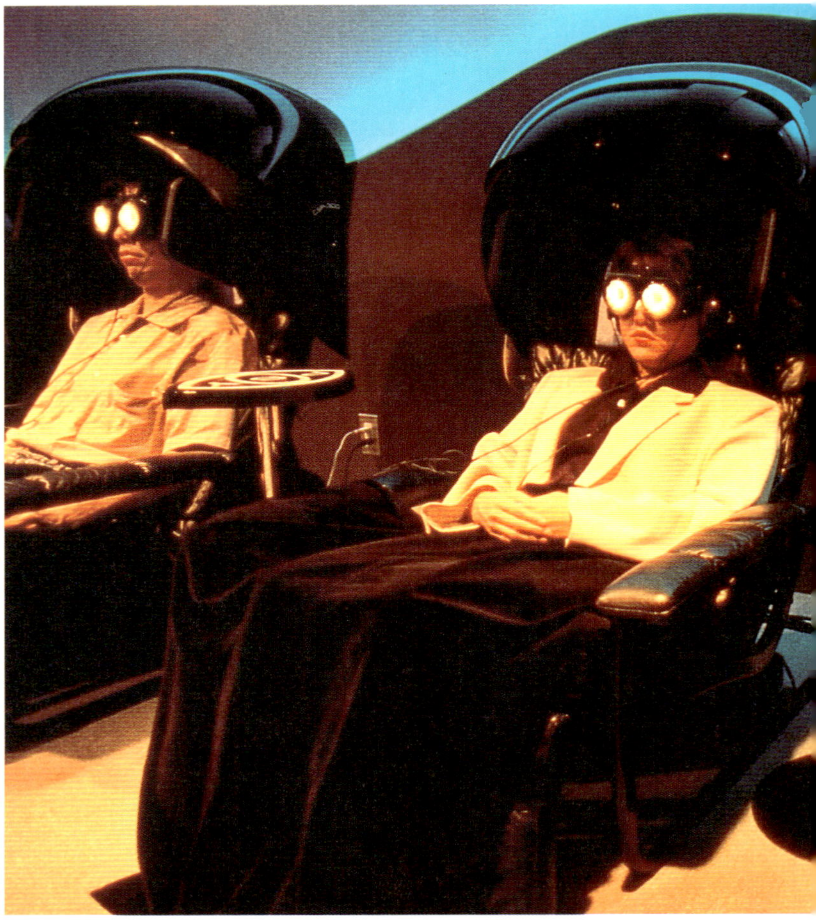

DOCTORS AND HOLISM

There are questions, though, as to how far holistic integration has been effected in the West through the medical profession. Many doctors and other allied health professionals have indeed now become interested in practising various forms of alternative medicine, including those with Eastern links, not least in holistic health centres. In addition, some Western doctors have formed associations restricted to a medical membership to advance the study of various specific fields of alternative therapy.[F2] However, in bringing Eastern and Western health traditions together in this manner, alternative practices have often been adopted by doctors in such a way that they are detached from their holistic roots and redefined as biomedical techniques. This is certainly true of acupuncture, which is increasingly employed by doctors in the West, but the effectiveness of which is mainly explained in terms of orthodox Western neurophysiological theories about the production of endorphins, rather than in terms of its classic Oriental rationale. In medical hands, acupuncture is also primarily used as an analgesic to suppress pain, not as a treatment for the broad range of conditions and illnesses for which it is typically employed in China.[S4]

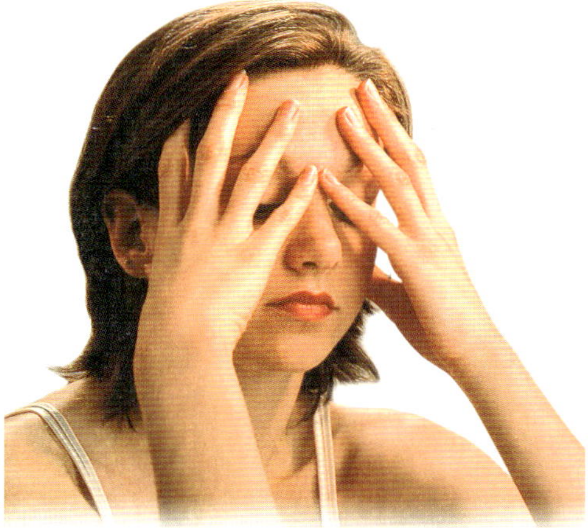

LEFT Holistic health-care centres now offer patients a diverse choice of therapies: orthodox clininal medicine is available alongside professionally organized alternative therapies and instruction in self-help techniques such as meditation and yoga.

It is also debatable to what extent leading medical figures in some Western countries are committed to advancing this position – in moving towards more holistic forms of integrated practice. In the case of alternative medicine, for instance, the most recent report of the British Medical Association in *1993*, although more favourably disposed to such therapies than previously, goes on to emphasize not only that doctors must remain responsible for patients, but also that alternative practitioners should include aspects of the orthodox medical curriculum, such as anatomy and physiology, in their programmes and training.[B4] This follows the experience of osteopaths in the United States, where the process of basing their curriculum on that of orthodox medical schools began several decades ago.[G2] Similar issues are posed by the continuing argument that randomized

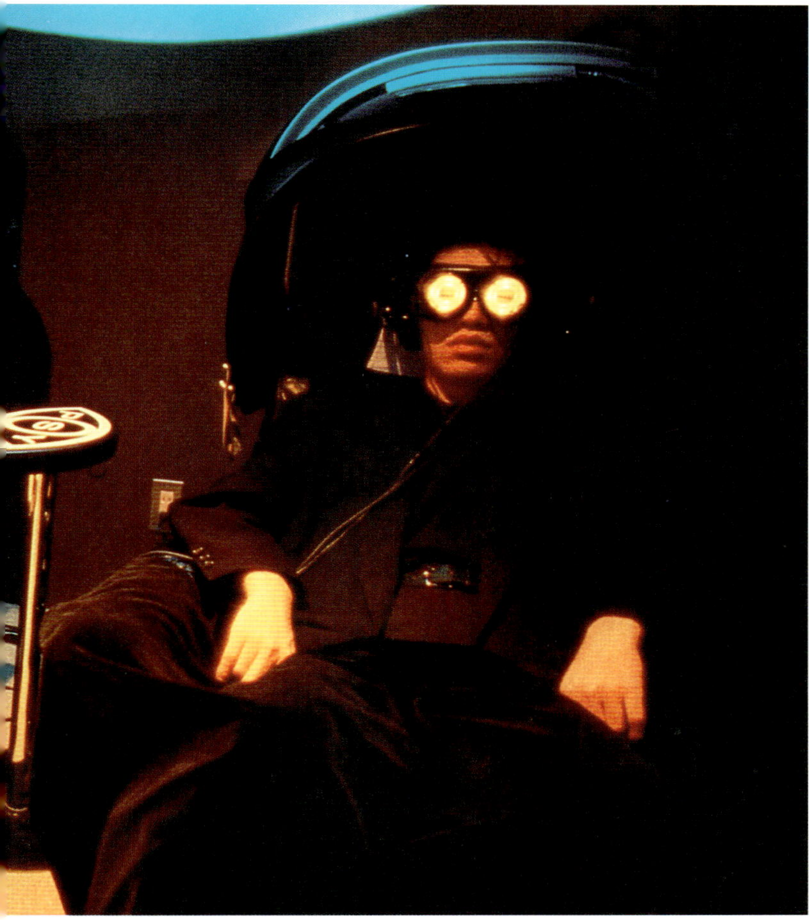

LEFT A group of people practising meditation with the assistance of electronic biofeedback monitors. Here, paradoxically, Western technology is brought to the service of a predominantly Eastern discipline.

controlled trials should be used as the 'gold standard' for assessing the value of alternative medicine in the West, as they are in biomedicine. This is not necessarily compatible with the notion of individually personalized treatment that is embedded in a more holistic, Eastern-style approach, which may require different methods of evaluation.[S2]

Such issues are also apparent in the reform of orthodox medicine more generally as it strives to become more holistic in face of the critique of high-technology medicine. There is, in fact, a tension between biomedical and holistic approaches here that has not yet been fully resolved, as highlighted by the classic work of Engel *(1977)*.[E3] This attempts to combine the influences of the family, community and the national dimensions of life with a narrow scientific notion of medicine in an integrated biopsychosocial model, leaving biomedicine as the overriding element in the equation. This mirrors the experience of many alternative practitioners when they are included within orthodox health-care teams. They, too, have frequently been subordinated within a framework of medical dominance, raising doubts about whether their approaches are really being employed in a balanced and integrated manner. These concerns are raised at a time when alternative therapists themselves seem to be increasingly seen by conventional doctors simply as another group of specialists in the health-care division of labour.[P1]

These points highlight that to date there has only been a limited convergence in the West of Eastern and Western health systems as far as the medical profession itself is concerned. To the extent that alternative forms of medicine embodying more holistic Eastern philosophies have been adopted since the mid-twentieth century, this has tended to come about on the medical profession's own terms. Although it is difficult to generalize across societies, after an initial period of resistance to such approaches, Western doctors have tended to favour a position of incorporation based heavily on biomedical orthodoxy, rather than an integration. This may again be interpreted as a stance reflecting the vested interests of professional elites in supporting the 'scientific' biomedical model in face of competition, in order to maintain and, in some cases, extend its position of dominance.

It is interesting to observe that Western doctors have tended to be most enthusiastic about employing alternative therapies when a monopoly of practice has been granted to them in the field concerned – as in the case of acupuncture in France and certain states in the United States in this period.[S4] This should not, however, blind the enquirer to the sometimes less than helpful influence of the major health corporations on the situation outside the professional domain. Nor should it obscure the fact that Western biomedicine and more holistic Eastern alternatives are increasingly coming together in Western societies. This is progressively occurring through the actions of the consumer and through interprofessional collaboration under the umbrella of medical orthodoxy – which is an encouraging development even if there is still some considerable way to go.

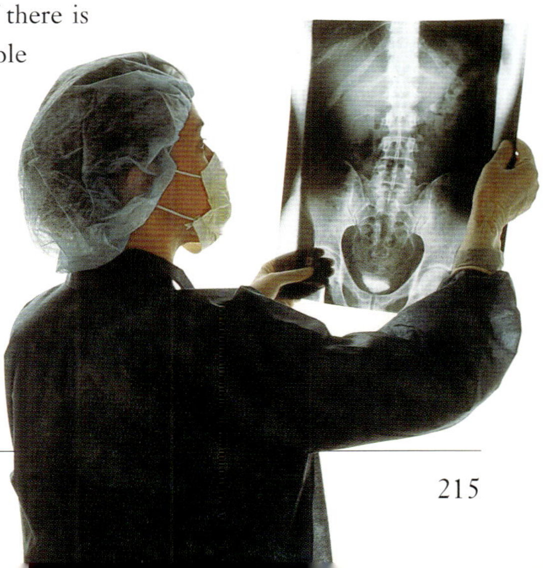

RIGHT Western doctors are embracing alternative therapies, albeit slowly. But this has generally come about because of market demand, rather than any deep-seated ideological commitment on their part.

THE IMPACT OF WESTERN BIOMEDICINE ON THE EAST

Health-care in the East today is characterized by a mosaic of differing holistic approaches. These centrally include the traditional systems of Ayurvedic and Chinese medicine that have been so influential in the West, as well as other related types of health care, which are strongly rooted traditional forms of medicine. It should not, however, be assumed that the East adopts a unified approach in terms of the knowledge and practice of these various medical traditions even today – for its culture is marked, perhaps more than the West, by its diversity in cultural as well as economic terms. Of course, ideas about health care have undeniably diffused through Oriental cultures. Tibetan medicine, which draws on a number of traditions, is a case in point. The personal physician to the Dalai Lama, for example, combines, among other things, the Chinese method of taking of pulses with Indian theories of medicine and Buddhist practices for his own concentration and purification – as well as a form of urine analysis derived from the medical practices of ancient Greece.[K2]

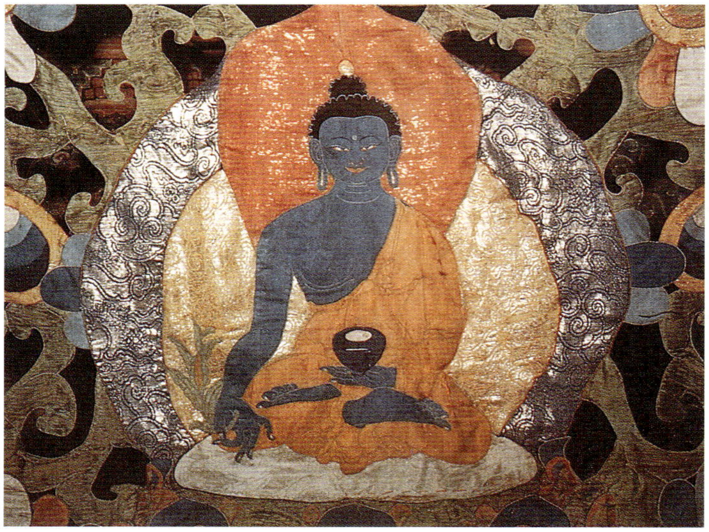

ABOVE The development of medicine in Tibet was particularly influenced by its close links to Buddhism. Novice monks studied medicine as part of their syllabus; healing the sick was encouraged because it helped develop a sense of compassion. This picture is of the Medicine Buddha.

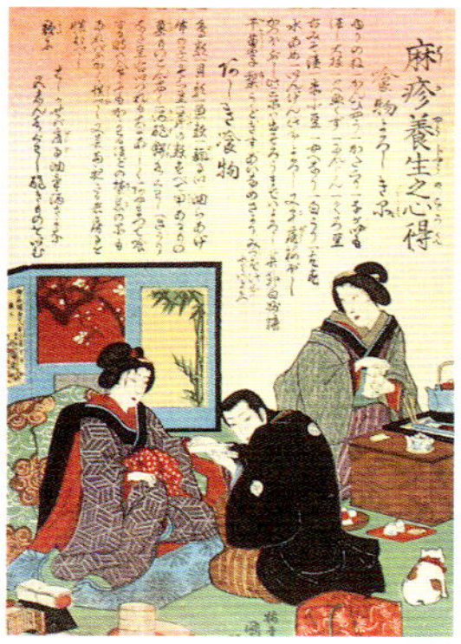

ABOVE A Japanese physician takes the pulse of his patient – a woodcut print of 1885 by Kunimasa entitled 'Dietary advice for patients with measles'.

This is the world, then, on which the Western health system has exerted its influence. The extent of this influence, particularly in relation to biomedicine, has undoubtedly been greater recently than in the period before the mid-twentieth century, when its application to the population at large tended to be very limited. It now offers more tangible benefits, as is illustrated by the use of essential Western drugs in primary health care in countries like Thailand and Malaysia, and the widespread employment of immunization for control of infectious disease.[T1] However, the impact of the West has also encouraged the use of a model of health care that is too heavily centred on hospital care. This is highlighted in third-world Eastern societies where the curative approach of biomedicine is of less importance than disease prevention, given the adverse social and environmental conditions in which many people live. In such situations, and without a well-defined public health structure, even positive aspects of biomedicine, such as vaccination programmes, only have a limited effect; they canreduce death rates, but without necessarily improving the quality of life.

A further dilemma is that the urban hospital focus so characteristic of less affluent societies has meant that in practice biomedical services in countries with a large rural population, like India, are only available to a small proportion of citizens. This is mirrored in the relative distribution of Western-style health personnel between the town and countryside. But if geographic factors usually limit and give rise to inequalities in the availability of biomedicine in such societies, so, too, do financial barriers in privatized areas of the health services for the impoverished majority. Access to biomedicine tends to be concentrated in the hands of more wealthy minorities as a luxury item of consumption in the private sector. This raises social issues paralleling to some degree those relating to the availability of certain forms of alternative medicine in the West.[D1]

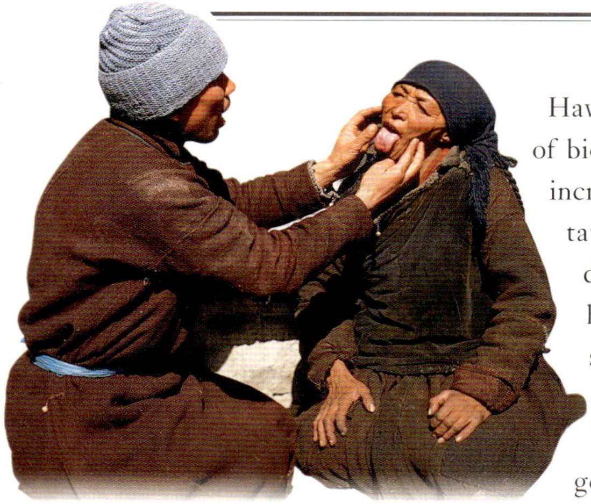

ABOVE An Indian village doctor examines the tongue of a patient by the side of a road. Western medicine has had little impact on such rural practitioners.

Having said this, the use of biomedical treatment is increasingly being facilitated through the development of state help and insurance schemes following the situation in the Western world, as governments in the East strive to ensure its provision for growing numbers of the population.[H3] In addition, Western patterns of medical education and training have now typically taken root indigenously in most Oriental societies – having developed initially in some areas from the rudimentary teaching system associated with colonialism and the presence of European practitioners. And while a significant number of doctors migrate to more affluent Western countries such as Britain, Germany and the United States, the number who stay to offer biomedical treatment has increased greatly in such Eastern societies.[D1] Indeed, these points of contact have broadened even further in more highly developed economies in the East, like that of Japan.[P6]

THE INFLUENCE OF BIG BUSINESS

Central to the growth of biomedicine in less economically advanced Eastern countries in the modern period has been the impact of Western multinational corporations, which are involved in the supply of medical equipment and hospital development. The most significant influence in this field has been multinational pharmaceutical companies.[G1] Such companies typically control most of the patents in the third-world countries with which they have contact. This explains why these nations represent an attractive and expanding market to them, often with a higher rate of profit on sales than in the West. While this has certainly helped to extend access to Western-style medicine, the multinational corporations have also frequently promoted high-technology hospitals at the expense of more basic health care for the broader population. This situation has also created additional hazards through the promotion of drugs with significant side effects, such as anabolic steroids and the antibiotic chloramphenicol. These are more likely to be recommended for less serious conditions in areas like south-east Asia, where many such potentially dangerous drugs are often available to the populace without the requirement of a prescription.[D1]

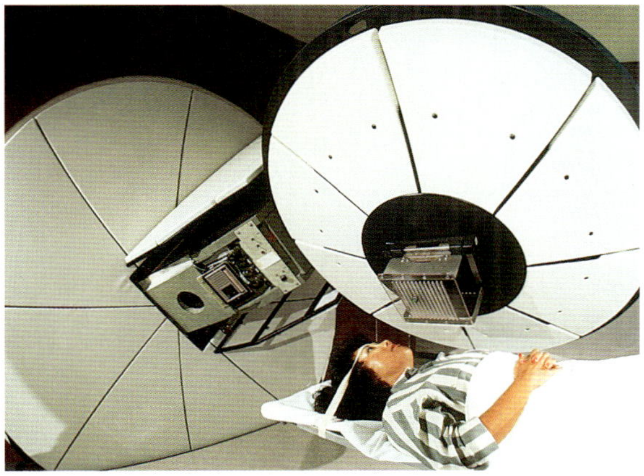

ABOVE Trainee doctors in China now study Western biomedicine in parallel with traditional indigenous forms of healing. Radiology and acupuncture are bedfellows in their hospitals.

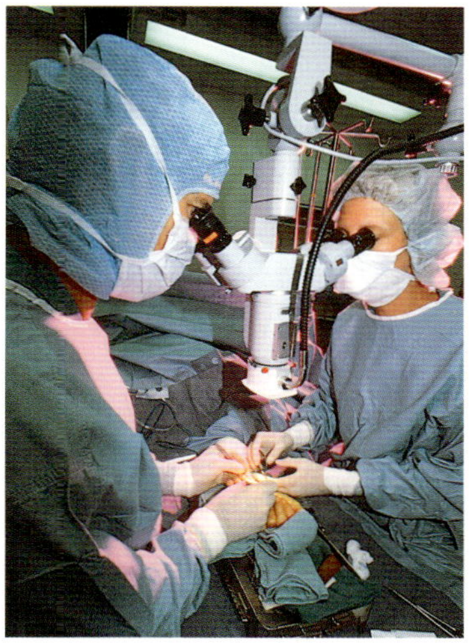

ABOVE Western-style high-tech hospitals have been established in the East, but they swallow huge amounts of the available resources, often at the expense of more basic health care.

In this situation it is reassuring that traditional Eastern health practices have so often survived alongside biomedicine, despite the fact that not all governments in third-world societies formally recognize traditional healers. The World Health Organization, in fact, has actively promoted such practices as a relatively inexpensive health resource in developing countries, in face of resistance from the drug industry and indeed certain sections of the Western medical establishment. This has been even more important in areas where traditional medicine is the only form of local health care available.[H3] One outcome has been that in societies like China and India medical students must now normally study Western biomedicine as part of their curriculum alongside their traditional health systems,[K2] even if these do not always assume the equal status that national political ideologies suggest.[R1] This, nonetheless, has significant implications for their practice. For example, in China, facilities for the practice of traditional Chinese medicine may be found alongside those for surgery and radiology in hospitals.

THE WORLD HEALTH ORGANIZATION AND TRADITIONAL MEDICINE

The World Health Organization has taken the following stance on traditional medicine in less developed societies, including those in the East. Its policy is founded on these six principles.

1. Give recognition to traditional practitioners and incorporate them into community development programmes.

2. Retrain traditional practitioners for appropriate use in primary health care.

3. Acquaint professional health personnel and students of modern systems with the principles of traditional medicine in order to promote dialogue, communication, mutual understanding and eventual integration.

4. Educate the community to believe that the provision of traditional remedies is not second-rate medicine.

5. Catalogue all medicinal plants in a country or region and disseminate this information.

6. Retain the traditional forms for prescriptions used in primary health care and carry out relevant research into traditional systems of medicine.

This statement on the promotion of traditional medicine was first made at a World Health Organization meeting in 1977, and has subsequently been reinforced on many occasions as a central part of its policy.[F2]

While medical students in Eastern societies can shut themselves off from traditional approaches to health care as a result of the overall balance of their training, viewing even those that are part of their national culture as irrational, or simply subsuming them under the biomedical umbrella, there are also now many focused educational programmes for traditional practitioners throughout the East.[T1] This means that Western-style medical practitioners are often far outnumbered by the traditional healers more commonly used by local populations. This applies not only to countries such as India, where there are some 400,000 Ayurvedic practitioners and 200,000 homeopaths, and Malaysia, where the 20,000 shamanistic bomohs numerically outstrip the 2,300 physicians,[F2] but also countries like South Africa, with 200,000 traditional healers as against 25,000 doctors of modern medicine.[K1] Although communication between such practitioners at both the collective and individual levels could often be enhanced in practice, the co-existence of biomedicine and traditional medicine – as in the West – again provides a framework for their integration.

BAREFOOT DOCTORS

There are situations in which both systems effectively meet in the person of the practitioner. One of the best examples is that of the barefoot doctors in China. These often little educated health-care workers are democratically elected on the basis of their willingness to train in theory and practice to serve the rural population. Most importantly in this context, their training includes both traditional and modern medicine and they combine the use of acupuncture, herbs and Western drugs in the primary-care setting in which they operate. This system has been broadly successful in China, even if it has not worked so well in such countries as India.[D1] The difficulties that can arise when traditional and Western systems of medicine come together in this way in the East are underlined by the gap between the principles of these systems. Western drugs provide rapid symptomatic relief, while the effects of traditional medicine take much longer to appear. This can lead – as it has done amongst the Bedouin people of the Middle East – to the destruction of ancient health traditions.[F2]

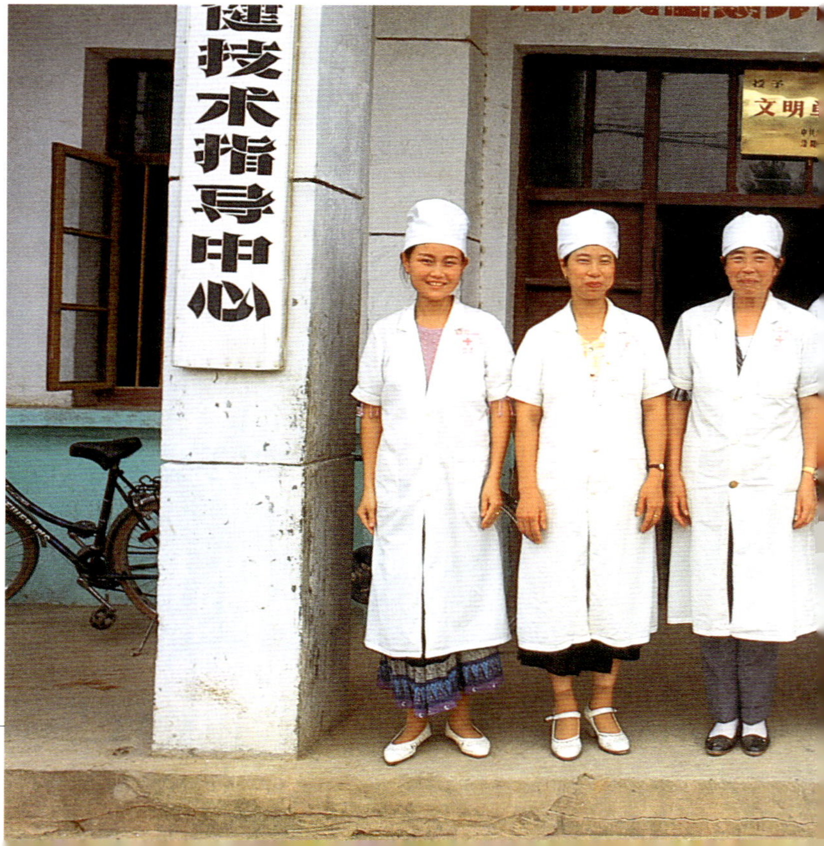

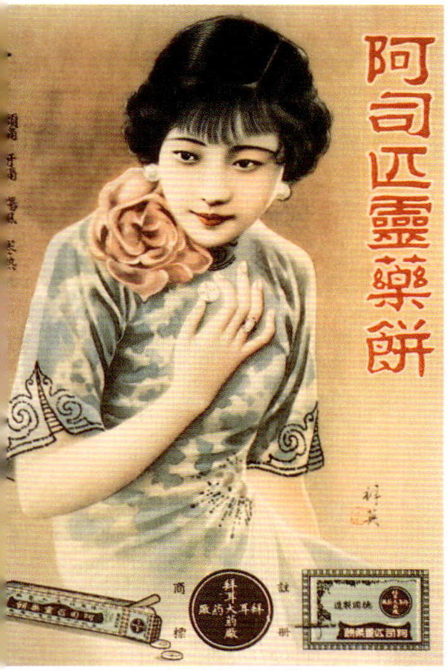

ABOVE West meets East: a 1935 Chinese advertising poster for aspirin marketed by its developers, the German pharmaceutical company Bayer.

CONVERGENCE

The example of the Chinese barefoot doctor clearly provides one model of how the Eastern and Western traditions can come together in the modern context. It should be noted, though, that the difficulties involved in integrating Eastern and Western practices are not exclusive to the East. They include the possibility of inappropriate combinations of medication being prescribed and problems of differential language use and communication. Nonetheless, the pragmatic benefits of integrating Eastern practices into Western medicine are plain. As an example, consider a case when traditional Chinese medicine might be used in preference to orthodox biomedicine – acupuncture analgesia may be viewed as a safer alternative to conventional anaesthesia for frail, elderly patients about to undergo the trauma of major surgery, or splints and massage could be used rather than the more conventional plaster cast to promote faster healing and to avoid the muscle wastage associated with setting fractured or broken bones.

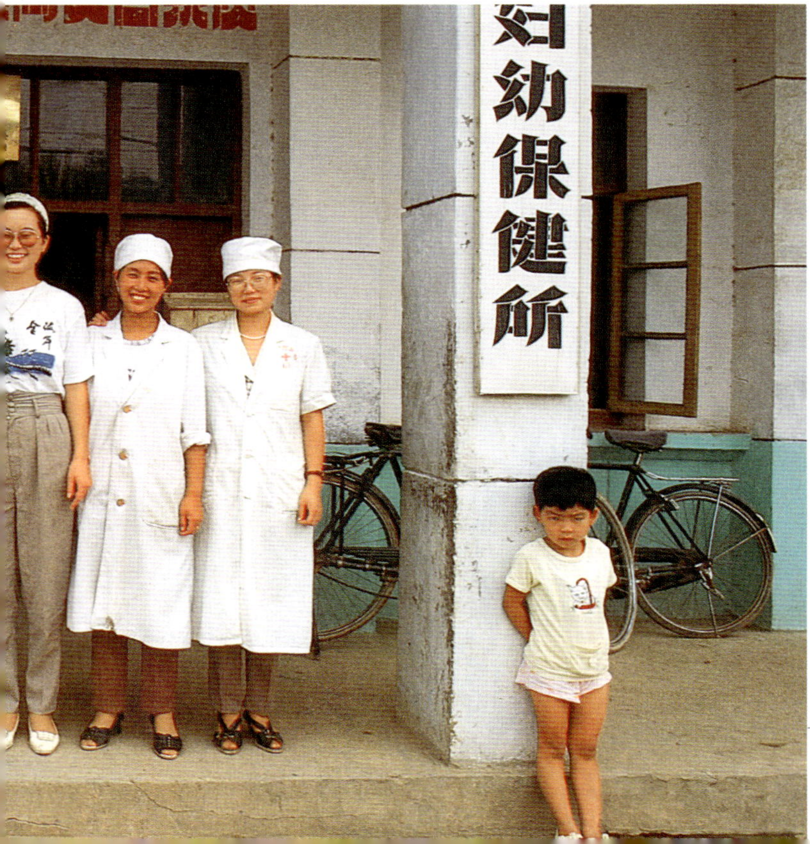

The advantages of being able to draw on more than one system in this way are highlighted by the following quotation from Dr Lu, a prominent Chinese doctor, reflecting the benefits of the present policy in China of uniting traditional and modern health-care practices.

> *'They are like chopsticks and a bowl – two ways of getting at the rice… Sometimes the sticks can probe deeper. At other times the embracing bowl fills the need. But in fact both methods serve each other'*
>
> CITED IN KAPTCHUK AND CROUCHER, *THE HEALING ARTS*[K2]

The analogies used in the West might be different, but the principle is the same – namely, that the coming together of Eastern and Western approaches to health care offers exciting opportunities for the consumer in the future across the globe. In Western societies these prospects are significant as the uniting of East and West also signals the re-emergence of the holistic tradition, following the rise of biomedicine over the past two centuries. Problems do remain. Despite the recent resurgence of a medical counterculture in Western Europe and North America, non-medically qualified alternative practitioners still do not adopt a universally holistic approach, the medical profession has not yet fully reformed itself in terms of the holistic revolution and the quality of relationship between these two groups needs to be developed further. What is clear, however, is that change is now rapidly occurring and that more holistic approaches, heavily influenced by Eastern medical traditions, are beginning to reassert themselves in a process that may well lead to the rehumanization of Western medical orthodoxy, as East meets West.

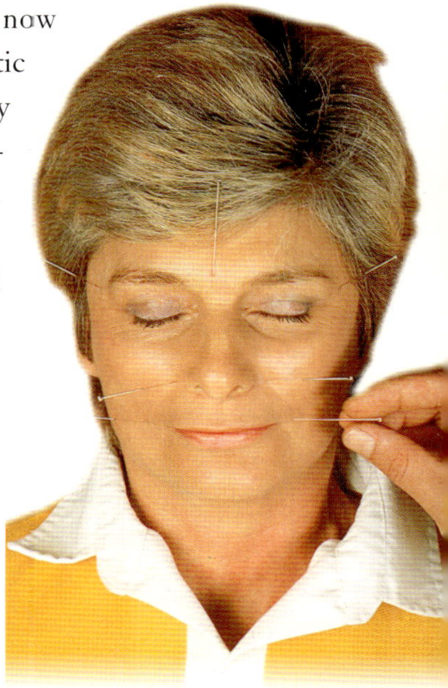

LEFT Staff of the Luoning Health Clinic in China combine the use of traditional Eastern and modern Western medicine.

RIGHT East meets West: acupuncture is now regularly used by many Westerners seeking relief from pain and chronic illness.

NOTES AND REFERENCES

CHAPTER ONE

❧ ADAMS, Francis, *The Genuine Works of Hippocrates*, London: Sydenham Society, 1849.

❧ BISHOP, WJ, *The Early History of Surgery*, London: Oldbourne, 1960.

❧ BROCK, Arthur John, *Galen on the Natural Faculties*, London: Heinemann, Loeb Classical Library, 1916.

❧ BULLOCH, William, *The History of Bacteriology*, London: Oxford University Press, 1938. Reprint 1960.

❧ CARTWRIGHT, F, *The Development of Modern Surgery*, London: Arthur Baker Ltd, 1967.

❧ CONRAD, LI *et al*, *The Western Medical Tradition 800 BC to AD 1800*, Cambridge University Press, 1995.

❧ COX, FEG (ed), *Illustrated History of Tropical Diseases*, London: Wellcome Trust, 1996.

❧ GWEI-DJEN, L & NEEDHAM, Joseph, *Celestial Lancets...*, Cambridge University Press, 1980.

❧ HASKINS, Charles Homer, *The Rise of the Universities*, New York: Cornell University Press, 1957.

❧ KEYNES, Geoffrey, *The Apologie and Treatise of Ambroise Paré*, London: Falcon Educational Books, 1951.

❧ LAMBERT, Royston, *Sir John Simon 1816–1904 and English Social Administration*, London: Macgibbon & Kee, 1963.

❧ MAJOR, Ralph H, *A History of Medicine*, Oxford: Blackwell, 1954.

❧ ROLLESTON, Humphry, *The Cambridge Medical School*, Cambridge University Press. 1932.

❧ SHRYOCK, Richard, *The Development of Modern Medicine*, University of Wisconsin Press, 1979.

❧ SIGERIST, Henry E, *The Great Doctors, A Biographical History of Medicine*, New York: Dover Publications, 1971.

CHAPTER TWO

❧ ACKERKNECHT, Erwin H, *A Short History of Medicine*, revised edition, Baltimore: Johns Hopkins University Press, 1982.

❧ BYNUM, WF, Porter, Roy, (eds), *Companion Encyclopaedia of the History of Medicine*, 2 vols, London: Routledge, 1993.

❧ FOUCAULT, Michel, *The Birth of the Clinic; an archaeology of medical perception*, translated from the French by AM Sheridan Smith, London: Tavistock Publications, 1973.

❧ KIPLE, KF, *The Cambridge World History of Human Diseases*, Cambridge: Cambridge University Press, 1993.

❧ PORTER, R, (ed), *The Cambridge Illustrated History of Medicine*, Cambridge: Cambridge University Press, 1996.

❧ REISER, Theodore, *Medicine and the Reign of Technology*, Cambridge: Cambridge University Press, 1978.

CHAPTER THREE

This chapter has drawn, directly and indirectly, on the work of many scholars. Hopefully, the list of secondary sources below acknowledges the principal names, if not necessarily all of each authors' relevant works. Although, quotations are generally from original works, a few have been taken from secondary sources in this bibliography.

❧ BYNUM, WF, Porter, R, (eds), *Companion encyclopedia of the history of medicine*. London: Routledge, 1993, 2 vols.

❧ CONRAD, LI, NEVE, M, NUTTON, V, PORTER, R, WEAR, A, *The western medical tradition*, Cambridge: Cambridge University Press, 1995.

❧ CRELLIN, JK, PHILPOTT, J, *Herbal medicine past and present*, Durham: Duke University Press, 2 vols.

❧ DEBUS, AG, *Science, medicine and society in the renaissance: essays to honor Walter Pagel*, New York: Science History Publications, 1972, vol 1.

❧ ESTES, JW, *The European reception of the first drugs from the new world*, Pharmacy in History, 1995; 37, 3-23.

❧ FOUST, CM, *Rhubarb, the wondrous drug*, Princeton: Princeton University Press, 1992.

❧ GORDON, C, *Sir John Pringle and the Apothecaries*, Pharmaceutical Historian, 1989; 19(4), 5-12 (quoted directly).

❧ GORDON, L, *A country herbal*, New York: Mayflower Books, 1980.

❧ GRIFFENHAGEN, GB, *The materia medica of Christopher Columbus*, Pharmacy in History, 1992; 34, 131-145.

❧ HEIN, WH, (ed) *Botanical drugs of the Americas in the old and new worlds*, Veröffentlichungen der Internationalen Gesellschaft fur Geschichte der Pharmazie, 1984, vol 53, various papers.

❧ HUNT, T, *The medieval surgery*, Woodbridge: The Boydell Press, 1992.

❧ JARCHO, S, *Quinine's predecessor*, Baltimore: The Johns Hopkins University Press, 1993.

❧ MACKINNEY, L, *Medical illustrations in medieval manuscripts*. London: Wellcome Historical Medical Library, 1965.

❧ MANNICHE, L, *An ancient Egyptian herbal*, Austin: University of Texas Press, 1989.

❧ MATTHEWS, LG, *The royal apothecaries*, London: Wellcome Historical Medical Library, 1967.

❧ MCVAUGH, MR, *Medicine before the plague: practitioners and their patients in the crown of Aragon, 1285-1345*, Cambridge: Cambridge University Press, 1993.

❧ MCVAUGH, MR and BALLESTER, LG, *Therapeutic method in the later middle ages: Arnau de Vilanova on medical contingency*, Caduceus, 1995; xi, 73-86 (quoted directly).

❧ NAGY, DG, *Popular medicine in seventeenth-century England*, Bowling Green, Ohio: Bowling Green State University Popular Press, 1988.

❧ NEEDHAM, J, GWEI-DJEN, L, *Science and civilisation in China*, Cambridge: Cambridge University Press, 1954-, various vols.

❧ NIJHUIS, K, *Greek doctors and Roman patients: a medical anthropological approach*, Pp. 49-63 in Ancient medicine in its socio-cultural context, van der Eijk, PJ, Horstmanshoff, HFJ, Schrijvers, PH, (eds), Amsterdam: Rodopi, 1995, vol 1.

❧ NUTTON, V, *The drug trade in antiquity*, Journal of the Royal Society of Medicine, 1985; 78, 138-145.

❧ NUTTON, V, *Murders and miracles: lay attitudes towards medicine in classical antiquity*, Pp 23-53 in Patients and practitioners: lay perceptions of medicine in pre-indutrial society, Porter, R, (ed), Cambridge: Cambridge University Press, 1985.

❧ ORTIZ DE MONTELLANO, BR, *Aztec medicine, health, and nutrition*, New Brunswick: Rutgers University Press, 1990.

❧ PALMER, R, *Medical botany in northern Italy in the renaissance*, Journal of the Royal Society of Medicine, 1985; 78, 149-157.

❧ PORTER, R, *Patients and practitioners: lay perceptions of medicine in pre-industrial society*, Cambridge: Cambridge University Press, 1985.

❧ POYNTER, FNL and BISHOP, WJ, *A seventeenth century doctor and his patients*, John Symcots 1592?-1662. Publications of the Bedfordshire Historical Record Society. 1951, vol 31.

❧ RAMSEY, M, *Professional and popular medicine in France*, 1770-1830. Cambridge: Cambridge University Press, 1988.

❧ RIDDLE, JM, *Dioscorides on Pharmacy and Medicine*, Austin: University of Texas Press, 1985.

❧ RINPOCHE, R, KUNZANG, J, *Tibetan medicine: illustrated in original texts*, London: Wellcome Institute of the History of Medicine, 1973.

❧ SCHMITZ, R, *The pomander. Pharmacy in History*, 1989; 31, 86-90.

❧ SIRAISI, NG, *Medieval & Early renaissance medicine: an introduction to knowledge and practice*, Chicago: The University of Chicago Press, 1990.

❧ STRABO, W Hortulus, Trans. R Payne, Pittsburgh: Hunt Botanical Library, 1966 (quoted directly).

❧ VEITH, I, *The yellow emperor's classic of internal medicine*. Birmingham: The Classics of Medicine Library, 1988.

❧ WEAR, A, FRENCH, RK, LONIE, IM, (eds), *The medical renaissance of the sixteenth century*, Cambridge: Cambridge University Press, 1985. Various papers.

❧ WEBSTER, C, (ed), *Health, medicine and mortality in the sixteenth century*, Cambridge: Cambridge University Press, 1979.

❧ WILCOX, J, and RIDDLE, JM, *Qustā Ibn Luqā's Physical ligatures and the recognition of the placebo effect*, Medieval Encounters, 1995; 1, 1-50.

CHAPTER FOUR

❧ [1] BARROW, John, *Travels in China, Containing Descriptions, Observations, And Comparisons, Made And Collected In The Course Of A Short Residence At The Imperial Palace Of Yuen-Min-Yuen, And On A Subsequent Journey Through The Country From Pekin To Canton. In Which It Is Attempted To Appreciate The Rank That This Extraordinary Empire May Be Considered To Hold In The Scale Of Civilized Nations*, London: T Cadell and W Davies, 1804.

❧ [2] GILLAN, Hugh, 'Mr Gillan's Observations on the State of Medicine, Surgery, and Chemistry in China', pp. 279-290 in JL Cranmer-Byng, (ed), *An Embassy to China: Being the Journal kept by Lord Macartney During his Embassy to the Emperor Ch'ien-lung 1793–1794*, London: Longmans, Green and Co., 1962.

❧ [3] TRAWICK, Margaret, 'Death and Nurturance in Indian Systems of Healing', pp. 129-159 in Leslie and Young, (eds), *Paths to Asian Medical Knowledge*, Oxford: University of California Press, 1992.

❧ [4] The traditional literature of Indian medicine is almost entirely written in the ancient language Sanskrit. Throughout this discussion of Indian medicine, I have used Dominik Wujastyk's new translations of the Sanskrit terms. For extended translations of Sanskrit texts, see Wujastyk, D, *Sanskrit Medical Writings*, forthcoming; and his essay 'Medicine in India' pp. 19-37 in Van Alphen and Aris, (eds), *Oriental Medicine: An Illustrated Guide to the Asian Arts of Healing*, London: Serindia Publications, 1995.

❧ [5] DESAI, PN, *Health and Medicine in the Hindu Tradition: Continuity and Cohesion*, New York: Crossroads Publishing Co., 1989; and Robert Svoboda, 'Theory and Practice of Ayurvedic Medicine', pp. 66-97 in Van Alphen and Aris, (eds), *Oriental Medicine: An Illustrated Guide to the Asian Arts of Healing*, London: Serindia Publications, 1995; to which texts I would advise interested readers to turn for further discussion of these topics.

❧ [6] UNSCHULD, Paul, *Medicine in China: A History of Ideas*, London: University of California Press, 1985, which I heartily recommend to curious readers.

❧ [7] VERCAMMEN, Dan, 'Theory and Practice of Chinese Medicine', pp. 156-195 in Van Alphen and Aris, (eds), *Oriental Medicine: An Illustrated Guide to the Asian Arts of Healing*, London: Serindia Publications, 1995.

❧ [8] This table is a slight modification of one in Ted Kaptchuck's *The Web That Has No Weaver*, New York: Congdon and Weed, 1983. Readers who wish to know more about the practice of Chinese medicine are advised to start with this detailed and readable book.

❧ [9] XUANJIE, Wang and MOFFETT, John, *Traditional Chinese Therapeutic Exercises – Standing Pole*, Beijing: Foreign Languages Press, 1994. My thanks to Nick Mabey for bringing this very clear exposition of Dao Yin and the Fundamental Substances to my attention.

❧ [10] XUANJIE, Wang and MOFFETT, John, ibid.

❧ [11] This and all other quotations attributed to Zhuang Zi are from *The Book of Master Zhuang*, quoted in Wang Xuanjie and John Moffett, op. cit., 1994.

❧ [12] This and all other quotations attributed to Ge Hong are from his *Bao Pu Zi*, quoted in Wang Xuanjie and John Moffett, op. cit., 1994

❧ [13] SVOBODA, Robert, 'Theory and Practice of Ayurvedic Medicine', 1995, as in note 5.

❧ [14] VOSSIUS, Isaac, *De Artibus et Scientiis Sinarum*, p. 76, 1685, quoted in Lu and Needham, *Celestial Lancets: A History and Rationale of Acupuncture*, Cambridge: Cambridge University Press, 1980, p. 286.

❧ [15] For more information about Mesmer and mesmerism, the reader is referred to George Bloch's *Mesmerism: A Translation of the original Scientific and Medical Writings of FA Mesmer*, Los Altos, California: William Kaufmann Inc, 1980, from which all quotations are taken, and to the introduction to this volume, written by ER Hilgard. For more on the politics of mesmerism, see R Darnton, *Mesmerism and the end of the Enlightenment in France*, Cambridge: Harvard University Press, 1968.

❧ [16] For a quick if partisan rendering of the history of homeopathy and homeopathic ideas, see Elizabeth Danciger's *The Emergence of Homeopathy: Alchemy into Medicine*, London: Century Paperbacks, 1987. It is rich in well translated quotations from Hahnemann and his intellectual predecessors. For a somewhat more academic and decidedly more specific approach, see (for example) Martin Kaufnam, *Homeopathy in America*, London: Johns Hopkins Press, 1971.

CHAPTER FIVE

❧ COPE, Z, *A History of the Acute Abdomen*, London: Oxford University Press, 1965.

❧ ELLIS, H, *Surgical Case Histories from the Past*, London: Royal Society of Medicine Press, 1994.

❧ ELLIS, H, *Operations That Made History*, London: Greenwich Medical Publications, 1996.

❧ RUTKOW, WIM, *Surgery, An Illustrated History*, St Louis: Mosby Year Books, 1993.

❧ ZIMMERMAN, LM and VEITH, I, *Great Ideas in the History of Surgery*, second edition, New York: Dover Publications, 1967.

CHAPTER SIX

❧ [1] ELLENBERGER, Henri, *The Discovery of the Unconscious: The History and Evolution of Dynamic Psychiatry*, New York: Basic Books, 1970, p. 4.

❧ [2] GOLDSTEIN, Jan, *Console and Classify: The French Psychiatric Profession in the Nineteenth Century*, Cambridge: Cambridge University Press, 1987, p. 83.

❧ [3] PORTER, Roy, 'Barely Touching: A Social Perspective on Mind and Body', in GS Rousseau (ed), *The Languages of Psyche. Mind and Body in Enlightenment Thought*, Berkeley: University of California Press, 1990, p. 55.

❧ [4] ibid., p.67.

❧ [5] GOLDSTEIN, Jan, op. cit.

❧ [6] BYNUM, WF, 'Rationales for Therapy in British Psychiatry, 1780–1835', in A Scull (ed), *Madhouses, Mad-doctors, and Madmen*, Philadelphia: University of Pennsylvania Press, 1981, p. 37.

❧ [7] PORTER, 'Barely Touching', p. 69.

❧ [8] SCULL, Andrew, 'Psychiatry and Social Control in the Nineteenth and Twentieth Centuries', *History of Psychiatry 2*, 1991, p. 110.

❧ [9] DIGBY, Anne, *Madness, Morality and Medicine: A Study of the York Retreat, 1796–1914*, Cambridge: Cambridge University Press, 1985, p. 6.

❧ [10] ibid., p. 4.

❧ [11] ibid., p. 42.

❧ [12] PORTER, 'Barely Touching', p. 68.

❧ [13] LYUBIMOV A, quoted in Ellenberger, *Discovery of the Unconscious*, p. 95.

❧ [14] See HARRINGTON, Anne, 'Hysteria, Hypnosis, and the Lure of the Invisible: The Rise of Neo-Mesmerism in fin-de-siècle French Psychiatry' in *The Anatomy of Madness* (ed. WF Bynum, Roy Porter and Michael Shepherd), 3 vols. London: Routledge, 1989, pp. 226–46. vol. 3.

❧ [15] quoted in VEITH, Ilza, *Hysteria. The History of a Disease*, Chicago: University of Chicago Press, 1965, p. 246.

[16] HARRIS, Ruth, *Murders and Madness: Medicine, Law, and Society in the fin de siècle,* Oxford: Oxford University Press, 1989, chapter 5.

[17] quoted in Ellenberger, *The Discovery of the Unconscious,* p. 87.

[18] ACKERKNECHT, Erwin H, *A Brief History of Psychiatry,* (tr. Sula Wolff), 2nd ed., New York, 1968, p. 82.

[19] SCHINDLER, Thomas-Peter, *'Psychiatrie im Wilhelminischen Deutschland im Spiegel der Verhandlungen des "Vereins der deutschen Irrenärzte"* (ab 1903 'Deutscher Verein für Psychiatrie)', Diss. Med., Freie Universität Berlin, 1990, p. 90.

[20] Scull, op. cit., p. 159.

[21] quoted in Sander Gilman, *Seeing the Insane: A Cultural History of Madness and Art in the Western World,* New York: Wiley, 1992, p. 124.

[22] quoted in Gilman, op. cit., p. 176.

[23] Martha Li Chiu, 'Insanity in Imperial China: A Legal Case Study', in A Kleinman and Tsung-Yi Lin, (eds), *Normal and Abnormal Behavior in Chinese Culture,* London: Reidel, 1981, p. 75.

[24] PEARSON, Veronica, 'The Development of Modern Psychiatric Services in China, 1891–1949', *History of Psychiatry* ii, 1991, p. 133.

[25] STEKEL, Wilhelm, *The Autobiography of Wilhelm Stekel: The Life Story of a Pioneer Psychoanalyst,* New York: Liveright, 1950, p. 161.

CHAPTER SEVEN

ACHTERBERG, Jeanne, *Imagery in Healing. Shamanism and Modern Medicine,* Boston: New Science Library, 1985.

ACKERKNECHT, Erwin J, *Medicine and Ethnology,* Baltimore: Johns Hopkins University Press, 1971.

ARIES, Philippe, *Western Attitudes Toward Death. From the Middle Ages to the Present,* Baltimore: Johns Hopkins University Press, 1974.

APPLE, Rima D, (ed), *Women, Health, and Medicine in America. A Historical Handbook,* New York: Garland Publishing, Inc, 1990.

ARMSTRONG, David and Elizabeth Metzger Armstrong, *The Great American Medicine Show,* New York: Prentice Hall, 1991.

BELL, Whitfield J Jr., *The Colonial Physician and Other Essays,* New York: Science History Publications, 1975.

BLOCH, Marc, *The Royal Touch. Sacred Monarchy and Scrofula in England and France,* Montreal: McGill University Press, 1973.

BOWERS, John Z, *Western Medical Pioneers in Feudal Japan,* Baltimore: Johns Hopkins University Press, 1970.

BUSHNELL, OA, *The Gifts of Civilization. Germs and Genocide in Hawai'i,* Honolulu: University of Hawai'i Press, 1993.

BYNUM, WF and Roy Porter, (eds), *Medical Fringe and Medical Orthodoxy 1750-1850,* London: Croom Helm, 1987.

CLENDENING, Logan, *Source Book of Medical History,* New York: Dover, 1960.

DALLY, Ann, *Women Under the Knife: A History of Surgery,* London: Hutchinson Radius, 1991.

DARNTON, Robert, *Mesmerism and the End of the Enlightenment in France,* Cambridge, Massachusetts: Harvard University Press, 1968.

DONAHUE, M Patricia, *Nursing, the Finest Art,* St Louis: CV Mosby Company, 1985.

DUFFY, John, *The Healers. A History of American Medicine,* Urbana: University of Illinois Press, 1979.

EDELSTEIN, Ludwig, *Ancient Medicine,* Baltimore: Johns Hopkins University Press, 1967.

FULLER, Robert C, *Alternative Medicine and American Religious Life,* Oxford: Oxford University Press, 1989.

GARRISON, Fielding H, *An Introduction to the History of Medicine,* 4th ed., Philadelphia: WB Saunders, 1929.

GEVITZ, Norman, *Other Healers. Unorthodox Medicine in America,* Baltimore: Johns Hopkins University Press, 1988.

HAND, Wayland D, (ed), *American Folk Medicine,* Berkeley: University of California Press, 1976.

HERTZLER, Arthur E, *The Horse and Buggy Doctor,* NY: Harper & Bros., 1938.

HUDSON, Robert P, *Disease and Its Control. The Shaping of Modern Thought,* Westport, Connecticut: Greenwood Press, 1983.

LAGUERE, Michel, *Afro-Caribbean Folk Medicine,* South Hadley, Massachusetts: Bergin & Garvey Publishers, Inc., 1987.

MAJNO, Guido, *The Healing Hand. Man and Wound in the Ancient World,* Cambridge, Massachusetts: Harvard University Press, 1975.

MAJOR, Ralph H, *Classic Descriptions of Disease.* 3rd ed., Springfield, Illinois: Charles C Thomas, 1945.

MBITI, John S, *African Religions & Philosophy,* 2nd ed., Oxford: Heinemann Educational Publishers, 1990.

MEAD, Kate Campbell Hurd-, *A History of Women in Medicine,* Haddam, Connecticut: Haddam Press, 1938.

MORANTZ-SANCHEZ, Regina Markall, *Sympathy and Science. Women Physicians in American Medicine,* Oxford: Oxford University Press, 1985.

PERRONE Bobette, H Henrietta Stockel, and Victoria Krueger, *Medicine Women, Curanderas, and Women Doctors,* Norman: University of Oklahoma Press, 1989.

PORTER, Roy, *Health For Sale: Quackery in England 1660-1850,* Manchester: Manchester University Press, 1989.

PORTER, Roy and PORTER, Dorothy, *Patient's Progress: Doctors and Doctoring in Eighteenth-Century England,* Cambridge: Polity Press, 1989.

RANDI, James, *The Faith Healers,* Amherst, NY: Prometheus Books, 1989.

RICHARDSON, Ruth, *Death, Dissection and the Destitute. A Political History of the Human Corpse,* London: Routledge & Kegan Paul, 1987.

ROSEN, George, *A History of Public Health,* New York: MD Publications, 1958.

ROSENBERG, Charles E, *Framing Disease. Studies in Cultural History,* New Brunswick, New Jersey: Rutgers University Press, 1992.

SAVITT, Todd L, *Medicine and Slavery. The Disease of Health Care of Blacks in Antebellum Virginia,* Urbana: University of Illinois Press, 1978.

SHORTER, Edward, *Bedside Manners: The Troubled History of Doctors and Patients,* New York: Simon and Schuster, 1985.

SIGERIST, Henry E, *The Great Doctors. A Biographical History of Medicine,* New York: WW Norton, 1933.

SIGERIST, Henry E, *A History of Medicine,* 2 vols, Oxford: Oxford University Press, 1951-1961.

TEMKIN, Owsei, *The Double Face of Janus and Other Essays in the History of Medicine,* Baltimore: Johns Hopkins University Press, 1977.

UNSCHULD, Paul U, *Medicine in China. A History of Ideas,* Berkeley: University of California Press, 1985.

VEITH, Ilza, *Huang Ti Nei Ching Su Wen. The Yellow Emperor's Classic of Internal Medicine,* Berkeley: University of California Press, 1949.

VOGEL, Virgil L, *American Indian Medicine,* Norman: University of Oklahoma Press, 1970.

WARNER, John Harley, *The Therapeutic Perspective. Medical Practice, Knowledge, and Identity in America, 1820-1885,* Cambridge, Massachusetts: Harvard University Press, 1986.

WEAR, Andrew, (ed), *Medicine in Society,* Cambridge: Cambridge University Press, 1992.

WILSON, Philip K, (ed), *Childbirth. Changing Ideas and Practices in Britain and America 1600 to the Present,* 5 vols, New York: Garland Publishing, Inc, 1996.

CHAPTER EIGHT

Each of the books in this list has been given a letter/number code. These correspond to the superscript codes that appear as attributions throughout the chapter.

[A1] ALDRIDGE, D, 'Unconventional medicine in Europe', *Advances: Journal of Mind-Body Health,* 10, 52–60, 1994.

[A2] ALSTER, K, *The Holistic Health Movement,* University of Alabama Press, Tuscaloosa, 1989.

[B1] BAKX, K, 'The "eclipse" of folk medicine in Western society', *Sociology of Health and Illness,* 13, 20–38, 1991.

[B2] BERLANT, J L, *Profession and Monopoly: A Study of Medicine in the United States and Great Britain,* University of California Press, Berkeley, 1975.

[B3] British Medical Association, *Report of the Board of Science and Education on Alternative Therapy,* BMA, London, 1986.

[B4] British Medical Association, *Complementary Medicine: New Approaches to Good Practice,* BMA, London, 1993.

[B5] BURROWS, J G, *AMA: Voice of American Medicine,* Johns Hopkins University Press, Baltimore, 1963.

[C1] CAMPBELL, A, *Natural Health Handbook,* New Burlington Books, London, 1991.

[C2] CANT, S and SHARMA, U, 'The reluctant profession – homoeopathy and the search for legitimacy', *Work, Employment and Society,* 9, 743–62, 1995.

[C3] CHOPRA, D, *Boundless Energy,* Ryder, London, 1995.

[C4] CHOW, EPY, 'Traditional Chinese medicine: a holistic system', in Salmon, JW (ed), *Alternative Medicines: Popular and Policy Perspectives,* Tavistock, London, 1985.

[C5] CLARKE, JN, *Health, Illness and Medicine in Canada,* McClelland & Stewart, Toronto, 1990.

[C6] COBURN, D & BIGGS, L, Chiropractic: legitimation or medicalization?', in Coburn, D, D'Arcy, C, Torrance, G and New, P (eds), *Health and Canadian Society,* Fitzhenry & Whiteside, Richmond Hill, Ontario, 1992.

[C7] COWARD, R, *The Whole Truth: The Myth of Alternative Medicine,* Faber & Faber, London, 1989.

[D1] DOYAL, L, *The Political Economy of Health,* Pluto Press, London, 1979.

[E1] EAGLE, R, *A Guide to Alternative Medicine,* British Broadcasting Corporation, London, 1980.

[E2] EISENBERG, D, KESSLER, R, FOSTER, C, NORLOCK, F, CALKINS, D and DELBANCO, T, 'Unconventional medicine in the United States: prevalence, costs, and patterns of use', *New England Journal of Medicine,* 328, 246–52, 1993.

[E3] ENGEL, G, 'The need for a new medical model: a challenge for biomedicine', *Science,* 196, 129–36, 1977.

[F1] FISHER, P and WARD, A 'Complementary medicine in Europe', *British Medical Journal,* 309, 107–10, 1994.

[F2] FULDER, S, *The Handbook of Complementary Medicine,* 2nd edition, Oxford University Press, Oxford, 1988.

[G1] GESLER, W, 'The global pharmaceutical industry: health, development and business', in Phillips, D and Verhasselt, Y, (eds), *Health and Development,* Routledge, London, 1994.

[G2] GEVITZ, N, 'Osteopathic medicine: from deviance to difference', in Gevitz, N, (ed); *Other Healers: Unorthodox Medicine in America,* Johns Hopkins University Press, Baltimore, 1988.

[G3] GORDON, J S, 'Holistic health centers in the United States', in Salmon, JW (ed), *Alternative Medicines: Popular and Policy Perspectives,* Tavistock, London, 1985.

[G4] GORDON, J S, *Holistic Medicine,* Chelsea House Publishers, New York, 1988.

[H1] HICKS, A, *Principles of Chinese Medicine,* Thorsons, London, 1996.

[H2] HUGGON, T and TRENCH, A, 'Brussels post-1992: protector or persecutor', in Saks, M (ed), *Alternative Medicine in Britain,* Clarendon Press, Oxford, 1992.

[H3] HYMA, B and RAMESH, A, 'Traditional medicine: its extent and potential for incorporation into modern national health systems', in Phillips, D, and Verhasselt, Y, (eds), *Health and Development,* Routledge, London, 1994.

[I1] ILLICH, I, *Limits to Medicine,* Penguin, Harmondsworth, 1976.

[I2] ILLICH, I, 'Pathogenesis, immunity and the quality of public health: medical nemesis revisited', *The Journal of Contemporary Health,* 4, 30–31, 1996.

[I3] INGLIS, B, *Natural Medicine,* Fontana, London, 1980.

[J1] JEWSON, N, 'The disappearance of the sick-man from medical cosmology 1770–1870', *Sociology,* 10, 225–44, 1976.

[K1] KALE, R, 'Traditional healers in South Africa: a parallel health care system', *British Medical Journal,* 310, 1182–85, 1995.

[K2] KAPTCHUK, T and CROUCHER, M, *The Healing Arts: A Journey through the Faces of Medicine,* British Broadcasting Corporation, London, 1986.

[K3] KAUFMAN, M, 'Homeopathy in America: the rise and fall and persistence of a medical heresy', in Gevitz, N, (ed), *Other Healers: Unorthodox Medicine in America,* Johns Hopkins University Press, Baltimore, 1988.

[L1] LARNER, C, 'Healing in pre-industrial Britain', in Saks, M (ed), *Alternative Medicine in Britain,* Clarendon Press, Oxford, 1992.

[L2] LYNG, S, *Holistic Health and Biomedical Medicine: A Countersystem Analysis,* SUNY Press, New York, 1990.

[M1] MCKEE, J, 'Holistic health and the critique of Western medicine', *Social Science and Medicine,* 26, 775–84, 1988.

[N1] NICHOLLS, P, *Homeopathy and the Medical Profession,* Croom Helm, London, 1988.

[P1] PETERS, D, 'Sharing responsibility for patient care: doctors and complementary practitioners', in Budd, S and Sharma, U, (eds), *The Healing Bond: The Patient-Practitioner Relationship and Therapeutic Responsibility,* Routledge, London, 1995.

[P2] PHILLIPS, A and RAKUSEN, J, *Our Bodies Ourselves,* 3rd edition, Penguin, Harmondsworth, 1996.

[P3] PIETRONI, P, *The Greening of Medicine,* Victor Gollancz, London, 1991.

[P4] PORTER, R, *Disease, Medicine and Society in England 1550–1860,* Macmillan, London, 1987.

[P5] PORTER, R, *Health for Sale: Quackery in England 1660–1850,* Manchester University Press, Manchester, 1989.

[P6] POWELL, M and ANESAKI, M, *Health Care in Japan,* Routledge, London, 1990.

[R1] ROSENTHAL, M, 'Political process and the integration of traditional and western medicine in the People's Republic of China', *Social Science and Medicine,* 15A, 599–613.

[R2] ROSZACK, T, *The Making of a Counter Culture,* Faber & Faber, London, 1970.

[R3] ROTHSTEIN, WG, 'The botanical movements and orthodox medicine', in Gevitz, N (ed), *Other Healers: Unorthodox Medicine in America,* Johns Hopkins University Press, Baltimore, 1988.

[S1] SAKS, M, 'Introduction', in Saks, M (ed), *Alternative Medicine in Britain,* Clarendon Press, Oxford, 1992.

[S2] SAKS, M, 'The alternatives to medicine', in Gabe, J, Kelleher, D, and Williams, G (eds), *Challenging Medicine,* Routledge, London, 1994.

[S3] SAKS, M, 'Educational and professional developments in acupuncture in Britain: an historical and contemporary overview', *European Journal of Oriental Medicine,* 1, 32–34, 1995a.

[S4] SAKS, M, *Professions and the Public Interest: Medical Power, Altruism and Alternative Medicine,* Routledge, London, 1995b.

[S5] SAKS, M, 'From quackery to complementary medicine: the shifting boundaries between orthodox and unorthodox medical knowledge', in Cant, S and Sharma, U, (eds), *Complementary and Alternative Medicines: Knowledge in Practice,* Free Association Books, London, 1996.

[S6] SAKS, M, 'Alternative therapies: are they holistic?', *Complementary Therapies in Nursing and Midwifery,* 3, 4–8, 1997.

[S7] SHARMA, U, *Complementary Medicine Today: Practitioners and Patients,* Routledge, London, 1992.

[S8] STANWAY, A, *Complementary Medicine: A Guide to Natural Therapies,* Penguin, Harmondsworth, 1994.

[T1] TARIMO, E and CREESE, A, (eds), *Achieving Health for All by the Year 2000,* World Health Organization, Geneva, 1990.

[T2] THOMAS, K J, CARR, J, WESTLAKE, L and WILLIAMS, B T, 'Use of non-orthodox and conventional health care in Great Britain', *British Medical Journal,* 302, 207–10, 1991.

[V1] VINCENT, J, 'Self-help groups and health care in contemporary Britain', in Saks, M, (ed), *Alternative medicine in Britain,* Clarendon Press, Oxford, 1992.

[W1] WALLIS, R and MORLEY, P, 'Introduction', in Wallis, R and Morley, P (eds), *Marginal Medicine,* Peter Owen, London, 1976.

[W2] WARDWELL, W, *Chiropractic: History and Evolution of a New Profession,* Mosby, St Louis, 1992.

[W3] WARDWELL, W, 'Alternative medicine in the United States', *Social Science and Medicine,* 38, 1061–68, 1994.

INDEX

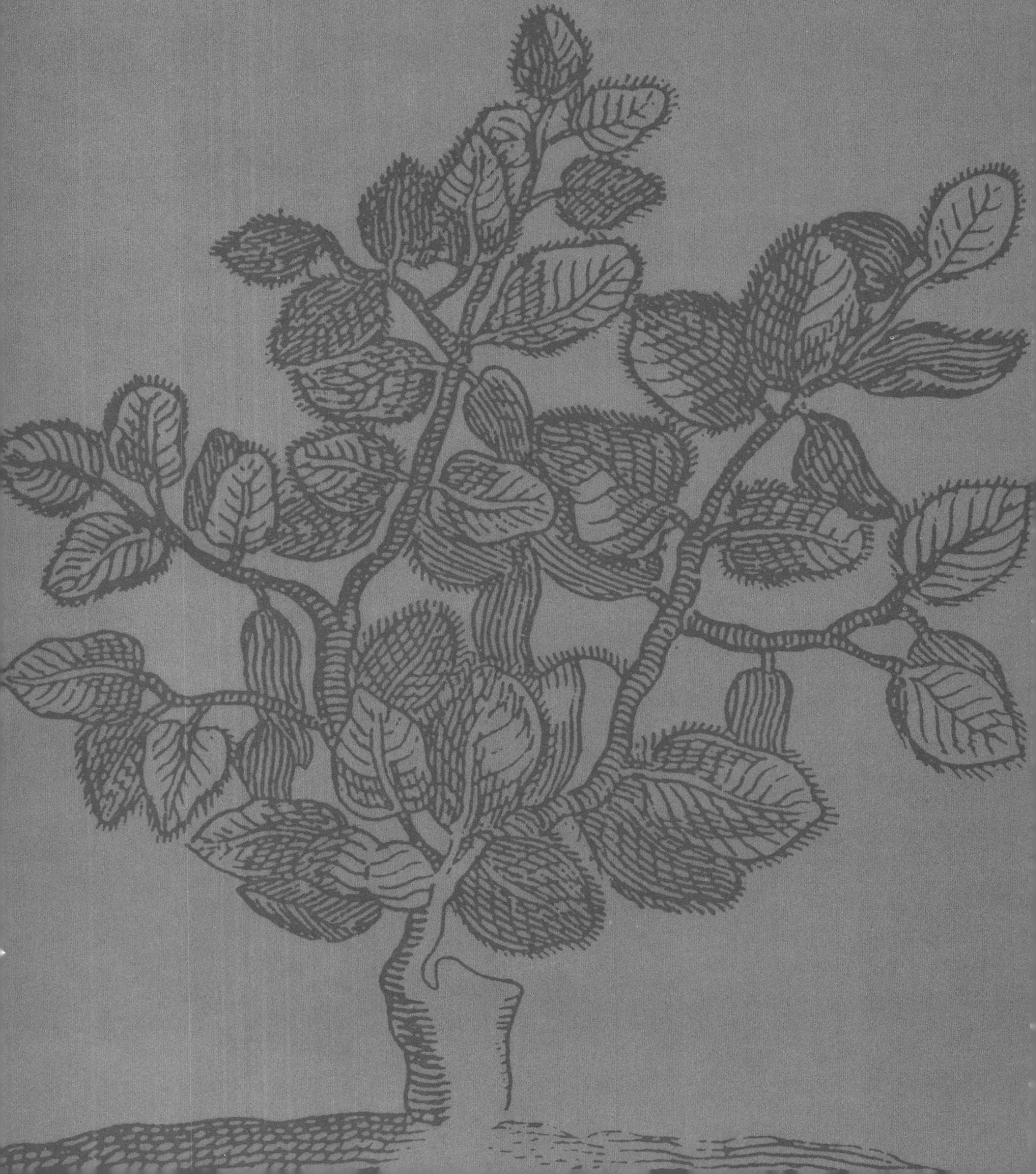